Seaweeds Secondary Metabolites

Seaweeds Secondary Metabolites

Successes in and/or Probable Therapeutic Applications

Special Issue Editor

Diana Cláudia Pinto

MDPI • Basel • Beijing • Wuhan • Barcelona • Belgrade • Manchester • Tokyo • Cluj • Tianjin

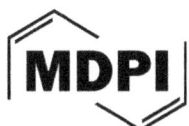

Special Issue Editor
Diana Cláudia Pinto
Universidade de Aveiro
Portugal

Editorial Office
MDPI
St. Alban-Anlage 66
4052 Basel, Switzerland

This is a reprint of articles from the Special Issue published online in the open access journal *Marine Drugs* (ISSN 1660-3397) (available at: https://www.mdpi.com/journal/marinedrugs/special_issues/seaweedssecmet).

For citation purposes, cite each article independently as indicated on the article page online and as indicated below:

LastName, A.A.; LastName, B.B.; LastName, C.C. Article Title. *Journal Name* **Year**, *Article Number*, Page Range.

ISBN 978-3-03928-300-2 (Pbk)
ISBN 978-3-03928-301-9 (PDF)

© 2020 by the authors. Articles in this book are Open Access and distributed under the Creative Commons Attribution (CC BY) license, which allows users to download, copy and build upon published articles, as long as the author and publisher are properly credited, which ensures maximum dissemination and a wider impact of our publications.

The book as a whole is distributed by MDPI under the terms and conditions of the Creative Commons license CC BY-NC-ND.

Contents

About the Special Issue Editor vii

Preface to "Seaweeds Secondary Metabolites" ix

Susana Santos, Tiago Ferreira, José Almeida, Maria J. Pires, Aura Colaço, Sílvia Lemos, Rui M. Gil da Costa, Rui Medeiros, Margarida M. S. M. Bastos, Maria J. Neuparth, Helena Abreu, Rui Pereira, Mário Pacheco, Isabel Gaivão, Eduardo Rosa and Paula A. Oliveira
Dietary Supplementation with the Red Seaweed *Porphyra umbilicalis* Protects against DNA Damage and Pre-Malignant Dysplastic Skin Lesions in HPV-Transgenic Mice
Reprinted from: *Mar. Drugs* **2019**, *17*, 615, doi:10.3390/md17110615 1

Mariagiulia Minetti, Giulia Bernardini, Manuele Biazzo, Gilles Gutierrez, Michela Geminiani, Teresa Petrucci and Annalisa Santucci
Padina pavonica Extract Promotes In Vitro Differentiation and Functionality of Human Primary Osteoblasts
Reprinted from: *Mar. Drugs* **2019**, *17*, 473, doi:10.3390/md17080473 15

Giulia Bernardini, Mariagiulia Minetti, Giuseppe Polizzotto, Manuele Biazzo and Annalisa Santucci
Pro-Apoptotic Activity of French Polynesian *Padina pavonica* Extract on Human Osteosarcoma Cells
Reprinted from: *Mar. Drugs* **2018**, *16*, 504, doi:10.3390/md16120504 29

Myeongjoo Son, Seyeon Oh, Chang Hu Choi, Kook Yang Park, Kuk Hui Son and Kyunghee Byun
Pyrogallol-Phloroglucinol-6,6-Bieckol from *Ecklonia cava* Attenuates Tubular Epithelial Cell (TCMK-1) Death in Hypoxia/Reoxygenation Injury
Reprinted from: *Mar. Drugs* **2019**, *17*, 602, doi:10.3390/md17110602 49

Su Hui Seong, Pradeep Paudel, Hyun Ah Jung and Jae Sue Choi
Identifying Phlorofucofuroeckol-A as a Dual Inhibitor of Amyloid-β_{25-35} Self-Aggregation and Insulin Glycation: Elucidation of the Molecular Mechanism of Action
Reprinted from: *Mar. Drugs* **2019**, *17*, 600, doi:10.3390/md17110600 59

Pradeep Paudel, Aditi Wagle, Su Hui Seong, Hye Jin Park, Hyun Ah Jung and Jae Sue Choi
A New Tyrosinase Inhibitor from the Red Alga *Symphyocladia latiuscula* (Harvey) Yamada (Rhodomelaceae)
Reprinted from: *Mar. Drugs* **2019**, *17*, 295, doi:10.3390/md17050295 77

Philipp Dörschmann, Kaya Saskia Bittkau, Sandesh Neupane, Johann Roider, Susanne Alban and Alexa Klettner
Effects of Fucoidans from Five Different Brown Algae on Oxidative Stress and VEGF Interference in Ocular Cells
Reprinted from: *Mar. Drugs* **2019**, *17*, 258, doi:10.3390/md17050258 91

Xuezhen Zhou, Mengqi Yi, Lijian Ding, Shan He and Xiaojun Yan
Isolation and Purification of a Neuroprotective Phlorotannin from the Marine Algae *Ecklonia maxima* by Size Exclusion and High-Speed Counter-Current Chromatography
Reprinted from: *Mar. Drugs* **2019**, *17*, 212, doi:10.3390/md17040212 111

Sara García-Davis, Ezequiel Viveros-Valdez, Ana R. Díaz-Marrero, José J. Fernández, Daniel Valencia-Mercado, Olga Esquivel-Hernández, Pilar Carranza-Rosales, Irma Edith Carranza-Torres and Nancy Elena Guzmán-Delgado
Antitumoral Effect of Laurinterol on 3D Culture of Breast Cancer Explants
Reprinted from: *Mar. Drugs* **2019**, *17*, 201, doi:10.3390/md17040201 . . . . **119**

Gonçalo P. Rosa, Wilson R. Tavares, Pedro M. C. Sousa, Aida K. Pagès, Ana M. L. Seca and Diana C. G. A. Pinto
Seaweed Secondary Metabolites with Beneficial Health Effects: An Overview of Successes in In Vivo Studies and Clinical Trials
Reprinted from: *Mar. Drugs* **2020**, *18*, 8, doi:10.3390/md18010008 . . . . **135**

Valentina Jesumani, Hong Du, Muhammad Aslam, Pengbing Pei and Nan Huang
Potential Use of Seaweed Bioactive Compounds in Skincare—A Review
Reprinted from: *Mar. Drugs* **2019**, *17*, 688, doi:10.3390/md17120688 . . . . **171**

Tosin A. Olasehinde, Ademola O. Olaniran and Anthony I. Okoh
Macroalgae as a Valuable Source of Naturally Occurring Bioactive Compounds for the Treatment of Alzheimer's Disease
Reprinted from: *Mar. Drugs* **2019**, *17*, 609, doi:10.3390/md17110609 . . . . **191**

Maria Dolores Torres, Noelia Flórez-Fernández and Herminia Domínguez
Integral Utilization of Red Seaweed for Bioactive Production
Reprinted from: *Mar. Drugs* **2019**, *17*, 314, doi:10.3390/md17060314 . . . . **209**

Paul Cherry, Supriya Yadav, Conall R. Strain, Philip J. Allsopp, Emeir M. McSorley, R. Paul Ross and Catherine Stanton
Prebiotics from Seaweeds: An Ocean of Opportunity?
Reprinted from: *Mar. Drugs* **2019**, *17*, 327, doi:10.3390/md17060327 . . . . **243**

Adriana C.S. Pais, Jorge A. Saraiva, Sílvia M. Rocha, Armando J.D. Silvestre and Sónia A.O. Santos
Current Research on the Bioprospection of Linear Diterpenes from *Bifurcaria bifurcata*: From Extraction Methodologies to Possible Applications
Reprinted from: *Mar. Drugs* **2019**, *17*, 556, doi:10.3390/md17100556 . . . . **279**

About the Special Issue Editor

Diana Cláudia Pinto studied chemistry at the University of Aveiro (Portugal) where she graduated in Chemistry in 1991. In 1996 she received her PhD in Chemistry and then joined the Department of Chemistry where she is currently professor of Organic and Medicinal Chemistry. She is an expert in organic synthesis, including the development of new strategies towards the synthesis of bioactive heterocyclic compounds. Over the years, her research has also been focused on natural products chemistry. Specifically, extraction, purification, structural elucidation of natural compounds, and chemical profiles of terrestrial and marine resources.

Preface to "Seaweeds Secondary Metabolites"

Seaweed use in gastronomy is common in Asian countries, but its consumption is increasing in other countries because its nutritional values are being established. Nowadays, scientific studies are more focused on the potential of seaweed to promote health benefits and prevent several diseases. In fact, their anticancer, anti-inflammatory, and anti-hypertensive activities have been established. The relationship between those health effects and the secondary metabolites produced has been less explored, and in vivo studies are still scarce. This book provides readers with an understanding of how seaweeds and/or their secondary metabolites can be used to combat some diseases. Simultaneously, some new isolation techniques are also addressed. Seaweeds Secondary Metabolites: Successes in and/or Probable Therapeutic Applications is an excellent resource for students and researchers in natural products chemistry and health-related fields, as well as a source of in-depth information about the health promoting value of seaweed.

Diana Cláudia Pinto
Special Issue Editor

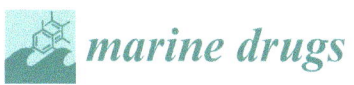

Article

Dietary Supplementation with the Red Seaweed *Porphyra umbilicalis* Protects against DNA Damage and Pre-Malignant Dysplastic Skin Lesions in HPV-Transgenic Mice

Susana Santos [1,2], Tiago Ferreira [1,2], José Almeida [1,2], Maria J. Pires [1,2], Aura Colaço [1,3], Sílvia Lemos [1,2], Rui M. Gil da Costa [2,4,5], Rui Medeiros [5,6,7,8], Margarida M. S. M. Bastos [4], Maria J. Neuparth [9], Helena Abreu [10], Rui Pereira [10], Mário Pacheco [11], Isabel Gaivão [12], Eduardo Rosa [2,13] and Paula A. Oliveira [1,2,*]

[1] Department of Veterinary Sciences, University of Trás-os-Montes and Alto Douro (UTAD), 5001-801 Vila Real, Portugal; suusanacoelhosantos@gmail.com (S.S.); tiagoterras55@gmail.com (T.F.); josecfralmeida@gmail.com (J.A.); joaomp@utad.pt (M.J.P.); acolaco@utad.pt (A.C.); silviaalexandralemos@gmail.com (S.L.)
[2] Centre for the Research and Technology of Agro-Environmental and Biological Sciences (CITAB), 5001-801 Vila Real, Portugal; rmcosta@fe.up.pt (R.M.G.d.C.); erosa@utad.pt (E.R.)
[3] Animal and Veterinary Research Center (CECAV), 5001-801 Vila Real, Portugal
[4] LEPABE—Laboratory for Process Engineering, Environment, Biotechnology and Energy, Faculty of Engineering, University of Porto, Rua Dr. Roberto Frias, 4200-465 Porto, Portugal; mbastos@fe.up.pt
[5] Molecular Oncology and Viral Pathology Group, IPO-Porto Research Center (CI-IPOP), Portuguese Institute of Oncology of Porto (IPO-Porto), 4200-072 Porto, Portugal; ruimmms@gmail.com
[6] Faculty of Medicine, University of Porto (FMUP), 4200-450 Porto, Portugal
[7] CEBIMED, Faculty of Health Sciences, Fernando Pessoa University, 4200-150 Porto, Portugal
[8] LPCC Research Department, Portuguese League against Cancer (NRNorte), 4200-172 Porto, Portugal
[9] Research Center in Physical Activity, Health and Leisure (CIAFEL), Faculty of Sports, University of Porto, 4200-450 Porto, Portugal; mneuparth@hotmail.com
[10] ALGAplus, Lda., PCI-Creative Science Park, 3830-352 Ílhavo, Portugal; helena.abreu@algaplus.pt (H.A.); rui.pereira@algaplus.pt (R.P.)
[11] Department of Biology and CESAM, University of Aveiro, 3810-193 Aveiro, Portugal; mpacheco@ua.pt
[12] Department of Genetic and Biotechnology, CECAV, UTAD, 5001-801 Vila Real, Portugal; igaivao@utad.pt
[13] Department of Agronomy, UTAD, 5001-801 Vila Real, Portugal
[*] Correspondence: pamo@utad.pt; Tel.: +351-259350000; Fax: +351-259325058

Received: 7 October 2019; Accepted: 24 October 2019; Published: 29 October 2019

Abstract: Some diet profiles are associated with the risk of developing cancer; however, some nutrients show protective effects. *Porphyra umbilicalis* is widely consumed, having a balanced nutritional profile; however, its potential for cancer chemoprevention still needs comprehensive studies. In this study, we incorporated *P. umbilicalis* into the diet of mice transgenic for the human papillomavirus type 16 (HPV16), which spontaneously develop pre-malignant and malignant lesions, and determined whether this seaweed was able to block lesion development. Forty-four 20-week-old HPV$^{+/-}$ and HPV$^{-/-}$ mice were fed either a base diet or a diet supplemented with 10% seaweed. At the end of the study, skin samples were examined to classify HPV16-induced lesions. The liver was also screened for potential toxic effects of the seaweed. Blood was used to study toxicological parameters and to perform comet and micronucleus genotoxicity tests. *P. umbilicalis* significantly reduced the incidence of pre-malignant dysplastic lesions, completely abrogating them in the chest skin. These results suggest that *P. umbilicalis* dietary supplementation has the potential to block the development of pre-malignant skin lesions and indicate its antigenotoxic activity against HPV-induced DNA damage. Further studies are needed to establish the seaweed as a functional food and clarify the mechanisms whereby this seaweed blocks multistep carcinogenesis induced by HPV.

Keywords: K14HPV16; genotoxicity assay; papillomavirus; cancer

1. Introduction

Seaweeds are an important nutritional resource in many parts of the world and have various health-promoting biological activities [1,2]. Frequent consumption of seaweeds in South-East Asian countries has been associated with low incidence rates of chronic diseases, such as cancer [3,4]. Seaweeds contain high amounts of vitamins, fibers, and minerals, potentially contributing to a balanced diet if consumed regularly [5]. They are also a source of bioactive compounds with antioxidant, antitumor, anti-inflammatory and antiviral bioactivities [1,6], which make seaweeds popular functional foods for disease prevention [7,8]. In fact, some seaweeds contain natural compounds with significant pharmacological potential for cancer prevention and treatment [9,10]. *Porphyra umbilicalis* (Bangiophyceae) is an intertidal red seaweed (Rhodophyta), and its genome has already been disclosed, contributing to clarify the evolution of red seaweeds [11]. *P. umbilicalis* is used as food and is particularly appreciated for its unusually high protein content, vitamins, and fibers [12]. In a per-portion comparison, 100 g of wet weight of *P. umbilicalis* contains more total fiber (3.8 g) than apples and bananas, 2.0 g and 3.1 g, respectively. Regarding the presence of vitamins, 8 g of *P. umbilicalis* contains 9 mg of vitamin C [5]. Among other uses, *P. umbilicalis* was found to improve the nutritional profile of meat preparations, increasing its antioxidant properties [13]. Cofrades et al. [12] demonstrated that this seaweed presents significant benefits to human health, being itself a functional food. However, to our knowledge, the potential of *P. umbilicalis* in the prevention of cancer has never been evaluated.

Many cancers are associated with infection by oncogenic viruses, most commonly, human papillomavirus (HPV) [14]. High-risk HPVs are responsible for 630,000 new cancer cases per year, mainly cervical cancer but also other anogenital cancers and some oropharyngeal carcinomas [15]. The most common high-risk HPVs are HPV16 and 18, associated with 73% of HPV-related cancer cases [15]. Compounds from seaweeds, like carrageenan from Rhodophyta, showed remarkable preventive effects against HPV infection [16,17]. Recently, *Fucus vesiculosus* (Ochrophyta) showed significant in vitro activity against HPV-positive oropharyngeal cancer [18]. The present study addresses, for the first time, the potential of *P. umbilicalis* as a functional food to block the development of HPV-induced pre-malignant dysplastic lesions through its incorporation into the diet of HPV16-transgenic (K14HPV16) mice [19]. These animals develop multi-step cutaneous lesions induced by the HPV16 oncogenes, from hyperplastic foci through dysplastic patches to invasive squamous cell carcinomas, and may be used to test chemopreventive strategies [20,21]. K14HPV16 mice also show a debilitating syndrome, characterized by systemic inflammation, stunted growth, and chronic hepatitis, which progresses to overt cachexia with age [22]. We took advantage of these features to confirm whether *P. umbilicalis* could help countering this syndrome or would actually raise any safety issues by aggravating any toxicological parameters.

2. Results

2.1. General Findings

At the end of the experiment, all animal survived, and none showed signs of distress. There were no significant differences in body weight between groups at any time point, and food intake was similar throughout the experiment (data not shown). Higher water consumption was observed in groups II and IV of transgenic animals (7.80 g ± 1.43 and 7.06 g ± 0.79, respectively), compared to groups I and III of wild-type animals (5.11 g ± 1.14 and 3.61 g ± 0.46, respectively). Thus, significant differences were not observed among groups ($p > 0.05$). The relative weight of internal organs is reported in Table 1.

There was a statistically significant decrease ($p = 0.016$) in the relative weight of lungs between group I and group III.

Table 1. Relative weight of organs in the experimental groups (mean ± standard error).

	Liver	Right Kidney	Left Kidney	Spleen	Lung	Heart	Bladder	Thymus
Group I (HPV16$^{-/-}$, *Porphyra umbilicalis*)	0.0541 ± 0.0049	0.0060 ± 0.0002	0.0058 ± 0.0003	0.0040 ± 0.0002	0.0052 ± 0.0002 [1]	0.0037 ± 0.0002	0.0006 ± 0.0001	0.0010 ± 0.0001
Group II (HPV16$^{+/-}$, *P. umbilicalis*)	0.0670 ± 0.0015	0.0067 ± 0.0002	0.0065 ± 0.0001	0.0063 ± 0.0007	0.0063 ± 0.0003	0.0046 ± 0.0002	0.0010 ± 0.0001	0.0011 ± 0.0001
Group III (HPV16$^{-/-}$, base diet)	0.0574 ± 0.0012	0.0057 ± 0.0002	0.0062 ± 0.0002	0.0047 ± 0.0002	0.0063 ± 0.0003	0.0042 ± 0.0002	0.0003 ± 0.0002	0.0012 ± 0.0002
Group IV (HPV16$^{+/-}$, base diet)	0.0717 ± 0.0019	0.0069 ± 0.0002	0.0068 ± 0.0002	0.0083 ± 0.0010	0.0071 ± 0.0002	0.0051 ± 0.0002	0.0008 ± 0.0001	0.0014 ± 0.0001

[1] $p = 0.016$ statistically different from group III.

2.2. HPV-Induced Lesions and Hepatic Histology

Histological analysis of skin chest and ear samples are reported in Table 2. *P. umbilicalis*-supplemented-diet group II showed epidermal hyperplasia in 100% of the mice, while base diet-fed group IV only showed 36.4% of epidermal hyperplasia. Therefore, there were statistically significant differences concerning the skin chest among supplemented and not supplemented animals ($p = 0.004$). On the other hand, the *P. umbilicalis*-supplemented-diet group II mice did not show epidermal dysplasia, while 63.6% of non-supplemented mice showed epidermal dysplasia. Regarding ear samples results, there were no statistically significant differences between the supplemented and the non-supplemented groups. Figure 1 shows skin histological samples for (a) normal skin, (b) epidermal hyperplasia, and (c) epidermal dysplasia. On histological analysis, all mice showed normal hepatic morphology (data not shown).

Table 2. Incidence of histological lesions in skin chest and ear samples in the experimental groups.

	Skin Chest Incidence/n (%)			Ear Incidence/n (%)		
	Normal	Epidermal Hyperplasia	Epidermal Dysplasia	Normal	Epidermal Hyperplasia	Epidermal Dysplasia
Group I (HPV16$^{-/-}$, *P. umbilicalis*)	11/11 (100.0%)	0/11 (0%)	0/11 (0%)	11/11 (100.0%)	0/11 (0%)	0/11 (0%)
Group II (HPV16$^{+/-}$, *P. umbilicalis*)	0/11 (0%)	11/11 (100.0%)	0/11 (0%)	0/11 (0%)	7/9 (77.8%)	2/9 (22.2%)
Group III (HPV16$^{-/-}$, base diet)	11/11 (100.0%)	0/11 (0%)	0/11 (0%)	11/11 (100.0%)	0/11 (0%)	0/11 (0%)
Group IV (HPV16$^{+/-}$, base diet)	0/11 (0%)	4/11 [1] (36.4%)	7/11 (63.6%)	0/11 (0%)	4/11 (36.4%)	7/11 (63.6%)

[1] $p = 0.004$, statistically different from group II.

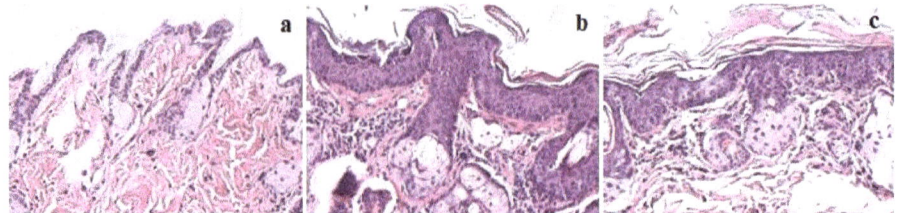

Figure 1. Skin histology samples of female FVB/n mice, magnification 200×, hematoxylin and eosin (H&E) staining: (**a**) Normal skin histology in wild-type groups (I and III); (**b**) Epidermal hyperplasia in K14human papillomavirus(HPV)16 transgenic mice; (**c**) Epidermal dysplasia in K14HPV16 transgenic mice.

2.3. Serum Biochemical Parameters

The serum biochemical parameters are registered in Table 3. There were no significant differences between *P. umbilicalis*-supplemented-diet and base diet-fed groups.

Table 3. Serum biochemical parameters (mean ± standard error).

	Group I (HPV16$^{-/-}$, *P. umbilicalis*)	Group II (HPV16$^{+/-}$, *P. umbilicalis*)	Group III (HPV16$^{-/-}$ Base Diet)	Group IV (HPV16$^{+/-}$ Base Diet)
Albumin (g/L)	28.65 ± 1.37	30.43 ± 0.93	29.78 ± 1.71	30.37 ± 0.96
Total proteins (g/L)	45.95 ± 1.72	50.32 ± 2.24	51.34 ± 4.07	49.62 ± 1.12
Glucose (mg/dL)	222.29 ± 11.16	197.65 ± 15.97	195.70 ± 15.99	198.07 ± 13.36
Aspartate aminotransferase (U/L)	35.63 ± 4.03	40.89 ± 5.65	37.28 ± 4.70	38.85 ± 3.54
Alanine aminotransferase (U/L)	59.34 ± 5.17	65.66 ± 7.16	44.74 ± 3.76	51.82 ± 3.70
Gamma glutamyltransferase (U/L)	31.75 ± 3.17	40.07 ± 7.67	48.61 ± 6.11	60.78 ± 8.35

2.4. Comet Assay

The *P. umbilicalis*-supplemented-diet transgenic group II showed a significantly lower basal genetic damage index (GDI) compared with the base diet-fed group IV ($p = 0.006$). There were no statistically significant differences concerning formamidopyrimidine DNA glycosylase (FPG) incubation (GDI$_{FPG}$) among groups (Figure 2), but the *P. umbilicalis*-supplemented-diet group I displayed significantly ($p = 0.001$) lower net enzyme-sensitive sites (NSS$_{FPG}$), compared with the base diet-fed group III (Figure 3). Higher ($p < 0.001$) NSS$_{FPG}$ levels were detected in *P. umbilicalis*-supplemented-diet transgenic group II, compared with group IV (base diet).

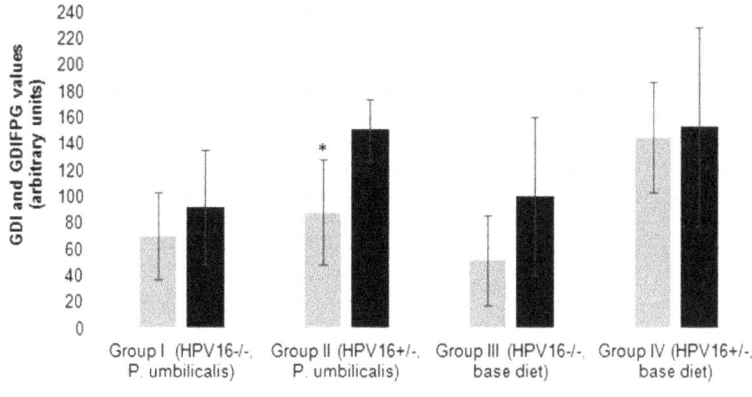

Figure 2. Mean values of non-specific genetic damage index (GDI, grey) and oxidative genetic damage index resulted from the assay with an extra step of digestion with formamidopyrimidine DNA glycosilase (FPG, GDI$_{FPG}$, black), measured in peripheral blood cells of female FVB/n mice ($n = 11$ for each group). Asterisk ('*') represents statistically significant differences ($p = 0.006$) relative to non-specific DNA damage (grey) in group II, in comparison to the control group IV (grey). Bars represent the standard deviation.

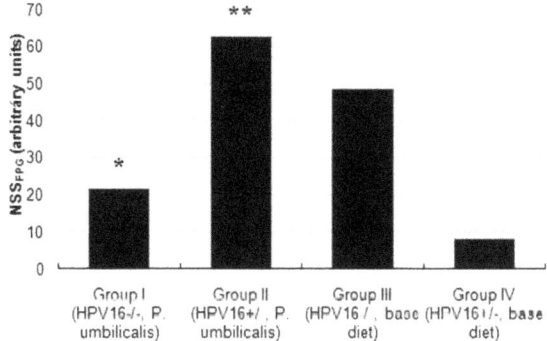

Figure 3. Values of net FPG-sensitive sites from the comet assay with an additional FPG step to detect oxidized purine bases. '*' represents statistically significant difference ($p = 0.001$) in group I, in relation to group III; '**' represents statistically significant difference ($p < 0.001$) in group II, in relation to group IV ($n = 11$ for each group).

2.5. Micronucleus Test

The micronucleus (MN) frequencies were slightly lower in the *P. umbilicalis*-supplemented-diet group I compared with the base diet-fed group III. The same applies to the *P. umbilicalis*-supplemented-diet group II that showed a lower MN frequency compared to the base diet-fed group IV (Figure 4), although these differences did not reach statistical significance.

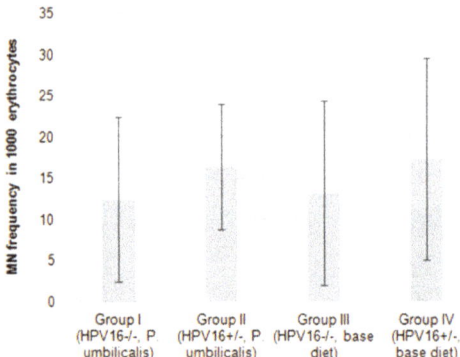

Figure 4. Mean frequency of micronuclei in 1000 erythrocytes of female mice FVB/n during the experimental study ($n = 22$ for each group). Bars represent the standard deviation.

3. Discussion

Cancers induced by high-risk HPVs remain among the most frequent and deadly, especially in developing countries, where the implementation of vaccination and screening programs have been less successful [15]. In fact, effective prevention efforts are critical to reduce the incidence of many types of cancer, either by withdrawing risk factors (e.g., oncogenic viruses and tobacco toxins) or by screening and treating pre-malignant lesions. A growing body of data suggests that some foods and nutrients also contribute to preventing the development of cancer [23]. Seaweeds are recognized as an important component of balanced diets in many world regions, and some species have shown anticancer activity. In general, addition of *P. umbilicalis* to food increases the concentration of some minerals (K, Ca, Mg, Mn, and Fe), amino acids, and consequently total protein [12]. Also, *P. umbilicalis* is a rich source of polyunsaturated fatty acids which are precursor of various cell components, allowing to maintain cellular homeostasis [13,24]. However, *P. umbilicalis*, a widely consumed red seaweed, has not yet been studied for its chemopreventive activity against cancer.

Here, we report the first data showing that *P. umbilicalis* is able to block the development of pre-malignant lesions in a mouse model of HPV16-induced cancer. In K14HPV16 transgenic mice, the *cytokeratin 14* (*K14*) gene promoter/enhancer is used to specifically target the expression of all the HPV16 early region genes, including the key drivers of malignant transformation E6 and E7, to epithelial basal cells in keratinized squamous epithelia [25]. The HPV16 E6 and E7 oncoproteins induce the degradation of the cellular p53 and retinoblastoma (pRb) proteins, allowing unchecked proliferation, survival, and accumulation of genetic mutations and driving carcinogenesis [26,27]. In consequence, this animal model develops multi-step lesions of the skin [21]. Our group and others have characterized these lesions and shown that their development may be blocked pharmacologically, using investigational and commercial drugs [20,22,28]. HPV16 causes cancers in mucosal surfaces such as the cervix rather than the skin, but skin lesions in this model closely follow the same histological and molecular pattern of multi-step carcinogenesis observed in cervical cancer [29,30]. In the present study, *P. umbilicalis* dietary supplementation completely abrogated the progression of hyperplastic epidermal lesions to the dysplastic stage in chest skin. Thus, we observed an increase of hyperplastic epidermal lesions from 36.4 to 100% in transgenic mice supplemented with *P. umbilicalis* in comparison with the control group. This suggests that *P. umbilicalis* was effective in preventing the progression of HPV16-induced lesions in this animal model. In the ear skin, this effect was less dramatic: supplementation with *P. umbilicalis* resulted in a decrease the incidence of dysplasia from 63.6 to 22.2%. Previous studies have shown that lesions in the chest and the ear progress along similar pre-malignant epidermal hyperplasia and dysplasia to form invasive squamous cell carcinomas (SCCs) and that SCCs originating from the chest skin are poorly differentiated and tend to metastasize to regional lymph nodes, while SCCs from the ear skin are well differentiated and only invade locally [19]. It is interesting to notice that *P. umbilicalis* preferentially inhibited the development of the most aggressive type of lesions from the chest, rather than that of the well-differentiated SCCs arising from the ear skin. The present study employed a short-term approach for *P. umbilicalis* supplementation, and additional studies are needed to confirm its long-term effects. While it is possible that long-term supplementation may enhance the protective effects of this seaweed, it is also possible that these effects may wane over time. *P. umbilicalis*, being a rich source of polyphenols, has a broad range of biological activities including anti-inflammatory, immune-modulatory, antioxidant, cardiovascular protective, and anti-cancer actions [13,31]. Polyphenols show a beneficial influence on skin aging and dermal diseases (cancer) [32]. A combination of vitamins A, C, and E with natural extracts obtained from *P. umbilicalis* can show significant effects in skin protection against UV radiation, preventing DNA damage and inflammation, and can also act on cell renewal [33]. Inflammation is associated with the development and malignant progression of most cancers [34]. Therefore, its control has a negative impact on tumor development. As we previously reported, K14HPV16 mice showed increased numbers of tumor-associated leukocytes compared with wild-type animals [35]. In fact, multiple studies have shown that the development of lesions in these animals depends on tumor-associated inflammation and that the administration of anti-inflammatory drugs is able to block tumor progression [22,28,30,35–37]. Our results support the hypothesis that dietary supplementation with *P. umbilicalis* may have chemopreventive effects against pre-malignant lesions induced by HPV16 and associated with inflammation. Another interesting possibility is that *P. umbilicalis* might be able to reduce the activity of the *cytokeratin 14* gene promoter, thereby decreasing the expression of the HPV16 transgenes and slowing down the development of lesions. Elucidating the mechanisms underlying this chemoprevention should be the focus of future studies on this red seaweed. We also wished to confirm that dietary supplementation with *P. umbilicalis* was safe, especially in the presence of a chronic debilitating condition. The present results do not show any influence of *P. umbilicalis* over animals' behavior or the clinico-physiological variables analyzed, such as food intake and body weight. There were also no changes in the intermediate and hepatic metabolism associated with *P. umbilicalis*, at both the biochemical and the histological level. This is particularly interesting, as this model was previously shown to develop chronic hepatitis easily, as part of a wasting syndrome characterized by chronic systemic inflammation, presumably in response to the lesions induced by HPV16 transgenes [22]. The reduced relative mass of the lung in animals treated with *P. umbilicalis* of the group I is likely due to the presence of different amounts of residual blood following cardiac puncture. Two genotoxicity assays were used to study possible mutagenic risks posed by *P. umbilicalis*, i.e., the comet assay, also known as single-cell gel electrophoresis (SCGE), and the MN test [38]. The use of both assays allows the gathering of complementary information, as DNA damage detected by the comet assay occurs earlier, is rather short-lived, and does not require cell division to become evident. On the contrary, the MN test detects DNA-strand breaks that are not repaired and persist beyond mitosis, giving rise to clastogenic lesions or to aneuploidy [39–41]. *P. umbilicalis* reduced non-specific GDI in HPV16-transgenic mice. Relatively to the oxidative damage revealed by FPG treatment, there was a side effect consisting in the stimulation of the antioxidant system. It has been shown that some foods with antioxidant action induce a slight increase in reactive oxygen species (ROS) to activate the antioxidant system and thus strengthen the defenses against stronger exogenous genotoxic stimuli [42]. Concerning wild-type mice, the seaweed had no effect over the non-specific GDI but significantly reduced oxidative DNA damage. Importantly, the MN test did not reveal any significant differences between groups, although there was a trend for HPV16-transgenic mice to show slightly higher MN frequencies. Overall, these results suggest that *P. umbilicalis* does not induce any genotoxicity. The seaweed may even have DNA protective effects in specific contexts, and the results observed in wild-type and HPV16-transgenic animals deserve further study. Currently, there is only very limited knowledge concerning the DNA protective or damaging effects of seaweeds, and some recent studies in *Drosophila melanogaster* suggested that some seaweed species may provide protection against different genotoxic insults [43].

4. Material and Methods

4.1. Animals

K14HPV16 transgenic mice were generously donated by Drs. Jeffrey Arbeit and Douglas Hanahan from the University of California, through the National Cancer Institute Mouse Repository (USA). In these animals, expression of the whole early region of HPV16 is controlled and directed to basal epithelial cells by the *cytokeratin 14* gene promoter [29]. Forty-four female mice on an FVB/n background (22 transgenic HPV16$^{+/-}$ mice and 22 wild-type HPV16$^{-/-}$ mice) at 20 weeks of age were used. By 20 weeks of age, these animals start undergoing a critical change in their lesions, which progress from a purely hyperplastic stage to a more advanced, dysplastic stage [29,30]. Preventing this transition theoretically blocks further progression towards malignancy, so we chose to act within this time frame. The animals were genotyped as previously described [25]. This experimental assay was approved by the University of Trás-os-Montes and Alto Douro Ethics committee (approval no. 10/2013) and the Portuguese Veterinary Authorities (approval no. 0421/000/000/2014).

4.2. Diet Preparation

Porphyra umbilicalis was harvested from Mindelo beach (41°18′36.8″N 8°44′25.9″W), Vila do Conde, Portugal (October 2015). This seaweed was taken to the ALGAplus company, Ílhavo, Portugal, where it was dried for 24 h in a controlled-temperature chamber (25 °C), to 10–12% humidity. Then, the seaweed was milled and incorporated at 10% (w/w) into a standard mouse diet (Diet Standard 4RF21, Ultragene, Italy). The chosen concentration (10%) was based on research performed with *D. melanogaster* [44]. The seaweed and the base diet were finely milled, mixed, and granulated to form new pellets (2 mm in diameter), using an industrial mixer and adding 6.67% (v/w) of water. The base diet for the control groups was milled and granulated without including *P. umbilicalis*. The newly made pellets were dried at 40 °C during 48 h and stored at 4 °C until used.

4.3. Experimental Conditions

The animals were maintained in accordance with the Portuguese (Portaria 1005/92 dated October the 23rd) and European (EU Directive 2010/63/EU) legislation, under controlled conditions of temperature (23 ± 2 °C), light–dark cycle (12 h light/12 h dark), and relative humidity (50 ± 10%). The animals were identified individually and housed in hard polycarbonate cages (Eurostandard Tipo IV 1354G, Tecniplast, Italy; Eurostandard Tipo IV S 1500U, Tecniplast, Italy) using corncob bedding (Ultragene, Santa Comba Dão, Portugal) and environmental enrichment with paper rolls. Water and food access were provided ad libitum.

4.4. Experimental Design

The animals were divided into four groups: group I (HPV16$^{-/-}$, $n = 11$) and group II (HPV16$^{+/-}$, $n = 11$) received *P. umbilicalis*-supplemented diet, while group III (HPV16$^{-/-}$, $n = 11$) and group IV (HPV16$^{+/-}$, $n = 11$) received the base diet, during 22 consecutive days. Animal body weight, body condition, behavior, mental status, grooming, ears and whiskers, mucosae, posture, respiratory and cardiac frequency, hydration status, answer to external stimuli, and feces were monitored weekly, along with water and food consumption. At the end of the experiment, all animals were sacrificed by xylazine–ketamine overdose followed by cardiac puncture exsanguination, according to FELASA guidelines [45]. A complete necropsy of the animals was performed, and the internal organs (liver, right and left kidney, spleen, lung, heart, bladder, and thymus) were collected. Skin samples (chest and ear) and internal organs (liver) were collected for histological analysis.

4.5. Histological Analysis

The left ear was collected and longitudinally sectioned for histological analysis. Chest skin was harvested from the lower cervical to the diaphragmatic zone, forming a square of approximately 1 cm². Skin samples from the chest and ear and liver samples were fixed in 10% neutral buffered formalin and processed for hematoxylin and eosin (H&E) staining to classify HPV-induced cutaneous lesions and any toxic hepatic lesions attributable to *P. umbilicalis*. Skin samples were classified as normal, epidermal hyperplasia, or epidermal dysplasia. Normal epidermis was characterized by the presence of only 1 or 2 cellular layers and a keratin layer, while hyperplastic and dysplastic lesions showed over 3 cellular layers. Additionally, dysplastic lesions showed marked nuclear pleomorphism and suprabasal mitotic figures. Liver samples were classified as normal liver, grade I hepatitis, grade II hepatitis, and grade III hepatitis, as previously described [22].

4.6. Biochemical Analysis of Serum

Blood samples were collected by cardiac puncture and centrifuged at 1400× g for 15 min to isolate serum. The concentration of glucose, albumin, and total protein, as well as alanine aminotransferase (ALT), aspartate aminotransferase (AST), and gamma glutamyltransferase (GGT) were determined through spectrophotometric methods using an autoanalyzer (Prestige 24i, Cormay PZ), in order to detect potential metabolic disorders and hepatotoxic effects.

4.7. Genotoxicity Assays

4.7.1. Comet Assay

The alkaline comet assay (pH > 13) was performed as previously described [46,47]. Briefly, slides were precoated with normal-melting-point (NMP) agarose. For each animal, 4 slides were prepared (2 for performing the assay with the repair enzyme and the other 2 for the assay without the enzyme). Approximately 10 µL of blood was diluted in 200 µL of ice-cold phosphate-buffered saline (PBS) in a 0.5 mL microtube to prepare a cell suspension. Twenty µL of cell suspension was mixed with 70 µL of 1% low-melting-point (LMP) agarose, and 8 drops were placed onto the 4 precoated slides (2 replicates per slide). The slides were immersed in a lysis solution and rinsed three times. In order to specifically measure oxidatively damaged DNA, namely, 8-oxoguanines and other altered purines, 2 slides were incubated for 30 min with formamidopyrimidine DNA glycosylase (FPG), a DNA lesion-specific repair enzyme which converts oxidized purines into DNA single-strand breaks, donated by Professor Andrew Collins (University of Oslo, Norway). Slides with and without FPG treatment were gently immersed in a freshly prepared alkaline electrophoresis solution to allow DNA unwinding. Subsequently, the cells were electrophoresed in the same solution for 30 min at 25 V and a current of 300 mA. Following electrophoresis, the cells were immersed in PBS followed by distilled water, dehydrated in 70% and absolute ethanol, and air-dried. For visual scoring, DNA was stained with 1 µg/mL of 4,6-diamidino-2-phenylindole (DAPI) solution (Sigma-Aldrich Chemical Company, Spain) and visualized using a fluorescent microscope (OLYMPUS R XC10, U-RFL-T). The relative fluorescence intensity of head and tail (extent of DNA migration) was used as an indicator of DNA damage. One hundred comets (50 comets per gel) were evaluated to obtain a GDI in a scale ranging between 0 and 400 arbitrary units. Scores for GDI_{FPG} were subtracted from those for GDI to quantify the NSS_{FPG}.

4.7.2. Micronucleus Test

The MN test was performed as previously reported [48]. Briefly, MN frequency in erythrocytes was evaluated through blood smears on glass slides. Two slides were prepared for each animal. The preparations were air-dried, fixed in methanol for 10 min, and stained in 5% Giemsa for 30 min. One thousand erythrocytes and the respective micronuclei were counted per slide (2000 cells for each animal) under an optical microscope (Nikon Eclipse E100). The MN frequencies were presented as mean ± SD for each experimental group.

4.8. Statistical Analysis

Relative organ weights were calculated as the ratio of the organ weight to the animal's bodyweight. The data were analyzed using IBM SPSS software, version 25. The statistical approach used analysis of variance (ANOVA), followed a Bonferroni test. A Chi-squared test was performed for the histological lesions. Student's *t* tests were performed for the comet and micronucleus assays. In all tests, we compared the HPV$^{-/-}$ and the HPV$^{+/-}$ groups fed with different diets (*P. umbilicalis*-supplemented animals and base diet-fed animals). So, group I compared to group III and group II to group IV. Differences were considered statistically significant in all the analyses when $p < 0.05$.

5. Conclusions

Red seaweed *P. umbilicalis* reduced the incidence of dysplastic cutaneous lesions induced by HPV16 in this model, suggesting that dietary supplementation with this seaweed in the concentration used may have beneficial chemopreventive effects. Results also indicate that the tested level of *P. umbilicalis* supplementation was safe and did not induce toxicity under the current experimental conditions.

Author Contributions: R.M.G.d.C., I.G. and P.A.O. designed the experiments; S.S., T.F., J.A., S.L., M.J.N., M.J.P., A.C., R.M.G.d.C. and P.A.O. conducted the experiments with live animals, participated in animals sacrifice and samples processing; H.A. and R.P. performed the harvesting, identification and dehydration of *Porphyra umbilicalis*; S.S., T.F., J.A., S.L., R.M., M.M.S.M.B., R.M.G.d.C., I.G. and P.A.O. participated in data analysis; S.S., T.F., J.A., S.L., R.M.G.d.C., R.M.G.d.C., R.M., I.G., M.P., M.M.S.M.B., M.J.N., E.R. and P.A.O. wrote the manuscript; R.M.G.d.C., I.G. and P.A.O. supervised and conducted the experiments; R.M.G.d.C. and P.A.O. funding acquisition.

Funding: This work was supported by National Funds by FCT—Portuguese Foundation for Science and Technology, under the projects UID/AGR/04033/2019, UID/EQU/00511/2019 - Laboratory for Process Engineering, Environment, Biotechnology and Energy – LEPABE funded by national funds through FCT/MCTES (PIDDAC); Project "LEPABE-2-ECO-INNOVATION" – NORTE-01-0145-FEDER-000005, funded by Norte Portugal Regional Operational Programme (NORTE 2020), under PORTUGAL 2020 Partnership Agreement, through the European Regional Development Fund (ERDF) and Interreg Program for the financial support of the Project IBERPHENOL, Project Number 0377_IBERPHENOL_6_E, co-financed by European Regional Development Fund (ERDF) through POCTEP 2014-2020.

Conflicts of Interest: The authors declare no conflict of interest.

References

1. Shalaby, E.A. Algae as promising organisms for environment and health. *Plant Signal. Behav.* **2011**, *6*, 1338–1350. [CrossRef] [PubMed]
2. Cofrades, S.; Benedí, J.; Garcimartin, A.; Sánchez-muniz, F.J.; Jimenez-colmenero, F. A comprehensive approach to formulation of seaweed-enriched meat products: From technological development to assessment of healthy properties. *Food Res. Int.* **2017**, *99*, 1084–1094. [CrossRef] [PubMed]
3. Brownlee, I.; Fairclough, A.; Hall, A.; Paxman, J. The potential health benefits of seaweed and seaweed extract. In *Seaweed: Ecology, Nutrient Composition and Medicinal Uses*; Pomin, V.H., Ed.; Nova Science: Hauppauge, NY, USA, 2012; pp. 119–136.
4. Brown, E.M.; Allsopp, P.J.; Magee, P.J.; Gill, C.I.; Nitecki, S.; Strain, C.R.; Mcsorley, E.M. Seaweed and human health. *Nutr. Rev.* **2014**, *72*, 205–216. [CrossRef] [PubMed]
5. MacArtain, P.; Gill, C.I.R.; Brooks, M.; Campbell, R.; Rowland, I.R. Nutritional value of edible seaweeds. *Nutr. Rev.* **2007**, *65*, 535–543. [CrossRef] [PubMed]
6. Pereira, L. A review of the nutrient composition of selected edible seaweeds. In *Seaweed: Ecology, Nutrient Composition and Medicinal Uses*, 1st ed.; Pomin, V.H., Ed.; Nova Science: Hauppauge, NY, USA, 2011; pp. 15–47.

7. Cardoso, S.M.; Pereira, O.R.; Seca, A.M.L.; Pinto, D.C.G.A.; Silva, A.M.S. Seaweeds as preventive agents for cardiovascular diseases: From nutrients to functional foods. *Mar. Drugs* **2015**, *13*, 6838–6865. [CrossRef] [PubMed]
8. Déléris, P.; Nazih, H.; Bard, J.M. Seaweeds in Human Health. In *Seaweed in Health and Disease Prevention*; Academic Press, Elsevier: Cambridge, MA, USA, 2016; pp. 319–367.
9. Gutiérrez-Rodríguez, A.G.; Juárez-Portilla, C.; Olivares-Bañuelos, T.; Zepeda, R.C. Anticancer activity of seaweeds. *Drug Discov. Today* **2018**, *23*, 434–447. [CrossRef] [PubMed]
10. Rocha, D.H.A.; Seca, A.M.L.; Pinto, D.C.G.A. Seaweed Secondary Metabolites In Vitro and In Vivo Anticancer Activity. *Mar. Drugs* **2018**, *16*, 410. [CrossRef]
11. Brawley, S.H.; Blouin, N.A.; Ficko-Blean, E.; Wheeler, G.L.; Lohr, M.; Goodson, H.V.; Jenkins, J.W.; Blaby-Haas, C.E.; Helliwell, K.E.; Chan, C.X.; et al. Insights into the red algae and eukaryotic evolution from the genome of *Porphyra umbilicalis* (Bangiophyceae, Rhodophyta). *Proc. Natl. Acad. Sci. USA* **2017**, *114*, E6361–E6370. [CrossRef]
12. Cofrades, S.; López-Lopez, I.; Bravo, L.; Ruiz-Capillas, C.; Bastida, S.; Larrea, M.T.; Jiménez-Colmenero, F. Nutritional and antioxidant properties of different brown and red Spanish edible seaweeds. *Food Sci. Technol. Int.* **2010**, *16*, 361–370. [CrossRef]
13. López-López, I.; Bastida, S.; Ruiz-Capillas, C.; Bravo, L.; Larrea, M.T.; Sánchez-Muniz, F.; Cofrades, S.; Jiménez-Colmenero, F. Composition and antioxidant capacity of low-salt meat emulsion model systems containing edible seaweeds. *Meat Sci.* **2009**, *83*, 492–498. [CrossRef]
14. Gaglia, M.M.; Munger, K. More than just oncogenes: Mechanisms of tumorigenesis by human viruses. *Curr. Opin. Virol.* **2018**, *32*, 48–59. [CrossRef] [PubMed]
15. De Martel, C.; Plummer, M.; Vignat, J.; Franceschi, S. Worldwide burden of cancer attributable to HPV by site, country and HPV type. *Int. J. Cancer* **2017**, 1–22. [CrossRef] [PubMed]
16. Wang, S.X.; Zhang, X.S.; Guan, H.S.; Wang, W. Potential anti-HPV and related cancer agents from marine resources: An overview. *Mar. Drugs* **2014**, *12*, 2019–2035. [CrossRef] [PubMed]
17. Pereira, L. Biological and therapeutic properties of the seaweed polysaccharides. *Int. Biol. Rev.* **2018**, *2*, 1–50.
18. Blaszczak, W.; Lach, M.S.; Barczak, W.; Suchorska, W.M. Fucoidan Exerts Anticancer Effects Against Head and Neck Squamous Cell Carcinoma In Vitro. *Molecules* **2018**, *23*, 3302. [CrossRef]
19. Coussens, L.M.; Hanahan, D.; Arbeit, J.M. Genetic predisposition and parameters of malignant progression in K14- HPV16 transgenic mice. *Am. J. Pathol.* **1996**, *149*, 1899–1917.
20. Medeiros-Fonseca, B.; Mestre, V.F.; Colaço, B.; Pires, M.J.; Martins, T.; Gil da Costa, R.M.; Neuparth, M.J.; Medeiros, R.; Moutinho, M.S.S.; Dias, M.I.; et al. *Laurus nobilis* (laurel) aqueous leaf extract's toxicological and anti-tumor activities in HPV16-transgenic mice. *Food Funct.* **2018**, *9*, 4419–4428. [CrossRef]
21. Santos, J.M.O.; Fernandes, M.; Araújo, R.; Sousa, H.; Ribeiro, J.; Bastos, M.M.S.M.; Oliveira, P.A.; Carmo, D.; Casaca, F.; Silva, S.; et al. Dysregulated expression of microRNA-150 in human papillomavirus-induced lesions of K14-HPV16 transgenic mice. *Life Sci.* **2017**, *175*, 31–36. [CrossRef]
22. Gil da Costa, R.M.; Aragão, S.; Moutinho, M.; Alvarado, A.; Carmo, D.; Casaca, F.; Silva, S.; Ribeiro, J.; Sousa, H.; Ferreira, R.; et al. HPV16 induces a wasting syndrome in transgenic mice: Amelioration by dietary polyphenols via NF-κB inhibition. *Life Sci.* **2017**, *169*, 11–19. [CrossRef]
23. Minkiewicz, P.; Turło, M.; Iwaniak, A. Free Accessible Databases as a Source of Information about Food Components and Other Compounds with Anticancer Activity—Brief Review. *Molecules* **2019**, *24*, 789. [CrossRef]
24. Calder, P.C.; Grimble, R.F. Polyunsaturated fatty acids, inflammation and immunity. *Eur. J. Clin. Nutr.* **2002**, *56*, S14–S19. [CrossRef] [PubMed]
25. Paiva, I.; Gil da Costa, R.M.; Ribeiro, J.; Sousa, H.; Bastos, M.; Faustino-Rocha, A.; Oliveira, P.A.; Medeiros, R. A role for MicroRNA-155 expression in microenvironment associated to HPV-induced carcinogenesis in K14-HPV16 transgenic mice. *PLoS ONE* **2015**, *10*, e0116868. [CrossRef] [PubMed]
26. Shirnekhi, H.K.; Kelley, E.P.; Deluca, J.G.; Herman, J.A.; Bloom, K.S. Spindle assembly checkpoint signaling and sister chromatid cohesion are disrupted by HPV E6-mediated transformation. *Mol. Biol. Cell* **2017**, *28*, 2035–2041. [CrossRef] [PubMed]
27. Reshmi, G.; Pillai, M.R. Interplay Between HPV Oncoproteins and MicroRNAs in Cervical Cancer. *IntechOpen* **2012**, 347–360.

28. Santos, C.; Neto, T.; Ferreirinha, P.; Sousa, H.; Ribeiro, J.; Bastos, M.M.S.M.; Faustino-Rocha, A.I.; Oliveira, P.A.; Medeiros, R.; Vilanova, M.; et al. Celecoxib promotes degranulation of CD8 + T cells in HPV-induced lesions of K14-HPV16 transgenic mice. *Life Sci.* **2016**, *157*, 67–73. [CrossRef]
29. Arbeit, J.M.; Munger, K.; Howley, P.M.; Hanahan, D. Progressive squamous epithelial neoplasia in K14-human papillomavirus type 16 transgenic mice. *J. Virol.* **1994**, *68*, 4358–4368. [PubMed]
30. Smith-McCune, K.; Zhu, Y.-H.; Hanhan, D.; Arbeit, A. Cross-species comarison of angiogenesis during the premalignant stages of squamous carcinogenesis in the human cervix and K14-HPV16 transgenic mice. *Cancer Res.* **1997**, *57*, 1294–1300.
31. Hussain, T.; Tan, B.; Yin, Y.; Blachier, F.; Tossou, M.C.B.; Rahu, N. Oxidative Stress and Inflammation: What Polyphenols Can Do for Us? *Oxidative Med. Cell. Longev.* **2016**, *2016*, 1–9. [CrossRef]
32. Działo, M.; Mierziak, J.; Korzun, U.; Preisner, M.; Szopa, J.; Kulma, A. The Potential of Plant Phenolics in Prevention and Therapy of Skin Disorders. *Int. J. Mol. Sci.* **2016**, *17*, 160. [CrossRef]
33. Mercurio, D.G.; Wagemaker, T.A.L.; Alves, V.M.; Benevenuto, C.G.; Gaspar, L.R.; Campos, P.M.B.G.M. In vivo photoprotective effects of cosmetic formulations containing UV filters, vitamins, *Ginkgo biloba* and red algae extracts. *J. Photochem. Photobiol. B* **2015**, *153*, 121–126. [CrossRef]
34. Fernandes, J.V.; Fernandes, T.A.A.D.M.; de Azevedo, J.C.V.; Cobucci, R.N.O.; de Carvalho, M.G.F.; Andrade, V.S.; De Araújo, J.M.G. Link between chronic inflammation and human papillomavirus-induced carcinogenesis (Review). *Oncol. Lett.* **2015**, *9*, 1015–1026. [CrossRef] [PubMed]
35. Ferreira, T.; Campos, S.; Silva, M.G.; Ribeiro, R.; Santos, S.; Almeida, J.; Pires, M.J.; Gil da Costa, R.M.; Córdova, C.; Nogueira, A.; et al. The Cyclooxigenase-2 Inhibitor Parecoxib Prevents Epidermal Dysplasia in HPV16-Transgenic Mice: Efficacy and Safety Observations. *Int. J. Mol. Sci.* **2019**, *20*, 3902. [CrossRef] [PubMed]
36. Santos, J.M.O.; Moreira-Pais, A.; Neto, T.; Peixoto da Silva, S.; Oliveira, P.A.; Ferreira, R.; Mendes, J.; Bastos, M.M.S.M.; Lopes, C.; Casaca, F.; et al. Dimethylaminoparthenolide reduces the incidence of dysplasia and ameliorates a wasting syndrome in HPV16-transgenic mice. *Drug Dev. Res.* **2019**, *80*, 824–830. [CrossRef] [PubMed]
37. Peirone, C.; Mestre, V.F.; Medeiros-Fonseca, B.; Colaço, B.; Pires, M.J.; Martins, T.; Gil da Costa, R.M.; Neuparth, M.J.; Medeiros, R.; Bastos, M.M.S.M.; et al. Ozone therapy prevents the onset of dysplasia in HPV16-transgenic mice—A preclinical efficacy and safety study. *Biomed. Pharmacother.* **2018**, *104*, 275–279. [CrossRef] [PubMed]
38. Kang, S.H.; Kwon, J.Y.; Lee, J.K.; Seo, Y.R. Recent Advances in In Vivo Genotoxicity Testing: Prediction of Carcinogenic Potential Using Comet and Micronucleus Assay in Animal Models. *J. Cancer Prev.* **2013**, *18*, 277–288. [CrossRef] [PubMed]
39. Cotelle, S.; Fe, J.F. Comet Assay in Genetic Ecotoxicology: A Review. *Environ. Mol. Mutagen.* **1999**, *255*, 246–255. [CrossRef]
40. Guilherme, S.; Gaivão, I.; Santos, M.A.; Pacheco, M. European eel (*Anguilla anguilla*) genotoxic and pro-oxidant responses following short-term exposure to Roundup®—A glyphosate-based herbicide. *Mutagenesis* **2010**, *25*, 523–530. [CrossRef]
41. Llana-Ruiz-Cabello, M.; Puerto, M.; Maisanaba, S.; Guzmán-Guillén, R.; Pichardo, S.; Cameán, A.M. Use of micronucleus and comet assay to evaluate evaluate the genotoxicity of oregano essential oil (*Origanum vulgare* L. Virens) in rats orally exposed for 90 days. *J. Toxicol. Environ. Heal.* **2018**, *81*, 525–533.
42. Droge, W. Free Radicals in the Physiological Control of Cell Function. *Siol. Rev.* **2002**, *82*, 47–95. [CrossRef]
43. Marques, A.; Ferreira, J.; Abreu, H.; Pereira, R.; Rego, A.; Serôdio, J.; Christa, G.; Gaivão, I.; Pacheco, M. Searching for antigenotoxic properties of marine macroalgae dietary supplementation against endogenous and exogenous challenges. *J. Toxicol. Environ. Heal.* **2018**, *81*, 939–956. [CrossRef]
44. Ferreira, J.; Marques, A.; Abreu, H.; Pereira, R.; Rego, A.; Gaivão, I. Red seaweeds *Porphyra umbilicalis* and *Grateloupia turuturu* display antigenotoxic and longevity-promoting potential in *Drosophila melanogaster*. *Eur. J. Phycol.* **2019**. [CrossRef]
45. Forbes, D.; Blom, H.; Kostomitsopulos, N.; Moore, G.; Perretta, G. *Euroguide: On the Accommodation and Care of Animals Used for Experimental and Other Scientific Purposes*; FELASA: London, UK, 2007.
46. Shaposhnikov, S.; Azqueta, A.; Henriksson, S.; Meier, S.; Gaivão, I.; Huskisson, N.H.; Smart, A.; Brunborg, G.; Nilsson, M.; Collins, A.R. Twelve-gel slide format optimised for comet assay and fluorescent in situ hybridisation. *Toxicol. Lett.* **2010**, *195*, 31–34. [CrossRef] [PubMed]

47. Guilherme, S.; Santos, M.A.; Gaivão, I.; Pacheco, M. DNA and chromosomal damage induced in fish (*Anguilla anguilla* L.) by aminomethylphosphonic acid (AMPA)—The major environmental breakdown product of glyphosate. *Environ Sci Pollut Res.* **2014**, *21*, 8730–8739. [CrossRef] [PubMed]
48. Sierra, L.M.; Gaivão, I. Genotoxicity and DNA Repair: A Practical Approach. In *Humana Press*; Springer: Oviedo, Spain; Vila Real, Portugal, 2014; pp. 103–113.

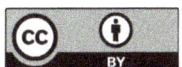

© 2019 by the authors. Licensee MDPI, Basel, Switzerland. This article is an open access article distributed under the terms and conditions of the Creative Commons Attribution (CC BY) license (http://creativecommons.org/licenses/by/4.0/).

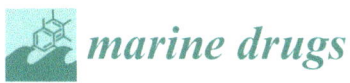

Article

Padina pavonica Extract Promotes In Vitro Differentiation and Functionality of Human Primary Osteoblasts

Mariagiulia Minetti [1,2], Giulia Bernardini [1], Manuele Biazzo [2], Gilles Gutierrez [2], Michela Geminiani [1], Teresa Petrucci [1] and Annalisa Santucci [1,*]

1. Dipartimento di Biotecnologie, Chimica e Farmacia (Dipartimento di Eccellenza 2018-2022), Università degli Studi di Siena, via Aldo Moro 2, 53100 Siena, Italy
2. Institute of Cellular Pharmacology (ICP Ltd.), F24, Triq Valletta, Mosta Technopark, Mosta MST 3000, Malta
* Correspondence: annalisa.santucci@unisi.it; Tel.: +39-0577234958; Fax: +39-0577234254

Received: 24 July 2019; Accepted: 12 August 2019; Published: 15 August 2019

Abstract: Marine algae have gained much importance in the development of nutraceutical products due to their high content of bioactive compounds. In this work, we investigated the activity of *Padina pavonica* with the aim to demonstrate the pro-osteogenic ability of its extract on human primary osteoblast (HOb). Our data indicated that the acetonic extract of *P. pavonica* (EPP) is a safe product as it did not show any effect on osteoblast viability. At the same time, EPP showed to possess a beneficial effect on HOb functionality, triggering their differentiation and mineralization abilities. In particular EPP enhanced the expression of the earlier differentiation stage markers: a 5.4-fold increase in collagen type I alpha 1 chain (COL1A1), and a 2.3-fold increase in alkaline phosphatase (ALPL), as well as those involved in the late differentiation stage: a 3.7-fold increase in osteocalcin (BGLAP) expression and a 2.8-fold in osteoprotegerin (TNFRSF11B). These findings were corroborated by the enhancement in ALPL enzymatic activity (1.7-fold increase) and by the reduction of receptor activator of nuclear factor-κB ligand (RANKL) and osteoprotegerin (OPG) ratio (0.6-fold decrease). Moreover, EPP demonstrated the capacity to enhance the bone nodules formation by 3.2-fold in 4 weeks treated HOb. Therefore, EPP showed a significant capability of promoting osteoblast phenotype. Given its positive effect on bone homeostasis, EPP could be used as a useful nutraceutical product that, in addition to a healthy lifestyle and diet, can be able to contrast and prevent bone diseases, especially those connected with ageing, such as osteoporosis (OP).

Keywords: *Padina pavonica*; marine algae; osteoporosis; bone metabolism; bone health; nutraceutical

1. Introduction

Bone is a specialized form of connective tissue and its functions include locomotion, protection and mineral homeostasis. Osteoblasts, osteocytes, and bone lining cells are bone-forming cells, whereas osteoclasts are involved in the bone resorption process. The retention of homeostasis is based on the balance between these opposite activities. Therefore, bone is a very dynamic tissue due to the continuous balance between mineralization and resorption processes, that guarantee tissue homeostasis and functions [1]. With ageing, a net loss of bone is observed due to the increment of the resorptive activity of osteoclasts that is not balanced by novel bone tissue formation. This condition leads to pathological processes, such as osteoporosis (OP), a devastating bone disease [2] characterized by thinning of the tissue, changes in skeletal architecture, and significant increase of fracture risks. OP affects both women and men (even if it is more frequently observed in postmenopausal women), and the healthy and socio-economic issues connected to this pathology are expected to grow due to the increase of life expectancy. Due to the inefficiencies of current treatment options and related side effects, alternative therapies and preventive agents are highly desirable [3]. Osteogenic bioactive compounds have been isolated from many marine organisms, mainly macroalgae, such as brown algae *Sargassum horneri* and *Undaria pinnatifida*, so that OP could benefit from a novel and more efficient marine-based treatment. Compounds from marine organism are known to have a wide range of osteogenic effects, including stimulation of osteoblast functions and mineralization, as well as suppression of osteoclast activity [3,4].

Many previous studies have focused on the beneficial protective effects of seaweeds on human health and against chronic disease as they represent a source of unique bioactive compounds, such as proteins, peptides and amino acids, lipids and fatty acids, sterols, polysaccharides, oligosaccharides, phenolic compounds, photosynthetic pigments, vitamins, and minerals [5,6].

For the extraction of all the above-mentioned compounds, many different methods and solvents have been used. The process parameters of each method and the solvent must be chosen and optimized in order to obtain the extracts with the targeted bioactive compounds [7]. Parameters such as techniques, solvent, temperature, and raw material are known to notably affect the yield of extracted compounds from a quantitative and a qualitative point of view [6,8]. As the demand of macroalgae in the development of PUFA-related dietary supplements is growing, Kumari P. et al. performed a comparison of different lipid and fatty acid extraction and derivatization methods [9].

P. pavonica is a marine brown seaweed, a member of the Dictyotaceae family that is widespread throughout the world in warm temperate to tropical locations, including North Carolina to Florida in the United States, the Gulf of Mexico, throughout the Caribbean and tropical Atlantic and the Eastern Atlantic, Mediterranean, and Adriatic Seas [10]. In marine biology, *P. pavonica* is used above all as sensor or marker to study pollution levels in the sea and, in general, in the marine environment [11]. Regarding the functional and positive influence of *P. pavonica* on human health, sterols, lipids, polysaccharides, carotenoids, polyphenols, and fibers are the main bioactive compounds found in *Padina* species [12].

In a previous in vivo study conducted on 40 postmenopausal women and based on the initial founding by Gilles Gutierrez [13], *P. pavonica* demonstrated the ability to increase bone mineral density (BMD) and to exert a positive effect on collagen control (ICP Ltd., personal communication based on the study performed by Professor Mark Brincat). Nevertheless, based on our literature research, in vitro biochemical and molecular evaluation supporting osteogenic beneficial effects from *P. pavonica* extracts are nonexistent Therefore, in this study, we aimed to demonstrate the activity of EPP on bone homeostasis, providing the first report on French Polynesian *P. pavonica* effects on HOb metabolism. In particular, we undertook biochemical and molecular analyses to demonstrate if this vegetal substance may increase the uptake and the fixation of calcium by osteoblasts, and thus can induce a mass increment of bone tissue.

2. Results

2.1. Chemical Composition and Antioxidant Capacity of EPP

EPP was chemically characterized for its total phenolic, flavonoid, and tannin content [6]. The total phenolic, flavonoid, and tannin contents of the seaweed were 27.0, 54.8, and 54.3 mg per g of extract, respectively, corresponding to 0.81, 1.64, and 1.63 mg per g of dry material, respectively. The antioxidant activity resulted as 256 ± 2 µmol of Fe^{2+} per g of extract.

EPP was also examined for its lipid content by GC-MS [6]. Hydrocarbons represented 79.88% of the total extract, among which 68.83% corresponded to fatty acids (FAs), 0.19% corresponded to squalene, and 10.86% to other hydrocarbon species (Figure 1). Sterols represented 8.37% of the extract and included fucosterol and cholesterol at percentages of 7.40% and 0.97%, respectively (Figure 1). GC-MS analysis was also performed with a different sample preparation approach consisting in a saponification and an extraction by dispersive liquid-liquid microextraction (DLLME) of EPP, in order to analyze the most lipophilic compounds. This analysis mostly confirmed the presence of several already identified compounds (Figure 1).

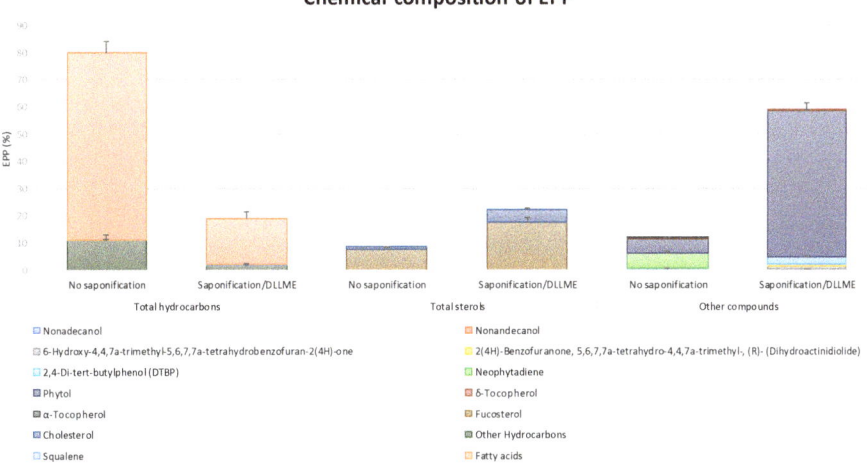

Figure 1. *Padina pavonica* extract (EPP) lipid content by GC-MS. For the analysis of the most lipophilic compounds, EPP was submitted to saponification and DLLME. Experiments were performed in triplicate. Data are presented as mean ± SD.

EPP's FA profile (Figure 2) showed that the presence of saturated FAs (SFAs) corresponded to 43.45% of total EPP (63.13% of total FAs). Among these, the most abundant FA was palmitic acid with a total percentage of 34.15%, followed by stearic (3.25%), pentadecanoic (1.95%), arachidic (0.74%), myristic (0.43%), lauric (0.47%), and behenic (0.04%) acids. Monounsaturated FAs (MUFAs) made up 23.67% of total EPP (34.40% of total FAs). The most abundant MUFA was palmitelaidic acid (16:1 n-7 E, 7.82%), followed by oleic acid (18:1 n-9, 7.79%) and palmitoleic acid (16:1 n-7 Z, 6.29%). Polyunsaturated FAs (PUFAs) corresponded to 1.70% of EPP (2.47% of total FAs). The main PUFA found in EPP was arachidonic acid (20:4 n-6, 0.64%), followed by linoleic (18:2 n-6, 0.53) and eicosapentanoic acid (20:5 n-3 0.24%) [6].

2.2. EPP Effects on HOb Viability

EPP did not exhibit significant effects on HOb viability at the concentrations used (1, 10, 20 µg/mL) after 24 h treatment (Figure 3). We detected a minor effect on HOb viability only at the highest concentrations tested. Therefore, having verified that EPP had no remarkable toxic effects at the concentrations tested, we focused on analyzing its functional activity on HOb.

2.3. Expression Analysis of Bone Differentiation Markers

To evaluate the effect of EPP at the molecular level, we extracted RNAs from EPP-treated cells and performed RT-qPCR analysis of osteoblastic-specific genes. Expression of genes coding for osteocalcin (BGLAP), osteoprotegerin (TNFRSF11B), collagen type I alpha 1 chain (COL1A1), alkaline phosphatase (ALPL) and Sox9 after 24 h of treatment with EPP at different concentrations (1, 10, and 20 µg/mL) was assessed. These mRNA species were chosen for our study as they represent recognized markers of the different osteoblast differentiation stages. Sox9 mRNA was also monitored as a transcription factor involved in cartilage growth during chondrogenesis. At the molecular level, Sox9 directly interacts with RUNX2, a transcription activator of osteoblast-specific genes, decreasing RUNX2 binding to its target sequences and inhibiting its activity. During osteochondroprogenitor cells' differentiation toward the osteoblastic phenotype, Sox9 expression levels decrease and RUNX2 increases [14].

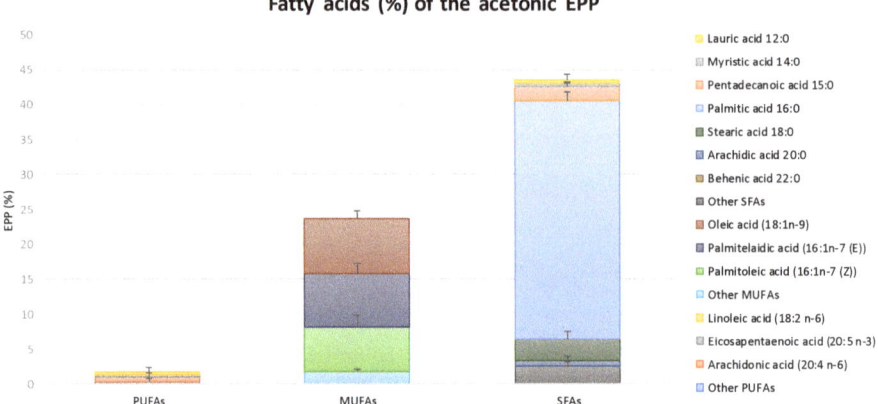

Figure 2. *Padina pavonica* extract (EPP) fatty acids (FAs) profile: PUFAs (polyunsaturated FAs), MUFAs (monounsaturated FAs) and SFAs (saturated FAs). Experiments were performed in triplicate. Data are presented as mean ± SD.

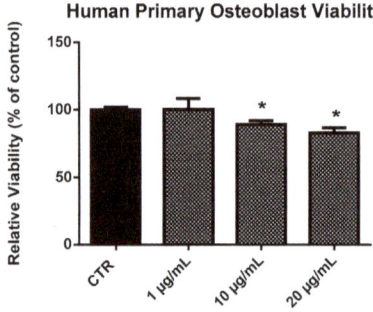

Figure 3. Viability of human primary osteoblasts (HOb) following 24 h treatment with EPP. Experiments were performed in triplicate. Data are expressed as percentage of control and presented as mean ± SD. Statistically significant differences from untreated control are denoted by * $p < 0.05$.

2.3.1. BGLAP

EPP treatment induced an increment of *BGLAP* expression in HOb at all the concentrations tested (Figure 4). In particular, a nearly two-fold increase of *BGLAP* was observed at 1 and 10 µg/mL, and of around 3.7-fold at 20 µg/mL.

2.3.2. TNFRSF11B

EPP treatment induced an increase of *TNFRSF11B* expression in HOb. In particular, all the concentrations tested induced statistically significant increase of the gene expression: 1.7-fold at 1 µg/mL, 2.8-fold at 10 µg/mL, and nearly two-fold at 20 µg/mL (Figure 5).

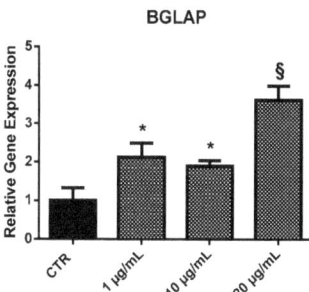

Figure 4. Relative expression of the *BGLAP* gene from HOb following 24 h treatment with EPP. Untreated cells were used as controls. Experiments were performed in triplicate. Results are shown as a mean of fold change in gene expression ± SD using untreated osteoblasts as a control. Statistically significant differences from untreated control are denoted by * $p < 0.05$ or § $p < 0.01$.

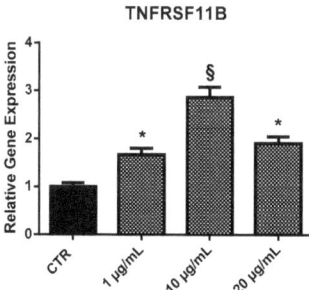

Figure 5. Relative expression of the *TNFRSF11B* gene from HOb following 24 h treatment with EPP. Experiments were performed in triplicate. Results are shown as a mean of fold change in gene expression ±SD using untreated osteoblasts as a control. Statistically significant differences from untreated control are denoted by * $p < 0.05$ or § $p < 0.01$.

2.3.3. COL1A1

COL1A1 was expressed in larger amounts in EPP-treated HOb in respect to control (Figure 6). EPP treatment induced a dose-dependent increase in *COL1A1* expression: 2.7-fold at 1 µg/mL, 3.8 at 10 µg/mL, and 5.4-fold at 20 µg/mL.

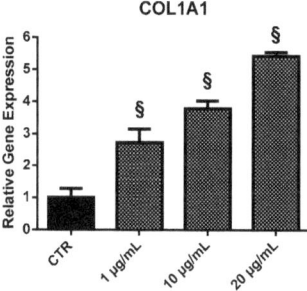

Figure 6. Relative expression of the *COL1A1* gene from HOb following 24 h treatment with EPP. Experiments were performed in triplicate. Results are shown as a mean of fold change in gene expression ± SD using untreated osteoblasts as a control. Statistically significant differences from untreated control are denoted by § $p < 0.01$.

2.3.4. ALPL

HOb showed an increase expression of *ALPL* following EPP treatment (Figure 7). The expression of the gene was enhanced by nearly 1.9-fold at 1 µg/mL, 2.3-fold at 10 µg/mL, and nearly two-fold at 20 µg/mL.

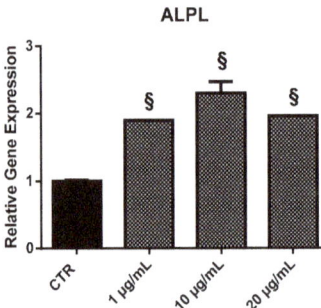

Figure 7. Relative expression of the *ALPL* gene from HOb following 24 h treatment with EPP. Experiments were performed in triplicate. Results are shown as a mean of fold change in gene expression ± SD using untreated osteoblasts as a control. Statistically significant differences from untreated control are denoted by § $p < 0.01$.

2.3.5. Sox9

EPP treatment of HOb resulted in a dose-dependent reduction of *Sox9* expression compared to control (Figure 8): 0.8-fold at 1 µg/mL, 0.4-fold at 10 µg/mL, and 0.3-fold at 20 µg/mL.

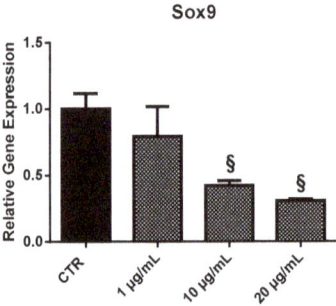

Figure 8. Relative expression of the *Sox9* gene from HOb following 24 h treatment with EPP. Experiments were performed in triplicate. Results are shown as a mean of fold change in gene expression ± SD using untreated osteoblasts as a control. Statistically significant differences from untreated control are denoted by § $p < 0.01$.

2.4. Receptor Activator of Nuclear Factor-κB Ligand (RANKL) and Osteoprotegerin (OPG) Ratio (RANKL/OPG Ratio)

The RANKL/OPG ratio is the main determinant of bone mass and better reflects the bone remodeling condition [15]. In EPP-treated HOb, we detected a reduction in RANKL/OPG ratio with increasing EPP concentrations (Figure 9). In particular, EPP at 20 µg/mL caused a reduction in RANKL/OPG ratio of nearly 0.6-fold compared to untreated HOb (CTR).

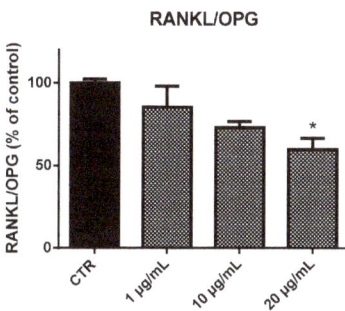

Figure 9. RANKL/OPG levels in HOb following 96 h treatment with EPP. Experiments were performed in triplicate. Data are expressed as percentage of control and presented as mean ± SD. Statistically significant differences from untreated control are denoted by * $p < 0.05$.

2.5. Alkaline Phosphatase (ALPL) Activity

ALPL activity was detected following 96 h treatment with EPP. Compared with control cell cultures, EPP treatment significantly upregulated ALPL activity in HOb (Figure 10). In particular, EPP treatment at 1, 10, and 20 µg/mL led to an increase in ALPL enzymatic activity of 1.25, 1.5, and 1.7-fold over the control, respectively.

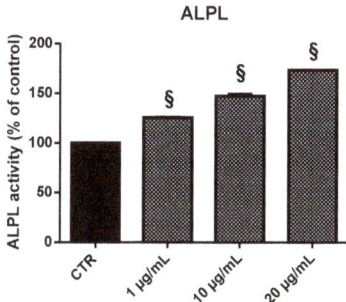

Figure 10. ALPL activity in HOb following 96 h treatment with EPP. Experiments were performed in triplicate. Data are expressed as percentage of control and presented as mean ± SD. Statistically significant differences from untreated control are denoted by § $p < 0.01$.

2.6. Bone Nodule Formation and Mineralization

Detecting the formation of mineralized nodules in EPP-treated HOb cultures has provided a means to assess mature osteoblast cells' function and the status of the cultures.

EPP treatment of HOb for 3 or 4 weeks induced the deposition of mineralized nodules (Figure 11a). The nodules appeared three-dimensional under a phase contrast microscope and continued to grow until the end of the culture period.

Quantifying the mineralized nodules after 3 weeks indicated no significant difference in HOb treated with EPP at 1 and 10 µg/mL compared to the control, whereas 20 µg/mL EPP induced a 2.6-fold increase in calcium deposition (Figure 11b). At 4 weeks EPP treatment, a larger increase in calcium deposition was observed at all the concentrations of EPP tested: 1.4-fold at 1 µg/mL, 3.1-fold at 10 µg/mL, and 3.2-fold at 20 µg/mL (Figure 11c).

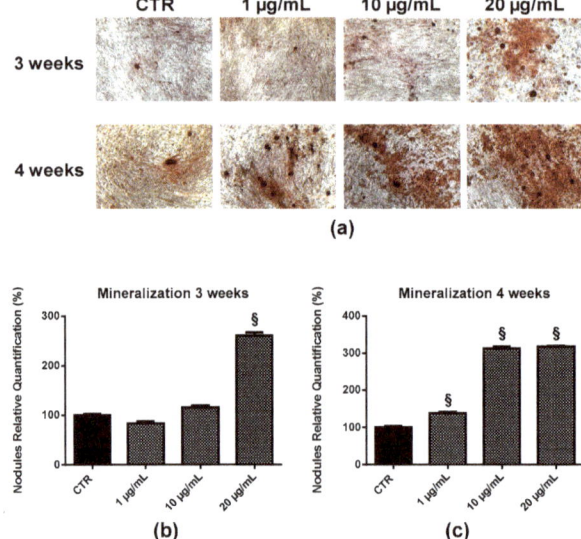

Figure 11. Detection (**a**) and quantification (**b**,**c**) of mineralized nodules formed in HOb cultured for 3 weeks (**b**) or 4 weeks (**c**) in the presence of EPP at different concentrations. Experiments were performed in triplicate. Bars represent mean ± SD. Original magnification: 10×.

3. Discussion

OP is a silent disease which leads to feeble quality of life and increased mortality in aged people, especially in postmenopausal women [16]. The balance between bone resorption and bone formation is the key point in bone homeostasis and health and an imbalance of these events causes OP. Loss of bone matrix and mass and microarchitectural deterioration are the main features of OP that increase the rate of fractures [16]. Nowadays, finding the proper treatment for bone-related disease is a matter of great interest. Due to the inefficiencies of current treatment options and related side effects, alternative therapies and preventive agents are highly desirable [3]. Since natural products are showing lower side effects and are more suitable for long-term use, they are quickly replacing traditional synthetic drugs [16].

Osteogenic bioactive compounds have been isolated from many marine organisms, mainly macroalgae, such as brown algae *Sargassum horneri* and *Undaria pinnatifida*, so that OP could benefit from a novel and more efficient marine-based treatment. Compounds from marine organisms are known to have a wide range of osteogenic effects, including stimulation of osteoblast functions and mineralization, as well as suppression of osteoclast activity [3,4].

Marine algae have been demonstrated to be strong candidates for the extraction and enforcement of novel drugs [17] and in recent years, significant development has been achieved in the isolation of these active compounds with several activities, such as anticancer, anti-inflammation, antioxidant, and having an inhibitory effect on ROS generation [18].

Numerous macroalgae have shown potent cytotoxic activities and some authors have suggested the utilization of algae as a chemopreventive agent against several cancers. Among these, extracts from *Laurencia viridis* and *Portieria horemanii*, containing dehydro-thrsiferol and halomon, have been tested in preclinical trials [19,20]. Recently, the methanolic extract of *P. pavonica* from the Adriatic Sea (Montenegro) was demonstrated to possess antitumoral activities on human cervical and breast cancer cell lines [21], inducing high DNA damage and cell growth inhibition due to apoptosis. Moreover, we previously demonstrated the proapoptotic activity of French Polynesian *P. pavonica* extract on human osteosarcoma cells. These finding suggests that EPP could be of special interest for developing novel therapeutic agents for osteosarcoma, a rare highly malignant bone cancer, whose cells phenotypically present an early stage of differentiation [2].

Extract or bioactive compounds from macroalgae have been shown to possess a noticeable effect on regulation of bone metabolism as proved by enhanced bone mass, trabecular bone volume, number and thickness and lower trabecular separation, resulting in a higher bone strength [17]. Such anti-OP effects seem to be mediated via antioxidant or anti-inflammatory pathways and their downstream signaling mechanisms, leading to osteoblast mineralization and osteoclast lack of activity [17].

Seaweeds not only consist of organic bio-active compounds such as phenols, flavonoids and tannins, fatty acids, polysaccharides, proteins, and fibers, but they are also a valuable source of minerals such as calcium, magnesium, and other bone-supporting elements [22]. Mineral-rich extracts have been isolated from the red marine algae *Lithothamnion calcareum* and tested as a dietary supplement for prevention of bone mineral loss [22]. The extract of the brown algae *Sargassum horneri* has been demonstrated to possess an anabolic effect on bone elements, due to its capacity to stimulate bone deposition and inhibit bone degradation in rat femoral tissues in vitro and in vivo [23].

The effect of algae such as *Undaria pinnatifida*, *Sargassum horneri*, *Eisenia bicyclis*, *Cryptonemia scmitziana*, *Gelidium amasii*, and *Ulva pertusa Kjellman* on bone calcification have been studied. Results showed that bone calcium content was significantly increased [22,24].

The methanol extract of brown algae *Ecklonia cava* has been used for in vitro arthritis treatment [25].

Nevertheless, very few compounds have been analyzed and reported for bone-related disease treatment and the effect of marine algae extracts on bone metabolism has not yet been entirely clarified. Still much research work is needed for further elucidations.

In this work, we investigated the proanabolic activity of *P. pavonica* on HOb by monitoring the effects of EPP on cell viability, differentiation, and mineralization.

EPP was previously characterized for its chemical composition; in particular, we determined the total phenolic, flavonoid, and tannin content, antioxidant activity, lipid composition, and fatty acid profile [6].

Regarding the effect of the brown algae *P. pavonica* on bone metabolism, in a previous in vivo study, the activity of a marine algae-derived molecules on bone density and collagen synthesis markers were investigated. Briefly, 40 postmenopausal women were recruited and randomly treated with different dose of *P. pavonica*. Every 3 months, physical examination, including bone densitometry and collagen markers measurement, was conducted. At the end of the 12-month period, an ultrasound scan and cervical cytology analysis were conducted. *P. pavonica* demonstrated the ability to increase BMD measured in lumbar spine and femur neck compared to the untreated group. Regarding collagen analysis, procollagen I C-end terminal peptides and pyridinium crosslinks were investigated as markers of bone formation and bone resorption, respectively. Results revealed that *P. pavonica* may have a positive effect on collagen control. Finally, *P. pavonica* did not appear to affect other estrogen-sensitive organs such as the endometrium or vaginal mucosa. Steroid structure compounds were suggested as the active molecules responsible for the observed effects. Such results led to the hypothesis of a selective estrogen receptor modulator-like molecules (ICP Ltd., personal communication based on the study performed by Professor Mark Brincat).

Nevertheless, based on our literature research, in vitro biochemical and molecular evaluation supporting beneficial osteogenic effects of *P. pavonica* extracts are nonexistent. Hence, in this study, for the first time, the biological activity of EPP was evaluated on HOb.

Overall, our data indicate that EPP is a safe product regarding cell viability, showing no toxicity against HOb. RT-qPCR was used to examine the expression of ALPL, collagen type I alpha 1 chain, osteoprotegerin, and osteocalcin. These mRNA species were chosen for our study as they represent recognized markers of the different osteoblast differentiation stages. COL1A1 and ALPL characterized the earlier stage; in the late stage, matrix mineralization occurs when the organic structure is supplemented with osteocalcin, which stimulates deposition of mineral substances [26]. EPP exhibited the capacity to increase the expression of the earlier differentiation-stage markers

(COL1A1 and ALPL) as well as those involved in terminally osteoblastic differentiation (BGLAP and TNFRSF11B). In accordance with these findings, EPP also showed the ability to increase ALPL enzymatic activity. Sox9 mRNA was also monitored. Sox9 is a chondrocyte-specific transcription factor and it is required for prechondrogenic cell condensation and prechondrocyte and chondroblast differentiation [27]. The SOX9 and RUNX2 expression ratio is crucial in determining the shift in equilibrium toward osteogenesis or chondrogenesis [28]. RUNX2 regulates downstream genes that determine the osteoblast phenotype and controls the expression of osteogenic marker genes such as ALPL, Osteopontin (OPN), Osterix (OSX), COL1A1, Bone sialoprotein (BSP), and BGLAP [28].

Zhou G. et al. [14] in their study identified a transcriptional repressor function of Sox9 on RUNX2 acting during chondrogenic cell fate commitment and chondrogenesis. There are evidences on the dominance of Sox9 function over RUNX2 during the early first step in the progenitor cell fate decision between osteoblastic vs. chondrogenic lineages. It has been shown that Sox9 misexpression repressed RUNX2 function and diverted cell fate from bone to cartilage in the craniofacial region [14]. Based on these evidences, we selected Sox9 as a marker for the osteoblast phenotype maintenance in order to prevent osteoblasts from shifting toward the chondrogenic lineage. Regarding EPP treatment, a decrease in Sox9 expression was detected in treated osteoblast culture compared to untreated culture.

RANK, RANKL, and OPG have a fundamental role in bone remodeling and the RANKL/OPG ratio is the main determinant of bone mass and better reflects the bone remodeling condition [29]. Our results showed that EPP upregulated OPG expression in HOb compared to the control culture. OPG acts as nonfunctional receptor to compete with the osteoclast activation receptor RANK for its ligand RANKL. Therefore, EPP showed an indirect inhibition effect on osteoclast activation. Finally, results showed a decrement in RANKL/OPG ratio as a demonstration of EPP capacity to inhibit bone resorption.

In the final step, the mineralizing ability of EPP was evaluated by Ca^{2+} deposition assay through an Alizarin red S (ARS) staining assay. EPP was found to significantly enhance mineralized nodule formation in osteoblast cultures. After 3 or 4 weeks, considering the tested concentrations of EPP (1, 10, 20 µg/mL), the extract did not have toxic effects on the cultures as cells were still vital, visibly attached, and occupying the entire bottom of the plate as compared with those of the control group. Mineralized nodules were observed in cells cultured in the absence of common mineralization agents such as dexamethasone and betaglycerophosphate, demonstrating the remarkably ability of the EPP to induce mineralization and indicating that this product serves as a suitable mineralized-nodule-inducing factor. Calcium level is crucial in the strengthening of bone and bone homeostasis. Regarding the therapeutic potential of marine algae in calcium-mineralization of osteoblasts, some phlorotannins have been identified as bioactive components in *Ecklonia* sp. [30].

Since there have been no previous reports, to our knowledge, this work can be considered the first to demonstrate the osteogenic capacity of *P. pavonica* extract in vitro. In the present study, we have shown EPP to be able to increase the deposition of mineralized organic matrix by osteoblasts through an increase of osteoblastic differentiation. The present study is the first to investigate the direct effects of EPP on bone-forming osteoblasts, providing evidences both at the molecular and cellular level. We demonstrated that EPP has a strong modulatory effect on the expression of osteoblast-specific markers such as: COL1A1, ALPL, BGLAP, TNFRSF11B genes, ALPL enzymatic activity, as well as on the RANKL/OPG ratio and on formation of mineralized bone nodules in long-term HOb cultures. This is important with regard to developing materials for bone repair or bone tissue engineering/regeneration, or active nutritional supplements.

4. Materials and Methods

4.1. Chemical Composition of EPP

EPP was produced and chemically characterized as previously described [6]. Briefly, EPP was produced by Soxhlet extraction using acetone as the solvent, starting from algae collected in French

Polynesia in June 2014. EPP was first tested for its total phenolic, flavonoid, and tannin content through spectrophotometric assay (Folin–Ciocalteu method, aluminum chloride colorimetric method, Broadhurst vanillin–HCl method, respectively) [6]. The determination of the antioxidant activity of the extract was performed using the method of FRAP assay [6]. Finally, EPP was examined for its lipid content by GC-MS. For the analysis of the most lipophilic compounds, EPP was subjected to saponification and dispersive liquid-liquid microextraction (DLLME) [6].

4.2. Isolation and Culture of HOb

HOb were isolated from the trabecular bone of adult knee samples obtained with ethical approval and informed consent during routine replacement surgery. Trabecular bone fragments were widely washed in PBS pH 7.4 to remove blood and bone marrow, and then transferred to culture containing DMEM (PAN Biotech) supplemented with 10% v/v fetal bovine serum (FBS) (Ultra-low endotoxin, Euroclone), and 1% v/v penicillin–streptomycin. Cultures were incubated at 37 °C in a humidified atmosphere of 5% CO_2. Bone fragments were maintained in culture by removing the conditioned medium and replacing it with a fresh one, every 2 weeks. After 3–6 weeks in culture, a cellular confluent monolayer of Hob had grown out from the bone fragments (E1 culture) [31].

4.3. Cell Culture and Treatment

HOb were seeded at a density of 3000 cells/well into a 96-well multiplate for MTT assay, or at a density of 15,000 cells/well into a 24-well multiplate for ARS assay or total RNA extraction, and cultured in DMEM supplemented with 10% v/v FCS and 1% v/v penicillin–streptomycin. Subconfluent cells were treated with EPP obtained as previously described [6] at 1 µg/mL, 10 µg/mL, and 20 µg/mL and using DMSO as control, for 24 h for MTT assay or RNA extraction and for 96 h for RANKL and OPG ELISA kit. Alternatively, for ARS assay, confluent cells were treated at the same EPP concentrations for 3 or 4 weeks; fresh medium (containing EPP or DMSO) was replaced twice a week.

4.4. MTT Assay

Cell viability was determined after 24 h of treatment. Culture medium was removed and cells were incubated with MTT in white DMEM for 3.5 h. After incubation time, Formazan salts were dissolved in DMSO and absorbance was evaluated by a microplate reader with at 550 nm.

4.5. RT-qPCR

Each cultured construct was independently collected after 24 h of treatment. Total RNA extraction and cDNA synthesis were obtained using the FastLane Cell cDNA kit (Qiagen, Milano, Italy) with a TProfessional Basic Thermocycler (Biometra, Cinisello Balsamo-Milano, Italy), following manufacturer's instruction. The RT-qPCR analyses were then performed with a RotorGene 6000 (Qiagen, Milano, Italy) using the SYBR®GreenERTM qPCR SuperMix Universal kit (Invitrogen Thermo Fisher, Monza, Italy). Target genes were amplified using specific primer pairs obtained from KiCqStart™ Primers (Sigma Aldrich, Milano, Italy). For each sample, the quality of the PCR product was tested by melting curve analysis. The results were expressed as fold change (increase or decrease) in expression of the treated sample in relation to the untreated sample. Glyceraldehyde-3-phosphate dehydrogenase (GAPDH) was used as reference gene to control for experimental variability and the level of mRNA expression was normalized to GAPDH mRNA. RT-qPCR analysis was performed in duplicate on samples taken from three independent cultures (i.e., six measurements for each gene).

4.6. ALPL Assay

After 96 h treatment, ALPL activity was quantified following the method described by Lowry and modified by Tsai [32]. Briefly, cells were washed with PBS and cells were lysed with 100 µL of 0.1% SDS. A total of 100 µL of the lysate was incubated with 250 µL p-nitrophenyl phosphate in glycine buffer at 37 °C for 30 min. The enzymatic reaction was stopped by adding 100 µL of ice-cold 3 M NaOH, and the amount of p-nitrophenol liberated was measured spectrophotometrically (405 nm). Each experiment was performed in triplicate and results were normalized to cell protein content.

4.7. Quantitative Detection of RANKL and OPG

OPG and RANKL release into the culture medium were measured after 96 h of treatment using their respective ELISA kit (Abcam, Cambridge, UK) following the manufacturer's instructions. Optical density was read at 450 nm wavelength.

4.8. Nodules Formation and Mineralization Assay

Mineralized nodules formation and degree of mineralization were determined in HOb cells treated with EPP at 1 µg/mL, 10 µg/mL, and 20 µg/mL and using DMSO as control, for 3 or 4 weeks, fresh medium (containing EPP or DMSO) was replaced twice a week. After 3 or 4 weeks treatment, cells were submitted to ARS staining as described [33]. Briefly, cells were fixed with 70% v/v cold ethanol for 1 h and stained with 40 mM ARS stain in dH$_2$O (pH 4.1) at RT for 20 min. Cells were washed five times with dH$_2$O and two times with cold PBS. Mineralized ARS-positive nodules present in each well were visualized using inverted microscope. For the quantification of mineralization, ARS was extracted with 10% cetylpyridinium chloride (CPC) in PBS for 1 h, followed by absorbance measurement at 550 nm.

4.9. Statistical Analysis

Experiments were performed in triplicate. Data were expressed as mean ± SD. Statistical significance of differences was determined by ANOVA analysis, with a Bonferroni post hoc test. Statistically significant differences from untreated control are denoted by * $p < 0.05$ or § $p < 0.01$. Differences were considered significant at $p < 0.05$ (Graphpad; San Diego, CA, USA).

Author Contributions: Conceptualization, A.S. and M.B.; Methodology, M.M. and G.B.; Validation: M.G. and T.P.; Formal Analysis, M.B.; Investigation, M.M.; M.G. and T.P.; Resources, M.B. and G.G.; Writing-Original Draft Preparation, M.M. and G.B.; Writing-Review & Editing, A.S.; Visualization, G.B. and M.M.; Supervision, A.S. and M.B.

Funding: This research received no external funding.

Acknowledgments: The Department of Biotechnology, Chemistry and Pharmacy has been granted by the Minister of Education, University and Research (MIUR) as "Department of Excellence 2018–2022".

Conflicts of Interest: The authors declare no conflict of interest.

References

1. Kim, B.J.; Koh, J.M. Coupling factors involved in preserving bone balance. *Cell. Mol. Life Sci.* **2019**, *76*, 1243–1253. [CrossRef] [PubMed]
2. Bernardini, G.; Braconi, D.; Spreafico, A.; Santucci, A. Post-genomics of bone metabolic dysfunctions and neoplasias. *Proteomics* **2012**, *12*, 708–721. [CrossRef] [PubMed]
3. Carson, M.A.; Clarke, S.A. Bioactive Compounds from Marine Organisms: Potential for Bone Growth and Healing. *Mar. Drugs* **2018**, *16*, 340. [CrossRef] [PubMed]
4. Cho, Y.S.; Jung, W.-K.; Kim, J.-A.; Choi, I.-W.; Kim, S.-J. Beneficial effects of fucoidan on osteoblastic MG63 cell differentiation. *Food Chem.* **2009**, *116*, 990–994. [CrossRef]
5. Hamed, I.; Özogul, F.; Özogul, Y.; Regenstein, J.M. Marine Bioactive Compounds and Their Health Benefits: A Review. *Compr. Rev. Food Sci. Food Saf.* **2015**, *14*, 446–465. [CrossRef]
6. Bernardini, G.; Minetti, M.; Polizzotto, G.; Biazzo, M.; Santucci, A. Pro-Apoptotic Activity of French Polynesian Padina pavonica Extract on Human Osteosarcoma Cells. *Mar. Drugs* **2018**, *16*, 504. [CrossRef]
7. Cikoš, A.M.; Jokić, S.; Šubarić, D.; Jerković, I. Overview on the Application of Modern Methods for the Extraction of Bioactive Compounds from Marine Macroalgae. *Mar. Drugs* **2018**, *16*, 348. [CrossRef]

8. Amaro, H.M.; Fernandes, F.; Valentão, P.; Andrade, P.B.; Sousa-Pinto, I.; Malcata, F.X.; Guedes, A.C. Effect of Solvent System on Extractability of Lipidic Components of Scenedesmus obliquus (M2-1) and *Gloeothece* sp. on Antioxidant Scavenging Capacity Thereof. *Mar. Drugs* **2015**, *13*, 6453–6471. [CrossRef]
9. Kumari, P.; Reddy, C.R.; Jha, B. Comparative evaluation and selection of a method for lipid and fatty acid extraction from macroalgae. *Anal. Biochem.* **2011**, *415*, 134–144. [CrossRef]
10. Orlando-Bonaca, M.; Lipej, L.; Orfanidis, S. Benthic macrophytes as a tool for delineating, monitoring and assessing ecological status: The case of Slovenian coastal waters. *Mar. Pollut. Bull.* **2008**, *56*, 666–676. [CrossRef]
11. Ofer, R.; Yerachmiel, A.; Shmuel, Y. Marine macroalgae as biosorbents for cadmium and nickel in water. *Water Environ. Res.* **2003**, *75*, 246–253. [CrossRef] [PubMed]
12. Behmer, S.T.; Olszewski, N.; Sebastiani, J.; Palka, S.; Sparacino, G.; Sciarrno, E.; Grebenok, R.J. Plant phloem sterol content: Forms, putative functions, and implications for phloem-feeding insects. *Front. Plant Sci.* **2013**, *4*, 370. [CrossRef] [PubMed]
13. Gutierrez, G. Compositions of Padina Algae or Their Extracts, and Their Pharmaceutical, Food Compositions, or Use for the Culture of Molluscs or Arthropods. European Patent EP 655250, 1995.
14. Zhou, G.; Zheng, Q.; Engin, F.; Munivez, E.; Chen, Y.; Sebald, E.; Krakow, D.; Lee, B. Dominance of SOX9 function over RUNX2 during skeletogenesis. *Proc. Natl. Acad. Sci. USA* **2006**, *103*, 19004–19009. [CrossRef] [PubMed]
15. Corrado, A.; Neve, A.; Macchiarola, A.; Gaudio, A.; Marucci, A.; Cantatore, F.P. RANKL/OPG Ratio and DKK-1 Expression in Primary Osteoblastic Cultures from Osteoarthritic and Osteoporotic Subjects. *J. Rheumatol.* **2013**, *40*, 684–694. [CrossRef] [PubMed]
16. Chaugule, S.; Indap, M.; Chiplunkar, S. Marine Natural Products: New Avenue in Treatment of Osteoporosis. *Front. Mar. Sci.* **2017**, *4*, 384. [CrossRef]
17. Senthilkumara, K.; Venkatesana, J.; Kim, S.K. Marine derived natural products for osteoporosis. *Biomed. Prev. Nutr.* **2014**, *4*, 1–7. [CrossRef]
18. Kiuru, P.; D'Auria, M.V.; Muller, C.D.; Tammela, P.; Vuorela, H.; Yli-Kauhaluoma, J. Exploring marine resources for bioactive compounds. *Planta Med.* **2014**, *80*, 1234–1246. [CrossRef]
19. Taskin, E.; Caki, Z.; Ozturk, M. Assessment of in vitro antitumoral and antimicrobial activities of marine algae harvested from the eastern Mediterranean sea. *Afr. J. Biotechnol.* **2010**, *9*, 4272–4277. [CrossRef]
20. Devery, R.; Miller, A.; Stanton, C. Conjugated linoleic acid and oxidative behavior in cancer cells. *Biochem. Soc. Transact.* **2001**, *29*, 341–344. [CrossRef]
21. Stanojković, T.P.; Šavikin, K.; Zdunić, G.; Kljajić, Z.; Grozdanić, N.; Antić, J. In vitro antitumoral Activities of Padina pavonia on human cervix and breast cancer cell Lines. *J. Med. Plant Res.* **2013**, *7*, 419–424. [CrossRef]
22. Venkatesan, J.; Kim, S.K. Osteoporosis treatment: Marine algal compounds. *Adv. Food Nutr. Res.* **2011**, *64*, 417–427. [CrossRef] [PubMed]
23. Matsumoto, T.; Hokari, Y.; Hashizume, M.; Yamaguchi, M. Effect of Sargassum horneri extract on circulating bone metabolic markers: Supplemental intake has an effect in healthy humans. *J. Health Sci.* **2008**, *54*, 50–55. [CrossRef]
24. Yamaguchi, M.; Hachiya, S.; Hiratuka, S.; Suzuki, T. Effect of marine algae extract on bone calcification in the femoral-metaphyseal tissues of rats: Anabolic effect of Sargassum horneri. *J. Health Sci.* **2001**, *47*, 533–538. [CrossRef]
25. Ryu, B.; Li, Y.; Qian, Z.-J.; Kim, M.-M.; Kim, S.-K. Differentiation of human osteosarcoma cells by isolated phlorotannins is subtly linked to COX-2, iNOS, MMPs, and MAPK signaling: Implication for chronic articular disease. *Chem. Biol. Interact.* **2009**, *179*, 192–201. [CrossRef] [PubMed]
26. Rutkovskiy, A.; Stensløkken, K.-O.; Vaage, I.-J. Osteoblast Differentiation at a Glance. *Med. Sci. Monit. Basic Res.* **2016**, *22*, 95–106. [CrossRef]
27. Smits, P.; Dy, P.; Mitra, S.; Lefebvre, V. Sox5 and Sox6 are needed to develop and maintain source, columnar, and hypertrophic chondrocytes in the cartilage growth plate. *J. Cell Biol.* **2004**, *164*, 747–758. [CrossRef]
28. Thiagarajan, L.; Abu-Awwad, H.A.M.; Dixon, J.E. Osteogenic Programming of Human Mesenchymal Stem Cells with Highly Efficient Intracellular Delivery of RUNX2. *Stem Cells Transl. Med.* **2017**, *6*, 2146–2159. [CrossRef]
29. Hofbauer, L.C.; Schoppet, M. Clinical implications of the osteoprotegerin/RANKL/RANK system for bone and vascular diseases. *JAMA* **2004**, *292*, 490–495. [CrossRef]

30. Nguyen, M.H.; Jung, W.K.; Kim, S.K. Marine algae possess therapeutic potential for Ca-mineralization via osteoblastic differentiation. *Adv. Food Nutr. Res.* **2011**, *64*, 429–441. [CrossRef]
31. Spreafico, A.; Frediani, B.; Capperucci, C.; Chellini, F.; Paffetti, A.; D'Ambrosio, C.; Bernardini, G.; Mini, R.; Collodel, G.; Scaloni, A.; et al. A proteomic study on human osteoblastic cells proliferation and differentiation. *Proteomics* **2006**, *6*, 3520–3532. [CrossRef] [PubMed]
32. Tsai, S.-W.; Liou, H.-M.; Lin, C.-J.; Kuo, K.-L.; Hung, Y.-S.; Weng, R.-C.; Hsu, F.-Y. MG63 Osteoblast-Like Cells Exhibit Different Behavior when Grown on Electrospun Collagen Matrix versus Electrospun Gelatin Matrix. *PLoS ONE* **2012**, *7*, e31200. [CrossRef] [PubMed]
33. Laschi, M.; Bernardini, G.; Geminiani, M.; Ghezzi, L.; Amato, L.; Braconi, D.; Millucci, L.; Frediani, B.; Spreafico, A.; Franchi, A.; et al. Establishment of Four New Human Primary Cell Cultures from Chemo-Naïve Italian Osteosarcoma Patients. *J. Cell Physiol.* **2015**, *230*, 2718–2727. [CrossRef] [PubMed]

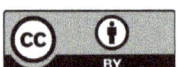

© 2019 by the authors. Licensee MDPI, Basel, Switzerland. This article is an open access article distributed under the terms and conditions of the Creative Commons Attribution (CC BY) license (http://creativecommons.org/licenses/by/4.0/).

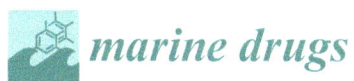

Article

Pro-Apoptotic Activity of French Polynesian *Padina pavonica* Extract on Human Osteosarcoma Cells

Giulia Bernardini [1], Mariagiulia Minetti [1,2], Giuseppe Polizzotto [2], Manuele Biazzo [2] and Annalisa Santucci [1,*]

[1] Dipartimento di Biotecnologie, Chimica e Farmacia (Dipartimento di Eccellenza 2018–2022), Università degli Studi di Siena, via Aldo Moro 2, 53100 Siena, Italy; bernardini@unisi.it (G.B.); minetti2@student.unisi.it (M.M.)
[2] Institute of Cellular Pharmacology (ICP Concepts Ltd.), F24, Triq Valletta, Mosta Technopark, MST 3000 Mosta, Malta; giuseppe@icpconcepts.com (G.P.); manuele@icpconcepts.com (M.B.)
* Correspondence: annalisa.santucci@unisi.it; Tel.: +39-0577234958; Fax: +39-0577234254

Received: 7 November 2018; Accepted: 11 December 2018; Published: 13 December 2018

Abstract: Recently, seaweeds and their extracts have attracted great interest in the pharmaceutical industry as a source of bioactive compounds. Studies have demonstrated the cytotoxic activity of macroalgae towards different types of cancer cell models, and their consumption has been suggested as a chemo-preventive agent against several cancers such as breast, cervix and colon cancers. Reports relevant to the chemical properties of brown algae *Padina* sp. are limited and those accompanied to a comprehensive evaluation of the biological activity on osteosarcoma (OS) are non existent. In this report, we explored the chemical composition of French Polynesian *Padina pavonica* extract (EPP) by spectrophotometric assays (total phenolic, flavonoid and tannin content, and antioxidant activity) and by gas chromatography-mass spectrometry (GC-MS) analysis, and provided EPP lipid and sterols profiles. Several compounds with relevant biological activity were also identified that suggest interesting pharmacological and health-protecting effects for EPP. Moreover, we demonstrated that EPP presents good anti-proliferative and pro-apoptotic activities against two OS cell lines, SaOS-2 and MNNG, with different cancer-related phenotypes. Finally, our data suggest that EPP might target different properties associated with cancer development and aggressiveness.

Keywords: *Padina pavonica*; osteosarcoma; apoptosis; algae; chemo-preventive agent; phytol; fucosterol; fatty acid

---

1. Introduction

Recently, seaweeds and their extracts have attracted great interest in the pharmaceutical industry as a source of bioactive compounds [1].

A number of studies have demonstrated the cytotoxic activity of macroalgae towards different types of cancer cell models and certain authors have suggested the consumption of algae as a chemo-preventive agent against several cancers. In particular, brown algae have demonstrated to be rich in unsaturated fatty acids, which block growth and systemic spread of human breast cancer, polysaccharides and terpenoids which are considered as promising bioactive molecules with anticancer activity [2,3]. *Padina pavonica* is representative of brown algae which can be found throughout the world from warm temperate to tropical locations, including: North Carolina to Florida in the United States, the Gulf of Mexico, throughout the Caribbean and tropical Atlantic and the Eastern Atlantic, Mediterranean and Adriatic Seas [4]. There are several species of algae belonging to the genus *padina*. The main chemical classes of compounds found in padina species are represented by: sterols, lipids, polysaccharides, carotenoids, polyphenols and fibers [5]. However, in addition to the name and the geographical spread, changes can be noted also in its biochemical composition.

Although Osteosarcoma (OS) is a rare disease comprising less than 1% of cancers diagnosed in the United States, it is the most common primary malignant bone tumor in adolescents and young adults. OS accounts for 8.9% of cancer-related deaths and carry an overall 5-year survival rate of 60–70% despite modern treatment protocols that combine chemotherapy and surgery [6,7]. Chemotherapy has been established as a critical component of OS therapy, but its adverse side effects associated with the drug resistance developed by tumors, lead to the urgent need for new and specific anticancer agents.

In this study, we aimed to demonstrate the antitumoral activity of the extract of *Padina pavonica* (EPP) on human OS cells in order to provide the molecular evidences supporting the development of EPP-based products usable as a potential chemo-preventive agent against OS.

2. Results

2.1. Chemical Composition and Antioxidant Capacity of Padina pavonica Extract

The extract of *Padina pavonica* (EPP) under investigation was produced by Soxhlet extraction using acetone as solvent, starting fronds of mature from algae collected in French Polynesia in June 2014.

EPP was first chemically characterized for its total phenolic, flavonoid and tannin content through spectrophotometric assays. The total phenolic, flavonoid and tannin contents of the seaweed were 27.0, 54.8, and 54.3 mg per g of extract, respectively, corresponding to 0.81, 1.64 and 1.63 mg per g of dry material, respectively. The antioxidant activity was evaluated by ferric reducing antioxidant power (FRAP) assay and resulted as 25.6 ± 0.2 µmol of Fe^{2+}/100 mg of extract.

EPP was also examined for its lipid content by GC-MS. Hydrocarbons represented the 79.88% of the total extract, among which 68.83% corresponded to fatty acids (FAs), 0.19% corresponded to squalene and 10.86% to other hydrocarbon species (Table 1).

Table 1. Chemical composition (%) of EPP.

	EPP (%)
	Hydrocarbons
Fatty acids	68.83
Squalene	0.19
Other hydrocarbons	10.86
Total hydrocarbons	**79.88**
	Sterols
Cholesterol	0.97
Fucosterol	7.40
Total sterols	**8.37**
	Other compounds
α-Tocopherol	0.17
δ-Tocopherol	0.19
Phytol	5.27
Neophytadiene	5.56
2,4-di-*tert*-butylphenol (DTBP)	0.18
2(4H)-Benzofuranone, 5,6,7,7a-tetrahydro-4,4,7a-trimethyl-, (R)-(Dihydroactinidiolide)	0.37

Sterols represented the 8.37% of the extract and included fucosterol and cholesterol in a percentage of 7.40% and 0.97%, respectively (Table 1). We also calculated the ratio between fucosterol and cholesterol (F:C) which corresponded to 7.6:1. Other noteworthy compounds identified were: α- and δ-tocopherol, which corresponded to 0.17 and 0.19% respectively, phytol (5.27%), neophytadiene, a terpene compound that amounted to 5.56%, 2,4-di-*tert*-butylphenol (0.18%) and dihydroactinidiolide (0.37%) (Table 1).

GC-MS analysis was also performed with a different sample preparation approach consisting in saponification and subsequent extraction by dispersive liquid-liquid microextraction (DLLME) of EPP, in order to analyse the most lipophilic compounds. This analysis mostly confirmed the presence of several already identified compounds (Table 2), such as: phytol (53.85%), fucosterol (17.57%), palmitic acid (12.00%), cholesterol (4.57%), 2,4-di-tert-butylphenol (2.99%), stearic acid (3.40%), oleic acid (0.59%), dihydroactinidiolide (0.62%), squalene (0.19%) and δ-tocopherol (0.27%), and n-nonadecanol-1 (0.20%).

Table 2. EPP composition (%) following saponification and DLLME.

	EPP (%)
	Hydrocarbons
Fatty acids	17.11
Squalene	0.19
Other hydrocarbons	1.65
Total hydrocarbons	**18.95**
	Sterols
Cholesterol	4.57
Fucosterol	17.57
Total sterols	**22.14**
	Other compounds
δ-Tocopherol	0.27
Phytol	53.85
2,4-di-*tert*-butylphenol (DTBP)	2.99
6-Hydroxy-4,4,7a-trimethyl-5,6,7,7a-tetrahydrobenzofuran-2(4*H*)-one	0.99
2(4*H*)-Benzofuranone, 5,6,7,7a-tetrahydro-4,4,7a-trimethyl-, (R)-(Dihydroactinidiolide)	0.62
n-Nonadecanol-1	0.20

EPPs FAs profile showed the presence of FAs with aliphatic chains ranging from 12 up to 22 carbon atoms (Table 3). Saturated FAs (SFAs) corresponded to 43.45% of total EPP (63.13% of total FAs). Among these, the most abundant FA was palmitic acid with a total percentage of 34.15%, followed by stearic (3.25%), pentadecanoic (1.95%), arachidic (0.74%), myristic (0.43%), lauric (0.47%) and behenic (0.04%). Monounsaturated FAs (MUFAs) were 23.67% of total EPP (34.40% of total FAs). The most abundant MUFA was palmitelaidic acid (16:1 *n*-7 E, 7.82%) followed by oleic acid (18:1 *n*-9, 7.79%) and palmitoleic acid (16:1 *n*-7 Z, 6.29%). Polyunsaturated FAs (PUFAs) corresponded to 1.70% of EPP (2.47% of total FAs). The main PUFAs found in EPP was arachidonic acid (20:4 *n*-6, 0.64%) followed by linoleic (18:2 *n*-6, 0.53) and eicosapentanoic acid (20:5 *n*-3 0.24%). We also calculated the ratio between *n*-6 and *n*-3 PUFAs which corresponded to 5.61.

Table 3. Fatty acids (%) of EPP.

Fatty Acids (FAs)	EPP (%)
Saturated fatty acids (SFAs)	
Lauric acid 12:0	0.47
Myristic acid 14:0	0.43
Pentadecanoic acid 15:0	1.95
Palmitic acid 16:0	34.15
Stearic acid 18:0	3.25
Arachidic acid 20:0	0.74
Behenic acid 22:0	0.04
Other SFAs	2.42
Total SFAs	**43.45**

Table 3. Cont.

Fatty Acids (FAs)	EPP (%)
Monounsaturated fatty acids (MUFAs)	
Oleic acid (18:1 n-9)	7.79
Palmitelaidic acid (16:1 n-7 (E))	7.82
Palmitoleic acid (16:1 n-7 (Z))	6.29
Other MUFAs	1.76
Total MUFAs	23.67
Polyunsaturated fatty acids (PUFAs)	
Linoleic acid (18:2 n-6)	0.53
Eicosapentanoic acid (20:5 n-3)	0.24
Arachidonic acid (20:4 n-6)	0.64
Other PUFAs	0.29
Total PUFAs	1.70
Total n-6 PUFAs	1.36
Total n-3 PUFAs	0.24
Ratio n-6/n-3	5.61

2.2. EPP Effects on OS Cell Viability and Proliferation

EPP inhibited SaOS-2 cell viability in a dose and time dependent trend with an IC_{50} after 24 h treatment of 152.2 ± 7.7 µg/mL (Figure 1). These results were confirmed also after 48 h treatment.

On MNNG cells EPP showed a more pronounced effect on cell viability in respect of SaOS-2 cells, with a IC_{50} of 87.75 ± 18.57 µg/mL after 24 h treatment and a more remarkable effect was detected after 48 h treatment.

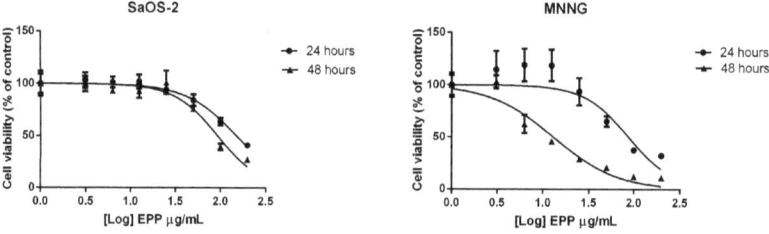

Figure 1. IC_{50} of EPP after 24 and 48 h treatment on SaOS-2 and MNNG. IC_{50} was calculated using Graphpad. Cell viability was expressed as percentage in respect to control and EPP concentrations (3.1, 6.25, 12.5, 25, 50, 100 and 200 µg/mL) were reported in a logarithmic scale.

EPP induced a decrease of proliferation in SaOS-2 and MNNG cells in a dose-dependent manner (Figure 2). A reduction of cells proliferation of about 51%, 70% and 82% was observed for SaOS-2 when treated for 24 h with EPP at $IC_{50}/2$, IC_{50} and $2*IC_{50}$ (as calculated by cell viability assay for SaOS-2) respectively. Analogously, in MNNG cells we observed a reduction in cells count of about 30%, 77% and 89% when treated for 24 h with EPP at $IC_{50}/2$, IC_{50} and $2*IC_{50}$ (as calculated by cell viability assay for MNNG) respectively.

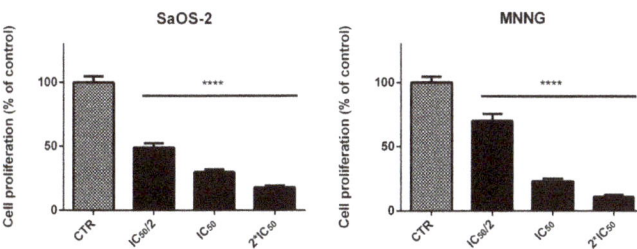

Figure 2. SaOS-2 and MNNG cell proliferation after 24 h treatment with EPP at $IC_{50}/2$, IC_{50} and $2*IC_{50}$ in starved conditions determined by the Scepter 2.0 cell counter. Data are expressed as percentage in respect to control and presented as mean ± SD, **** $p < 0.0001$.

2.3. EPP Effects on OS Cell and Nuclear Morphology

Bright-field images showed noticeable morphological changes in both OS cell lines, moving from control to the highest concentration of EPP (Figure 3A). After 24 h treatment with EPP at IC_{50} and $2*IC_{50}$, cells lost their original elongated shape and become rounding and blebbing. A reduction in cell number and dimension, as well as cytoplasm condensation were also observed in both SaOS-2 and MNNG cells, representing a clear sign of the activity of the treatment.

To evaluate whether EPP exhibited cytotoxicity through apoptosis in both OS cell lines, a DAPI staining analysis was performed to observe nuclear morphological changes (Figure 3B). Such analysis demonstrated that the exposure of OS cells to EPP induced apoptosis in a dose dependent manner; indeed, both SaOS-2 and MNNG cells showed loss of regular shape and well-defined boundaries. Moreover, at the highest concentration tested ($2*IC_{50}$), EPP exhibited a more remarkable apoptotic effect against MNNG than SaOS-2 with greater nuclear fragmentation, chromatin condensation and nuclear blebbing.

These evidences were confirmed by the high percentage of late apoptotic MNNG cells rather than SaOS-2 cells (*par.* 2.4).

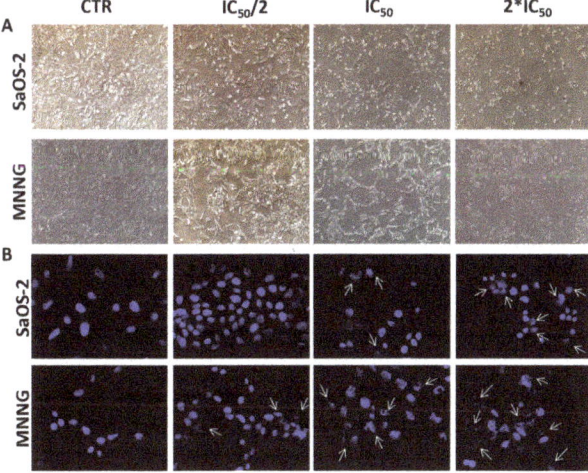

Figure 3. (**A**) Bright-field images of SaOS-2 and MNNG OS cells line after 24 h treatment with EPP at $IC_{50}/2$, IC_{50} and $2*IC_{50}$ or DMSO 0.3% as negative control. Cells are shown at ×10 magnification. (**B**) Nuclear morphological changes and DNA damage assessment in SaOS-2 and MNNG cells OS cells line after 24 h treatment with EPP at $IC_{50}/2$, IC_{50} and $2*IC_{50}$ using DMSO 0.3% as negative control. Arrows indicate nuclear fragmentation, which can be considered a biochemical hallmark of apoptosis. Cells are shown at ×63 magnification.

2.4. EPP Induces Apoptosis in OS Cells

The exposure of SaOS-2 and MNNG cells to EPP resulted in dose-dependent increase of the percentage of small diameter cells (6–9 µm), compared to control (Figure 4). The gradual increase in the percentage of cells in the small particle fraction after treatment with different concentrations of EPP can be regarded as an index of late cell apoptosis.

To confirm the pro-apoptotic effect of EPP, we performed the Annexin V-FITC/propidium iodide (PI) assay on SaOS-2 and MNNG cells treated with EPP (at their relative $IC_{50}/2$, IC_{50} and $2*IC_{50}$) for 6 h (Figure 5A,B and Table 4). SaOS-2 apoptotic cells were, roughly, completely absent in the untreated culture, as expected for cancer cells: $88.04 \pm 3.33\%$ of non-apoptotic (AnV−/PI−), 11.17 ± 2.94 of early apoptotic (AnV+/PI−) and $0.79 \pm 0.47\%$ of late apoptotic (AnV+/PI+). When cells were treated with progressively higher concentrations of EPP, the number of early apoptotic and late apoptotic cells increased in a dose-dependent manner ($IC_{50}/2$: $21.80 \pm 8.31\%$ of AnV+/PI− and $31.83 \pm 8.20\%$ of AnV+/PI+; IC_{50}: $10.46 \pm 1.07\%$ of AnV+/PI and $83.43 \pm 2.76\%$ AnV+/PI+; $2*IC_{50}$: $9.60 \pm 3.53\%$ of AnV+/PI and $90.40 \pm 3.53\%$ of AnV+/PI+). MNNG cells (Figure 5A,B) had a quite similar trend, finding a very low percentage of apoptotic cells ($6.08 \pm 2.84\%$) in the untreated culture and an increasing percentage of early and late apoptotic cells with progressively higher concentrations of EPP ($IC_{50}/2$: $2.05 \pm 1.26\%$ of AnV+/PI− and $72.46 \pm 9.12\%$ of AnV+/PI+; IC_{50}: $2.99 \pm 2.12\%$ of AnV+/PI and 90.34 ± 4.27 AnV+/PI+; $2*IC_{50}$: 5.63 ± 5.63 of AnV+/PI and $93.67 \pm 5.32\%$ of AnV+/PI+). On MNNG cells, EPP demonstrated a greater pro-apoptotic effect. In fact, in MNNG cells treated with $IC_{50}/2$, we detected a greater percentage of late apoptotic cells in respect of SaOS-2 challenged with the same EPP concentration (AnV+/PI+: $72.46 \pm 9.12\%$ and $31.83 \pm 8.20\%$, respectively).

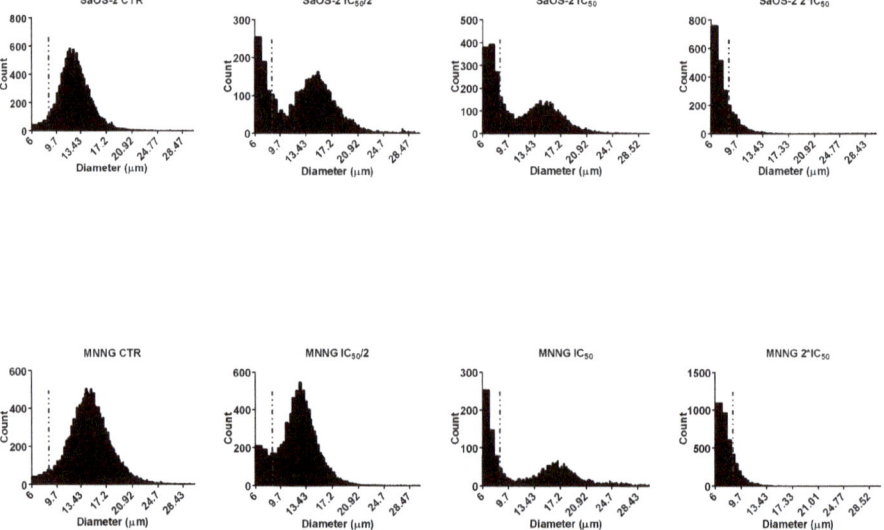

Figure 4. Diameter distributions of SaOS-2 and MNNG cells after 24 h treatment with EPP at $IC_{50}/2$, IC_{50} and $2*IC_{50}$ as measured by Scepter 2.0 cell counter. The cells were classified into small (diameter: 6–9 µm) or large (diameter 9–24 µm) fractions depending on the gating range.

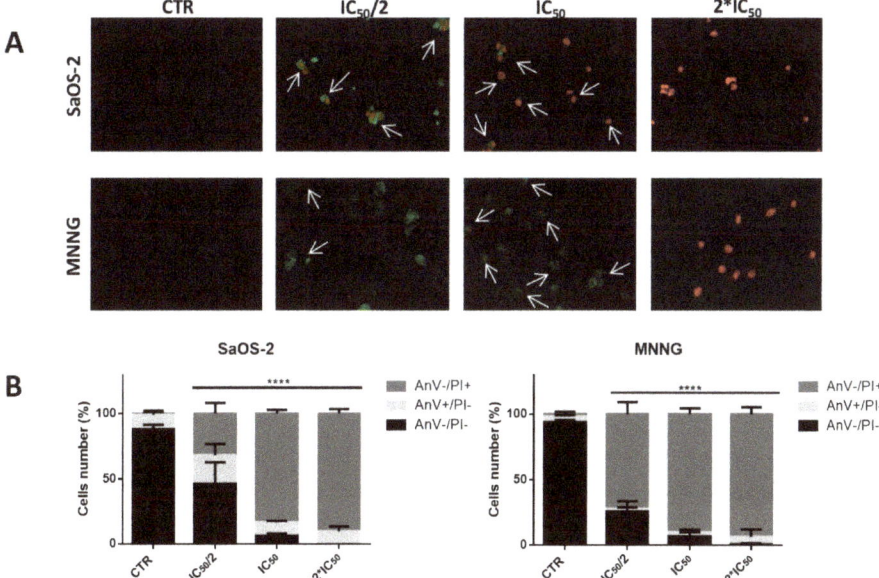

Figure 5. (**A**) Apoptosis assessment using Annexin V-FITC/PI staining and fluorescent microscopy of SaOS-2 and MNNG OS cells line treated with EPP/Acetone ($IC_{50}/2$, IC_{50}, $2*IC_{50}$) for 6 h. Viable cells did not show any kind of coloration (Anv−/PI−). Cells stained in green (AnV+/PI−) were considered as early apoptotic cells, while cells stained both in green and red (Anv+/PI−) were considered as late apoptotic cells. Cells are shown at ×40 magnification. Arrows indicate co-localization. (**B**) Histograms show the percentage of non-apoptotic(AnV−/PI−), early apoptotic (AnV+/PI−) and late apoptotic (AnV+/PI+) cells in respect to control. The quantitative assessment of apoptosis was obtained observing merged images. Results were obtained from three different experiments in triplicate, **** $p < 0.0001$.

Table 4. Apoptosis in SaOS-2 and MNNG OS cells treated with EPP at $IC_{50}/2$, IC_{50} and $2*IC_{50}$ after 6 h treatment. Percentage (±SD) of non-apoptotic (AnV−/PI−), early apoptotic (AnV+/PI−) and late apoptotic (AnV+/PI+) cells are reported. Results were obtained from three different experiments in triplicate. Results were obtained from three different experiments in triplicate. p-values were calculated, by one-way ANOVA with post hoc Dunnett test, comparing the percentages of non-apoptotic cells (AnV−/PI−) in control and treated conditions, **** $p < 0.0001$.

SaOS-2 OS Cells	Non-Apoptotic AnV−/PI− (%) ± SD	Early Apoptotis AnV+/PI− (%) ± SD	Late Apoptotis AnV+/PI+ (%) ± SD	p-Value
CTR	88.04 ± 3.33	11.17 ± 2.94	0.79 ± 0.47	
$IC_{50/2}$	46.36 ± 16.31	21.80 ± 8.31	31.83 ± 8.20	****
IC_{50}	6.11 ± 1.72	10.46 ± 1.07	83.43 ± 2.76	****
$2*IC_{50}$	0.00	9.60 ± 3.53	90.40 ± 3.53	****
MMNG OS Cells	Non-apoptotic AnV−/PI− (%) ± SD	Early Apoptotis AnV+/PI− (%) ± SD	Late Apoptotis AnV+/PI+ (%) ± SD	p-Value
CTR	93.90 ± 1.54	4.30 ± 1.06	1.78 ± 1.78	
$IC_{50/2}$	25.48 ± 8.11	2.05 ± 1.26	72.46 ± 9.12	****
IC_{50}	6.67 ± 2.89	2.99 ± 2.12	90.34 ± 4.27	****
$2*IC_{50}$	0.69 ± 0.69	5.63 ± 5.63	93.67 ± 5.32	****

To study if caspases activation was involved in EPP-induced apoptosis, we finally evaluated the activation of caspase-3 by western blot analysis. The immunoreactive band of cleaved caspase-3 increased in a dose-dependent manner after 6 h treatment with EPP (Figure 6). In SaOS-2 cell lines we detected a 2.6 and 7.1-fold increase in the activation of caspase-3 when treated with EPP at IC_{50} and $2*IC_{50}$ respectively. On the contrary in MNNG cells, we observed a dose-dependent increase in the activation of caspase-3. The immunoreactive band was significantly higher than SaOS-2 already after treatment with the lowest concentration of EPP (2.4-fold at $IC_{50}/2$) and increased over the other two concentrations (3.2-fold at IC_{50} and 3.7-fold at $2*IC_{50}$).

Lower panel: Graph reports the decrease of procaspase-3 and the increase of cleaved caspase-3 in a dose dependent manner after 6 h of treatment with $IC_{50}/2$, IC_{50} and $2*IC_{50}$ EPP. Values are calculated as a ratio of band volume of procaspase-3 or caspase-3 over band volume of GAPDH.

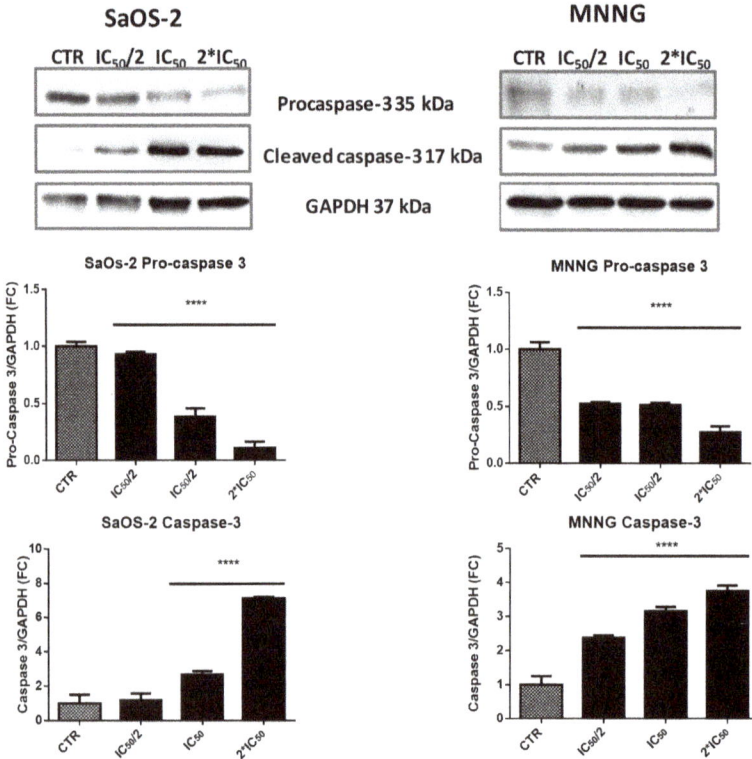

Figure 6. EPP treated SaOS-2 and MNNG OS cells line western blotting images of procaspase-3, cleaved caspase-3 and GAPDH. Data are expressed as fold-change in respect to control and presented as mean ± SD. Results were obtained from three different experiments in triplicate, **** $p < 0.0001$.

3. Discussion

Recently, natural bioactive compounds derived from marine organisms, especially those obtained from seaweeds, have received greater attention. Their high level of biodiversity makes them a considerable reservoir for active compounds as they are able to produce a great variety of secondary metabolites characterized by a wide range of biological activities. Many previous studies demonstrated the remarkable benefits of seaweeds on human health and protection against chronic disease [8] due to their content in proteins, lipids and fatty acids, polysaccharides and antioxidant compounds. It has been demonstrated that fatty acids extracted from marine algae block growth and spread of human breast cancer [9]. In addition, polysaccharides and terpenoids from brown algae have demonstrated to be promising bioactive molecules with anticancer activity [3].

In this work, for the first time the acetonic extract of *Padina pavonica* (EPP), a brown seaweed collected from French Polynesia, was chemically characterized and demonstrated to have a strong pro-apoptotic effect on human OS cells.

Reports relevant to the chemical properties of brown algae *Padina* sp. are limited and those providing a detailed description of the chemical profile accompanied to a comprehensive evaluation of the biological activity for *Padina pavonica* from French Polynesia are nonexistent.

We first characterized EPP for its total phenolic, flavonoid and tannin content, providing the first chemical report on French Polynesian *Padina pavonica*.

In our extract, total phenolic compounds amounted to 27 mg per g of extracts (0.81 mg per g of dry material). Considering the acetone as the solvent used for the extraction, our is a remarkable quantity if compared to total phenolic compounds found by Khaled et al. in Lebanese *Padina pavonica* (10.76 mg per g of the methanolic extract) [10] and by CAF et al. in Turkish Mediterranean *Padina pavonica* (0.96 mg per g of the aqueous extract and 1.76 mg per g of the methanolic extract) [11]. Pinteus et al. in *Padina pavonica* from Portugal, found values of 44.61 and 10.48 mg per g of extract when using methanol and dichloromethane respectively as extraction solvents [12]. In their work Hlila et al. determined the total phenolic content of aqueous and acetonic extract of Tunisian *Padina pavonica*, with values corresponding to 57.34 and 90.61 mg per g of extract, respectively [13].

Phenolic compounds, one of the most important class of natural compounds, are commonly found in brown algae where they exert a protective effect toward adverse environmental conditions. They have been reported to possess several biological activities including anti-oxidant, anti-bacterial and anti-allergic and anti-diabetes, and to be involved in the protection against several human diseases such as cancer, coronary heart disease, inflammatory and neurodegenerative diseases and aging [14,15].

With regard to flavonoid content, *Padina pavonica* from French Polynesia appeared to be rich in flavonoids, showing a value of 54.8 mg per g of extract. This is a relevant data if compared to previous report for Australian *Padina* sp., which reported a total flavonoid content of 20.74 mg per g of ethanol extract [16]. Flavonoids are an important class of phenolic compounds, that contribute to the antioxidant activity of algae extracts.

About tannin content, their concentrations vary greatly among different species of brown seaweeds, as well as among different geographical areas [12]. The tannin content of our extract (54.3 mg per g) appeared similar to that showed by Dang et al., who founded a tannin content of 56.17 ± 0.22 mg per g of the Australian *Padina* sp. extract [16].

Previous studies reported the antioxidant activity of some brown algae measured with the FRAP method. Agregán et al. measured the in vitro antioxidant activity of aqueous extracts of three brown seaweed from the Atlantic Ocean, in the area of Camariñas, Spain. They found FRAP values of 7.52, 51.66 and 26.93 µmol/g of extract for *Ascophyllum nodosum*, *Fucus vesiculosus* and *Bifurcaria bifurcata*, respectively [14]. Kelman et al. quantified the antioxidant activity of methanol extracts from 37 samples of algae, comprising 30 species of Hawaiian algae from 27 different genera. They showed that the brown algae as a group had the highest mean antioxidant activity among Hawaiian algae with a mean FRAP value of 3.55 ± 3.16 µM/µg extract [15]. The antioxidant activity of our extract from French Polynesia *Padina pavonica* appeared in line with the previous works on brown algae, given that acetone is not the chosen solvent for the extraction of antioxidant compounds.

Different *Padina* species possess different sterol compositions. In French Polynesian *Padina pavonica* we tested, fucosterol appeared to be exceptionally high (7.40% of EPP) in respect of cholesterol (0.97% of EPP), leading to a ratio between fucosterol and cholesterol (F:C) of 7.6:1. Comparing our sterols pattern with literature data, we can see that F:C for *Padina pavonica* from French Polynesia is higher than what previously found in the Aegean Sea *Padina pavonica*, 0.7:1 [17], Adriatic Sea *Padina pavonica*, 0.3:1 [2] and in Turkish Mediterranean Sea *Padina pavonica* [11]. The differences found in the sterol composition could be attributed to differences in the ecological conditions, life cycle of the algae and seasonal variations. [2,18,19]. Fucosterol is the main phytosterol in brown algae [20]. Many studies have described the biological and pharmacological effects of fucosterol including antidiabetic, antioxidant, anti-inflammatory, ability to reduce blood cholesterol levels in in hyper- and normocholesterolemic subjects. Fucosterol has been demonstrated to possess pro-apoptotic activity toward several cancer cell lines (colon carcinoma [21], breast carcinoma [22], promyelocytic leukemia [21]) by promoting activation of caspase-3 [20]. These data strongly suggest the potential anti-cancer activity of EPP, analogously with what reported for *Turbinaria ornata* sterols [21] or fucosterol from *Turbinaria conoides* [23]. Furthermore, fucosterol has bone regenerative effects as demonstrated by in vivo and vitro studies [24]. In an estrogen-deficient ovariectomized (OVX) animal model, oral administration of fucosterol ameliorated several bone-quality parameters (bone mineral density, bone microarchitecture and BV/TV ratio, osteocalcin and CTx serum biomarkers [24]. At cell level, fucosterol increased MG63 osteoblast-like cells proliferation, alkaline phosphatase activity and mineralization capacity, while preventing osteoclasts differentiation and RANK expression [24–26].

Several terpenes and terpenoid compounds were identified in *P. pavonica*. Terpenoids are considered as promising bioactive molecules in the search for anticancer drugs, due to their effect in inhibiting mitotic cell division [27]. Various diterpenes have been identified in several species of the genus *Cystoseira* with antitumoral and antioxidant activities [9]. Among these, squalene appears to influence several biochemical and physiological activities which are interesting for the treatment of cancer [28], it can suppress the growth of tumor cells, partially prevent the development of chemically-induced cancer and cause regression of some already existing tumors [29]. A rich squalene diet enhances chemoterapeutic activity by increasing immune system efficiency and by lowering blood cholesterol content [28,29]. Squalene supplementation stimulates the reticuloendothelial system, resulting in a marked increase in cellular and non-specific immune function [28]. Evidence suggests that squalene might assist in maintaining white cell counts during radiation treatment [28], and, in animal models, supplementation is associated with prolonged survival time subsequent to exposure to lethal doses of radiation [28]. Squalene's ability to inhibit ornithine decarboxylase (ODC) is also of significant interest in cancer prevention and treatment [29]. Cancer cells are known to utilize polyamines as growth substrates, and since ODC is a rate-limiting enzyme in the generation of many of the polyamines, ongoing cancer research has been, and is currently, investigating agents with the ability to interfere with this enzyme's activity [28].

In EPP, phytol—an acyclic monounsaturated diterpene alcohol and constituent of chlorophyll—was found in a remarkable amount. The anticancer activity of phytol against several tumor cell lines in vitro has been assessed [30–32], as well as its capacity to induce the apoptosis in hepatocellular carcinoma cells [33] and in human gastric adenocarcinoma AGS [34].

Other identified compounds with relevant biological activity are: neophytadiene, dihydroactinidiolide, 2,4-di-*tert*-butylphenol (DTBP) and n-Nonadecanol-1. Neophytadiene, is a terpene compound that possess a strong bactericidal, antifungal, antipyretic, analgesic, antioxidant and anti-inflammatory properties [35]; dihydroactinidiolide has cytotoxic effects against five human carcinoma cell lines and one melanoma cell line [36,37]; DTBP was found to possess potent antioxidant effect [38,39] in addition to fungicidal and cytotoxic activity against HeLa cancer cell line [40]. Finally, n-Nonadecanol-1, one of the major detected component in *Ceratonia siliqua* pods essential oil, demonstrated a strong cytotoxic effect against two cancer human cell lines, HeLa and MCF-7 [41].

As far as the FAs composition, palmitic acid appears to be the predominant FA in our extract, as in Dictyotales order brown algae [2,11,17,42,43]. Palmitic acid has been reported to have to have antioxidant, hypocholesterolmic nematicide, pesticide, antiandrogenic flavor, hemolytic and 5-alpha reductase inhibitor activity. In French Polynesian *Padina pavonica*, a significant percentage of oleic and palmitoleic acid was also detected. Oleic acid attracted attention as the Mediterranean diet, characterized by high olive oil (rich in oleic acid) consumption, has been linked to a protective effect against cancer [44]. A wide range of studies have been conducted on breast cancer, where a potential protective effect of oleic acid has been described [45,46]. In addition, epidemiological studies suggest that olive oil may have a protective effect on colorectal cancer development [47]. In this regard, animal studies have also shown that dietary olive oil prevented the development of colon carcinomas in rats, confirming that olive oil may have chemopreventive properties against colon carcinogenesis [48,49]. Oleic acid has been reported to act synergistically with cytotoxic drugs, enhancing their antitumor effect [50,51]. Eventually, palmitoleic has been demonstrated to possess antitumor effect on Ehrlich ascites tumor [52].

Although C_{18} and C_{20} PUFAs are reported to be characteristic of brown algae [2,53], the concentrations of PUFAs in our *Padina pavonica* appeared unusually low compared to PUFAs composition of Turkish Mediterranean Sea *Padina pavonica* [11], *Padina boryana* from the Saudi Arabian coast [2], or *Padina pavonica* from Jordan [53] and other characterized brown algae from the Bohai Sea [54]. By contrast, in our material, SFAs represented the prevalent percentage of total FAs (63.85% of total FAs and 41.03% of total EPP).

The differences in EPP chemical profiles observed between present and literature data can be explained on the basis of environmental and experimental conditions. Several parameters are known to influence the composition of phenolic compounds or FAs produced by the same species of algae: stage of algal growth, harvest season, geographic location, genetic diversity etc. [11,13]. As an example, higher amount of high-quality phenolic compounds is generated during the hot climate and during the early stage of the growth in order to prevent the photooxidative damage and sea grazers [13]. In addition, also the extraction methodology (techniques, solvent, temperature, raw material) notably affect the yield of extracted compounds from a quantitative and a qualitative point of view [55].

As far as it regards the anti-OS activity of EPP, anti-OS effects of *Padina pavonica* from French Polynesia has not been clearly studied yet. Therefore, this is the first work that tests and demonstrates the anti-OS properties of *Padina pavonica* from French Polynesia.

According to our results, EPP presents good anti-proliferative and pro-apoptotic activities against two osteosarcoma cell lines, namely MNNG and SaOS-2. These two cell lines were chosen based on their intrinsic properties, as they have opposite cancer-related phenotypes. According to Lauvrak [56], MNNG cells have been defined as very aggressive in terms of tumorigenicity, colony forming ability, migration/invasion and proliferation capacity; on the contrary, SaOS-2 cells have been classified as poorly aggressive. Moreover, these two cell lines possess a different p53 mutation status, being MNNG p53 mutant and SaOS-2 p53-null [57]. This approach let us speculate on a possible mechanism of action of EPP. In the present study EPP was found to be much more active against MNNG that SaOS-2 cells suggesting that EPP may upregulate p53 expression [58] and thus induce p53-dependent apoptosis in human OS cells by the activation of extrinsic pathways. Finally, we evaluated EPP toxicity in human primary osteoblasts and found that these cells were significantly less affected by the antiproliferative and pro-apoptotic activities of EPP (data not shown)

In literature there are several works that confirm the antitumoral activities for *Padina pavonica*. The dichloromethane extract of *Padina pavonica* was found to be cytotoxic towards the KB tumor cell line. An oxysterol, (hydroperoxy-24 vinyl-24 cholesterol), was identified as being responsible for this activity [59]. Likewise, the cytotoxic and apoptotic effects of *Padina pavonica* methanol extract against human cervix (HeLa) and breast cancer (MDA-MB-453) cell lines have been reported [60]. The observed anticancer activity could be connected to the rich content of phenolics, in particular the antiproliferative effects of polyphenols were reported to be due to the regulation of apoptosis, decreased Bcl-2 levels and increased Bax, Caspase-8 and Caspase-10 levels, and Fas death receptor signalling [61]. Moreover, glycosides, sulfated polysaccharides and carotenoids of the brown seaweed were found to act as potential chemoterapeutic or chemopreventive agents through the induction of caspases or cell cycle arrest [60,62–65]. In agreement with the works above mentioned and considering the present characterization of EPP (Tables 1–3), we might assume that the main constituents responsible for the antitumoral effect—that we observed in our work—may be identified in fucosterol, in two terpenoid compounds, such as dihydroactinidiolide and phytol, of which EPP was found to be rich, and in oleic acid. Notwithstanding, it should be also considered that macroalgae extracts are complex matrices and that biological activities of such extracts might not be closely related to a specific compound but rather to the mixture of components that can act synergistically. Therefore, any biological activity can be hardly explained with the analysis of a specific algae component.

4. Materials and Methods

4.1. Collection of Padina pavonica and Preparation of the Algae Extract (EPP)

The algae (*Padina pavonica* (Linnaeus) Thivy) were collected from the coastal area of Moorea, French Polynesia, in June 2014. Fronds of mature plants (20 mm) were harvested and then rinsed with water to remove salt and the associated debris. The cleaned material was air-dried and stored in a dehumidified chamber to remove the residual moisture. Once completely dried, the algae material was ground into a fine powder and extracted with acetone in a Soxhlet extractor. After that, the mixture was filtered through filter paper and the filtrate was collected. The solution was dried by rotary evaporator and the resulting material was kept in the refrigerator until the analyses.

4.2. Total Phenolic Content

The quantitative assay of the total phenolic compounds was determined by the Folin-Ciocalteu method [66]. A stock standard solution of 0.5 mg/mL gallic acid was prepared in 95% methanol, and then working standard solutions were prepared in the range 0.05–0.45 mg/mL. 100 µL of standard/sample (5 mg/mL in DMSO) were mixed to 200 µL of 10% Folin-Ciocalteu reagent in DI water and 700 µL of 0.7 M Na_2CO_3. Each solution was prepared in triplicate. The samples and the standards were incubated for 30 min in the dark. The absorbance was red at 765 nm using a Tecan Spark 20M multimode microplate reader. The total phenolic content was expressed as mg gallic acid per gram of extract.

4.3. Total Flavonoid Content

The determination of the content of flavonoid compounds was carried out according to the aluminum chloride colorimetric method [67]. A stock standard solution of 1 mg/mL of quercetin was prepared in methanol, and then working standard solutions were prepared in the range of 0.05–0.30 mg/mL. 500 µL of standard/sample (1 mg/mL in DMSO) were mixed to 100 µL of 10% $AlCl_3$ in 1 M potassium acetate and 3.3 mL of methanol. Each solution was prepared in triplicate. After 30 min of incubation, the absorbance was measured at 430 nm using a Tecan Spark 20M multimode microplate reader. The results were expressed as mg of quercetin per gram of extract.

4.4. Total Condensed Tannins Content

The determination of the content of condensed tannins was performed according to the Broadhurst vanillin-HCl method [68]. A stock standard solution of 1 mg/mL of catechin was prepared in methanol, and then working standard solutions were prepared in the range of 0.05–0.30 mg/mL. 500 µL of standard/sample (2 mg/mL in DMSO) were mixed to 3 mL of 4% vanillin solution in methanol and 1.5 mL of concentrated HCl. Each solution was prepared in triplicate. The samples and the standard were incubated for 15 min in the dark. The absorbance was red at 765 nm using a Tecan Spark 20M multimode microplate reader. The results were expressed as mg of catechin per gram of extract.

4.5. FRAP Scavenging Ability for the Antioxidant Activity

The determination of the antioxidant activity of the extract was performed on the method of FRAP assay [69], based on the redox reaction of the reduced oxidant Fe(III) complexed by TPTZ (2,4,6-Tris(2-pyridyl)-s-triazine). The FRAP reagent for the calibration curve was prepared mixing 0.3 M acetate buffer (pH 3.6), 0.01 M TPTZ and DI water in proportion 10:1:1, respectively. A 0.001 M $FeSO_4 \cdot 7H_2O$ solution in DI water was used as standard for the calibration levels. The sample was analyzed mixing 100 µL of the extract solution at 5 mg/mL in DMSO with 900 µL of DI water and 2 mL of FRAP reagent, obtained mixing 0.3 M acetate buffer, 0.01 M TPTZ and a 0.02 M $FeCl_3 \cdot 6H_2O$ solution in proportion 10:1:1, respectively. All the reagents were prepared fresh. Each solution was prepared in triplicate. All the solutions were incubated for 30 min in the dark. Then the absorbance was measured at 593 nm using a Tecan Spark 20M multimode microplate reader. The scavenging ability was expressed as µmol of Fe^{2+} per 100 mg of extract.

4.6. GC-MS Analysis

5 mg of EPP were dissolved in 50 µL of pyridine and 75 µL of bis(trimethylsilyl)trifluoroacetamide (BSTFA). The mixture was heated at 80 °C for 30 min and analysed by GC/MS and finally 3 µL were injected manually in the GC-MS.

For the analysis of the most lipophilic compounds, EPP was submitted to saponification and dispersive liquid-liquid microextraction (DLLME) [70] before the derivatization step. Briefly, 30 mg of EPP were dispersed in 2 mL of methanol; 1 mL of 2 M methanolic KOH was added and the mixture was heated in a water bath for 1 h at 80 °C shaking vigorously every 15 min. Then 1.2 mL of 1 M HCl was added and the mixture was vortex-mixed. An aliquot of 400 µL was transferred to a glass centrifuge tube and 1.6 mL of DI water was added. The DLLME was performed injecting rapidly 1 mL of a mixture of acetone (900 µL) and chloroform (100 µL) into the glass tube. The tube was closed and gently shaken by hand for 1 min. After that the tube was centrifuged at 3000 rpm for 5 min and the lower phase was collected with a microsyringe. An aliquot of 50 µL of the collected phase was mixed with 30 µL of pyridine and 30 µL of BSTFA and heated in a water bath for 30 min at 80 °C. An aliquot of 3 µL was injected manually in the GC-MS.

Analysis was performed with an Agilent 6890 Series gas chromatograph (Santa Clara, CA, USA) coupled with an Agilent 5973 quadrupole mass analyser (Santa Clara, CA, USA) equipped with the MSD ChemStation software (software version D.03.00). A Phenomenex ZB-5MS plus (30 m × 0.25 mm × 0.25 µm) column (Torrance, CA, USA) was used. The oven temperature was programmed as follow: the initial column temperature of 90 °C (1 min) was increased to 110 °C at a rate of 5 °C/min; then it was increased to 233 °C at a rate of 10 °C/min and held for 5 min; then it was increased to 300 °C at a rate of 20 °C/min and held for 5 min and then it was increased to 325 °C at a rate of 10 °C/min and held for 10 min. The total run time was 40.65 min. Helium was used as a carrier gas at a flow rate of 1.4 mL/min. The split ratio was 50:1 and the injector temperature was 285 °C. For electron ionization (EI) we used the ionization voltage 70 eV. The temperatures used were 150 °C for the MS Quad and 230°C for the MS Source. Full scan mass spectra were acquired at the mass range of 35–550 Da.

The identification of the compounds in the GC-MS chromatograms was based on a comparison of the electron ionization (EI) spectra with the NIST MS library database and, in addition, the study of the mass spectrum of each peak was carried out to further elucidate the identification of the compounds with a higher probability. Standards of fucosterol and cholesterol were also analysed to obtain the exact retention time for the identification. Considering the instrumental technique used, the discrimination between isomers was not possible in certain cases.

4.7. Cell Cultures

Human OS SaOS-2 (ATCC-HTB-85) and MNNG (ATCC-CRL-1547) cells were obtained from American Type Culture Collection (ATCC, Manassas, VA, USA) and cultured as described [71–73] in DMEM containing 10% v/v FBS, 100 mg/mL penicillin and 100 mg/mL streptomycin. Cultures were maintained at 37 °C in a humidified atmosphere of 5% CO_2. Comparative analysis was performed with cell populations at the same generation.

4.8. Cell Viability and Proliferation

SaOS-2 and MNNG cells were seeded in a 96-well plate at a density of 8×10^3 or 3×10^3 cells/well, respectively, and cultured until sub-confluence (70–75% confluence). Cells were serum starved (FBS 0.1%) for 24 h and then treated with different concentrations of EPP (3.1, 6.25; 12.5, 25, 50 100 and 200 µg/mL) in starvation medium. Controls were performed treating cells with DMSO 0.2% v/v, corresponding to the higher concentration of the compound. After 24 h of treatment, cells were washed with sterile PBS and MTT was added to a final concentration of 1 mg/mL. After a 3.5 h incubation, cells were lysed with 100 µL DMSO. The absorbance was measured at 550 nm and percentage of cell viability was calculated relative to control and EPP half-maximal inhibitory concentration (IC_{50}) was calculated by GraphPad Prism software. The experiment was repeated three times.

Cell proliferation was evaluated by cell counting with Scepter™ 2.0 Cell Counter (Merck Millipore, Burlington, MA, USA). SaOS-2 and MNNG cells were seeded in 24-well plate at a density of 4×10^4 and 3×10^4 cells/well, respectively, and cultured until sub-confluence (70–75% confluence). Cells were serum starved (FCS 0.1%) for 24 h and then treated with different concentrations of EPP corresponding to $IC_{50}/2$, IC_{50} and $2*IC_{50}$ in starvation medium. After 24 h of treatment, cells were washed with sterile PBS and detached by trypsin. Cells were collected in clean tubes and counted, percentage of cell proliferation was calculated relative to control.

4.9. Cell Morphology

Cell morphology of SaOS-2 and MNNG cells was recorded with bright field microscopy (Zeiss AxioLabA1, Oberkochen, Germany). Cell morphology images were collected after 24 h treatment with EPP at different concentrations ($IC_{50}/2$, IC_{50} and $2*IC_{50}$) in starved conditions (FCS 0.1%).

4.10. Nuclear Staining with 4′, 6-Diamidine Phenylindole (DAPI)

SaOS-2 and MNNG cells were seeded in 8-well chambered slide at a density of 8×10^3 and 6×10^3 cells/well respectively. After treatment with EPP for 24 h, the slides were washed with PBS and fixed in 70% ethanol for 30 min. Finally, the slides were washed twice with PBS and mounted with fluoroshield mounting medium containing DAPI. Images were captured by fluorescence microscopy (Zeiss AxioLabA1, Oberkochen, Germany).

4.11. Cell Diameter Analysis

As proved by Tahara et al. [74] the Scepter 2.0 cell counter could be used to evaluate apoptosis in an accurate and reproducible way by measuring cell diameter. Cell size distributions were shown as histograms on the monitor of the Scepter™ 2.0 Cell Counter, and these data were analyzed with the Scepter™ 2.0 Software Pro computer software. Before the cell diameter were analyzed, the upper and lower gates of the counter were adjusted manually to eliminate small particles. Data regarding cell diameter are presented as the mean ± standard deviation (SD) values of triplicated experiments.

4.12. Annexin V/Propidium Iodide Assay

Apoptosis was detected in SaOS-2 and MNNG cells treated with EPP for 6 h, by FITC Annexin V/Dead Cell Apoptosis Kit (Molecular Probes; Invitrogen Corp., Eugene, OR, USA) following manufactures protocol. A total of 300 cells from each sample were scored by using a fluorescence microscope (Zeiss AXIO LAB AI, Oberkochen, Germany) and were assessed as viable cells (AnV−/PI−), early apoptotic cells (AnV+/PI−), late apoptosis (AnV+/PI+) and necrotic cells (AnV−/PI+).

4.13. Western Blot Analysis

After treatment with EPP, cells were washed with sterile PBS, lysed with RIPA buffer, added with phosphate and protease inhibitors, and then disrupted by sonication for 5 min in an ice bath. Protein concentration was assessed by BCA protein assay. 20 µg of protein were resolved by 12% SDS–PAGE and transferred onto nitrocellulose membrane. The membrane was blocked in TBS, 0.1% Tween 20, 5% *w/v* nonfat dry milk at 4 °C with gentle shaking, ON. The membrane was incubated with anti-caspase 3 (rabbit polyclonal IgG, 1:1000 Cell Signaling) and anti-GAPDH HRP-conjugated (1:50,000) primary antibodies, in the same buffer, ON at 4 °C. The blot was washed three times with PBS and incubated with anti-rabbit HRP-conjugated secondary antibody

(Sigma-Aldrich, Saint Louis, MO, USA) 1:80,000 for 1 h at room temperature. The membrane was washed three times with PBS and immunoreactive bands were detected using ECL (Luminata Crescendo, Merck Millipore, Burlington, MA, USA) and images acquired by LAS4000 (GE Healthcare, Chicago, IL, USA). The optical densities of immunoreactive bands were analysed by ImageQuant TL software (GE Healthcare, Chicago, IL, USA, V 7.0) using GAPDH as a loading normalizing factor. The experiment was performed in triplicate.

4.14. Statistical Analysis

Experiments were performed in triplicate. Data were expressed as mean ± SD. Differences between the values were tested for statistical analysis of variance (ANOVA) using two-tailed Student's t-test. The values of $p < 0.05$ were considered to be statistically different to control.

5. Conclusions

The extract of brown algae *Padina pavonica* under investigation exhibited an interesting pharmacological potential with relevant health-protecting effects. Our findings confirmed this macroalgae as a promising and unlimited source of new functional food ingredients and bioactive compounds. Moreover, this study provides convincing and integrated evidences that EPP possesses anti-cancer properties towards osteosarcoma cell lines and can be used as a nutraceutical tool to prevent bone-related diseases or to support the current treatment protocols for osteosarcoma.

Author Contributions: Conceptualization, A.S., G.B. and M.B.; Methodology, M.M.; Validation, G.P.; Formal Analysis, M.B.; Investigation, G.B., M.M. and G.P.; Resources, M.B.; Writing-Original Draft Preparation, M.M. and G.B.; Writing-Review & Editing, A.S.; Visualization, G.B. and M.M.; Supervision, A.S. and M.B.

Funding: This research received no external funding.

Acknowledgments: The authors thank Emanuele G. Pirrone for technical assistance. The Department of Biotechnology, Chemistry and Pharmacy has been granted by the Minister of Education, University and Research (MIUR) as "Department of Excellence 2018–2022".

Conflicts of Interest: The authors declare no conflict of interest.

References

1. Pereira, R.C.; Costa-Lotufo, L.V. Bioprospecting of bioactives from seaweeds: Potential, obstacles and alternatives. *Braz. J. Pharmacog.* **2012**, *22*, 894–905. [CrossRef]
2. Kamenarska, Z.; Gasic, M.J.; Zlatovic, M.; Rasovic, A.; Sladic, D.; Kljajic, Z.; Stefanov, K.; Seizova, K.; Najdenski, H.; Kujumgiev, A.; et al. Chemical composition of the brown alga *Padina pavonia* (L.) Gaill. from the Adriatic Sea. *Bot. Mar.* **2002**, *45*, 339–345. [CrossRef]
3. Taskin, E.; Caki, Z.; Ozturk, M. Assessment of in vitro antitumoral and antimicrobial activities of marine algae harvested from the eastern Mediterranean sea. *Afr. J. Biotechnol.* **2010**, *9*, 4272–4277. [CrossRef]
4. Orlando-Bonaca, M.; Lipej, L.; Orfanidis, S. Benthic macrophytes as a tool for delineating, monitoring and assessing ecological status: The case of Slovenian coastal waters. *Mar. Pollut. Bull.* **2008**, *56*, 666–676. [CrossRef] [PubMed]
5. Behmer, S.T.; Olszewski, N.; Sebastiani, J.; Palka, S.; Sparacino, G.; Sciarrno, E.; Grebenok, R.J. Plant phloem sterol content: Forms, putative functions, and implications for phloem-feeding insects. *Front. Plant Sci.* **2013**, *4*, 370. [CrossRef] [PubMed]
6. Bernardini, G.; Laschi, M.; Geminiani, M.; Santucci, A. Proteomics of osteosarcoma. *Expert Rev. Proteom.* **2014**, *11*, 331–343. [CrossRef] [PubMed]
7. Bernardini, G.; Braconi, D.; Spreafico, A.; Santucci, A. Post-genomics of bone metabolic dysfunctions and neoplasias. *Proteomics* **2012**, *12*, 708–721. [CrossRef]
8. Hamed, I.; Özogul, F.; Özogul, Y.; Regenstein, J.M. Marine Bioactive Compounds and Their Health Benefits: A Review. *Compr. Rev. Food Sci. Food Saf.* **2015**, *14*, 446–465. [CrossRef]

9. Zubia, M.; Fabre, M.S.; Kerjean, V.; Le Lann, K.; Stiger-Pouvreau, V.; Fauchon, M.; Deslandes, E. Antioxidant and antitumor activities of some Phaeophyta from Brittany Coasts. *Food Chem.* **2009**, *116*, 693–701. [CrossRef]
10. Khaled, N.; Hiba, M.; Asma, C. Antioxidant and Antifungal activities of *Padina pavonica* and *Sargassum vulgare* from the Lebanese Mediterranean Coast. *Adv. Environ. Biol.* **2012**, *6*, 42–48.
11. Caf, F.; Yilmaz, Ö.; Durucan, F.; Özdemir, N.S. Biochemical components of three marine macroalgae (*Padina pavonica*, Ulva lactuca and *Taonia atomaria*) from the levantine sea coast of antalya, Turkey. *J. Biodivers. Environ. Sci.* **2015**, *6*, 401–411.
12. Pinteus, S.; Silva, J.; Alves, C.; Horta, A.; Fino, N.; Rodrigues, A.I.; Mendes, S.; Pedrosa, R. Cytoprotective effect of seaweeds with high antioxidant activity from the Peniche coast (Portugal). *Food Chem.* **2017**, *218*, 591–599. [CrossRef] [PubMed]
13. Hlila, M.B.; Hichri, A.O.; Mahjoub, M.A.; Mighri, Z.; Mastouri, M. Antioxidant and antimicrobial activities of *Padina pavonica* and *Enteromorpha* sp. from the Tunisian Mediterranean coast. *J. Coast. Life Med.* **2017**, *5*, 336–342. [CrossRef]
14. Agregán, R.; Munekata, P.E.; Domínguez, R.; Carballo, J.; Franco, D.; Lorenzo, J.M. Proximate composition, phenolic content and in vitro antioxidant activity of aqueous extracts of the seaweeds *Ascophyllum nodosum*, *Bifurcaria bifurcata* and *Fucus vesiculosus*. Effect of addition of the extracts on the oxidative stability of canola oil under accelerated storage conditions. *Food Res. Int.* **2017**, *99*, 986–994. [CrossRef] [PubMed]
15. Kelman, D.; Kromkowski Posner, E.; McDermid, K.J.; Tabandera, N.K.; Wright, P.R.; Wright, A.D. Antioxidant Activity of Hawaiian Marine Algae. *Mar. Drugs* **2012**, *10*, 403–416. [CrossRef] [PubMed]
16. Dang, T.T.; Bowyer, M.C.; Van Altena, I.A.; Scarlett, C.J. Comparison of chemical profile and antioxidant properties of the brown algae. *Int. J. Food Sci. Technol.* **2018**, *53*, 174–181. [CrossRef]
17. Kanias, G.D.; Skaltsa, H.; Tsitsa, E.; Loukis, A.; Bitis, J. Study of the correlation between trace elements, sterols and fatty acids in brown algae from the Saronikos Gulf of Greece. *Fresenius' J. Anal. Chem.* **1992**, *344*, 334–339. [CrossRef]
18. Petkov, G.; Furnadzieva, S.; Popov, S. Petrol-induced changes in the lipid and sterol composition of three microalgae. *Phytochemistry* **1992**, *31*, 1165–1166. [CrossRef]
19. Combaut, G.; Yacoubou, A.; Piovetti, L.; Kornprobst, J.M. Sterols of the Senegalese brown alga *Padina vickersiae*. *Phytochemistry* **1985**, *24*, 618–619. [CrossRef]
20. Abdul, Q.A.; Choi, R.J.; Jung, H.A.; Choi, J.S. Health benefit of fucosterol from marine algae: A review. *J. Sci. Food Agric.* **2016**, *96*, 1856–1866. [CrossRef]
21. Sheu, J.H.; Wang, G.H.; Sung, P.J.; Chiu, Y.H.; Duh, C.Y. Cytotoxic sterols from the formosan brown alga *Turbinaria ornata*. *Planta Med.* **1997**, *63*, 571–572. [CrossRef] [PubMed]
22. Khanavi, M.; Gheidarloo, R.; Sadati, N.; Ardekani, M.R.S.; Nabavi, S.M.B.; Tavajohi, S.; Ostad, S.N. Cytotoxicity of fucosterol containing fraction of marine algae against breast and colon carcinoma cell line. *Pharmacogn. Mag.* **2012**, *8*, 60–64. [CrossRef] [PubMed]
23. Sheu, J.H.; Wang, G.H.; Sung, P.J.; Duh, C.Y. New cytotoxic oxygenated fucosterol from the brown alga *Turbinaria conoides*. *J. Nat. Prod.* **1999**, *62*, 224–227. [CrossRef] [PubMed]
24. Lee, D.G.; Park, S.Y.; Chung, W.S.; Park, J.H.; Shin, H.S.; Hwang, E.; Kim, I.H.; Yi, T.H. The bone regenerative effects of fucosterol in in vitro and in vivo models of postmenopausal osteoporosis. *Mol. Nutr. Food Res.* **2014**, *58*, 1249–1257. [CrossRef] [PubMed]
25. Huh, G.W.; Lee, D.Y.; In, S.J.; Lee, D.G.; Park, S.Y.; Yi, T.H.; Kang, H.C.; Seo, W.D.; Baek, N.I. Fucosterols from *Hizikia fusiformis* and their proliferation activities on osteosarcoma-derived cell MG63. *J. Korean Soc. Appl. Biol. Chem.* **2012**, *55*, 551–555. [CrossRef]
26. Bang, M.H.; Kim, H.H.; Lee, D.Y.; Han, M.W.; Baek, Y.S.; Chung, D.K.; Baek, N.I. Anti-osteoporotic activities of fucosterol from sea mustard (*Undaria pinnatifida*). *Food Sci. Biotechnol.* **2011**, *20*, 343–347. [CrossRef]
27. Smit, A.J. Medicinal and Pharmaceutical Uses of Seaweed Natural Products: A Review. *J. Appl. Phycol.* **2004**, *16*, 245–262. [CrossRef]
28. Kelly, G.S. Squalene and its potential clinical uses. *Altern. Med. Rev.* **1999**, *4*, 29–36. [PubMed]
29. Kendel, M.; Wielgosz-Collin, G.; Bertrand, S.; Roussakis, C.; Bourgougnon, N.; Bedoux, G. Lipid Composition, Fatty Acids and Sterols in the Seaweeds *Ulva armoricana*, and *Solieria chordalis* from Brittany (France): An Analysis from Nutritional, Chemotaxonomic, and Antiproliferative Activity Perspectives. *Mar. Drugs* **2015**, *13*, 5606–5628. [CrossRef] [PubMed]

30. Lee, K.I.; Rhee, S.H.; Park, K.Y. Anticancer activity of phytol and eicosatrienoic acid identified from Perilla leaves. *J. Korean Soc. Food Sci. Nutr.* **1999**, *28*, 1107–1112.
31. Jiang, R.; Sun, L.; Wang, Y.; Liu, J.; Liu, X.; Feng, H.; Zhao, D. Chemical composition, and cytotoxic, antioxidant and antibacterial activities of the essential oil from ginseng leaves. *Nat. Prod. Commun.* **2014**, *9*, 865–868. [PubMed]
32. Pejin, B.; Kojic, V.; Bogdanovic, G. An insight into the cytotoxic activity of phytol at in vitro conditions. *Nat. Prod. Res.* **2014**, *28*, 2053–2056. [CrossRef] [PubMed]
33. Kim, C.W.; Lee, H.J.; Jung, J.H.; Kim, Y.H.; Jung, D.B.; Sohn, E.J.; Lee, J.H.; Woo, H.J.; Baek, N.I.; Kim, Y.C.; et al. Activation of Caspase-9/3 and Inhibition of Epithelial Mesenchymal Transition are Critically Involved in Antitumor Effect of Phytol in Hepatocellular Carcinoma Cells. *Phytother. Res.* **2015**, *29*, 1026–1031. [CrossRef] [PubMed]
34. Song, Y.W.; Cho, S.K. Phytol induces apoptosis and ROS-mediated protective autophagy in human gastric adenocarcinima AGS cells. *Biochem. Anal. Biochem.* **2015**, *4*, 211. [CrossRef]
35. Venkataraman, B.; Samuel, L.A.; Pardha Saradhi, M.; Narashimharao, B.; Naga Vamsi Krishna, A.; Sudhakar, M.; Radhakrishnan, T.M. Antibacterial, antioxidant activity and GC-MS analysis of Eupatorium odoratum. *Asian J. Pharm. Clin. Res.* **2012**, *5*, 99–106.
36. Sri Nurestri, A.M.; Sim, K.S.; Norhanom, A.W. Phytochemical and Cytotoxic Investigations of *Pereskia grandifolia* Haw. (Cactaceae) Leaves. *J. Biol. Sci.* **2009**, *9*, 488–493. [CrossRef]
37. Rigano, D.; Russo, A.; Formisano, C.; Cardile, V.; Senatore, F. Antiproliferative and cytotoxic effects on malignant melanoma cells of essential oils from the aerial parts of *Genista sessilifolia* and *G. tinctoria*. *Nat. Prod. Commun.* **2010**, *5*, 1127–1132. [PubMed]
38. Kusch, P.; Deininger, S.; Specht, S.; Maniako, R.; Haubrich, S.; Pommerening, T.; Kong Thoo Lin, P.; Hoerauf, A.; Kaiser, A. 2,5 In vitro and in vivo antimalarial activity assays of seeds from *Balanites aegyptiaca*: Compounds of the extract show growth inhibition and activity against plasmodial aminopeptidase. *J. Parasitol. Res.* **2011**, *2011*. [CrossRef] [PubMed]
39. Yoon, M.A.; Jeong, T.S.; Park, D.S.; Xu, M.Z.; Oh, H.W.; Song, K.B.; Lee, W.S.; Park, H.Y. Antioxidant effects of quinoline alkaloids and 2,4-di-tert-butylphenol isolated from *Scolopendra subspinipes*. *Biol. Pharm. Bull.* **2006**, *29*, 735–739. [CrossRef] [PubMed]
40. Varsha, K.K.; Devendra, L.; Shilpa, G.; Priya, S.; Pandey, A.; Nampoothiri, K.M. 2,4-Di-tert-butyl phenol as the antifungal, antioxidant bioactive purified from a newly isolated *Lactococcus* sp. *Int. J. Food Microbiol.* **2015**, *211*, 44–50. [CrossRef]
41. Hsouna, A.B.; Trigui, M.; Mansour, R.B.; Jarraya, R.M.; Damak, M.; Jaoua, S. Chemical composition, cytotoxicity effect and antimicrobial activity of *Ceratonia siliqua* essential oil with preservative effects against *Listeria* inoculated in minced beef meat. *Int. J. Food Microbiol.* **2011**, *148*, 66–72. [CrossRef] [PubMed]
42. Aknin, M.; Dogbevi, K.; Samb, A.; Kornprobst, J.M.; Gaydou, E.M.; Miralles, J. Fatty acid and sterol composition of eight algae from the Senegalese coast. *Comp. Biochem. Physiol.* **1992**, *102*, 841–843. [CrossRef]
43. Tabarsa, M.; Rezaei, M.; Ramezanpour, Z.; Robert Waaland, J.; Rabiei, R. Fatty acids, amino acids, mineral contents, and proximate composition of some brown seaweeds. *J. Phycol.* **2012**, *48*, 285–292. [CrossRef] [PubMed]
44. Carrillo, C.; Cavia Mdel, M.; Alonso-Torre, S.R. Antitumor effect of oleic acid; mechanisms of action: A review. *Nutr. Hosp.* **2012**, *27*, 1860–1865. [CrossRef] [PubMed]
45. Chajes, V.; Thiebaut, A.C.; Rotival, M.; Gauthier, E.; Maillard, V.; Boutron-Ruault, M.C.; Joulin, V.; Lenoir, G.M.; Clavel-Chapelon, F. Association between serum trans-monounsaturated fatty acids and breast cancer risk in the E3N-EPIC Study. *Am. J. Epidemiol.* **2008**, *167*, 1312–1320. [CrossRef] [PubMed]
46. Sianipar, N.F.; Purnamaningsih, R.; Rosaria. Bioactive compounds of fourth generation gamma-irradiated *Typhoniumflagelliforme* Lodd. mutants based on gas chromatography-mass spectrometry. In *IOP Conference Series: Earth and Environmental Science*; IOP Publishing Ltd.: Bristol, UK, 2016; Volume 41, p. 012025. [CrossRef]

47. Stoneham, M.; Goldacre, M.; Seagroatt, V.; Gill, L. Olive oil, diet and colorectal cancer: An ecological study and a hypothesis. *J. Epidemiol. Community Health* **2000**, *54*, 756–760. [CrossRef] [PubMed]
48. Bartoli, R.; Fernández-Banares, F.; Navarro, E.; Castella, E.; Mane, J.; Alvarez, M.; Pastor, C.; Cabre, E.; Gassull, M. Effect of olive oil on early and late events of colon carcinogenesis in rats: Modulation of arachidonic acid metabolism and local prostaglandin E2 synthesis. *Gut* **2000**, *46*, 191–199. [CrossRef] [PubMed]
49. Schwartz, B.; Birk, Y.; Raz, A.; Madar, Z. Nutritional-pharmacological combinations—A novel approach to reducing colon cancer incidence. *Eur. J. Nutr.* **2004**, *43*, 221–229. [CrossRef] [PubMed]
50. Shaikh, I.A.; Brown, I.; Wahle, K.W.; Heys, S.D. Enhancing cytotoxic therapies for breast and prostate cancers with polyunsaturated fatty acids. *Nutr. Cancer* **2010**, *62*, 284–296. [CrossRef] [PubMed]
51. Menéndez, J.A.; del Mar Barbacid, M.; Montero, S.; Sevilla, E.; Escrich, E.; Solanas, M.; Cortés-Funes, H.; Colomer, R. Effects of gamma-linolenic acid and oleic acid on paclitaxel cytotoxicity in human breast cancer cells. *Eur. J. Cancer* **2001**, *37*, 402–413. [CrossRef]
52. Ito, H.; Kasama, K.; Naruse, S.; Shimura, K. Antitumor effect of palmitoleic acid on Ehrlich ascites tumor. *Cancer Lett.* **1982**, *17*, 197–203. [CrossRef]
53. Wahbeh, M.I. Amino acid and fatty acid profiles of four species of macroalgae from Aqaba and their suitability for use in fish diets. *Aquaculture* **1997**, *159*, 101–109. [CrossRef]
54. Li, X.; Fan, X.; Han, L.; Lou, Q. Fatty acids of some algae from the Bohai Sea. *Phytochemistry* **2002**, *59*, 157–161. [CrossRef]
55. Amaro, H.M.; Fernandes, F.; Valentão, P.; Andrade, P.B.; Sousa-Pinto, I.; Malcata, F.X.; Guedes, A.C. Effect of solvent system on extractability of lipidic components of Scenedesmus obliquus (M2-1) and Gloeothece sp. on antioxidant scavenging capacity thereof. *Mar. Drugs* **2015**, *13*, 6453–6471. [CrossRef]
56. Lauvrak, S.U.; Munthe, E.; Kresse, S.H.; Stratford, E.W.; Namløs, H.M.; Meza-Zepeda, L.A.; Myklebost, O. Functional characterisation of osteosarcoma cell lines and identification of mRNAs and miRNAs associated with aggressive cancer phenotypes. *Br. J. Cancer* **2013**, *109*, 2228–2236. [CrossRef] [PubMed]
57. Roepke, M.; Diestel, A.; Bajbouj, K.; Walluscheck, D.; Schonfeld, P.; Roessner, A.; Schneider-Stock, R.; Gali-Muhtasib, H. Lack of p53 augments thymoquinone-induced apoptosis and caspase activation in human osteosarcoma cells. *Cancer Biol. Ther.* **2007**, *6*, 160–169. [CrossRef]
58. Mahmoud, A.M.; Abdella, E.M.; El-Derby, A.M.; Abdella, E.M. Protective Effects of *Turbinaria ornata* and *Padina pavonia* against Azoxymethane-Induced Colon Carcinogenesis through Modulation of PPAR Gamma, NF-κB and Oxidative Stress. *Phytother. Res.* **2015**, *29*, 737–748. [CrossRef]
59. Ktari, L.; Guyot, M. A cytotoxic oxysterol from the marine alga *Padina pavonica* (L.) Thivy. *J. Appl. Phycol.* **1999**, *11*, 511–513. [CrossRef]
60. Stanojković, T.P.; Šavikin, K.; Zdunić, G.; Kljajić, Z.; Grozdanić, N.; Antić, J. In vitro antitumoral Activities of *Padina pavonia* on human cervix and breast cancer cell Lines. *J. Med. Plant Res.* **2013**, *7*, 419–424. [CrossRef]
61. Jaganathan, S.K.; Mandal, M. Antiproliferative effects of honey and of its polyphenols: A review. *J. Biomed. Biotechnol.* **2009**, *2009*, 1–13. [CrossRef]
62. Zhang, Z.; Teruya, K.; Yoshida, T.; Eto, H.; Shirahata, S. Fucoidan extract enhances the anti-cancer activity of chemotherapeutic agents in MDA-MB-231 and MCF-7 breast cancer cells. *Mar. Drugs* **2013**, *11*, 81–98. [CrossRef] [PubMed]
63. Kim, E.J.; Park, S.Y.; Lee, J.Y.; Park, J.H. Fucoidan present in brown algae induces apoptosis of human colon cancer cells. *BMC Gastroenterol.* **2010**, *10*, 96. [CrossRef] [PubMed]
64. Konishi, I.; Hosokawa, M.; Sashima, T.; Kobayashi, H.; Miyashita, K. Halocynthiaxanthin and fucoxanthinol isolated from *Halocynthia roretzi* induce apoptosis in human leukemia, breast and colon cancer cells. *Comp. Biochem. Physiol. C Toxicol. Pharmacol.* **2006**, *142*, 53–59. [CrossRef] [PubMed]
65. Yu, R.X.; Hu, X.M.; Xu, S.Q.; Jiang, Z.J.; Yang, W. Effects of fucoxanthin on proliferation and apoptosis in human gastric adenocarcinoma MGC-803 cells via JAK/STATsignal pathway. *Eur. J. Pharmacol.* **2011**, *657*, 10–19. [CrossRef] [PubMed]
66. Song, F.L.; Gan, R.Y.; Zhang, Y.; Xiao, Q.; Kuang, L.; Li, H.B. Total Phenolic Contents and Antioxidant Capacities of Selected Chinese Medicinal Plants. *Int. J. Mol. Sci.* **2010**, *11*, 2362–2372. [CrossRef] [PubMed]
67. Chang, C.C.; Yang, M.H.; Wen, H.-M.; Chern, J.C. Estimation of total flavonoid content in propolis by two complementary colorimetric methods. *J. Food Drug Anal.* **2002**, *10*, 178–182.

68. Broadhurst, R.B.; Jones, W.T. Analysis of Condensed Tannins Using Acidified Vanillin. *J. Sci. Food Agric.* **1978**, *29*, 788–794. [CrossRef]
69. Benzie, I.F.; Strain, J.J. The ferric reducing ability of plasma (FRAP) as a measure of "antioxidant power": The FRAP assay. *Anal. Biochem.* **1996**, *239*, 70–76. [CrossRef]
70. Rezaee, M.; Assadia, Y.; Milani Hosseini, M.R.; Aghaee, E.; Ahmadi, F.; Berijani, S. Determination of organic compounds in water using dispersive liquid–liquid microextraction. *J. Chromatogr. A* **2006**, *1116*, 1–9. [CrossRef]
71. Bernardini, G.; Geminiani, M.; Gambassi, S.; Orlandini, M.; Petricci, E.; Marzocchi, B.; Laschi, M.; Taddei, M.; Manetti, F.; Santucci, A. Novel smoothened antagonists as anti-neoplastic agents for the treatment of osteosarcoma. *J. Cell. Physiol.* **2018**, *233*, 4961–4971. [CrossRef]
72. Laschi, M.; Bernardini, G.; Geminiani, M.; Ghezzi, L.; Amato, L.; Braconi, D.; Millucci, L.; Frediani, B.; Spreafico, A.; Franchi, A.; et al. Establishment of Four New Human Primary Cell Cultures from Chemo-Naïve Italian Osteosarcoma Patients. *J. Cell. Physiol.* **2015**, *230*, 2718–2727. [CrossRef] [PubMed]
73. Laschi, M.; Bernardini, G.; Geminiani, M.; Manetti, F.; Mori, M.; Spreafico, A.; Campanacci, D.; Capanna, R.; Schenone, S.; Botta, M.; et al. Differentially activated Src kinase in chemo-naïve human primary osteosarcoma cells and effects of a Src kinase inhibitor. *Biofactors* **2017**, *43*, 801–811. [CrossRef] [PubMed]
74. Tahara, M.; Inoue, T.; Miyakura, Y.; Horie, H.; Yasuda, Y.; Fujii, H.; Kotake, K.; Sugano, K. Cell diameter measurements obtained with a handheld cell counter could be used as a surrogate marker of G2/M arrest and apoptosis in colon cancer cell lines exposed to SN-38. *Biochem. Biophys. Res. Commun.* **2013**, *434*, 753–759. [CrossRef] [PubMed]

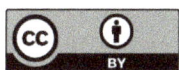

© 2018 by the authors. Licensee MDPI, Basel, Switzerland. This article is an open access article distributed under the terms and conditions of the Creative Commons Attribution (CC BY) license (http://creativecommons.org/licenses/by/4.0/).

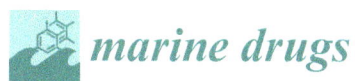

Article

Pyrogallol-Phloroglucinol-6,6-Bieckol from *Ecklonia cava* Attenuates Tubular Epithelial Cell (TCMK-1) Death in Hypoxia/Reoxygenation Injury

Myeongjoo Son [1,2,†], Seyeon Oh [2,†], Chang Hu Choi [3], Kook Yang Park [3], Kuk Hui Son [3,*] and Kyunghee Byun [1,2,*]

1. Department of Anatomy & Cell Biology, Gachon University College of Medicine, Incheon 21936, Korea; mjson@gachon.ac.kr
2. Functional Cellular Networks Laboratory, College of Medicine, Department of Medicine, Graduate School and Lee Gil Ya Cancer and Diabetes Institute, Gachon University, Incheon 21999, Korea; seyeon8965@gachon.ac.kr
3. Department of Thoracic and Cardiovascular Surgery, Gachon University Gil Medical Center, Gachon University, Incheon 21565, Korea; cch624@gilhospital.com (C.H.C.); kkyypark@gilhospital.com (K.Y.P.)
* Correspondence: dr632@gilhospital.com (K.H.S.); khbyun1@gachon.ac.kr (K.B.); Tel.: +82-32-460-3666 (K.H.S); +82-32-899-6511 (K.B.)
† These authors contributed equally to this work.

Received: 25 September 2019; Accepted: 22 October 2019; Published: 24 October 2019

Abstract: The hypoxia/reoxygenation (H/R) injury causes serious complications after the blood supply to the kidney is stopped during surgery. The main mechanism of I/R injury is the release of high-mobility group protein B1 (HMGB1) from injured tubular epithelial cells (TEC, TCMK-1 cell), which triggers TLR4 or RAGE signaling, leading to cell death. We evaluated whether the extracts of *Ecklonia cava (E. cava)* would attenuate TEC death induced by H/R injury. We also evaluated which phlorotannin—dieckol (DK), phlorofucofuroeckol A (PFFA), pyrogallol phloroglucinol-6,6-bieckol (PPB), or 2,7-phloroglucinol-6,6-bieckol (PHB)—would have the most potent effect in the context of H/R injury. We used for pre-hypoxia treatment, in which the phlorotannins from *E. cava* extracts were added before the onset of hypoxia, and a post- hypoxia treatment, in which the phlorotannins were added before the start of reperfusion. PPB most effectively reduced HMGB1 release and the expression of TLR4 and RAGE induced by H/R injury in both pre- and post-hypoxia treatment. PPB also most effectively inhibited the expression of NF-kB and release of the inflammatory cytokines TNF-α and IL-6 in both models. PPB most effectively inhibited cell death and expression of cell death signaling molecules such as Erk/pErk, JNK/pJNK, and p38/pp38. These results suggest that PPB blocks the HGMB1–TLR4/RAGE signaling pathway and decreases TEC death induced by H/R and that PPB can be a novel target for renal H/R injury therapy.

Keywords: kidney; ischemia-reperfusion injury; *Ecklonia cava*; phlorotannins

---

1. Introduction

Ischemia/reperfusion (I/R) injury, which occurs when blood supply to tissues or organs is restored after ischemia, leads to more tissue damage than ischemia itself by enhancing the inflammatory reaction in the reperfused tissue [1].

Renal I/R injury is a major pathophysiology of acute kidney injury (AKI) and can induce AKI after kidney transplantation, partial nephrectomy, renal artery angioplasty, aortic aneurysm surgery, and elective urological surgery when blood supply to the kidney is stopped or decreased during surgery [2]. In addition to AKI, I/R injury leads to the loss of tubular epithelial cell (TEC) function, resulting in delayed graft function and acute or chronic rejection of the transplanted kidney [3]. To decrease the incidence of AKI after surgeries accompanied by I/R injury, treatments to decrease I/R injury should be developed.

High-mobility group protein B1 (HMGB1) is released from injured renal cells and activates Toll-like receptors (TLR), which trigger production of pro-inflammatory cytokines such as tumor necrosis factor-α (TNF-α) and transcription of nuclear factor kappa B (NF-κB) [4–6], finally leading to tissue injury after I/R injury in the kidney [7,8]. In I/R injury, TECs play a dual role as both injury initiators (by releasing HMGB1) and targets [9]. Receptor for advanced glycation end products (RAGE) also initiates pro-inflammatory signaling in I/R injury by binding HMGB1 in the liver and heart [10,11].

Ecklonia cava is a brown alga that contains phlorotannins, polyphenolic compounds that have multiple biological activities including anti-inflammatory [12,13] and antioxidant activities [14]. One study has shown that polyphenol extract from *E. cava* attenuated renal inflammation induced by a high-fat diet by decreasing pro-inflammatory signaling via TNF-α and NF-κB [15]. However, the effect of *E. cava* on I/R injury has not been studied.

Here, we evaluated whether phlorotannins from *E. cava* extract would attenuate TEC death induced by I/R injury. Commonly, renal hypoxia/reoxygenation (H/R) was established to simulate renal I/R injury in vitro [16,17] and we also used the H/R model. We used two treatment models: a pre-hypoxia model, in which the phlorotannins were added before the onset of hypoxia, and a post- hypoxia model, in which the phlorotannins were added before the start of reoxygenation. In addition, we evaluated which phlorotannin—dieckol (DK), phlorofucofuroeckol A (PFFA), pyrogallol phloroglucinol-6,6-bieckol (PPB), or 2,7-phloroglucinol-6,6-bieckol (PHB)—would have the most potent effect in the context of H/R injury.

2. Results and Discussion

2.1. Attenuation of HMGB1 Release from TECs after H/R Injury by the Phlorotannins from E. cava Extracts

In this study, we used mouse kidney tubular cells (TCMK-1) as TECs. In the pre-hypoxia model, the HMGB1 level was increased by H/R injury in both TEC lysate and supernatant (Figure 1A,B), suggesting that TECs injured by H/R increased the synthesis and release of HMGB1. HMGB1 levels in both the TEC lysate and supernatant were decreased by individual phlorotannins added before TECs were exposed to hypoxia. Among individual phlorotannins, PPB and DK showed the strongest attenuation effects.

In the post-hypoxia treatment model, the HMGB1 level increased by H/R injury was also decreased by adding *E. cava* extracts before reperfusion in both TEC lysate and supernatant. Among the 4 phlorotannins, the effect of DK and PPB was the most significant (Figure 1C,D).

HMGB1 is passively released in response to inflammatory stress or necrosis [18]. Our results showed that the HMGB1 release from TECs was increased after H/R injury and that this increase was attenuated by PPB most significantly among the 4 phlorotannins from *E. cava*.

2.2. TLR4 and RAGE Expression Induced by H/R Injury Is Attenuated Most Efficiently by PPB

TLR4 and RAGE expression in TECs induced by H/R injury were attenuated by the 4 phlorotannins in the pre-hypoxia treatment model, among them, PPB had the strongest effect on TLR4 and RAGE expression (Figure 2A–C,E). The patterns were the same in the post-hypoxia treatment (Figure 2A,B,D,F).

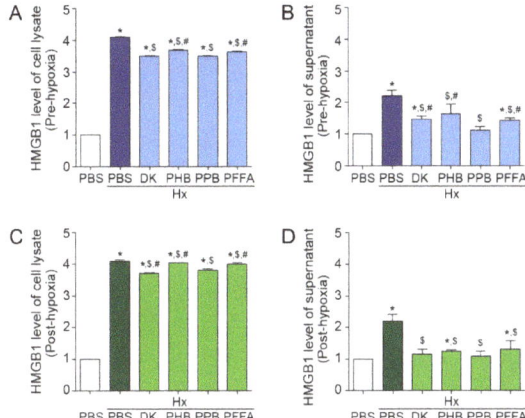

Figure 1. Inhibitory effects of phlorotannins from *E. cava* extract on HMGB1 synthesis and secretion in pre-hypoxia and post-hypoxia treatment (**A,B**) To examine the preventive effects of 4 phlorotannins from *E. cava* extract (DK, PHB, PPB, PFFA), they were added to mouse kidney tubular cells (TCMK-1) before hypoxia (pre-hypoxia treatment). (**C,D**) To examine the therapeutic effects of the 4 phlorotannins, they were added to TCMK-1 after hypoxia (post-hypoxia treatment). In each treatment model, (**A,C**) HMGB1 synthesis in cell lysate and (**B,D**) secretion levels in cell culture medium were measured by ELISA. All levels are normalized to those in cells treated with PBS under normoxic control conditions. Significance represented as: * $p < 0.05$ versus PBS, $ $p < 0.05$ versus Hx/PBS, # $p < 0.05$ versus Hx/PPB. DK, dieckol, PHB, 2,7-phloroglucinol-6,6-bieckol, PPB, pyrogallol-phloroglucinol-6,6-bieckol, PFFA, phlorofucofuroeckol A, HMGB1, high mobility group box 1.

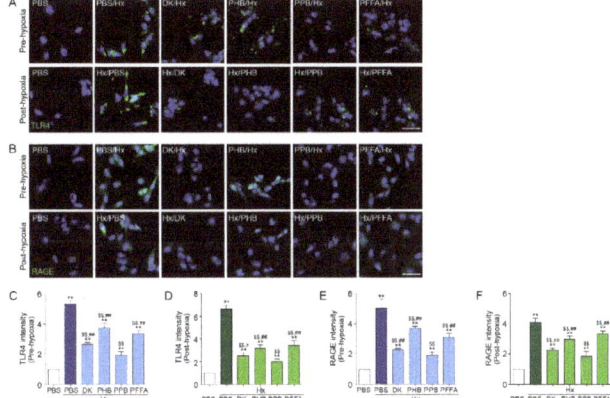

Figure 2. Inhibitory effects of phlorotannins from *E. cava* extract on TLR4 and RAGE expression in pre-hypoxia and post-hypoxia treatment using Mouse kidney tubular cells (TCMK-1) were treated with 4 phlorotannins (DK, PFFA, PPB, PHB) before hypoxia (pre-hypoxia model) or after hypoxia (post-hypoxia model). (**A,B**) Microscopic fluorescence images showing (**A**) TLR4 and (**B**) RAGE protein expression (green) in the pre-hypoxia treatment (upper rows) and post-hypoxia treatment (bottom rows). Nuclei were stained with DAPI (blue). Scale bar = 50 μm. (**C–F**) Quantification of (**C,D**) TLR4 and (**E,F**) RAGE expression using representative images from (**A**) and (**B**) in the pre-hypoxia treatment model and post-hypoxia treatment. Significance represented as: ** $p < 0.01$ versus PBS, $$ $p < 0.01$ versus Hx/PBS, # $p < 0.05$, ## $p < 0.01$ versus Hx/PPB. DK, dieckol, PHB, 2,7-phloroglucinol-6,6-bieckol, PFFA, phlorofucofuroeckol A, PPB, pyrogallol-phloroglucinol-6,6-bieckol, TLR4, Toll-like receptor 4, RAGE, receptor for advanced glycation end-products.

TLR4 [19] and RAGE [20] are the primary cell membrane receptors that bind HMGB1. In H/R injury, this binding leads to pro-inflammatory signaling pathway activation by TLR and RAGE.

2.3. Expression of NF-kB and Pro-Inflammatory Cytokines after H/R Injury Is Attenuated Efficiently by PPB

The level of NF-κB was increased in both the pre-hypoxia and post-hypoxia treatment models and was decreased by the 4 phlorotannins, with PPB showing the strong effect (Figure 3). The levels of TNF-α and IL-6 were also increased by H/R injury and were attenuated by adding the 4 phlorotannins, among which PPB showed a strong effect.

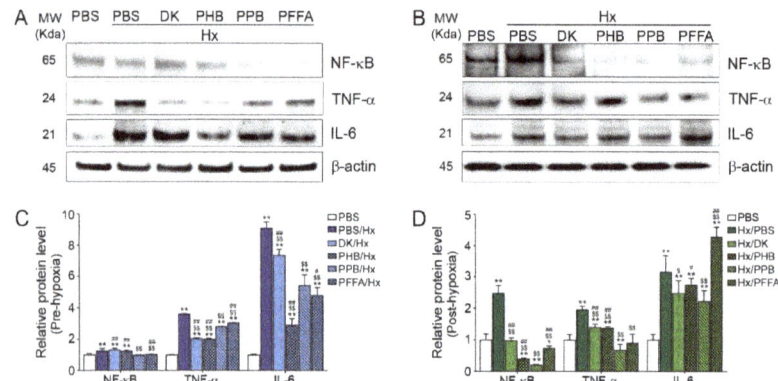

Figure 3. Inhibitory effects of phlorotannins from *E. cava* extract on NF-kB expression and pro-inflammatory cytokine expression in pre-hypoxia and post-hypoxia treatment Mouse kidney tubular cells (TCMK-1) were treated with 4 phlorotannins (DK, PFFA, PPB, PHB) before hypoxia (pre-hypoxia treatment) or after hypoxia (post-hypoxia treatment). NF-κB and the pro-inflammatory cytokines TNF-α and IL-6 were detected by immunoblotting in (**A**) pre-hypoxia and (**B**) post-hypoxia treatment and immunoblotting results are quantified and normalized to those in cells treated with PBS in (**C**) pre-hypoxia and (**D**) post-hypoxia treatment. Significance represented as: * $p < 0.05$, ** $p < 0.01$ versus PBS, $ $p < 0.05$, $$ $p < 0.01$ versus Hx/PBS, # $p < 0.05$, ## $p < 0.01$ versus Hx/PPB. DK, dieckol, Hx, Hypoxia, PHB, 2,7-phloroglucinol-6,6-bieckol, PFFA, phlorofucofuroeckol A, PPB, pyrogallol-phloroglucinol-6,6-bieckol, NF-kB, nuclear factor kappa light chain enhancer of activated B cells, TNF-α, tumor necrosis factor-alpha, IL-6, Interleukin-6.

During H/R injury, TLR4 initiates the inflammatory response by increasing the production of NF-κB-dependent cytokines such as TNF-α [5,6]. In addition, IL-6 is released upon TLR4 activation during H/R injury and amplifies inflammation [11,21]. The RAGE pathway also induces NF-κB activation and leads to an increase in TNF-α and IL-6 levels [22]. TNF-α and IL-6 induce tubular cell death during renal H/R injury [23].

2.4. TEC Apoptosis Induced by H/R Injury Is Attenuated Efficiently by PPB

TEC apoptosis induced by H/R injury was attenuated by adding the phlorotannin from *E. cava* extracts in both the pre-hypoxia and post-hypoxia treatments (Figure 4A–C).

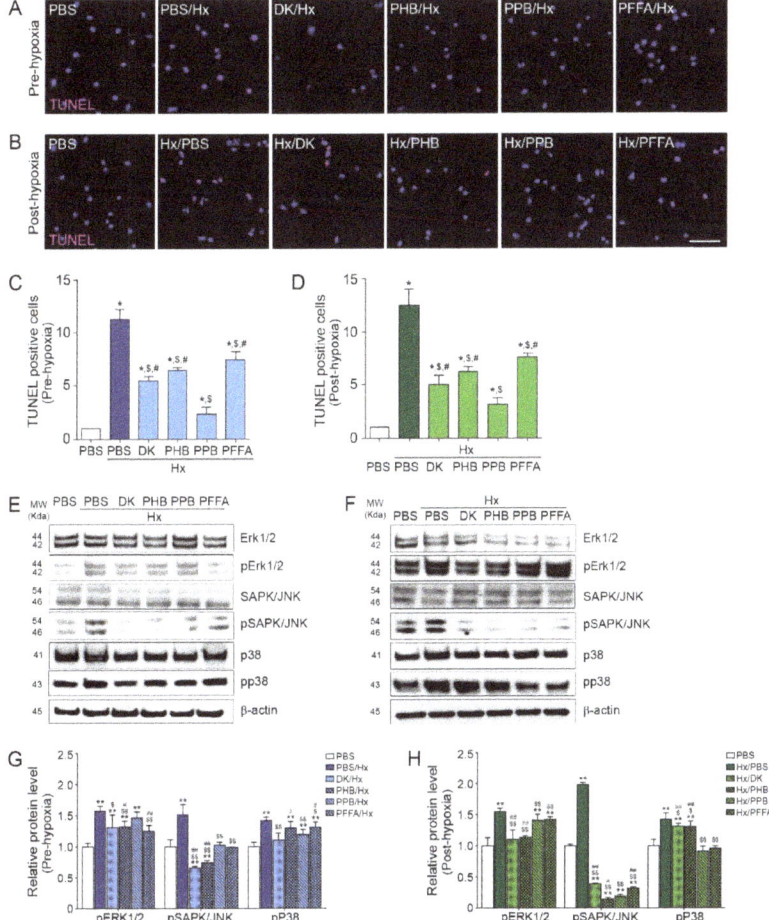

Figure 4. Inhibitory effects of phlorotannins from *E. cava* extract on apoptosis and apoptotic cell death–related MAPK pathway molecules in pre-hypoxia and post-hypoxia treatment Mouse kidney tubular cells (TCMK-1) were treated with the 4 phlorotannins (DK, PHB, PPB, PFFA) before hypoxia (pre-hypoxia treatment) or after hypoxia (post-hypoxia treatment). (**A,B**) Microscopic fluorescence images showing TUNEL-positive apoptotic cells (pink dot) and nuclei (blue, DAPI) in (**A**) the pre-hypoxia treatment and (**B**) post-hypoxia treatment. Scale bar = 50 μm. Quantification of TUNEL-positive apoptotic cells using representative images is shown in (**C**) the pre-hypoxia treatment and in (**D**) the post-hypoxia treatment. Apoptosis-related MAPK pathway molecules were detected by immunoblotting in (**E**) pre-hypoxia treatment and (**F**) post-hypoxia treatment. Apoptosis-related phosphorylated MAPKs expression are quantified using non-phosphorylated protein expression in (**G**) pre-hypoxia and (**H**) post-hypoxia treatment model. All levels are normalized to those in cells treated with PBS. Significance represented as: * $p < 0.05$, ** $p < 0.01$ versus PBS, $ $p < 0.05$, $$ $p < 0.01$ versus Hx/PBS, # $p < 0.05$, ## $p < 0.01$ versus Hx/PPB. DK, dieckol, Hx, Hypoxia, PHB, 2,7-phloroglucinol-6,6-bieckol, PFFA, phlorofucofuroeckol A, PPB, pyrogallol-phloroglucinol-6,6-bieckol, TUNEL, terminal deoxynucleotidyl transferase dUTP nick end labeling.

2.5. PPB Attenuated Cell Death Signals Induced by H/R Injury

The level of SAPK/JNK was increased in both the pre-hypoxia and post-hypoxia treatment models and was decreased by the 4 phlorotannins, with PPB showing the effect (Figure 4D–G). The extracellular signal-regulated kinases-1 and -2 (Erk1/2), the c-Jun N-terminal kinases (SAPK/JNK), and p38 mitogen-activated protein kinases (MAPKs) are involved in cell death induced by H/R injury [24]. ERK signaling is involved in injury and apoptosis of kidney cells during H/R injury [25–27]. Both p38 and JNK pathways induce tubular cell death and their inhibition reduces apoptosis and inflammation induced by H/R injury [28,29].

In our study, these cell death signals were increased by H/R injury in TEC and were attenuated most significantly by PPB in both the pre-hypoxia and post-hypoxia treatment models.

Previous one study shows that intraperitoneally administration of *E. cava* polyphenols at 10 mg/kg and 50 mg/kg decreased rat brain infarct size and neuronal cell apoptosis [30] and the other studies shows that 10 μg/mL or 1–50 μM only DK from *E. cava* have protective effects on oxidative stress-induced apoptosis in endothelial progenitor cells (EPCs) [31], primary cortical neurons and HT22 neurons [32]. However, this study tried to mimic renal ischemia reperfusion injury in vitro and validated effects on 4 phlorotannins including dieckol (DK), phlorofucofuroeckol A (PFFA), pyrogallol phloroglucinol-6,6-bieckol (PPB), or 2,7-phloroglucinol-6,6-bieckol (PHB) from *E. cava*.

3. Materials and Methods

3.1. Cell Culture

Mouse renal tubular epithelial cells, TCMK-1, were purchased from Korean Cell Line Bank (Seoul, Korea) and cultured in Dulbecco's Modified Eagle's medium (DMEM; Gibco, Waltham, MA, USA) containing 10% fetal bovine serum (FBS; Gibco) and 1% penicillin/streptomycin (Gibco) in a 5% CO_2 incubator (Thermo Fisher Scientific; Waltham, MA, USA) at 37 °C. Growth medium was changed every 2 days.

3.2. Hypoxia/Reoxygenation (H/R) Injury Cell Models

To examine the inhibitory effects of 4 phlorotannins DK, PHB, PFFA, and PPB from *E. cava* extract, we designed two types of H/R cell models using TCMK-1 cells, the experimental method and image scheme is shown in Figure S1.

3.2.1. Pre-Hypoxia Treatment Model

Four prepared phlorotannins (2.5 μg/mL) were added to the growth medium, which was used to treat TCMK-1 cells for 6 h before hypoxia. After treatment, the medium was completely removed, and the cells were washed thoroughly with PBS. Hypoxia medium contained 0.5% FBS and 1% penicillin/streptomycin in DMEM. The TCMK-1 cells were cultured in hypoxia medium with the 4 phlorotannins and exposed to gas mixture of 1% O_2, 5% CO_2, 94% N_2 for 14 h within hypoxia incubator chamber (Stemcell technologies, Cambridge, MA, USA). After flushing the hypoxia chamber with the desired gas mixture, the chamber seals tightly with clamp. After incubation, the hypoxia chamber was dismantled and the hypoxia medium was removed, and the cells were washed with PBS. The cells were cultured with fresh oxygenated medium containing FBS, 1% penicillin/streptomycin, 4 phlorotannins in a mixture of 20% O_2, 5% CO_2, 75% N_2 for 9 h, and then used for experiments. The experimental method and image scheme is shown in Figure S1.

3.2.2. Post-Hypoxia Treatment Model

TCMK-1 cells were cultured in growth medium for 6 h before hypoxia, growth medium was completely removed, and the cells were washed with PBS. Hypoxia exposure was performed following in Section 3.2.1 *'Pre-hypoxia treatment model'* of material and methods section. After the hypoxia treatment, the hypoxia chamber was dismantled and the hypoxia medium was removed, and the cells were washed with PBS. The cells were cultured with fresh oxygenated medium containing FBS, 1% penicillin/streptomycin, 4 phlorotannins in a mixture of 20% O_2, 5% CO_2, 75% N_2 for 9 h, and then used for experiments. The experimental method and image scheme is shown in Figure S1.

3.3. Immunostaining

TCMK-1 cells were seeded in an 8-well chamber slide (1×10^4 per chamber well) and incubated for 24 h. Growth medium was completely removed, the cells were rinsed with PBS and fixed with 4% paraformaldehyde for 15 min. To suppress non-specific binding, animal serum was used and the cells were incubated with anti-TLR4 (Abcam; Cambridge, UK, dilution rate 1:200) and anti-RAGE (Santa-cruz biotechnology; Starr County, TX, USA, dilution rate 1:100) antibodies for 24 h at 4°C. After incubation, the cells were rinsed with PBS and incubated with Alexa 488–conjugated secondary antibody (dilution, 1:500) in the dark for 1 h and rinsed with PBS again. To stain the nuclei, the cells were incubated with DAPI (Sigma-Aldrich) for 1 min. Fluorescence was detected by confocal microscopy (LSM 710; Carl Zeiss, Oberkochen, Germany).

3.4. Immunoblotting

For protein extraction, TCMK-1 cells were lysed using an EzRIPA lysis kit (ATTO, Tokyo, Japan) and centrifuged at $13,000 \times g$ for 20 min at 4 °C. The clear supernatants were collected, and protein concentration was determined by using a bicinchoninic acid assay kit (Thermo Fisher Scientific). Proteins (15 µg/lane) were separated by sodium dodecylsulfate-polyacrylamide gel electrophoresis (SDS-PAGE) in a 10% to 12% gradient gels and transferred to polyvinylidene fluoride membranes in a Semi-Dry transfer system (ATTO) at 25 V for 10 min. The membranes were blocked with 5% skimmed milk for 1 h, washed twice with Tris-buffered saline containing 0.1% Tween 20 (TBST), and incubated with primary antibodies at 4 °C for 24 h. The membranes were then washed with TBST twice, incubated with appropriate secondary antibodies for 1 h at room temperature, and washed with TBST again. Proteins of interest were detected using ECL Western Blotting Substrate (Thermo Scientific; Waltham, MA, USA) on a LAS-4000 imager (GE Healthcare, Uppsala, Sweden). Protein expression levels were quantified using Image J software (NIH; Bethesda, MD, USA) and the antibodies used are listed in Table S1.

3.5. Detection of Apoptotic Cells by TUNEL Staining

TUNEL staining was used to determine the effects of the 4 phlorotannins on apoptosis in both hypoxia treatment models. TCMK-1 cells were cultured in an 8-well chamber (3×10^5 well) and treated with 4 phlorotannins before and after hypoxia for 24 h each., Cells were fixed with freshly prepared 4% paraformaldehyde for 5 min at room temperature, permeabilized with 0.1% Triton X-100 and 0.1% sodium citrate in PBS at 4 °C for 2 min and stained with the TUNEL assay kit (Roche; Indianapolis, IN, USA) following the manufacturer's instructions. DAPI (Sigma-Aldrich) staining at room temperature for 5 min was used to visualize nuclei. Then, cover slips were mounted onto glass slides with Vectashield mounting medium (Vector Laboratories; San Francisco, CA, USA, H-1500) and examined under a confocal microscope (LSM 710). Apoptotic cells were analyzed with Zen 2009 software (Zeiss).

3.6. Enzyme-Linked Immunosorbent Assay (ELISA)

HMGB1 protein levels in cell lysates and culture supernatants of TCMK-1 cells exposed to hypoxia were measured by an indirect ELISA. A 96-well plate was coated with 0.6% sodium bicarbonate and 0.3% sodium carbonate in distilled water (pH 9.6) overnight at 4 °C. Each well was washed with 0.1% Triton X-100 in phosphate-buffered saline (TPBS), and remaining protein-binding sites were blocked with 5% skim milk at 4 °C overnight. The wells were washed with TPBS, and cell lysate and supernatant were added and incubated overnight at 4 °C. Unbound proteins were removed by washing with TPBS, and bound proteins were incubated with anti-HMGB1 antibody (Abcam, dilution rate 1:1000) for 24 h at 4 °C. After rinsing the plate with TPBS, the samples were incubated for 2 h at room temperature with horseradish peroxidase–conjugated anti-rabbit antibody (Vector, dilution rate 1:1000). After washing with TPBS, color was developed by incubating samples with 3,3′,5,5′-tetramethylbenzidine (Sigma-Aldrich) for 20 min. The reaction was stopped by adding 50 μL of 2 M H_2SO_4 to each well, and absorbance was measured at 450 nm using an ELISA plate reader (VERSA Max; Molecular Devices, San Jose, CA, USA).

3.7. Isolation of 4 Phlorotannins from E. cava

E. cava used this study were obtained from Aqua Green Technology Co., Ltd (Jeju, Korea). In briefly, E. cava were thoroughly washed with pure water and air-dried at room temperature for 48 h, the clean E. cava was ground and 50% ethyl alcohol was added followed by incubation at 85 °C for 12 h. The extracts of E. cava were filtered, concentrated, sterilized by heating at high temperatures above 85 °C for 40–60 min and then spray-dried. Phlorotannins were isolated following a published procedure [33]. In briefly, centrifugal partition chromatography (CPC) was performed using a two phase solvent system full of water/ethyl acetate/methyl alcohol/n-hexane (7:7:3:2, ratio v/v/v/v). The organic stationary phase was filled in the centrifugal partition chromatography column followed by pumping of the mobile phase into the column in descending mode at the same flow rate (2 mL per min) used for separation.

3.8. Statistical Analysis

The statistical analysis was conducted using SPSS version 22 software (IBM Co.; Armonk, NY, USA). In this study, statistical differences were compared among 6 groups (PBS, Hx/PBS, Hx/DK, Hx/PHB, Hx/PPB, Hx/PFFA) in pre-hypoxia and post-hypoxia treatment using the non-parametric Kruskal-Wallis test. For post-test, the difference between 2 groups was compared using the Mann-Whitney U test. All experiments were performed in triplicate, and results are presented as means ± standard deviation. * (asterisk) means comparing with PBS, $ comparing with Hx/PBS and # comparing with Hx/PPB. All the experiments were repeated three times.

4. Conclusions

In conclusion, PPB showed a protective effect against H/R injury of TECs. The PPB reduced HMGB1 release, which initiates TLR4 and RAGE activation. The decrease in TRL4 and RAGE signaling by PPB inhibited NF-κB activation, which leads to TNF-α and IL-6 release. Those cytokines are well-known inducers of TEC apoptosis after H/R injury. PPB reduced TNF-α and IL-6 release, and reduced cell death and cell death signaling molecules such as pErk1/2, pSAPK/JNK, and pP38, which suggested that PPB has a potential to prevent kidney H/R injury by inhibiting the HMGB1-TLR4 or RAGE pathway. Among the 4 phlorotannins, PPB had the strongest protective effect from H/R injury, in both the pre- and post-hypoxia models. Our data suggested that PPB treatment could be used to protect against I/R injury during kidney surgery before the blood supply to the kidney is stopped and even after ischemia, before the blood supply to the kidney is restored, the latter treatment might be as effective as when treatment with PPB is performed before the onset of ischemia.

Supplementary Materials: The following are available online at http://www.mdpi.com/1660-3397/17/11/602/s1, Table S1: List of antibodies for immunoblotting, Figure S1: Experimental scheme image of pre- and post-hypoxia treatment model in vitro.

Author Contributions: Data curation, M.S. and S.O.; Formal analysis, M.S., S.O. and K.Y.P.; Funding acquisition, K.B.; Investigation, C.H.C.; Project administration, K.H.S. and K.B.; Writing—original draft, M.S. and K.H.S.

Funding: This research was part of a project entitled 'Development of functional food products with natural materials derived from marine resources' (no. 20170285), funded by the Ministry of Oceans and Fisheries, Republic of Korea.

Acknowledgments: All authors thank Aqua Green Technology Co., LTD (Jeju, Korea) for assistance in preparing 4 phlorotannins from E. cava extract.

Conflicts of Interest: The authors have no conflict of interest to declare.

Abbreviations

DK: dieckol; Hx, hypoxia; H/R, hypoxia/ reoxygenation; I/R, ischemia/reperfusion; PFFA, phlorofucofuroeckol A; PHB, 2,7-phloroglucinol-6,6-bieckol; PPB, pyrogallol-phloroglucinol-6,6-bieckol; RAGE, receptor for advanced glycation end-products; TEC, kidney tubular epithelial cells; TLR4, Toll-like receptor 4; TUNEL, terminal deoxynucleotidyl transferase dUTP nick end labeling.

References

1. Eltzschig, H.K.; Eckle, T. Ischemia and reperfusion—From mechanism to translation. *Nat. Med.* **2011**, *17*, 1391–1401. [CrossRef]
2. Vargas, F.; Romecín, P.; García-Guillén, A.I.; Wangesteen, R.; Vargas-Tendero, P.; Paredes, M.D.; Atucha, N.M.; García-Estañ, J. Flavonoids in Kidney Health and Disease. *Front. Physiol.* **2018**, *24*, 394. [CrossRef]
3. Saat, T.C.; van den Akker, E.K.; IJzermans, J.N.; Dor, F.J.; de Bruin, R.W. Improving the outcome of kidney transplantation by ameliorating renal ischemia reperfusion injury: Lost in translation? *J. Transl. Med.* **2016**, *14*, 20. [CrossRef]
4. Yang, W.S.; Han, N.J.; Kim, J.J.; Lee, M.J.; Park, S.K. TNF-alpha Activates High-Mobility Group Box 1—Toll-Like Receptor 4 Signaling Pathway in Human Aortic Endothelial Cells. *Cell Physiol. Biochem.* **2016**, *38*, 2139–2151. [CrossRef]
5. Arumugam, T.V.; Okun, E.; Tang, S.C.; Thundyil, J.; Taylor, S.M.; Woodruff, T.M. Toll-like receptors in ischemia-reperfusion injury. *Shock* **2009**, *32*, 4–16. [CrossRef]
6. Bonventre, J.V.; Yang, L. Cellular pathophysiology of ischemic acute kidney injury. *J. Clin. Investig.* **2011**, *121*, 4210–4221. [CrossRef]
7. Chen, C.B.; Liu, L.S.; Zhou, J.; Wang, X.P.; Han, M.; Jiao, X.Y.; He, X.; Yuan, X.P. Up-Regulation of HMGB1 Exacerbates Renal Ischemia-Reperfusion Injury by Stimulating Inflammatory and Immune Responses through the TLR4 Signaling Pathway in Mice. *Cell Physiol. Biochem.* **2017**, *41*, 2447–2460. [CrossRef] [PubMed]
8. Wu, H.; Chadban, S.J. Roles of Toll-like receptors in transplantation. *Curr. Opin. Organ Transplant.* **2014**, *19*, 1–7. [CrossRef] [PubMed]
9. Smith, S.F.; Hosgood, S.A.; Nicholson, M.L. Ischemia-reperfusion injury in renal transplantation: 3 key signaling pathways in tubular epithelial cells. *Kidney Int.* **2019**, *95*, 50–56. [CrossRef] [PubMed]
10. Zeng, S.; Feirt, N.; Goldstein, M.; Guarrera, J.; Ippagunta, N.; Ekong, U.; Dun, H.; Lu, Y.; Qu, W.; Schmidt, A.M.; et al. Blockade of receptor for advanced glycation end product (RAGE) attenuates ischemia and reperfusion injury to the liver in mice. *Hepatology* **2004**, *39*, 422–432. [CrossRef] [PubMed]
11. Andrassy, M.; Volz, H.C.; Igwe, J.C.; Funke, B.; Eichberger, S.N.; Kaya, Z.; Buss, S.; Autschbach, F.; Pleger, S.T.; Lukic, I.K.; et al. High-mobility group box-1 in ischemia-reperfusion injury of the heart. *Circulation* **2008**, *117*, 3216–3226. [CrossRef] [PubMed]
12. Yang, Y.I.; Woo, J.H.; Seo, Y.J.; Lee, K.T.; Lim, Y.; Choi, J.H. Protective Effect of Brown Alga Phlorotannins against Hyperinflammatory Responses in Lipopolysaccharide-Induced Sepsis Models. *J. Agric. Food Chem.* **2016**, *64*, 570–578. [CrossRef] [PubMed]
13. Yang, Y.I.; Shin, H.C.; Kim, S.H.; Park, W.Y.; Lee, K.T.; Choi, J.H. 6,6′-Bieckol, isolated from marine alga Ecklonia cava, suppressed LPS-induced nitric oxide and PGE production and inflammatory cytokine expression in macrophages: The inhibition of NFkappaB. *Int. Immunopharmacol.* **2012**, *12*, 510–517. [CrossRef] [PubMed]
14. Lee, M.S.; Shin, T.; Utsuki, T.; Choi, J.S.; Byun, D.S.; Kim, H.R. Isolation and identification of phlorotannins from Ecklonia stolonifera with antioxidant and hepatoprotective properties in tacrine-treated HepG2 cells. *J. Agric. Food Chem.* **2012**, *60*, 5340–5349. [CrossRef] [PubMed]
15. Eo, H.; Park, J.E.; Jeon, Y.J.; Lim, Y. Ameliorative Effect of Ecklonia cava Polyphenol Extract on Renal Inflammation Associated with Aberrant Energy Metabolism and Oxidative Stress in High Fat Diet-Induced Obese Mice. *J. Agric. Food Chem.* **2017**, *65*, 3811–3818. [CrossRef] [PubMed]
16. Ying, X.; Daofang, J.; Jing, X.; Chensheng, F.; Zhenxing, Z.; Zhibin, Y.; Xiaoli, Z. Ischemic preconditioning attenuates ischemia/reperfusion-induced kidney injury by activating autophagy via the SGK1 signaling pathway. *Cell Death Dis.* **2018**, *9*, 338.

17. Sun, Y.; Xun, L.; Jin, G.; Shi, L. Salidroside protects renal tubular epithelial cells from hypoxia/reoxygenation injury in vitro. *J. Pharmacol. Sci.* **2018**, *137*, 170–176. [CrossRef]
18. Faraco, G.; Fossati, S.; Bianchi, M.E.; Patrone, M.; Pedrazzi, M.; Sparatore, B.; Moroni, F.; Chiarugi, A. High mobility group box 1 protein is released by neural cells upon different stresses and worsens ischemic neurodegeneration in vitro and in vivo. *J. Neurochem.* **2007**, *103*, 590–603. [CrossRef]
19. Tadie, J.M.; Bae, H.B.; Jiang, S.; Park, D.W.; Bell, C.P.; Yang, H.; Pittet, J.F.; Tracey, K.; Thannickal, V.J.; Abraham, E.; et al. HMGB1 promotes neutrophil extracellular trap formation through interactions with Toll-like receptor 4. *Am. J. Physiol. Lung Cell Mol. Physiol.* **2013**, *304*, L342–L349. [CrossRef]
20. Hori, O.; Brett, J.; Slattery, T.; Cao, R.; Zhang, J.; Chen, J.X.; Nagashima, M.; Lundh, E.R.; Vijay, S.; Nitecki, D.; et al. The receptor for advanced glycation end products (RAGE) is a cellular binding site for amphoterin. Mediation of neurite outgrowth and co-expression of rage and amphoterin in the developing nervous system. *J. Biol. Chem.* **1995**, *270*, 25752–25761. [CrossRef]
21. Kent, B.D.; Ryan, S.; McNicholas, W.T. Obstructive sleep apnea and inflammation: Relationship to cardiovascular co-morbidity. *Respir Physiol. Neurobiol.* **2011**, *178*, 475–481. [CrossRef] [PubMed]
22. Ohtsu, A.; Shibutani, Y.; Seno, K.; Iwata, H.; Kuwayama, T.; Shirasuna, K. Advanced glycation end products and lipopolysaccharides stimulate interleukin-6 secretion via the RAGE/TLR4-NF-κB-ROS pathways and resveratrol attenuates these inflammatory responses in mouse macrophages. *Exp. Ther. Med.* **2017**, *14*, 4363–4370. [CrossRef] [PubMed]
23. Bai, J.; Zhao, J.; Cui, D.; Wang, F.; Song, Y.; Cheng, L.; Gao, K.; Wang, J.; Li, L.; Li, S.; et al. Protective effect of hydroxysafflor yellow A against acute kidney injury via the TLR4/NF-κB signaling pathway. *Sci. Rep.* **2018**, *8*, 9173. [CrossRef] [PubMed]
24. Luo, F.; Shi, J.; Shi, Q.; Xu, X.; Xia, Y.; He, X. Mitogen-Activated Protein Kinases and Hypoxic/Ischemic Nephropathy. *Cell Physiol. Biochem.* **2016**, *39*, 1051–1067. [CrossRef] [PubMed]
25. Ka, S.O.; Hwang, H.P.; Jang, J.H.; Hyuk Bang, I.; Bae, U.J.; Yu, H.C.; Cho, B.H.; Park, B.H. The protein kinase 2 inhibitor tetrabromobenzotriazole protects against renal ischemia reperfusion injury. *Sci. Rep.* **2015**, *5*, 14816. [CrossRef]
26. Alderliesten, M.; de Graauw, M.; Oldenampsen, J.; Qin, Y.; Pont, C.; van Buren, L.; van de Water, B. Extracellular signal-regulated kinase activation during renal ischemia/reperfusion mediates focal adhesion dissolution and renal injury. *Am. J. Pathol.* **2007**, *171*, 452–462. [CrossRef]
27. Zhuang, S.; Schnellmann, R.G. A death-promoting role for extracellular signal-regulated kinase. *J. Pharmacol. Exp. Ther.* **2006**, *319*, 991–997. [CrossRef]
28. Hung, C.C.; Ichimura, T.; Stevens, J.L.; Bonventre, J.V. Protection of renal epithelial cells against oxidative injury by endoplasmic reticulum stress preconditioning is mediated by ERK1/2 activation. *J. Biol. Chem.* **2003**, *278*, 29317–29326. [CrossRef]
29. Stambe, C.; Atkins, R.C.; Tesch, G.H.; Kapoun, A.M.; Hill, P.A.; Schreiner, G.F.; Nikolic-Paterson, D.J. Blockade ofp38alpha MAPK ameliorates acute inflammatory renal injury in rat anti-GBM glomerulonephritis. *J. Am. Soc. Nephrol.* **2003**, *14*, 338–351. [CrossRef]
30. Kim, J.H.; Lee, N.S.; Jeong, Y.G.; Lee, J.H.; Kim, E.J.; Han, S.Y. Protective efficacy of an Ecklonia cava extract used to treat transient focal ischemia of the rat brain. *Anat. Cell Biol.* **2012**, *45*, 103–113. [CrossRef]
31. Lee, S.H.; Kim, J.Y.; Yoo, S.Y.; Kwon, S.M. Cytoprotective effect of dieckol on human endothelial progenitor cells (hEPCs) from oxidative stress-induced apoptosis. *Free Radic. Res.* **2013**, *47*, 526–534. [CrossRef] [PubMed]
32. Cui, Y.; Amarsanaa, K.; Lee, J.H.; Rhim, J.K.; Kwon, J.M.; Kim, S.H.; Park, J.M.; Jung, S.C.; Eun, S.Y. Neuroprotective mechanisms of dieckol against glutamate toxicity through reactive oxygen species scavenging and nuclear factor-like 2/heme oxygenase-1 pathway. *Korean J. Physiol. Pharmacol.* **2019**, *23*, 121–130. [CrossRef] [PubMed]
33. Lee, J.H.; Ko, J.Y.; Oh, J.Y.; Kim, C.Y.; Lee, H.J.; Kim, J.; Jeon, Y.J. Preparative isolation and purification of phlorotannins from Ecklonia cava using centrifugal partition chromatography by one-step. *Food Chem.* **2014**, *158*, 433–437. [CrossRef] [PubMed]

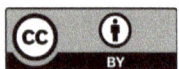

© 2019 by the authors. Licensee MDPI, Basel, Switzerland. This article is an open access article distributed under the terms and conditions of the Creative Commons Attribution (CC BY) license (http://creativecommons.org/licenses/by/4.0/).

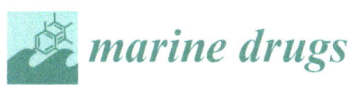

Article

Identifying Phlorofucofuroeckol-A as a Dual Inhibitor of Amyloid-β$_{25\text{-}35}$ Self-Aggregation and Insulin Glycation: Elucidation of the Molecular Mechanism of Action

Su Hui Seong [1], Pradeep Paudel [1], Hyun Ah Jung [2,*] and Jae Sue Choi [1,*]

[1] Department of Food and Life Science, Pukyong National University, Busan 48513, Korea; seongsuhui@naver.com (S.H.S.); phr.paudel@gmail.com (P.P.)
[2] Department of Food Science and Human Nutrition, Jeonbuk National University, Jeonju 54896, Korea
* Correspondence: jungha@jbnu.ac.kr (H.A.J.); choijs@pknu.ac.kr (J.S.C.); Tel.: +82-63-270-4882 (H.A.J.); +82-51-629-5845 (J.S.C.)

Received: 4 October 2019; Accepted: 20 October 2019; Published: 23 October 2019

Abstract: Both amyloid-β (Aβ) and insulin are amyloidogenic peptides, and they play a critical role in Alzheimer's disease (AD) and type-2 diabetes (T2D). Misfolded or aggregated Aβ and glycated insulin are commonly found in AD and T2D patients, respectively, and exhibit neurotoxicity and oxidative stress. The present study examined the anti-Aβ$_{25\text{-}35}$ aggregation and anti-insulin glycation activities of five phlorotannins isolated from *Ecklonia stolonifera*. Thioflavin-T assay results suggest that eckol, dioxinodehydroeckol, dieckol, and phlorofucofuroeckol-A (PFFA) significantly inhibit Aβ$_{25\text{-}35}$ self-assembly. Molecular docking and dynamic simulation analyses confirmed that these phlorotannins have a strong potential to interact with Aβ$_{25\text{-}35}$ peptides and interrupt their self-assembly and conformational transformation, thereby inhibiting Aβ$_{25\text{-}35}$ aggregation. In addition, PFFA dose-dependently inhibited D-ribose and D-glucose induced non-enzymatic insulin glycation. To understand the molecular mechanism for insulin glycation and its inhibition, we predicted the binding site of PFFA in insulin via computational analysis. Interestingly, PFFA strongly interacted with the Phe1 in insulin chain-B, and this interaction could block D-glucose access to the glycation site of insulin. Taken together, our novel findings suggest that phlorofucofuroeckol-A could be a new scaffold for AD treatment by inhibiting the formation of β-sheet rich structures in Aβ$_{25\text{-}35}$ and advanced glycation end-products (AGEs) in insulin.

Keywords: phlorotannin; amyloid-β aggregation; insulin glycation; dynamic simulation

1. Introduction

The aberrant aggregation of misfolded proteins within a biological system is responsible for various pathological conditions. Protein aggregates commonly form and accumulate during normal aging, and it remains unclear whether misfolded proteins are a cause or consequence of aging [1]. In any case, protein aggregates are the major hallmarks of numerous neurodegenerative and metabolic disorders, and many central nervous system pathologies are associated with protein aggregation, such as amyloid-β peptide (Aβ) and tau protein aggregates in Alzheimer's disease (AD), α-synuclein in Parkinson's disease (PD), and the huntingtin protein in Huntington's disease [2].

The Aβ peptide is a byproduct of proteolytic processing of the amyloid precursor protein, a transmembrane protein, by β- and γ-secretases. The initial cleavage of Aβ forms soluble and non-toxic monomers of varying lengths, the most common of which are the Aβ$_{1\text{-}40}$ and Aβ$_{1\text{-}42}$ peptides.

However, when the monomers combine into clusters, they form Aβ oligomers which go on to form insoluble fibrils known as β-sheets [3]. That process is known as amyloid aggregation, and it eventually produces insoluble plaques. Aβ self-assembly is a complicated multi-phase process governed by noncovalent interactions with a delicate balance of entropic and enthalpic contributions [4]. Many physical factors can contribute to the development of strains and in how the β-sheets pack and the strands H-bond to each other: temperature, pH, concentration, ionic strength, agitation conditions such as sonication, and the presence of seeds [5]. Conventionally, Aβ fibrils have been considered the neurotoxic species primarily responsible for AD, but recent correlational research with the symptoms of dementia has found that soluble oligomers are the most cytotoxic Aβ forms [6]. A healthy body produces Aβ proteins at physiological concentrations that are essential for normal memory function and synaptic plasticity [7]. However, those same proteins at the high levels seen in AD are associated with synaptic dysfunction and memory loss [8]. Therefore, inhibiting amyloid aggregation or disaggregating pre-aggregated amyloid peptide is one therapeutic approach to treating AD.

Insulin is a major hormone for regulating glucose homeostasis, and it can be non-enzymatically glycated by glucose and other reactive carbonyls under hyperglycemic conditions. Glycated insulin is less effective in controlling glucose homeostasis and stimulating glucose uptake than non-glycated insulin, and thus glycation might contribute to the insulin resistance and glucose intolerance of type 2 diabetes (T2D) [9]. Non-enzymatic protein glycation is an irreversible modification that begins with a chemical reaction between reducing sugars and primary amino groups, produces additional rearrangements to form a stable Amadori product, and eventually leads to the production of advanced glycation end-products (AGEs) [10]. An accumulation of AGEs is a feature of diabetic complications such as nephropathy [11], retinopathy [12], and atherosclerosis [13] and of neurodegenerative diseases such as AD. A receptor for advanced glycation end products (RAGE) is a multi-ligand transmembrane receptor expressed in several cell types that recognizes various ligands, including AGEs and Aβ. Cellular effects induced by protein glycation have been reported to be mediated by RAGE [10]. Previously, ribosylated insulin decreased cell viability and triggered death pathway through the activation of caspases-3 and -7, intracellular reactive oxygen species (ROS) production, and nuclear factor-κB (NF-κB) activation in NIH-3T3 mouse embryonic fibroblasts [10]. In addition, an AGEs–RAGE pathway triggers the pathogenesis of Aβ and tau hyperphosphorylation via activation of glycogen synthase kinase 3β and induces oxidative stress and neuro-inflammation via NF-κB activation [14]. Therefore, the inhibition of insulin glycation could be an important strategy for preventing AD, T2D, and diabetic complications.

Phlorotannins, which are polymers of phloroglucinol elements, are abundant in *Ecklonia* species of brown algae and have recently attracted much interest among neurodegeneration researchers. Due to the profound biological activities of marine-derived phlorotannins, including antioxidant and anti-inflammatory [15], antiviral [16], anti-cancer [17], anti-melanogenic [18], anti-adipogenic [19], and anti-diabetic [20] properties, research on their neuroprotective effects is emerging. Recently, we demonstrated that the molecular mechanism of the neuroprotective effects of eckol depended on monoamine oxidase-A inhibition and dopamine D_3/D_4 receptor agonism [21,22]. Similarly, dieckol and phlorofucofuroeckol-A (PFFA) showed MAOs-A/B inhibition, D_3R/D_4R receptor agonism, and $D_1/5HT_{1A}/NK_1$ receptor antagonism [23]. In addition, we discovered that the anti-AD activity of phlorotannins, including eckol, dioxinodehydroeckol, dieckol, and PFFA, occurred via inhibition of β-secretase and acetylcholinesterase [24,25].

Previously, Kang et al. reported that *n*-butanol fraction obtained from *Ecklonia cava* significantly inhibited the oligomerization and fibrillation of $Aβ_{1-42}$ [26]. Cho and coworkers reported that eckol and dieckol are abundant in the *n*-butanol fraction of *E. cava* ethanolic extract, with respective quantities of 37.55 and 115.0 mg/g [27]. However, no one has reported the effect of phlorotannins against Aβ self-aggregation.

It is both nutritionally and pharmaceutically important if phlorotannins derived from edible brown seaweeds can inhibit Aβ aggregation and insulin glycation because those processes are closely related to the pathogenesis of AD. Therefore, our main aim in this study was to characterize the inhibitory effects of various phlorotannins (Figure 1) against self-induced $Aβ_{25-35}$ aggregation and non-enzymatic insulin glycation and to provide molecular insights via molecular dynamics (MD) simulations of the inhibition of Aβ self-aggregation and insulin glycation. To the best of our knowledge, this study is the first to identify phlorotannins as dual inhibitors of both Aβ$_{25-35}$ self-aggregation and insulin glycation.

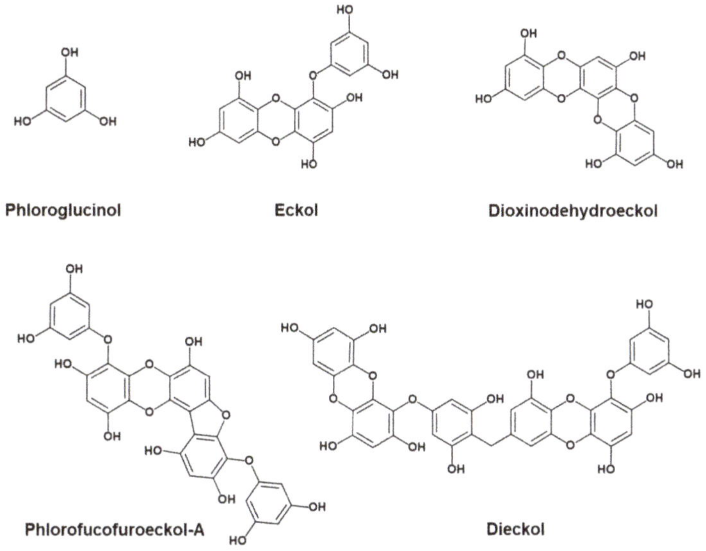

Figure 1. Structures of phlorotannins.

2. Results

2.1. Inhibition of Aβ$_{25-35}$ Self-Aggregation by Phlorotannins

We screened the inhibitory effects of five phlorotannins on Aβ$_{25-35}$ self-aggregation at a concentration of 10 µM using thioflavin-T fluorescence. To verify our experiments, we used curcumin as a standard compound. As shown in Figure 2A, thioflavin-T fluorescence decreased significantly in the presence of eckol ($p < 0.05$), dioxinodehydroeckol ($p < 0.001$), dieckol ($p < 0.001$), and PFFA ($p < 0.001$) at 10 µM. Among them, PFFA showed the strongest inhibitory effect with 80.00% ± 5.5% inhibition, followed by dieckol, dioxinodehydroeckol, and eckol with inhibitions of 66.98% ± 1.5%, 66.07% ± 2.5%, and 34.45% ± 1.5%, respectively. However, phloroglucinol showed no inhibitory effect on Aβ$_{25-35}$ self-aggregation even at 50 µM. As shown in Figure 2B, eckol, dioxinodehydroeckol, dieckol, and PFFA had dose-dependent inhibitory effects on Aβ$_{25-35}$ self-aggregation. We obtained the 50% inhibitory concentration (IC$_{50}$) of phlorotannins for Aβ$_{25-35}$ self-aggregation from the dose-activity graph and found it to be in the range of 6.18 to 34.36 µM (Table 1). Notably, PFFA, dieckol, and dioxinodehydroeckol exhibited lower IC$_{50}$ values (6.18 ± 0.18, 7.93 ± 0.16, and 8.31 ± 0.23 µM, respectively) than the standard compound, curcumin (10.73 ± 1.40 µM).

2.2. Inhibition of Insulin Glycation by Phlorotannins

Glycated bovine insulin was observed by fluorescence spectroscopy because AGEs are marked by a typical fluorescence emission at 410 nm (excitation at 320 nm). To verify our experimental condition, we used vanillin as a negative control for D-ribose-induced protein glycation [28] and rutin as a positive control for d-glucose-induced protein glycation [29].

As shown in Figure 2C, fluorescence intensity after a 1-week incubation of bovine insulin and D-ribose increased significantly compared to the blank group ($p < 0.001$). However, in the presence of

100 µM eckol, PFFA, or dieckol, a significant reduction of insulin glycation was detected, as indicated by a decline in fluorescence intensity. Those inhibitory activities of eckol, PFFA, and dieckol were dose-dependent, with IC$_{50}$ values of 258.54 ± 10.81, 29.50 ± 0.53, and 63.67 ± 3.83 µM, respectively (Figure 2D). Phloroglucinol and dioxinodehydroeckol showed weak or no inhibitory activity on D-ribose-induced insulin glycation at 100 µM, and the negative control (vanillin) showed no activity at 500 µM.

Similarly, fluorescence intensity after a 2-weeks incubation of insulin and D-glucose increased remarkably compared to the blank group (Figure 2E). In the presence of PFFA, fluorescence intensity was dose-dependently reduced with an IC$_{50}$ value of 43.55 ± 2.38 µM. In addition, phloroglucinol showed 40.02% inhibition at 100 µM. However, other phlorotannins showed no inhibitory activity on D-glucose-induced insulin glycation under the tested concentration.

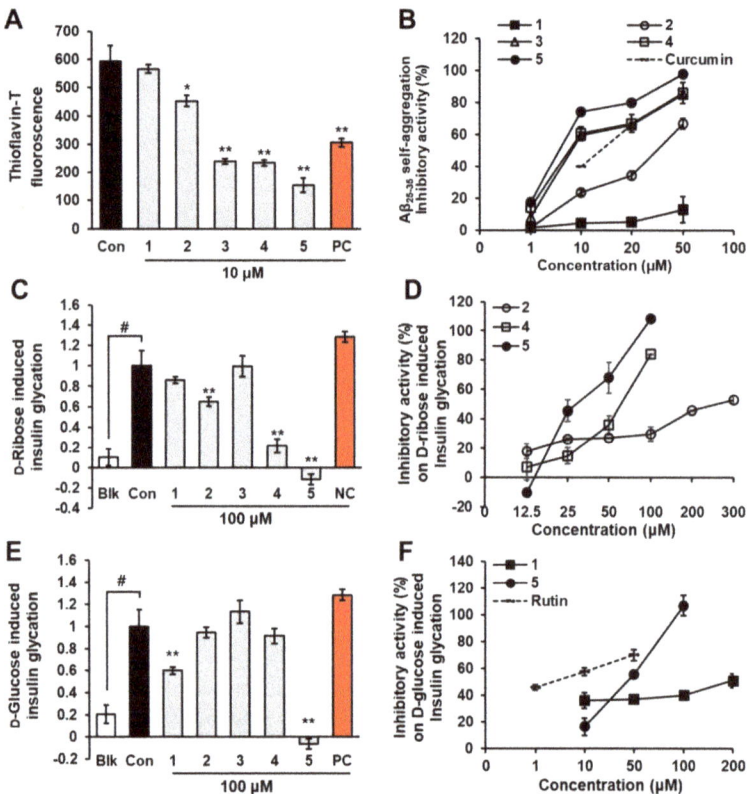

Figure 2. Effects of phloroglucinol (**1**), eckol (**2**), dioxinodehydroeckol (**3**), dieckol (**4**), and PFFA (**5**) on Aβ$_{25-35}$ self-aggregation (**A**) and insulin glycation (**C** and **E**). Dose-dependent inhibitory activity of phlorotannins on Aβ$_{25-35}$ self-aggregation (**B**) and insulin glycation (**D** and **F**). Values are expressed as mean ± SD (n = 3). # $p < 0.01$ indicates a significant difference from the blank group (Blk). * $p < 0.05$ and ** $p < 0.001$ indicate significant differences from the control group (Con). (Con: aggregated Aβ$_{25-35}$ (100 µM) for A; glycated insulin group for C and E, **1–5**: Aβ$_{25-35}$ + tested phlorotannins for A; insulin + D-ribose or D-glucose + tested phlorotannins for C and E, PC: curcumin for A; rutin for E, NC: vanillin).

2.3. Prevention of Lipid Peroxidation in Whole Rat Brain Homogenates by Phlorotannins

A combination of H_2O_2 and Fe^{2+} was used to initiate lipid peroxidation in the brain via Fenton's reaction [30]. We evaluated the inhibitory activity of phlorotannins on lipid peroxidation using Fe^{2+}-treated rat brain homogenates. In the control group, the malondialdehyde (MDA) level was significantly elevated compared with the blank group (not treated with Fe^{2+} or TBA; $p < 0.001$), as shown in Figure 3. However, the MDA level was significantly decreased in the presence of eckol, dioxinodehydroeckol, dieckol, PFFA, or Trolox (positive control). Among the tested phlorotannins, PFFA best prevented lipid peroxidation, with an EC_{50} value of 10.96 ± 0.16 µM, followed by dioxinodehydroeckol, dieckol, and eckol with respective EC_{50} values of 12.43 ± 1.50, 13.51 ± 0.38, and 38.64 ± 1.16 µM (Table 1). Interestingly, PFFA, dioxinodehydroeckol, and dieckol exhibited lower EC_{50} values than the positive control, Trolox ($EC_{50} = 49.01 \pm 3.50$ µM).

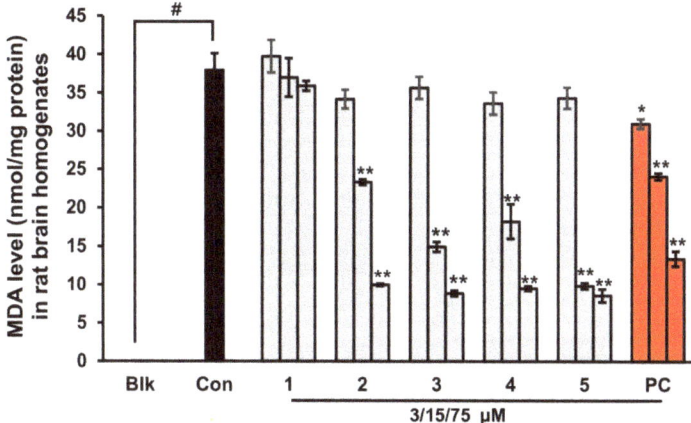

Figure 3. Effects of phloroglucinol (**1**), eckol (**2**), dioxinodehydroeckol (**3**), dieckol (**4**), and PFFA (**5**) on lipid peroxidation in whole rat brain homogenates. Values are expressed as mean $\pm$ SD ($n = 3$). * $p < 0.01$ and ** $p < 0.001$ indicate significant differences from the Con group (Blk: without Fe^{2+} or TBA, Con: with Fe^{2+} and TBA, **1**–**5**: with Fe^{2+}, TBA, and the tested phlorotannins, PC: Trolox).

Table 1. Effect of phlorotannins on $A\beta_{25-35}$ self-aggregation, bovine insulin glycation, and lipid peroxidation in rat brain homogenates.

Compounds	IC_{50} (µM) [a]			EC_{50} (µM) [a]
	$A\beta_{25-35}$ Aggregation	D-Ribose-Induced Insulin Glycation	D-Glucose-Induced Insulin Glycation	Lipid Peroxidation
Phloroglucinol	>100	>100	>100	>75
Eckol	34.36 ± 1.11	258.54 ± 10.81	>100	38.64 ± 1.16
Dioxinodehydroeckol	8.31 ± 0.23	>100	>100	12.43 ± 1.50
Dieckol	7.93 ± 0.16	63.67 ± 3.83	>100	15.48 ± 2.14
Phlorofucofuroeckol-A	6.18 ± 0.18	29.50 ± 0.53	43.55 ± 2.38	10.96 ± 0.16
Curcumin [b]	10.73 ± 1.40	-	-	-
Vanillin [c]	-	>500	-	-
Rutin [b]	-	-	5.19 ± 1.35	-
Trolox [b]	-	-	-	49.01 ± 3.50

[a] The 50% inhibition concentration (IC_{50}) and 50% effective concentrations (EC_{50}) are expressed as mean $\pm$ SD, $n = 3$. [b] Curcumin, rutin, and Trolox were used as a positive control for the $A\beta_{25-35}$ aggregation, D-glucose-induced insulin glycation and lipid peroxidation assays, respectively. [c] Negative control for the D-ribose-induced insulin glycation assay.

2.4. Docking Simulation for Phlorotannins on Aβ25-35

We conducted an in silico docking analysis to find the most stable binding site of the phlorotannins on Aβ25-35 (sequence GSNKGAIIGLM). The predicted binding site residues and maximum binding affinities for the phlorotannins are presented in Table 2. The five phlorotannins showed a negative binding energy to Aβ25-35 and docked near it. As shown in Figure 4e,f, dieckol and PFFA formed 5- and 7-hydrogen bonding interactions with Aβ25-35, respectively, along with pi-interactions between the aromatic rings of these compounds and hydrophobic residues such as Ala30–Ile31–Ile32. The aromatic ring of dioxinodehydroeckol (Figure 4D) formed many pi-interactions with Ala30 and Ile32. As shown in Figure 4C, the OH group of eckol formed three hydrogen bonds with the Gly25-Asn27 residues, and the aromatic ring of eckol interacted with Ile31 and Ala30 via pi-interactions. These results indicate that bulky compounds of more than three repeating phloroglucinol units interacted evenly with most Aβ25-35 residues. However, the phloroglucinol monomer is not expected to cause structural changes to Aβ25-35 because of its very small structure, although it did form hydrogen bonds with the Gly25, Asn27, and Ile32 residues of the peptide, as shown in Figure 4B. On the other hand, dioxinodehydroeckol and PFFA, which have two dibenzo-1,4-dioxin or dibenzofuran linkages, retain fewer rotatable bonds than the other phlorotannins, so they showed low torsion energies and stably interacted with the Aβ25-35 with a high binding affinity.

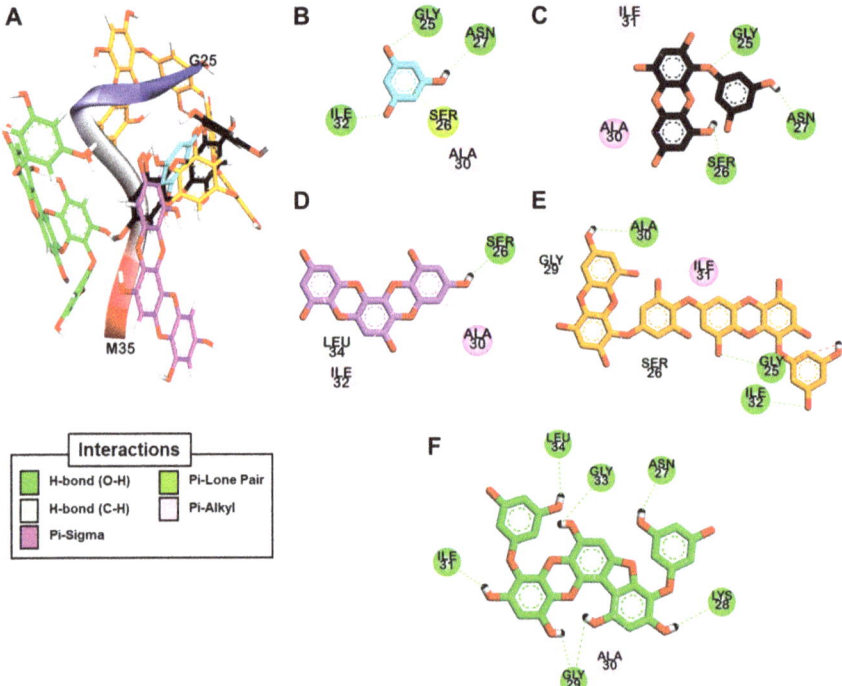

Figure 4. The best docked poses of phloroglucinol (cyan stick), eckol (black stick), dioxinodehydroeckol (purple stick), dieckol (orange stick), and PFFA (green stick) bound to the Aβ25-35 peptide (**A**) and a detailed 2D view of the phlorotannin–peptide interactions (**B–F**).

Table 2. Binding affinity and interacting residues of phlorotannins with human Aβ$_{25-35}$ and bovine insulin peptides from docking analysis.

Ligands	Binding Energy (kcal/mol)	Hydrogen Bonding Interactions	Other Interactions
		Target protein: human Aβ$_{25-35}$	
Phloroglucinol	−3.19	Gly25, Asn27, Ile32	Ala30 (Pi-Alkyl), Ser26 (Pi-Lone pair)
Eckol	−4.73	Gly25, Ser26, Asn27	Ile31 (Pi-Alkyl), Ala30 (Pi-sigma)
Dioxinodehydroeckol	−4.94	Ser26, Leu34	Ala30 (Pi-sigma, Pi-Alkyl), Ala30 (Pi-Alkyl), Ile32 (Pi-Alkyl)
Dieckol	−3.51	Gly25, Ile32, Ala30, Ser26, Gly29	Ile31 (Pi-sigma), Ile31 (Pi-Alkyl), Ile32 (Pi-Alkyl)
PFFA	−5.33	Gly29, Lys28, Asn27, Ile31, Leu34, Gly33	Ala30 (Pi-Alkyl)
		Target protein: bovine insulin	
PFFA	−5.03	Ser12 (A), Gln15 (A), Glu17 (A), Asn18 (A), Asn3 (B), Phe1 (B)	Tyr14 (Pi-Amide stacked)

2.5. Dynamic Simulation of Phlorotannins Inhibiting Aβ$_{25-35}$ Self-Aggregation

In the absence of inhibitors, the amorphous form of Aβ$_{25-35}$ changed into the β-sheet form with many internal hydrogen bonds between strands in a 150 mM NaCl aqueous solution during a 20 ns MD simulation (Figure 5A–C). We analyzed and visualized the evolution of the secondary structure during that 20 ns MD simulation using VMD. As shown in Figure 6A, the β-sheet began being generated at 5.9 ns and continued forming until 20 ns.

To understand the binding modes between Aβ and phlorotannins, we subjected the most stable phlorotannin–Aβ$_{25-35}$ complexes from the docking study to MD simulation.

As shown in Figure 7A, the MD simulation results suggest that eckol interacts favorably with the Asn27–Lys28–Gly29 residues of the peptide. After 20 ns, the hydroxyl moiety of the eckol formed strong hydrogen bonds with the Asn27 and Gly29 residues, and the aromatic ring of this compound interacted with Lys28 via an amide-pi stacked bond. Those interactions between the peptide and eckol increased the β-bridge content during the 20 ns MD simulation. However, unlike Aβ25-35 alone, no β-sheet was observed in the presence of eckol (Figure 6A).

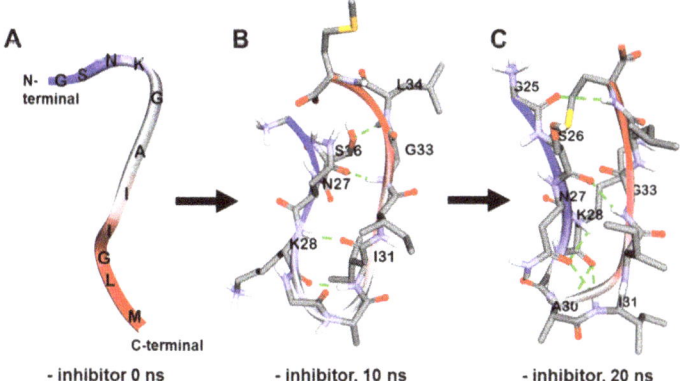

Figure 5. Molecular dynamics (MD) simulation trajectories of Aβ$_{25-35}$ peptide at times $t = 0$ (**A**), 10 (**B**), and 20 ns (**C**).

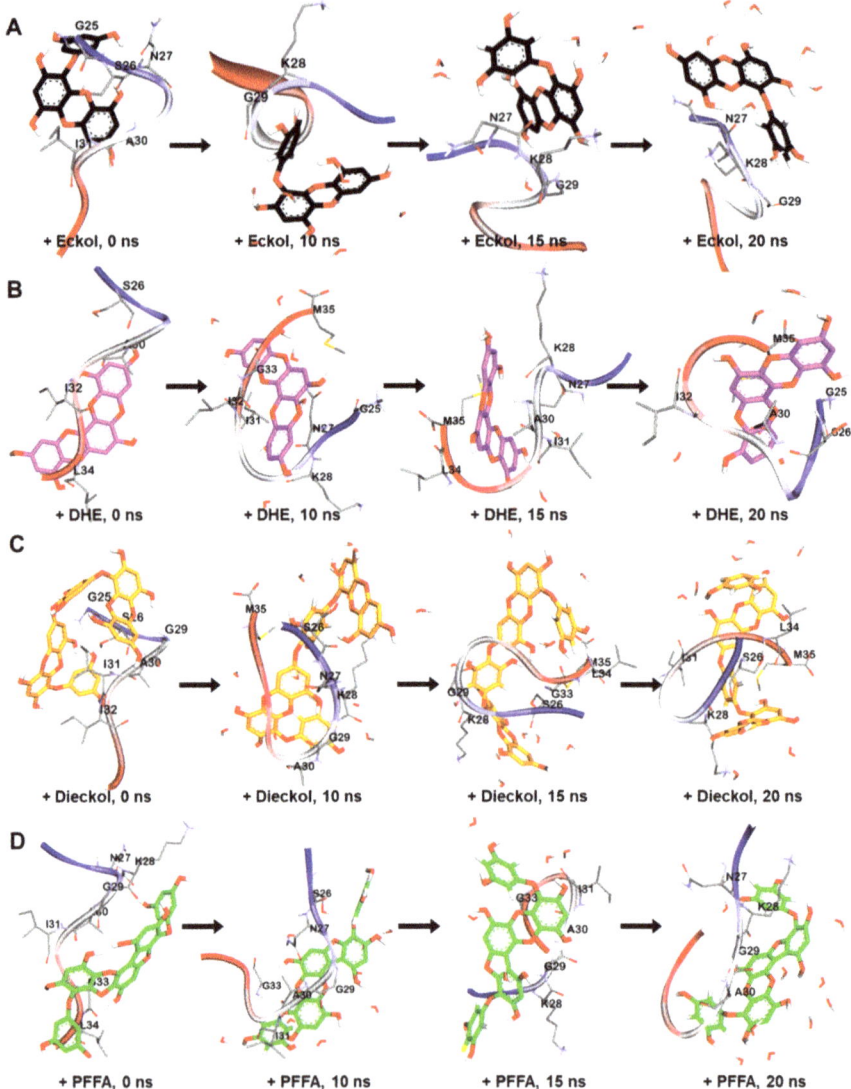

Figure 6. MD simulation trajectories of eckol (**A**), dioxinodehydroeckol (DHE, **B**), dieckol (**C**), and phlorofucofuroeckol-A (PFFA, **D**) bound to Aβ$_{25-35}$ peptide at times t = 0, 10, 15, and 20 ns.

Dioxinodehydroeckol formed many interactions with most of the peptide residues, which eliminated all β-structures, including β-sheet and β-bridge formations (Figure 6A). Although it did not interact with Met35 and Ile31, which are assumed to play a key role in the assembly and neurotoxicity of Aβ [31], in the best docked pose (Figure 4D), dioxinodehydroeckol continuously interacted with those residues via hydrophobic and hydrophilic bonds during the MD simulations. After 20 ns of simulation, dioxinodehydroeckol formed seven hydrogen bonds with the Ser26, Ile32, Gly25, and Met35 residues. In addition, the aromatic ring of this compound interacted with Ala30 and Met35 via several pi-interactions: pi-sigma, pi-sulfur, and pi-alkyl bonds (Figure 7B).

As shown in Figure 7C, dieckol strongly interacted with Met35 and Lys28 via hydrogen bonds during the simulations. In addition to Met35, dieckol continuously reacted with the Ser26, Lys28, Ile31, and Leu34 residues. After the 20 ns MD simulation, hetero oxygen atoms and the hydroxyl moiety of dieckol formed hydrogen bonds with Met35 and Lys28. Pi-interactions were also detected between the aromatic rings of dieckol and the Met35, Ile31, Leu34, Ser26, and Lys28 residues.

PFFA (Figure 7D) interacted favorably with the Ile31, Ala30, Gly29, and Gly33 residues during the simulations and effectively interrupted the self-assembly of Aβ$_{25-35}$. After the 20 ns simulation, this compound formed a hydrogen bond with Asn27 and a strong electrostatic interaction (pi-cation) with Lys28. In addition, hydrophobic interactions were observed between PFFA and the Gly29 and Lys28 residues. Furthermore, a secondary structure analysis revealed that the formation of a β-sheet decreased significantly in the presence of dieckol and PFFA, as shown in Figure 8A.

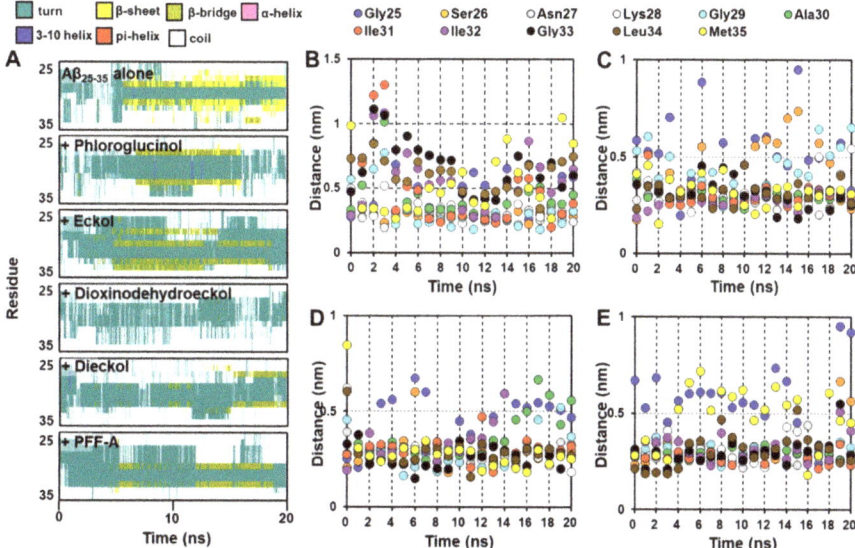

Figure 7. Evolution of secondary structures with time (ns) for Aβ$_{25-35}$ peptide with and without phlorotannins (**A**). Minimum distances (ns) between the residues in the Aβ$_{25-35}$ peptide and the phlorotannins (**B** for eckol, **C** for dioxinodehydroeckol, **D** for dieckol, and **E** for PFFA) during 20 ns MD simulations.

We also analyzed the minimum distances between each residue in the peptide and the phlorotannins during the 20 ns simulations. As shown in Figure 6B, dieckol, PFFA, and dioxinodehydroeckol moved to within 0.5 nm of the Aβ$_{25-35}$ during the simulations, whereas eckol moved to within 1.0 nm of the peptide. In addition, these four phlorotannins continuously interacted with Asn27 and Ile31 at a close distance during the 20 ns MD simulations. Dioxinodehydroeckol and dieckol interacted closely with Gly33, Leu34, and Met35. PFFA did not interact closely with Met, but it did compactly interact with other hydrophobic residues, including Ile31-Ile32-Gly33-Leu34. However, phloroglucinol could not access the Aβ$_{25-35}$ peptide until 3 ns into the 20 ns MD simulation even though the simulation began with a docked phloroglucinol–Aβ$_{25-35}$ complex (data not shown).

2.6. Docking Simulation for PFFA on Bovine Insulin

The most stable binding site of PFFA on the bovine insulin was analyzed using an in silico automated docking study. PFFA showed a negative binding energy (−5.03 kcal/mol) to the bovine insulin. As shown in Figure 8A and Table 2, the hydroxyl moieties of the PFFA interacted with Phe1 and Asn3 in chain B and Ser12, Gln15, Glu17, and Asn18 in chain A of the insulin via hydrogen bonds. In addition, the dibenzofuran ring of the PFFA interacted with Tyr14 in chain A via a pi-amide stacked interaction.

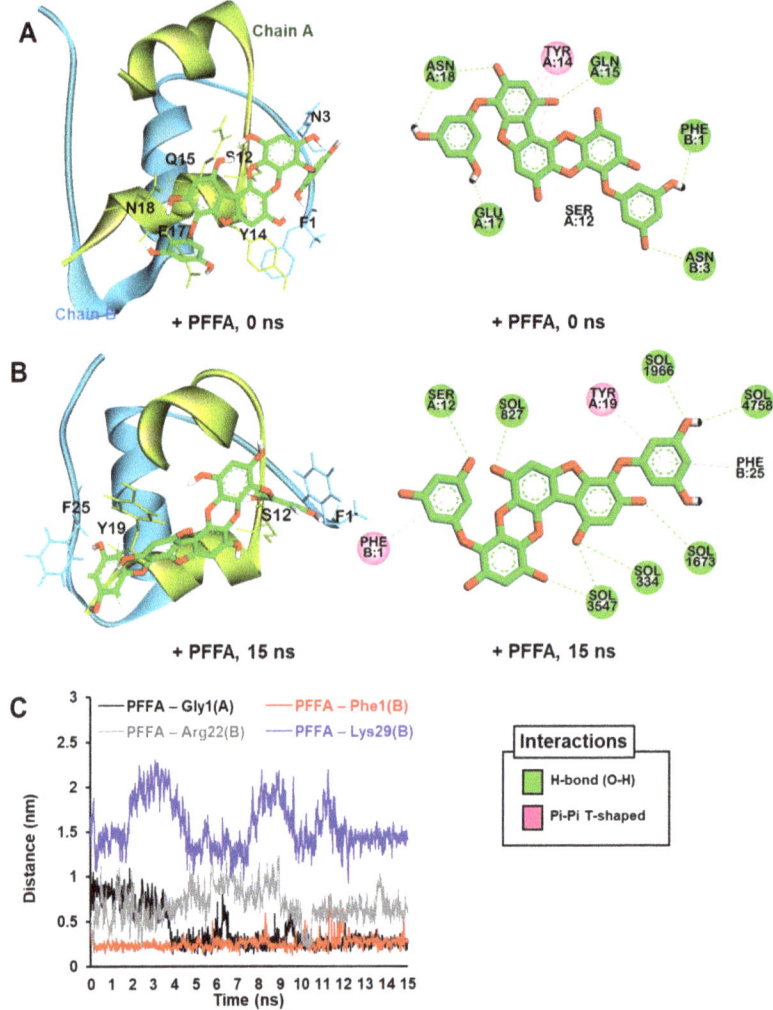

Figure 8. The best predicted pose from the molecular docking simulation for PFFA (green stick) binding to bovine insulin (**A**). The MD trajectories for PFFA bound to bovine insulin at 15 ns of the MD simulation (**B**). Water molecules are not shown in the 3D view for clarity. Hydrogen bonds, pi-donor hydrogen bonds, and pi-amide stacked interactions are shown as green, pale green, and pink dashed lines, respectively. Water molecules are labeled "SOL" in the 2D view. Minimum distances (nm) between the glycation site residues in the bovine insulin and PFFA during 15 ns MD simulations (**C**).

2.7. Dynamic Simulation of PFFA on Bovine Insulin

To understand the binding modes between insulin and PFFA, we subjected the most stable PFFA–insulin complex (Figure 8A) obtained from the docking study to MD simulation.

As shown in Figure 8B, the MD results reveal that PFFA moved slightly closer to Phe25 (chain B) over time, and the PFFA-insulin complex was finally stabilized by intra-interactions between PFFA and insulin residues, including Ser12 and Tyr19 in chain A and Phe1 and Phe25 in chain B.

Furthermore, minimum distances (nm) between PFFA and major glycation site residues including Phe1, Arg22, and Lys29 in chain B and Gly1 in chain A of insulin over MD run times are described in Figure 8C. PFFA formed stable interaction with Phe1 in chain B over the entire runs, whereas PFFA interacted with Gly1 in chain A via H-bond from 5 ns until 10 ns runs (data not shown). In addition, PFFA weakly interacted with Arg22 and could not reach near Lys29 residue during 15 ns MD runs.

3. Discussion

Phlorotannins, a natural polyphenol found abundantly in brown seaweeds (especially in the *Ecklonia* species), are known to have a diverse range of pharmacological activity. As neuroscience research progresses, the many neuroprotective effects of various phlorotannins are being reported, including inhibitory activity against enzymes linked to the pathogenesis of AD and PD [22,24,25,32], modulatory activity against G-protein coupled receptors related to neuronal diseases such as PD and psychological diseases [22,23], and free-radical scavenging activity [15]. Although some reports have indicated that phlorotannins have protective effects against the neurotoxicity of the $A\beta_{1-42}$ oligomer [32] or $A\beta_{25-35}$ peptides [33,34] in neuronal cell-lines, phlorotannins have not previously been studied as an inhibitor of $A\beta$ self-aggregation.

Soluble $A\beta$ oligomers and insoluble fibrils are known to bind several receptors at the cell surface, including the insulin receptor (IR), RAGE, α-7-nicotinic acetylcholine receptor, β2 adrenergic receptor, N-methyl-D-aspartic acid receptor, and toll-like receptor 2 [35]. Many of the signaling pathways initiated by those receptors converge into common downstream targets that are ultimately responsible for synaptic impairment, neurotoxicity, and cell death. The predominant forms of the $A\beta$ present in aggregates are $A\beta_{1-40}$ and $A\beta_{1-42}$. Aggregates of shorter fragments such as $A\beta_{25-35}$ result from the cleavage of soluble racemized $A\beta_{1-40}$ peptides and are observed in the brain tissue of AD patients [36]. The $A\beta_{25-35}$ fragment is the smallest that retains both the toxicity and aggregation properties of the full-length molecule [37]. In a previous study, $A\beta_{25-35}$ showed outstanding speed of aggregation and immediate cytotoxicity in vitro compared with other forms [38]. The $A\beta_{25-35}$ treated animals exhibit a statistically relevant cognitive impairment as well as alteration of the key markers of cell death and neurodegeneration [39]. Therefore, to evaluate whether phlorotannins could prevent the self-aggregation of $A\beta$, we tested their potency using $A\beta_{25-35}$ as the target.

As with previous reports [38], the thioflavin T fluorescence of $A\beta_{25-35}$ increased after 24 h' incubation compared with freshly prepared $A\beta_{25-35}$. However, the thioflavin T intensity decreased significantly when $A\beta_{25-35}$ was co-incubated with eckol, dioxinodehydroeckol, dicckol, or PFFA, though phloroglucinol showed no effect at the tested concentrations. Among them, PFFA (a pentamer of a phloroglucinol unit with both dibenzo-1,4-dioxin and dibenzofuran linkages), dieckol, and dioxinodehydroeckol (a trimer of phloroglucinol with two dibenzo-1,4-dioxin linkages) showed strong potency, with an IC_{50} range of 6.18 to 9.06 µM. Eckol, a trimer of phloroglucinol with a dibenzo-1,4-dioxin linkage, showed less activity than the others. These outcomes imply that having both dibenzo-1,4-dioxin and dibenzofuran linkages (or two dibenzo-1,4-dioxin linkages) in the phlorotannin scaffolds are essential to effectively prevent the self-assembly of $A\beta_{25-35}$.

Our molecular docking and MD simulation studies have clearly demonstrated the binding modes between the peptide and phlorotannins. After a 20 ns MD simulation, $A\beta_{25-35}$ alone showed β-sheet content and had β-turn content at Gly29-Ala30, in accord with the results of a previous study [40]. However, when bound to eckol, dioxinodehydroeckol, dieckol, or PFFA, the peptide had significantly less β-sheet content and existed in an amorphous state. The MD analysis revealed that these four phlorotannins commonly interacted with the Asn27 and Ile31 residues, though their interactions differed. Eckol and dioxinodehydroeckol favorably interacted with hydrophilic residues, including Asn27-Lys28-Gly29, whereas dieckol and PFFA mainly interacted with the C-terminus hydrophobic residues, including Ile31-Ile32-Gly33-Leu34-Met35. It was previously reported that Aβ$_{25-35}$ assemblies are mediated by side-chain to side-chain hydrogen interactions in the Asn27-Ile32 region. In addition, an experimental analysis conducted by Pike and coworkers confirmed that the Leu34-Met35 region is essential to Aβ aggregation, and Met35 is important for the neurotoxicity of Aβ$_{25-35}$/$_{1-40}$ [31,38]. Therefore, the different binding aspects of the phlorotannins could explain their different potency against Aβ$_{25-35}$ aggregations in vitro. However, it was reported that GROMOS force fields showed strongly biased results toward β-sheet structures [41] and the drug-binding sites of Aβ monomers and small oligomers are very transient [42], thus further extensive MD simulation using other CHARMM, AMBER99-ILDN, or AMBER14SB force fields, which showed good balanced results in structures as well as kinetics, should be conducted to confirm our MD results [42,43].

For many years, it was commonly believed that the brain was insensitive to insulin. However, it is now acknowledged that insulin has vital neuro-modulatory functions, such as the regulation of glucose homeostasis and roles in cognition, learning, and memory, which are impaired in AD [44]. In addition, insulin can prevent the formation of the Aβ$_{1-42}$ oligomer and ameliorate the Aβ$_{1-42}$-induced impairment of long-term potentiation in hippocampal slices [45]. But once insulin is glycated under hyperglycemic or diabetic conditions, it cannot bind IR or block Aβ aggregation, which produces a decline in IR-mediated signaling pathways and can facilitate Aβ-mediated brain damage [9,45]. Glucose is the most abundant reducing sugar in vivo with its plasma concentrations ranging from 70 to 140 mg/dL in healthy individuals, while two times higher in T2D patients [46]. In addition, abnormally high doses of D-ribose have been found in the urine of T2D patients [47], and ribosylated insulin was found to exhibit significant cytotoxicity in NIH-3T3 cells [10].

Although some reports have suggested that natural products, such as vanillin, rutin, quercetin, and pinocembrin, can act as insulin glycation inhibitors [28], studies about insulin glycation remain inadequate. Therefore, in this study, we evaluated the inhibitory effects of phlorotannins on D-glucose or D-ribose-induced non-enzymatic and irreversible glycation of bovine insulin, and we elucidated the molecular mechanism of action for insulin glycation and its inhibition by phlorotannins.

PFFA and dieckol showed remarkably potent inhibition of D-ribose induced insulin glycation at less than 100 μM. However, other phlorotannins showed weak or no activity at the tested concentrations. In the case of D-glucose induced insulin glycation assay, only PFFA showed significant inhibitory activity at 100 μM. Our results suggest that PFFA might be promising lead compounds against non-enzymatically glycated insulin–mediated pathogenesis.

Glucose-binding sites (Phe1, Val2, Leu17, Arg22, and Lys29 in chain B; Glu1 in chain A) on insulin had already been elucidated via in silico prediction and mass spectrometry studies [48,49]. Our docking and MD simulation analyses clearly show the binding modes between bovine insulin and PFFA. Phe1 in chain B of insulin, which is the major glycation site of insulin, connected strongly with PFFA via H-bond and pi-pi bonds during MD runs. Our computational prediction also indicated that PFFA could interact with Ser12, Tyr19, and Phe25 residues, which could inhibit insulin glycation by disturbing the interaction between glycation site of insulin and D-glucose (or D-ribose).

In the brain, Aβ plaques and AGEs can be major sources of oxidative stress [14,37]. Brains are highly susceptible to oxidative damage because their membranes contain high amounts of polyunsaturated and peroxidable fatty acids and have a high rate of oxygen consumption [50]. In our study, eckol, dioxinodehydroeckol, dieckol, and PFFA dose-dependently reduced MDA levels in whole rat brain tissue homogenate. Dioxinodehydroeckol, dieckol, and PFFA showed strong activity, and eckol had moderate potency. Thus, phlorotannins with more than three repeating phloroglucinol units are required to prevent lipid peroxidation. However, in the homogenates, destroying the structures and cells via a myriad of processes that is started cannot occur in the living organism and almost all unspecific antioxidants could inhibit this nonspecific peroxidation [51,52]. Therefore, further mechanism studies are required to confirm this activity.

AD drugs are required to enter the blood-brain barrier (BBB) to achieve therapeutic levels in the central nervous system (CNS). Pharmacokinetic parameter prediction study indicated that eckol penetrates the CNS moderately [22]. In addition, Kwak et al. reported that dieckol, with a number of hydroxyl groups and high molecular weight, effectively passed the BBB in rats upon intravenous injection [53]. Studies of PFFA in BBB permeability has not been implemented, but properties similar to dieckol may be anticipated. To strengthen the penetration property of BBB, several methods were developed using nanoparticles, aromatic substances (e.g., borneol), and chemical drug delivery systems [54]. Recently, Venkatesan et al. successfully biosynthesized the silver nanoparticles using *E. cava* [55]. Therefore, we are able to overcome the limitation of phlorotannins over BBB penetration.

We are the first to identify the inhibitory activity of phlorotannins as dual Aβ aggregation and insulin glycation inhibitors, and our computational study clearly shows the mechanism by which PFFA inhibits Aβ self-aggregation and bovine insulin glycation. However, further in vivo experiments are needed to verify this in vitro and in silico prediction.

In conclusion, our results show that dieckol and PFFA derived from marine brown algae strongly reduce $Aβ_{25-35}$ self-aggregation and non-enzymatic insulin glycation. In addition, we used docking and MD simulation studies to demonstrate the molecular mechanism by which the active phlorotannins inhibit Aβ aggregation and insulin glycation. Therefore, those phlorotannins can prevent neuronal damage by inhibiting the formation of β-sheet rich amyloid peptide structures and insulin glycation as well as by preventing lipid peroxidation, producing normal insulin and Aβ processing pathways. Taken together, our findings suggest that phlorotannins could be a promising therapeutic lead compound for the treatment of AD and T2D.

4. Materials and Methods

4.1. Chemicals and Reagents

Amyloid β-protein fragment 25–35 ($Aβ_{25-35}$), 1,1,1,3,3,3-hexafluoro-2-propanol, 1,1,3,3-tetramethoxypropane, Trolox, curcumin, D-ribose, D-glucose, vanillin, and insulin from bovine pancreas were purchased from Sigma-Aldrich (St. Louis, MO, USA). Sodium dodecyl sulfate (SDS) and thiobarbituric acid (TBA) were purchased from Biosesang (Seoul, Republic of Korea) and Tokyo Chemical Industry (Tokyo, Japan), respectively. All chemicals and solvents for column chromatography were of reagent grade from commercial sources and were used as received.

4.2. Preparation of Phlorotannins

Five phlorotannins—phloroglucinol, eckol, dioxinodehydroeckol, dieckol, and PFFA—were isolated from the ethyl acetate fraction of *E. stolonifera* ethanolic extract as described by Yoon et al. [23]. The cemical structures of the isolaed phlorotannins are shown in Figure 1.

4.3. Assay for $Aβ_{25-35}$ Self-Aggregation

A monomeric $Aβ_{25-35}$ solution was prepared using the method of Naldi and coworkers [56]. A 2.5 µL aliquot of various concentrations of the tested phlorotannins in 50 mM phosphate buffer (pH 7.4) with 100 mM NaCl was added to 72.5 µL of $Aβ_{25-35}$ sample (100 µM), and the mixture was incubated at 4 °C for 1 day. After incubation, 25 µM thioflavin T in 50 mM glycine-NaOH buffer (pH 8.5) was added to the reaction mixture. Fluorescence emission intensity was monitored at 490 nm ($λ_{exc}$ = 446 nm) using a fluorescence microplate reader (Gemini XPS, Molecular Devices, Sunnyvale, CA, USA). Curcumin was used as a standard compound.

4.4. Assay for Non-Enzymatic Insulin Glycation

The insulin from bovine pancreas was dissolved in third grade distilled water to a concentration of 6 mg/mL and acidified to pH 2.4 using phosphoric acid to produce monomeric insulin. Then the insulin solution was neutralized to pH 7.0 using 10 M NaOH. Non-enzymatic glycation of insulin was initiated by mixing the insulin solution, 0.5 M D-ribose (or 1.5 M D-glucose) in 50 mM NaH_2PO_4 buffer (pH 7.0), and 10% dimethyl sulfoxide (DMSO) or the test phlorotannins in a 1:8:1 ratio and incubating the mixture at 37 °C for 6 days (2 weeks for D-glucose induced insulin glycation). Vanillin was used as a negative control for D-ribose induced insulin glycation [27], whereas rutin was used as a positive control for D-glucose induced insulin glycation [28]. After incubation, the reaction mixture was measured at an excitation wavelength of 320 nm and emission wavelength of 410 nm using a fluorescence microplate reader (Gemini XPS).

4.5. Preparation of Rat Brain Homogenates

Whole rat brain homogenates were prepared from freshly killed Sprague Dawley rats (male, 6-months old) and provided by the Aging Tissue Bank of Pusan National University. One g of whole rat brain was homogenized in 10 mL of cold 20 mM sodium phosphate buffer containing 140 mM KCl (pH 7.4) and centrifuged at 1300× g for 15 min.

4.6. Lipid Peroxidation Assay

A TBA reactive species (TBARS) assay was used to evaluate the antioxidant activity of the phlorotannins in the rat brain homogenates [57]. An aliquot of the supernatant fraction of the homogenates was mixed with phlorotannins dissolved in 10% DMSO, freshly prepared ferric sulfate (250 μM), and distilled water in a 10:5:3:12 ratio, and then the reaction mixture was incubated at 37 °C for 1 h. The reaction was completed by adding a color reagent containing 0.8% TBA, 8.1% SDS, and a 7.5% (final concentration) acetic acid-NaOH solution (pH 3.4) in a 2:1:2 ratios. The mixture was boiled in a water bath for 1 h. After cooling, the reaction mixture was mixed with an equal volume of *n*-butanol and centrifuged at 1300× g for 10 min. The absorbance of the upper layer was measured at 532 nm using a spectrophotometer (Molecular Devices). The formation of TBARS was expressed as MDA nmol/mg protein using 1,1,3,3-tetramethoxypropane as a standard. Trolox was used as a positive control.

4.7. Molecular Docking Simulation

Docking simulations were carried out with AutoDock 4.2 [58]. The X-ray crystallographic structures of $A\beta_{25-35}$ and bovine insulin were obtained from the RCSB Protein Data Bank using codes 1QXC (model 1) [59] and 2ZP6, respectively. The chemical structures of the phlorotannins (phloroglucinol, eckol, eckstolonol, dieckol, and PFFA) were obtained from the PubChem database using codes 359, 145937, 10429214, 3008868, and 130976, respectively. The rotatable bonds were set by the Autodock tools, and all torsions were allowed to rotate during ligand preparation. Grid map files were generated using the Autogrid. For each phlorotannin-$A\beta_{25-35}$ or PFFA-insulin complex, 10 docking poses were generated using the default genetic algorithm (GA) parameters. Further, Lamarckian GA was used to compute ligand conformations. The pose with the lowest binding energy was selected as the final docking result. Docking results were visualized using Discovery Studio (v17.2, Accelrys, San Diego, CA, USA).

4.8. Molecular Dynamic simulation

All simulations in this study were done using the open source GROMACS 2018.1 package [60] with a force field of GROMOS96 43A1 [61]. The most stable phlorotannin-$A\beta_{25-35}$ and PFFA-insulin complexes obtained from the automated docking simulation were subjected to MD simulation. The type of N- (Gly25 for $A\beta_{25-35}$; Gly1 and Phe1 for insulin) and C-terminals (Met35 for $A\beta_{25-35}$; Asn21 and Ala30 for insulin) of the peptides were set as NH^{3+} and COO^-, respectively. Each phlorotannin-peptide complex was placed in a single cubic box and solvated using the spc216 water model. The system was neutralized with appropriate numbers of Na^+ and Cl^- ions using a 0.15 mM ion concentration (without an ion concentration for the PFFA-insulin complex). After that, the system was subjected to energy minimization by the steepest descent method with a maximum of 5000 steps and was optimized with the LINCS algorithm using 100 ps under constant volume and pressure [62]. Electrostatic interactions were calculated by the particle mesh Ewald process [63]. The pressure (1 bar) and temperature (300 K) of the system were controlled by the Parrinello–Rahman and V-rescale methods, respectively. The simulation results were scrutinized and visualized using Discovery Studio (v17.2, Accelrys, San Diego, CA, USA). The timeline for the secondary structure of Aβ_{25-35} peptide was investigated using visual molecular dynamics (VMD) [64].

4.9. Statistical Analysis

The 50% inhibitory concentration (IC$_{50}$) values (µM) obtained from the dose-inhibition curves are expressed as the mean ± SD (n = 3). The Student's *t*-test (two-tailed) was used to determine the significant differences between the blank and control or the phlorotannin-treated groups and control in Figures 2 and 3.

Author Contributions: In vitro and in silico assays, and writing—original draft preparation, S.H.S.; writing—editing, P.P.; writing—review and supervision, H.A.J. and J.S.C. All authors read and approved the final manuscript.

Funding: This research was supported by the Basic Science Research Program through the National Research Foundation of Korea (NRF) funded by the Ministry of Science (2012R1A6A1028677).

Conflicts of Interest: The authors declare no conflict of interest.

References

1. Cuanalo-Contreras, K.; Mukherjee, A.; Soto, C. Role of protein misfolding and proteostasis deficiency in protein misfolding diseases and aging. *Int. J. Cell Biol.* **2013**, *2013*, 638083. [CrossRef]
2. Owen, M.C.; Gnutt, D.; Gao, M.; Wärmländer, S.K.; Jarvet, J.; Gräslund, A.; Winter, R.; Ebbinghaus, S.; Strodel, B. Effects of in vivo conditions on amyloid aggregation. *Chem. Soc. Rev.* **2019**, *48*, 3946–3996. [CrossRef] [PubMed]
3. Matsuzaki, K.; Kato, K.; Yanagisawa, K. Ganglioside-mediated assembly of amyloid β-protein: Roles in Alzheimer's disease. *Prog. Mol. Biol. Transl. Sci.* **2018**, *156*, 413–434. [PubMed]
4. Ilie, I.M.; Caflisch, A. Simulation studies of amyloidogenic polypeptides and their aggregates. *Chem. Rev.* **2019**, *119*, 6956–6993. [CrossRef] [PubMed]
5. Nasica-Labouze, J.; Nguyen, P.H.; Sterpone, F.; Berthoumieu, O.; Buchete, N.V.; Coté, S.; Simone, A.D.; Doig, A.J.; Faller, P.; Garcia, A.; et al. Amyloid β protein and Alzheimer's disease: When computer simulations complement experimental studies. *Chem. Rev.* **2015**, *115*, 3518–3563. [CrossRef] [PubMed]
6. Smith, A.K.; Klimov, D.K. De novo aggregation of Alzheimer's Aβ25-35 peptides in a lipid bilayer. *Sci. Rep.* **2019**, *9*, 7161. [CrossRef] [PubMed]
7. Puzzo, D.; Privitera, L.; Leznik, E.; Fà, M.; Staniszewski, A.; Palmeri, A.; Arancio, O. Picomolar amyloid-β positively modulates synaptic plasticity and memory in hippocampus. *J. Neurosci.* **2008**, *28*, 14537–14545. [CrossRef]
8. Shankar, G.M.; Li, S.; Mehta, T.H.; Garcia-Munoz, A.; Shepardson, N.E.; Smith, I.; Brett, F.M.; Farrell, M.A.; Rowan, M.J.; Lemere, C.A. Amyloid-β protein dimers isolated directly from Alzheimer's brains impair synaptic plasticity and memory. *Nat. Med.* **2008**, *14*, 837. [CrossRef]
9. Boyd, A.C.; Abdel-Wahab, Y.H.; McKillop, A.M.; McNulty, H.; Barnett, C.R.; O'Harte, F.P.; Flatt, P.R. Impaired ability of glycated insulin to regulate plasma glucose and stimulate glucose transport and metabolism in mouse abdominal muscle. *Biochim. Biophys. Acta* **2000**, *1523*, 128–134. [CrossRef]
10. Iannuzzi, C.; Borriello, M.; Carafa, V.; Altucci, L.; Vitiello, M.; Balestrieri, M.L.; Ricci, G.; Irace, G.; Sirangelo, I. D-ribose-glycation of insulin prevents amyloid aggregation and produces cytotoxic adducts. *Biochim. Biophys. Acta* **2016**, *1862*, 93–104. [CrossRef]
11. Fukami, K.; Yamagishi, S.; Ueda, S.; Okuda, S. Role of AGEs in diabetic nephropathy. *Curr. Pharm. Des.* **2008**, *14*, 946–952. [CrossRef] [PubMed]
12. Stitt, A.W. AGEs and diabetic retinopathy. *Investig. Ophthalmol. Vis. Sci.* **2010**, *51*, 4867–4874. [CrossRef] [PubMed]
13. Schleicher, E.; Friess, U. Oxidative stress, AGE, and atherosclerosis. *Kidney Int. Suppl.* **2007**, *106*, S17–S26. [CrossRef] [PubMed]
14. Cai, Z.; Liu, N.; Wang, C.; Qin, B.; Zhou, Y.; Xiao, M.; Chang, L.; Yan, L.J.; Zhao, B. Role of RAGE in alzheimer's disease. *Cell. Mol. Neurobiol.* **2016**, *36*, 483–495. [CrossRef]

15. Kim, A.R.; Shin, T.S.; Lee, M.S.; Park, J.Y.; Park, K.E.; Yoon, N.Y.; Kim, J.S.; Choi, J.S.; Jang, B.C.; Byun, D.S.; et al. Isolation and identification of phlorotannins from *Ecklonia stolonifera* with antioxidant and anti-inflammatory properties. *J. Agric. Food Chem.* **2009**, *57*, 3483–3489. [CrossRef]
16. Artan, M.; Li, Y.; Karadeniz, F.; Lee, S.H.; Kim, M.M.; Kim, S.K. Anti-HIV-1 activity of phloroglucinol derivative, 6, 6′-biekol, from *Ecklonia cava*. *Bioorg. Med. Chem.* **2008**, *16*, 7921–7926. [CrossRef]
17. Kim, E.K.; Tang, Y.; Kim, Y.S.; Hwang, J.W.; Choi, E.J.; Lee, J.H.; Lee, S.H.; Jeon, Y.J.; Park, P.J. First evidence that *Ecklonia cava*-derived dieckol attenuates MCF-7 human breast carcinoma cell migration. *Mar. Drugs* **2015**, *13*, 1785–1797. [CrossRef]
18. Manandhar, B.; Wagle, A.; Seong, S.H.; Paudel, P.; Kim, H.-R.; Jung, H.A.; Choi, J.S. Phlorotannins with potential anti-tyrosinase and antioxidant activity isolated from the marine seaweed *Ecklonia stolonifera*. *Antioxidants* **2019**, *8*, 240. [CrossRef]
19. Kim, H.; Kong, C.S.; Lee, J.I.; Kim, H.; Baek, S.; Seo, Y. Evaluation of inhibitory effect of phlorotannins from *Ecklonia cava* on triglyceride accumulation in adipocyte. *J. Agric. Food Chem.* **2013**, *61*, 8541–8547. [CrossRef]
20. Kang, M.C.; Wijesinghe, W.A.J.P.; Lee, S.H.; Kang, S.M.; Ko, S.C.; Yang, X.; Kang, N.; Jeon, B.T.; Kim, J.; Lee, D.H.; et al. Dieckol isolated from brown seaweed *Ecklonia cava* attenuates type II diabetes in *db/db* mouse model. *Food Chem. Toxicol.* **2013**, *53*, 294–298. [CrossRef]
21. Jung, H.A.; Roy, A.; Jung, J.H.; Choi, J.S. Evaluation of the inhibitory effects of eckol and dieckol isolated from edible brown alga *Eisenia bicyclis* on human monoamine oxidases A and B. *Arch. Pharm. Res.* **2017**, *40*, 480–491. [CrossRef] [PubMed]
22. Paudel, P.; Seong, S.H.; Wu, S.; Park, S.; Jung, H.A.; Choi, J.S. Eckol as a potential therapeutic against neurodegenerative diseases targeting dopamine D3/D4 receptors. *Mar. Drugs* **2019**, *17*, 108. [CrossRef] [PubMed]
23. Seong, S.H.; Paudel, P.; Choi, J.W.; Ahn, D.H.; Nam, T.J.; Jung, H.A.; Choi, J.S. Probing multi-target action of phlorotannins as new monoamine oxidase inhibitors and dopaminergic receptor modulators with the potential for treatment of neuronal disorders. *Mar. Drugs* **2019**, *17*, 377. [CrossRef] [PubMed]
24. Jung, H.A.; Oh, S.H.; Choi, J.S. Molecular docking studies of phlorotannins from *Eisenia bicyclis* with BACE1 inhibitory activity. *Bioorg. Med. Chem. Lett.* **2010**, *20*, 3211–3215. [CrossRef] [PubMed]
25. Yoon, N.Y.; Chung, H.Y.; Kim, H.R.; Choi, J.E. Acetyl-and butyrylcholinesterase inhibitory activities of sterols and phlorotannins from *Ecklonia stolonifera*. *Fish. Sci.* **2008**, *74*, 200–207. [CrossRef]
26. Kang, I.J.; Jeon, Y.E.; Yin, X.F.; Nam, J.S.; You, S.G.; Hong, M.S.; Jang, B.G.; Kim, M.J. Butanol extract of *Ecklonia cava* prevents production and aggregation of beta-amyloid, and reduces beta-amyloid mediated neuronal death. *Food Chem. Toxicol.* **2011**, *49*, 2252–2259. [CrossRef] [PubMed]
27. Cho, S.; Yang, H.; Jeon, Y.J.; Lee, C.J.; Jin, Y.H.; Baek, N.I.; Kim, D.; Kang, S.M.; Yoon, M.; Yong, H.; et al. Phlorotannins of the edible brown seaweed *Ecklonia cava* Kjellman induce sleep via positive allosteric modulation of gamma-aminobutyric acid type A–benzodiazepine receptor: A novel neurological activity of seaweed polyphenols. *Food Chem.* **2012**, *132*, 1133–1142. [CrossRef]
28. Iannuzzi, C.; Borriello, M.; Irace, G.; Cammarota, M.; Di Maro, A.; Sirangelo, I. Vanillin affects amyloid aggregation and non-enzymatic glycation in human insulin. *Sci. Rep.* **2017**, *7*, 15086. [CrossRef]
29. Asgary, S.; Naderi, G.A.; Sarraf Zadegan, N.; Vakili, R. The inhibitory effects of pure flavonoids on in vitro protein glycosylation. *J. Herb. Pharmacother.* **2002**, *2*, 47–55. [CrossRef]
30. Braughler, J.M.; Duncan, L.A.; Chase, R.L. The involvement of iron in lipid peroxidation. Importance of ferric to ferrous ratios in initiation. *J. Biol. Chem.* **1986**, *261*, 10282–10289.
31. Pike, C.J.; Burdick, D.; Walencewicz, A.J.; Glabe, C.G.; Cotman, C.W. Neurodegeneration induced by beta-amyloid peptides in vitro: The role of peptide assembly state. *J. Neurosci.* **1993**, *13*, 1676–1687. [CrossRef] [PubMed]
32. Wang, J.; Zheng, J.; Huang, C.; Zhao, J.; Lin, J.; Zhou, X.; Naman, C.B.; Wang, N.; Gerwick, W.H.; Wang, Q.; et al. Eckmaxol, a phlorotannin extracted from *Ecklonia maxima*, produces anti-β-amyloid oligomer neuroprotective effects possibly via directly acting on glycogen synthase kinase 3β. *ACS Chem. Neurosci.* **2018**, *9*, 1349–1356. [CrossRef] [PubMed]
33. Ahn, B.R.; Moon, H.E.; Kim, H.R.; Jung, H.A.; Choi, J.S. Neuroprotective effect of edible brown alga *Eisenia bicyclis* on amyloid beta peptide-induced toxicity in PC12 cells. *Arch. Pharm. Res.* **2012**, *35*, 1989–1998. [CrossRef] [PubMed]

34. Lee, S.; Youn, K.; Kim, D.H.; Ahn, M.R.; Yoon, E.; Kim, O.Y.; Jun, M. Anti-neuroinflammatory property of phlorotannins from *Ecklonia cava* on Aβ25-35-induced damage in PC12 cells. *Mar. Drugs* **2019**, *17*, 7. [CrossRef]
35. Jarosz-Griffiths, H.H.; Noble, E.; Rushworth, J.V.; Hooper, N.M. Amyloid-β receptors: The good, the bad, and the prion protein. *J. Biol. Chem.* **2016**, *291*, 3174–3183. [CrossRef]
36. Larini, L.; Shea, J.E. Role of β-hairpin formation in aggregation: The self-assembly of the amyloid-β (25-35) peptide. *Biophys. J.* **2012**, *103*, 576–586. [CrossRef]
37. Millucci, L.; Ghezzi, L.; Bernardini, G.; Santucci, A. Conformations and biological activities of amyloid beta peptide 25-35. *Curr. Protein Pept. Sci.* **2010**, *11*, 54–67. [CrossRef]
38. Pike, C.J.; Walencewicz-Wasserman, A.J.; Kosmoski, J.; Cribbs, D.H.; Glabe, C.G.; Cotman, C.W. Structure-activity analyses of β-amyloid peptides: Contributions of the β25–35 region to aggregation and neurotoxicity. *J. Neurochem.* **1995**, *64*, 253–265. [CrossRef]
39. Reggiani, A.M.; Simoni, E.; Caporaso, R.; Meunier, J.; Keller, E.; Maurice, T.; Minarini, A.; Rosini, M.; Cavalli, A. In vivo characterization of ARN14140, a memantine/galantamine-based multi-target compound for Alzheimer's disease. *Sci. Rep.* **2016**, *6*, 1–11. [CrossRef]
40. Wei, G.; Shea, J.E. Effects of solvent on the structure of the Alzheimer amyloid-β (25-35) peptide. *Biophys. J.* **2006**, *91*, 1638–1648. [CrossRef]
41. Man, V.H.; He, X.; Derreumaux, P.; Ji, B.; Xie, X.Q.; Nguyen, P.H.; Wang, J. Effects of all-atom molecular mechanics force fields on amyloid peptide assembly: The case of Aβ16–22 dimer. *J. Chem. Theory Comput.* **2019**, *15*, 1440–1452. [CrossRef] [PubMed]
42. Nguyen, P.; Derreumaux, P. Understanding amyloid fibril nucleation and aβ oligomer/drug interactions from computer simulations. *ACC Chem. Res.* **2014**, *47*, 603–611. [CrossRef]
43. Doig, A.J.; Del Castillo-Frias, M.P.; Berthoumieu, O.; Tarus, B.; Nasica-Labouze, J.; Sterpone, F.; Nguyen, P.H.; Hooper, N.M.; Faller, P.; Derreumaux, P. Why is research on amyloid-β failing to give new drugs for Alzheimer's disease. *ACS Chem. Neurosci.* **2017**, *8*, 1435–1437. [CrossRef] [PubMed]
44. De Felice, F.G.; Lourenco, M.V.; Ferreira, S.T. How does brain insulin resistance develop in Alzheimer's disease? *Alzheimers Dement.* **2014**, *10*, S26–S32. [CrossRef] [PubMed]
45. Lee, C.C.; Kuo, Y.M.; Huang, C.C.; Hsu, K.S. Insulin rescues amyloid β-induced impairment of hippocampal long-term potentiation. *Neurobiol. Aging* **2009**, *30*, 377–387. [CrossRef] [PubMed]
46. American Diabetes Association. Screening for type 2 diabetes. *Diabetes Care* **2002**, *25*, S21–S24. [CrossRef]
47. Chen, X.; Su, T.; Chen, Y.; He, Y.; Liu, Y.; Xu, Y.; Wei, Y.; Li, J.; He, R. D-Ribose as a Contributor to Glycated Haemoglobin. *EBioMedicine* **2017**, *25*, 143–153. [CrossRef]
48. O'Harte, F.P.; Hojrup, P.; Barnett, C.R.; Flatt, P.R. Identification of the site of glycation of human insulin. *Peptides* **1996**, *17*, 1323–1330. [CrossRef]
49. Zoete, V.; Meuwly, M.; Karplus, M. Investigation of glucose binding sites on insulin. *Proteins* **2004**, *55*, 568–581. [CrossRef]
50. Cini, M.; Fariello, R.Y.; Bianchettei, A.; Moretti, A. Studies on lipid peroxidation in the rat brain. *Neurochem. Res.* **1994**, *19*, 283–288. [CrossRef]
51. Stocks, J.; Gutteridge, J.M.C.; Sharp, R.J.; Dormandy, T.L. Assay using brain homogenate for measuring the antioxidant activity of biological fluids. *Clin. Sci.* **1974**, *47*, 215–222. [CrossRef] [PubMed]
52. Wills, E.D. Mechanisms of lipid peroxide formation in animal tissues. *Biochem. J.* **1966**, *99*, 667–676. [CrossRef] [PubMed]
53. Kwak, J.H.; Yang, Z.; Yoon, B.; He, Y.; Uhm, S.; Shin, H.C.; Lee, B.H.; Yoo, Y.C.; Lee, K.B.; Han, S.Y.; et al. Blood-brain barrier-permeable fluorone-labeled dieckols acting as neuronal ER stress signaling inhibitors. *Biomaterials* **2015**, *61*, 52–60. [CrossRef] [PubMed]
54. He, Q.; Liu, J.; Liang, J.; Liu, X.; Li, W.; Liu, Z.; Ding, Z.; Tuo, D. Towards improvements for penetrating the blood–brain barrier—recent progress from a material and pharmaceutical perspective. *Cells* **2018**, *7*, 24. [CrossRef] [PubMed]
55. Venkatesan, J.; Kim, S.K.; Shim, M.S. Antimicrobial, antioxidant, and anticancer activities of biosynthesized silver nanoparticles using marine algae *Ecklonia cava*. *Nanomaterials* **2016**, *6*, 235. [CrossRef]
56. Naldi, M.; Fiori, J.; Pistolozzi, M.; Drake, A.F.; Bertucci, C.; Wu, R.; Mlynarczyk, K.; Filipek, S.; De Simone, A.; Andrisano, V. Amyloid β-peptide 25-35 self-assembly and its inhibition: A model undecapeptide system to gain atomistic and secondary structure details of the Alzheimer's disease process and treatment. *ACS Chem. Neurosci.* **2012**, *3*, 952–962. [CrossRef]

57. Seong, S.H.; Ali, M.Y.; Jung, H.A.; Choi, J.S. Umbelliferone derivatives exert neuroprotective effects by inhibiting monoamine oxidase A, self-amyloid β aggregation, and lipid peroxidation. *Bioorg. Chem.* **2019**, *92*, 10323. [CrossRef]
58. Goodsell, D.S.; Morris, G.M.; Olson, A.J. Automated docking of flexible ligands: Applications of AutoDock. *J. Mol. Recognit.* **1996**, *9*, 1–5. [CrossRef]
59. D'Ursi, A.M.; Armenante, M.R.; Guerrini, R.; Salvadori, S.; Sorrentino, G.; Picone, D. Solution structure of amyloid beta-peptide (25-35) in different media. *J. Med. Chem.* **2004**, *12*, 4231–4238. [CrossRef]
60. Abraham, M.J.; Murtola, T.; Schulz, R.; Páll, S.; Smith, J.C.; Hess, B.; Lindahl, E. GROMACS: High performance molecular simulations through multi-level parallelism from laptops to supercomputers. *SoftwareX* **2015**, *1*, 19–25. [CrossRef]
61. Daura, X.; Mark, A.E.; Van Gunsteren, W.F. Parametrization of aliphatic CH_n united atoms of GROMOS96 force field. *J. Comput. Chem.* **1998**, *19*, 535–547. [CrossRef]
62. Hess, B.; Bekker, H.; Berendsen, H.J.C.; Fraaije, J.G.E.M. LINCS: A linear constraint solver for molecular simulations. *J. Comput. Chem.* **1997**, *18*, 1463–1472. [CrossRef]
63. Darden, T.; York, D.; Pedersen, L. Particle mesh Ewald: An N_log(N) method for Ewald sums in large systems. *J. Chem. Phys.* **1993**, *98*, 10089–10092. [CrossRef]
64. Humphrey, W.; Dalke, A.; Schulten, K. VMD—Visual molecular dynamics. *J. Mol. Graph.* **1996**, *14*, 33–38. [CrossRef]

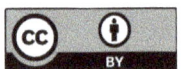

© 2019 by the authors. Licensee MDPI, Basel, Switzerland. This article is an open access article distributed under the terms and conditions of the Creative Commons Attribution (CC BY) license (http://creativecommons.org/licenses/by/4.0/).

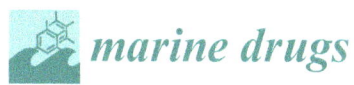

Article

A New Tyrosinase Inhibitor from the Red Alga *Symphyocladia latiuscula* (Harvey) Yamada (Rhodomelaceae)

Pradeep Paudel [1], Aditi Wagle [1], Su Hui Seong [1], Hye Jin Park [2], Hyun Ah Jung [3,*] and Jae Sue Choi [1,*]

[1] Department of Food and Life Science, Pukyong National University, Busan 48513, Korea; phr.paudel@gmail.com (P.P.); aditiwagle05@gmail.com (A.W.); seongsuhui@naver.com (S.H.S.)
[2] Department of Food Science and Nutrition, Changshin University, Gyeongsangnam-do 51352, Korea; parkhj@cs.ac.kr
[3] Department of Food Science and Human Nutrition, Chonbuk National University, Jeonju 54896, Korea
* Correspondence: jungha@jbnu.ac.kr (H.A.J.); choijs@pknu.ac.kr (J.S.C.); Tel.: +82-63-270-4882 (H.A.J.); +82-51-629-5845 (J.S.C.)

Received: 20 April 2019; Accepted: 15 May 2019; Published: 17 May 2019

Abstract: A marine red alga, *Symphyocladia latiuscula* (Harvey) Yamada (Rhodomelaceae), is a rich source of bromophenols with a wide array of biological activities. This study investigates the anti-tyrosinase activity of the alga. Moderate activity was demonstrated by the methanol extract of *S. latiuscula*, and subsequent column chromatography identified three bromophenols: 2,3,6-tribromo-4,5-dihydroxybenzyl methyl alcohol (**1**), 2,3,6-tribromo-4,5-dihydroxybenzyl methyl ether (**2**), and bis-(2,3,6-tribromo-4,5-dihydroxybenzyl methyl ether) (**3**). Bromophenols **1** and **3** exhibited potent competitive tyrosinase inhibitory activity against L-tyrosine substrates, with IC_{50} values of 10.78 ± 0.19 and 2.92 ± 0.04 µM, respectively. Against substrate L-3,4-dihydroxyphenylalanine (L-DOPA), compounds **1** and **3** demonstrated moderate activity, while **2** showed no observable effect. The experimental data were verified by a molecular docking study that found catalytic hydrogen and halogen interactions were responsible for the activity. In addition, compounds **1** and **3** exhibited dose-dependent inhibitory effects in melanin and intracellular tyrosinase levels in α-melanocyte-stimulating hormone (α-MSH)-induced B16F10 melanoma cells. Compounds **3** and **1** were the most effective tyrosinase inhibitors. In addition, increasing the bromine group number increased the mushroom tyrosinase inhibitory activity.

Keywords: *Symphyocladia latiuscula*; bromophenols; mushroom tyrosinase; B16F10; melanin

---

1. Introduction

Marine algae are widely used in a variety of cuisines [1] and are preferred by a growing number of consumers for their functional and nutraceutical properties [2,3]. The pharmaceutical industry has also developed a strong interest in algae [4,5], as have cosmetologists [6]. A major concern among the latter is hyperpigmentation, which is an abnormal darkening of the skin associated with excessive melanin production [7,8]. Although melanin is a pigment responsible for the photo-protective effect of skin, overproduction may lead to skin disorders [9]. Because tyrosinase is a rate-limiting step in melanin formation, identification of a strong tyrosinase inhibitor would be of significant value to hyperpigmentation research.

Melanogenesis describes the production of distinct melanin pigments by specialized cells called melanocytes, which are found within membrane-bound organelles known as melanosomes [10]. The embryonic precursors of melanocytes, i.e., melanoblasts, originate in neural crest cells [11].

Mature melanocytes are connected with keratinocytes through dendritic cells, which facilitate the transfer of melanin in neighboring keratinocytes cells, are responsible for skin pigmentation, and protect the skin from harmful ultraviolet radiation [12]. Melanocyte-specific markers, which are used to identify the expression of melanocyte cells in the melanogenesis process, include tyrosinase, tyrosinase-related protein 1 (TRP1), tyrosinase-related protein 2 (TRP2)/dopachrome tautomerase (DCT), pre-melanosome protein 17 (Pmel17/gp100), melan-A/melanoma antigen recognized by T-cells 1 (MART-1), and microphthalmia-associated transcription factor (MITF). In melanin synthesis, the rate-limiting step is catalyzed by tyrosinase, while TRP1 is responsible for the oxidation of 5,6-dihydroxyindole-2-carboxylic acid to a carboxylated indole quinone [13]. Moreover, TRP2/DCT enzymes catalyze the tautomerization of dopachrome into 5,6-dihydroxyindole-2-carboxylic acid, which can be detected in both melanocytes and melanoblasts [14,15]. Pmel17/gp100 is necessary for the formation of the structural matrix of stage II melanosomes [16]. MART-1, meanwhile, is specifically targeted to tumor-directed T-lymphocytes and is a probable target for immunotherapy of melanoma [17]. MITF is a major transcriptional factor in the regulation of melanocyte-specific genes encoding tyrosinase, TRP2/DCT, and MART-1 [18–20].

Melanin pigments common in humans include eumelanin (a brown-black pigment) and pheomelanin (a yellow/orange-red pigment). Melanin is produced from its precursor, L-tyrosine, through a series of enzymatic and chemical reactions. The first step of melanin biosynthesis, the oxidation of an L-tyrosine substrate, is catalyzed by the rate-limiting enzyme tyrosinase. This is followed by dopaquinone formation [21,22]. Autoxidation of dopaquinone leads to the formation of L-DOPA and dopachrome. L-DOPA acts as a co-factor in the reaction [23] and also as a substrate for tyrosinase. Eumelanin is subsequently formed through a series of oxidation reactions with dihydroxyindole and dihydroxyindole-2-carboxylic acid. Dopaquinone is condensed into cysteinyldopa or glutathionyldopa in the presence of cysteine or gluthathione, producing pheomelanin pigments. A heterogeneous pool of mixed-type melanins can also be formed through interactions between eumelanin and pheomelanin [22,24].

Recently, marine algae have gained considerable interest in the discovery of tyrosinase inhibitors. In a study conducted to find new anti-browning and whitening agents from marine sources, Cha et al. [25] screened 43 indigenous marine algae for tyrosinase inhibitory activity and found potent tyrosinase inhibitory activity of extracts from *Endarachne binghamiae*, *Schizymenia dubyi*, *Ecklonia cava*, and *Sargassum silquastrum*. However, *Symphyocladia latiuscula* (Harvey) Yamada was not in the list of the 43 studied algae. Of the total microalgae in marine source, brown algae account for approximately 59%, followed by red algae at 40% and green algae at less than 1% [26], and phlorotannins and halogenated compounds are predominant secondary metabolites with prominent biological activities. Lately, tyrosinase inhibitory potentials of phlorotannins from marine algae have emerged with great interest [27–29]. Similarly, due to various advantages of halogens in drug pharmacokinetics such as lipophilicity, cell membrane solubility, membrane binding, permeation, diffusion, and half-life, chemists are focusing on the synthesis of novel tyrosinase inhibitors, taking halogenation as a basic tool [30–32]. However, reports on natural halogenated compounds from marine sources are limited. Therefore, this study focuses on a red alga, *Symphyocladia latiuscula*, and its constituent, bromophenols (Figure 1), for anti-tyrosinase activity.

Symphyocladia latiuscula (Harvey) Yamada is a member of the Rhodomelaceae family predominantly distributed along the coasts of Korea, Japan, and northern China. It is a red alga rich in bromophenols with a wide range of bioactive properties [33]. Among the compounds found in *S. latiuscula* are antioxidants [34,35], free radicals scavengers [36–38], peroxynitrite scavengers [39], anti-inflammatory and antibacterial [40], antifungal [41,42], antiviral [43], cytoprotective [39], and anti-diabetes [44], along with aldose reductase inhibitors [45], Taq DNA polymerase inhibitors [46], and anti-proliferators [47]. However, anti-tyrosinase activity has not yet been investigated in detail.

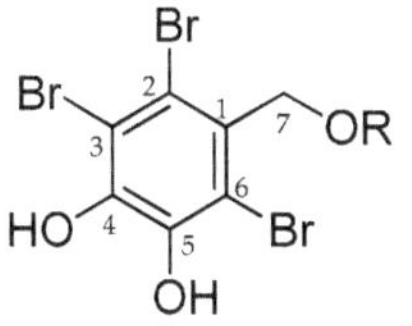

R = H; 2,3,6-tribromo-4,5-dihydroxybenzyl methyl alcohol (1)

R = CH₃; 2,3,6-tribromo-4,5-dihydroxybenzyl methyl ether (2)

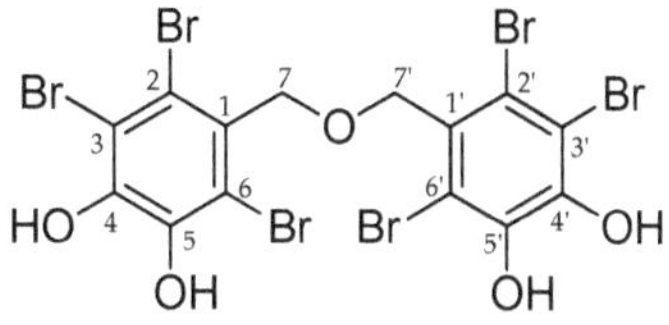

Bis-(2,3,6-tribromo-4,5-dihydroxybenzyl methyl ether) (3)

Figure 1. Structure of the compounds isolated from the ethyl acetate fraction of *S. latiuscula*.

2. Results

2.1. Effect of Bromophenols on Tyrosinase Activity

Mushroom tyrosinase inhibitory activity of MeOH extract of *S. latiuscula* demonstrated inhibition percentages of 39.58% and 86.47% at a concentration of 1000 and 250 μg/mL for L-tyrosine and L-DOPA, respectively. This result helped determine the compounds (Figure 1) responsible for the activity in the MeOH extract of *S. latiuscula*.

In L-tyrosine substrate, compound **3** demonstrated a potent mushroom tyrosinase inhibitory activity, with a half-maximal inhibitory concentration (IC_{50}) of 2.92 ± 0.04 μM, followed by compound **1** with 10.78 ± 0.04 μM. However, compound **2** exhibited weaker inhibition, with an IC_{50} value of 113.94 ± 0.75 μM (Table 1). Weak inhibition was also exhibited by compounds in L-DOPA substrate.

Table 1. Mushroom tyrosinase inhibitory potential of bromo-compounds from *S. latiuscula*.

Compounds	IC_{50} (μM) [a] (n = 3)		L-Tyrosine	
	L-Tyrosine	L-DOPA	K_i Value (μM) [b]	Inhibition Type [c]
1	10.78 ± 0.19 [h]	270.53 ± 2.04 [f]	10.59	Competitive
2	113.94 ± 0.75 [g]	>300	_ [d]	_ [d]
3	2.92 ± 0.04 [i]	110.91 ± 4.95 [g]	1.98	Competitive
Kojic acid [e]	3.17 ± 0.07 [i]	3.07 ± 0.04 [h]	_ [d]	_ [d]
Arbutin [e]	172.82 ± 4.71 [f]	>300	_ [d]	_ [d]

[a] The 50% inhibitory concentration (μM) expressed as mean ± SD of triplicate experiments; [b] The inhibition constant (K_i) was determined from secondary plots; [c] Inhibition type determined from Lineweaver-Burk plots; [d] Not determined; [e] Used as reference drug; [f–i] Means with different letters are significantly different with Duncan's test at $p < 0.05$.

2.2. Effect of Bromophenols on Enzyme Kinetic Inhibition

Changes in K_m values were observed on a double-reciprocal Lineweaver–Burk plot, which showed that compounds **1** and **3** induced competitive-type inhibition (Table 1, Figure 2). Furthermore, the secondary replot of K_{mapp}/V_{maxapp} and $1/V_{maxapp}$ versus compounds **1** and **3** was used to determine the binding constant of the inhibitor for free enzymes (K_{ic}). The K_{ic} ($\approx K_i$) values for compounds **1** and **3** were 10.59 and 1.98 μM.

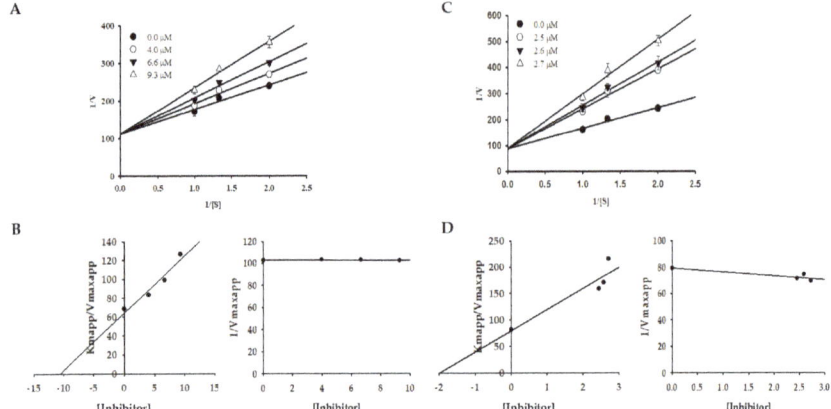

Figure 2. Lineweaver–Burk plots and the secondary plots of K_{mapp}/V_{maxapp} and $1/V_{maxapp}$ for the inhibition of tyrosinase by compounds **1** (**A**,**B**) and **3** (**C**,**D**) in the presence of different concentrations of substrate (L-tyrosine).

2.3. Molecular Docking Simulation on Tyrosinase Inhibition

To predict the binding site of the active compounds, a molecular docking simulation was performed. The binding energy, the number of hydrogen bonds, and the hydrogen-bond interaction, along with other interaction residues of the compounds and the reference compounds L-tyrosine (competitive inhibitor) and luteolin (allosteric inhibitor) are summarized in Table 2 and Figures 3 and 4. The most potent bromophenol, compound **3**, formed two hydrogen-bond interactions with Arg268 and peroxide ions (Per404) between the two copper ions. Furthermore, the complex was stabilized by His259, Asn260, Glu256, Met280, Val283, His263, Phe264, Ser282, Ala286, Val248, Met257, Val283, His85, His244, His259, His263, and Phe264 interacting residues (Figure 4C). Similarly, together with the three-hydrogen-bond interaction with Per404, Asn260, and His61, the compound **1**-tyrosinase complex was stabilized by Glu256, Met280, Val283, His263, Ala286, Val283, His85, Phe90, His244, His259, His263, and Phe264, as shown in Figure 4A. Likewise, only one hydrogen bond with peroxide ions was found with compound **2** (Figure 4B). The binding energies of −6.19, −6.29, and −7.81 kcal/mol were consumed by compounds **1**, **2**, and **3**, respectively.

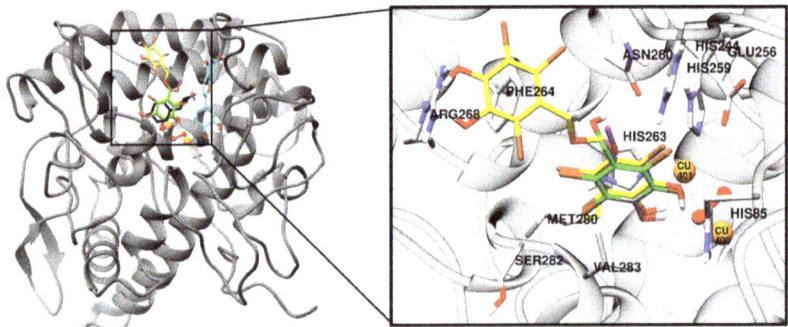

Figure 3. Molecular docking results of bromophenol compounds from *S. latiuscula* in the active site of oxy-form *Agaricus bisporus* tyrosinase (2Y9X) along with reference ligands. The chemical structure of compounds **1**, **2**, **3**, L-tyrosine, and luteolin are shown in green, purple, yellow, black, and cyan sticks, respectively. Bromine, oxygen, and nitrogen atoms are shown in brown, red, and blue, respectively. Copper and peroxide ions are shown in orange and red spheres, respectively.

Table 2. Binding energy and interacting residues of bromo-compounds from *S. latiuscula* against oxy-form *Agaricus bisporus* tyrosinase (2Y9X).

Compounds	Binding Energy (kcal/mol)	No. of H-Bonds	H-Bond Interactions	Other Interacting Residues
1	−6.19	3	Asn260, His61, and Per404 (O–H bond)	Glu256 and Met280 (O-Br bond), Val283 (Pi-Sigma), His263 (Pi-Pi Stacked), Ser282 (Amide-Pi Stacked), Ala286 and Val283 (Alkyl-Br), His85, Phe90, His244, His259, His263, and Phe264 (Pi-Br), Cu401, and 400 (van der Waals)
2	−6.29	1	Per404 (O–H bond)	Met280 (O-Br bond), Val283 (Pi-Sigma), His263 (Pi-Pi Stacked), Ala286 and Val283 (Alkyl-Br), His85, Phe90, His259, His263, and Phe264 (Pi-Br), Cu401, and 400 (van der Waals)
3	−7.81	2	Arg268 and Per404 (O–H bond)	His259 and Asn260 (C-O bond), Glu256 and Met280 (O-Br bond), Val283 (Pi-Sigma), His263 (Pi-Pi Stacked), Phe264 (Pi-Pi T-shaped), Ser282 (Amide-Pi Stacked), Ala286, Val248, Met257, and Val283 (Alkyl-Br), His85, His244, His259, His263, and Phe264 (Pi-Br), Cu401, and 400 (van der Waals)
L-Tyrosine [a]	−6.31	5	His244, Asn260, and Met280 (O–H bond), Glu256 (Salt-bridge)	Ala286 (Pi-Alkyl), Val283 (Pi-Sigma), His263 (Pi-Pi Stacked), Cu401, and 400, Per402 (van der Waals)
Luteolin [a]	−5.77	4	Cys83, Gly245, Ala246, and Val248 (O–H bond)	Val248 (Pi-Alkyl), His85 (Pi-Sigma), Glu322 (Pi-Anion)

[a] L-tyrosine and luteolin were used as reference catalytic and allosteric inhibitor, respectively.

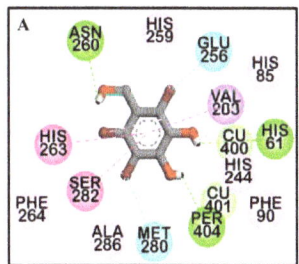 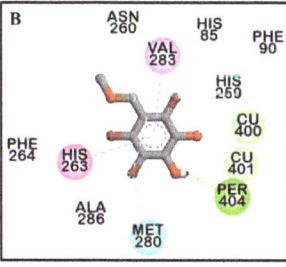 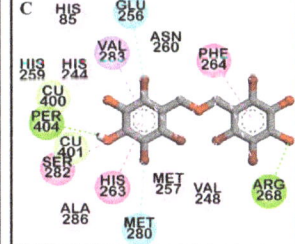

Figure 4. Molecular docking results of bromo-compounds **1** (**A**), **2** (**B**), and **3** (**C**) in the catalytic site of oxy-form *Agaricus bisporus* tyrosinase (2Y9X).

2.4. Effect of Bromophenols on Cell Viability of B16F10 Cells

To evaluate the toxicity of the bromophenols in B16F10 melanoma cells, cell viability upon bromophenol treatment only (Figure 5A) and/or co-treatment with 5 µM α-MSH for 48 h (Figure 5B) was determined using a 3-(4,5-dimethylthiazol-2-yl)-2,5-diphenyltetrazolium bromide (MTT) assay. The B16F10 melanoma cells were treated at a concentration of 25–100 µM of isolated bromophenols for 48 h. Bromophenol **2** showed no toxicity up to a concentration of 100 µM (approximately 100%

viable cells). However, compounds **1** and **3** displayed significant toxicity (74.6% and 86.9% viable cells, respectively). No toxicity was observed up to 50 μM concentration for all compounds. Consequently, a 25 μM sample concentration was used for further experiments.

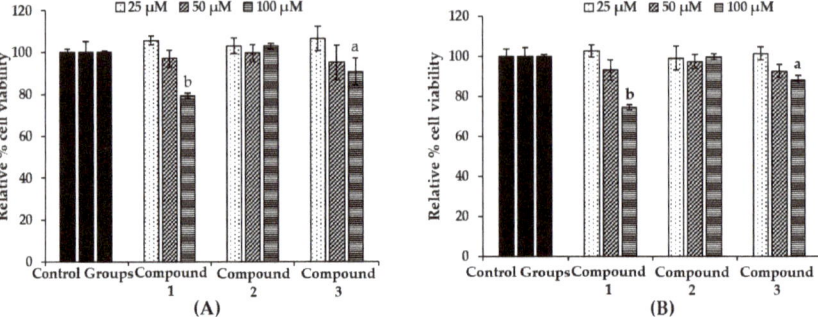

Figure 5. Effect of bromophenols **1–3** on cell viability in B16F10 cells (**A**) and co-treatment with 5 μM α-MSH (**B**). Cell viability was determined using the 3-(4,5-dimethylthiazol-2-yl)-2,5-diphenyl tetrazolium bromide (MTT) method. Cells were pretreated with the indicated concentrations (25, 50, and 100 μM) of test compounds for 48 h. Data shown represent mean ± SD of triplicate experiments.
[a] $p < 0.05$ and [b] $p < 0.01$ indicates significant differences from the control group.

2.5. Effect of Bromophenols on Melanin Content and Intracellular Tyrosinase Activity in B16F10 Cells

Melanin and intracellular tyrosinase (TYR) contents were measured after pretreatment of B16F10 melanoma cells with different concentrations (6.25, 12.5, and 25 μM) of the three bromophenols for 1 h, followed by 48 h of α-MSH treatment. After stimulating B16F10 cells with 5 μM α-MSH for 48 h, the melanin content rose to 151.72% (Figure 6A). However, treatment of bromophenols **1** and **3** reduced the melanin content in a dose-dependent manner. At a 25 μM concentration, compounds **1** and **3** reduced the melanin content to 115.94% and 98.68%, respectively. Arbutin at a 500 μM concentration reduced the content to 124.06%. In parallel with the enzyme assay, compound **2** showed no significant reduction in the melanin content. Because cellular tyrosinase enhances melanin overproduction, reduction of tyrosinase activity is an efficient strategy for the development of anti-melanogenic agents. A L-DOPA oxidation protocol was designed to examine the inhibitory activity of isolated bromophenols against tyrosinase in α-MSH-induced B16F10 melanoma cells, because L-tyrosine and L-DOPA are sequentially generated substrates that regulate melanogenesis and modulate melanocyte function through overlapping substrates. After 48 h of sample treatment, intracellular tyrosinase activity was measured. As shown in Figure 6B, with treatments **1** and **3**, intracellular tyrosinase activity decreased in a dose-dependent manner compared with controls. The level of intracellular tyrosinase after α-MSH treatment was 215.73%, which was reduced to 122.64% and 94.81% after treatment with 25 μM concentration of **1** and **3**, respectively. The activities of **1** and **3** were better than that of 500 μM arbutin, which reduced intracellular tyrosinase levels to 130.75%. As with melanin content, compound **2** did not show a significant reduction in intracellular tyrosinase level at tested concentrations.

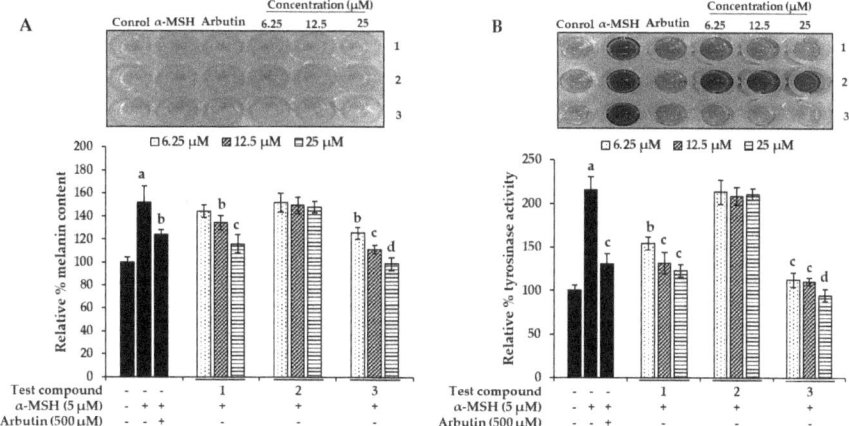

Figure 6. Effect of bromophenols **1–3** on extracellular melanin content (**A**) and cellular tyrosinase activity (**B**) in α-MSH-stimulated B16F10 cells. Cells were pretreated with the indicated concentrations (6.25, 12.5, and 25 μM) of bromophenols **1–3** for 1 h followed by exposure to α-MSH (5.0 μM) for 48 h in the presence or the absence of test bromophenols. Arbutin (500 μM) was used as a positive control. Values represent the mean ± SD of triplicate experiments. [a] $p < 0.01$ indicates significant differences from the control group; [b] $p < 0.05$, [c] $p < 0.01$ and [d] $p < 0.001$ indicate significant differences from the α-MSH treated group.

2.6. Effect of Bromophenols on Tyrosinase Expression

Increased tyrosinase activity enhances melanogenesis and hyperpigmentation, implying that downregulation of tyrosinase activity would theoretically represent an anti-pigmenting property. To evaluate the effect of bromophenols **1-3** on tyrosinase expression, the B16F10 cells were pre-treated with the bromophenols before stimulation with α-MSH, and the tyrosinase protein levels were examined using western blot analysis. As shown in Figure 7, treatment with compounds **1** and **3** at concentrations of 6.25, 12.5, and 25 μM for 48 h inhibited α-MSH-induced accumulation of tyrosinase proteins in a concentration-dependent manner.

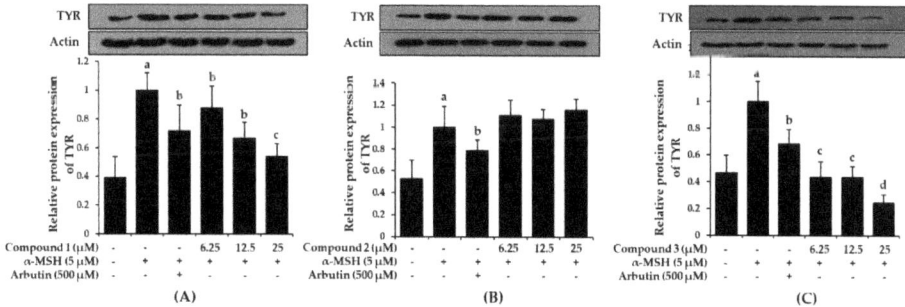

Figure 7. Effects of bromophenol **1** (**A**), **2** (**B**), and **3** (**C**) on cellular tyrosinase protein expression levels in α-MSH-stimulated B16F10 cells. Western blotting was performed, and protein band intensities were quantified by densitometric analysis. Upper panels display representative blots. Graphs under each bands represent the relative band density for tyrosinase (TYR) normalized to β-actin. Values represent the mean ± SD of three independent experiments; [a] $p < 0.001$ indicates significant differences from the control group; [b] $p < 0.05$, [c] $p < 0.01$ and [d] $p < 0.001$ indicate significant differences from the α-MSH treated group.

Compared with the normal control group, which had low levels of tyrosinase expression, the α-MSH-treated group demonstrated intensified tyrosinase expression levels. However, pre-treatment with arbutin and/or bromophenols **1** and **3** significantly reduced the expression levels. Compound **1** at 25 μM and compound **3** at 6.25 μM were more effective at downregulating tyrosinase expression than arbutin. Compound **2** did not reduce expression up to 25 μM.

3. Discussion

Use of cosmetics can lead to a variety of adverse effects and allergies in users sensitive to certain chemicals and other ingredients. To avoid unnecessary interactions and to reduce adverse effects of synthetic and semi-synthetic cosmetics, consumer preferences are shifting toward natural products. Marine species are an abundant source of chemical and bioactive compounds due to the variety of biological activities associated with marine organisms [48]. Many compounds derived from marine species with possible applications in the nutraceutical and cosmetics fields remain unexamined [49,50].

To meet the demand for new compounds that exhibit potent anti-tyrosinase activity, a preliminary screening of the methanolic extract of *S. latiuscula* was performed. The study revealed that a MeOH extract was associated with inhibition rates of 39.58% and 86.47% at concentrations of 1000 and 250 μg/mL for L-tyrosine and L-DOPA, respectively. A study performed by Seo and Yoo [51] reported inhibition rates of 84% and 60% against MeOH extract and a mixture of acetone and methylene chloride, respectively, using L-tyrosine as a substrate. In contrast, no inhibition was observed at a concentration of 500 μg/mL [27]. The possible reasons for the discrepancies among these experiments include the difference in concentrations of enzyme and substrate, incubation time, and environmental conditions. Based on the results, *S. latiuscula* extract was subjected to bio-assay guided fractionation, which yielded 2,3,6-tribromo-4,5-dihydroxybenzyl methyl alcohol (**1**), 2,3,6-tribromo-4,5-dihydroxybenzyl methyl ether (**2**), and bis-(2,3,6-tribromo-4,5-dihydroxybenzyl methyl ether) (**3**). For the first time, a mushroom tyrosinase inhibitory assay with an L-tyrosine substrate for the isolated compounds revealed compound **3** to be approximately twice and 23 times more potent than compounds **1** and **2**, respectively (Table 1). A similar tendency was observed for the L-DOPA substrate but with only moderate potency. This result highlights the dimeric form of compound **2**, specifically how the O-linkage of the 2,3,6-tribromo-4,5-dihydroxyl methyl ether element enhances mushroom tyrosinase inhibition. Moreover, an increased number for bromophenol moiety contributes to increased inhibition toward tyrosinase. The results were further verified by the observations of B16F10 melanoma cells, which had concentration-dependent inhibitory effects on melanin content and tyrosinase activity for compounds **1** and **3**. A similar tendency for reduction of tyrosinase expression levels by **1** and **3** was observed in a western blot analysis.

To shed light on the inhibition mode against tyrosinase, kinetic analysis for active compounds **1** and **3** using an L-tyrosine substrate was performed, supplemented by a molecular docking study. A double-reciprocal Lineweaver-Burk plot of compounds **1** and **3** for the oxidation of different concentrations of L-tyrosine demonstrated competitive inhibition of both compounds, as K_m changed while V_{max} was constant. Graphing 1/V versus 1/[S] produced a family of straight lines with diverse slopes, although the lines intersected on the Y-axis. The results showed that compounds **1** and **3** could only bind with free enzymes. An inhibition constant for the inhibitor binding with the free enzyme (K_{ic}) was obtained from the secondary plot as 10.59 and 1.98 μM.

To predict binding affinity, activity of the small molecules, and the interaction of the molecules, and to determine the optimal orientation of the protein–ligand complex with minimum energy, molecular docking tools can be applied. This helps reveal the underlying mechanism of the compound responsible for a particular bioactivity. A simulated docking study of the binding of the compounds to the catalytic site of tyrosinase (Figures 3 and 4) provided evidence of the competitive inhibition, as shown by a kinetic analysis (Figure 3). An H-bond interaction was formed by compound **1** as the fourth and fifth hydroxyl group interacted with the peroxide ion located between the two copper ions and His61, respectively, and the seventh hydroxyl group interacted with an Asn260 amino-acid residue. Moreover, the O-atom at the carboxylic moiety of Glu256 and Met280 interacted with the third- and the sixth-position bromine atoms. The complex was stabilized by hydrophobic interactions with Val283, His263, and Ser282 and halogen interactions with Ala286, Val283, His85, Phe90, His244, His259, His263, and Phe264 residues (Figure 4A). Although similar interactions were observed for compound 3, the strong H-bond interaction between Arg268 residue and the 4′-OH group of active compound 3 helped stabilize the compound 3-tyrosinase complex [52]. Because of the increase in the bromine moiety number, there was an increase in halogen interactions assisting the potent anti-tyrosinase activity (Figure 4C). A similar result was seen in tyrosine phosphatase 1B and α-glucosidase inhibition [44]. Although compound 2 lacked the H-bond interaction with the other amino-acid residues, a peroxide ion between the two copper atoms can explain its weak tyrosinase inhibitory activity (Figure 4B). The lower the value of binding energy shown by the compounds was, the more stable the complex formed between the ligand and targeted protein was. Binding energies of compounds 1–3 to tyrosinase was comparable. However, compound 2 showed ineffective anti-melanogenic activity. The probable reason for this discrepancy might be that, despite the fact that compound 2 was involved in van der Waals interactions with copper ions (Cu401 and 400) and H-bond interactions with a peroxide ion (Per404) at the active site, the complex was not stable. For 1 and 3, H-bond interactions with Asn260 and Arg268 and hydrophobic interaction with Ser282 most probably stabilized the complex, and these interactions were not observed for 2. However, this should be confirmed through molecular dynamic simulation. Moreover, as the present study reports just three compounds, the structural-activity relationship study might be incomplete. Therefore, in depth study of the structural-activity relationship with a larger number of bromophenols is warranted. The results confirm the strong activity exhibited by the compounds isolated from *S. latiuscula*, making the alga a possible source for depigmenting agents in cosmetology.

4. Materials and Methods

4.1. Chemicals and Reagents

L-Tyrosine, L-3,4-dihydroxyphenylalanine (L-DOPA), arbutin, mushroom tyrosinase enzyme (EC 1.14.18.1), and α-melanocyte-stimulating hormone (α-MSH) were obtained from Sigma Aldrich (St. Louis, MO, USA). Dulbecco's modified Eagle's medium (DMEM), fetal bovine serum (FBS), and penicillin-streptomycin were purchased from Gibco-BRL Life Technologies (Grand Island, NY, USA). Primary tyrosinase (TYR) antibodies, β-actin, and horseradish peroxidase-conjugated secondary antibodies were obtained from Santa Cruz Biotechnology Inc. (Santa Cruz, CA, USA). Dipotassium phosphate and monopotassium phosphate were obtained from Junsei Chemical Co. Ltd. (Tokyo, Japan) and Yakuri Pure Chemicals Co. Ltd. (Osaka, Japan), respectively. All other reagents and solvents were purchased from E. Merck, Fluka, and Sigma-Aldrich unless otherwise stated.

4.2. Algal Material

Leafy thalli of *S. latiuscula* (Harvey) Yamada collected from Cheongsapo, Busan, Korea, in January 2016 were authenticated by an algologist, Doctor K. W. Nam, at the Department of Marine Biology, Pukyong National University. A voucher specimen (No. 20160140) was deposited in the laboratory of professor J. S. Choi, Pukyong National University.

4.3. Extraction, Fractionation, and Isolation

Clean and dried leafy thalli of *S. latiuscula* (Harvey) Yamada (700 g) was extracted in methanol (MeOH) three times successively for 3 h at a time (5 L × 3 times) under reflux, followed by concentration until dry in vacuo at 40 °C to obtain 207.38 g of MeOH extract. The resulting MeOH extract was successively partitioned with different solvent soluble fractions. Details on partition, isolation, and identification of compounds are reported in Paudel et al. [44].

4.4. Mushroom Tyrosinase Inhibitory Assay

The inhibitory activity of mushroom tyrosinase was carried out using a spectrophotometric method described in [27] with slight modifications. In brief, 10 µL of samples/positive control (kojic acid) together with 50 mM of phosphate buffer (pH 6.5), 1 mM of substrate (L-tyrosine/L-DOPA) solution, and distilled water were mixed at a ratio of 10:10:9 in a 96-well plate. Then, 20 µL of tyrosinase was added and incubated at room temperature for between 10 and 30 minutes. Absorbance was measured at 490 nm after incubation.

4.5. Kinetic Study Against Mushroom Tyrosinase

The inhibition type was determined using a Lineweaver–Burk plot [53]. The apparent slope (K_{mapp}/V_{maxapp}) and intercept ($1/V_{maxapp}$) versus different inhibitor concentrations was used to determine the inhibition constant (K_i) [54]. Different kinetic parameters were obtained for different concentrations of the substrate (0.5, 0.75, and 1 mM) and inhibitors (compound 1—0.0, 4.0, 6.6, and 9.3 µM; compound 3—0, 2.5, 2.6, and 2.7 µM). Sigmaplot version 12.0 (SPSS Inc., Chicago, IL, USA) was employed to generate the plots.

4.6. Molecular Docking Simulation of Mushroom Tyrosinase

Molecular docking analysis was carried out using the procedure described [55] in AutoDock 4.2. Structures for L-tyrosine (6057) and luteolin (5280445) were obtained from the PubChem compound database. The three-dimensional (3D) structures of the bromophenol compounds were generated by Marvin Sketch (v17.1.30, ChemAxon, Budapest, Hungary). Docking results were visualized and analyzed using PyMOL (v1.7.4, Schrödinger, LLC, Cambridge, MA) and Discovery Studio (v16.1, Accelrys, San Diego, CA, USA).

4.7. Cell Culture and Viability Assay

B16F10 mouse melanoma cells obtained from American Type Culture Collection (Manassas, VA, USA) were maintained in 10% FBS in high-glucose DMEM containing 100 U/mL penicillin and 100 µg/mL streptomycin at 37 °C in a humidified atmosphere with 5% CO_2. Cytotoxicity was evaluated using a 3-(4,5-dimethylthiazol-2-yl)-2,5-diphenyltetrazolium bromide (MTT) assay. After 95% of confluence, B16F10 cells were seeded in a 96-well plate at 10,000 cells/well and incubated for 24 h in DMEM supplemented with 10% FBS. The cells were then fed fresh serum-free DMEM containing different concentrations (25 to 100 µM) of the test compounds and incubated for 48 h. After that, the cells were incubated with 100 µL of MTT at a concentration of 0.5 µg/mL in phosphate-buffered saline (PBS) for 2 h. Absorbance was measured at 490 nm by a microplate reader (Promega Corporation Instrument, USA) after 2 h of incubation. The viability of cells at 48 h upon co-treatment with α-MSH was evaluated by treating cells with 5 µM α-MSH 1 h after the treatment with test compounds.

4.8. Melanin Content Assay

Intracellular melanin content was determined according to a previously reported procedure [56] with minor modifications. Briefly, B16F10 cells were seeded in a 24-well plate at 2 × 10,000 cells/well and incubated for 24 h in DMEM containing 10% FBS. Cells were pretreated with 6.25, 12.5, and 25 µM test compounds for 1 h and stimulated with 5 µM α-MSH for 48 h. Arbutin (500 µM) was used as a positive control. The cells were washed with PBS and dissolved in 1 N NaOH containing 10% DMSO by boiling at 80 °C for 30 min. The cell lysates were centrifuged at 14,000 rpm for 20 min, and absorbance of the supernatant was measured at 405 nm. Melanin content was determined by normalizing the absorbance with total protein content.

4.9. Cellular Tyrosinase Assay

Intracellular tyrosinase inhibitory activity was evaluated by measuring the rate of oxidation of L-DOPA [57]. Briefly, $2 \times 10{,}000$ cells/well were seeded and incubated for 24 h in a 6-well plate and treated with various concentrations of bromophenols (6.25, 12.5, and 25 μM) or arbutin (500 μM) for 1 h, then stimulated with α-MSH (5 μM) for 48 h. The cells were washed with PBS and lysed with a radio immunoprecipitation assay buffer. The cell lysates were kept in a deep freezer ($-80\ ^\circ C$) for 1 h. After defrosting the cell lysates, the cellular extracts were purified by centrifugation at 14,000 rpm for 20 min at $4\ ^\circ C$, and the supernatant was used as cellular tyrosinase solution. A total of 80 μL of supernatant and 20 μL of L-DOPA (2 mg/mL) were added to a 96-well plate and incubated at $37\ ^\circ C$ for 45 min. Dopachrome formation was then measured spectrophotometrically at 450 nm using a microplate spectrophotometer (Molecular Devices). Intracellular tyrosinase activity was calculated as the percentage of control.

4.10. Determination of Tyrosinase Protein Levels via Western Blotting

After stimulating B16F10 cells with α-MSH in the presence or the absence of test bromophenols and arbutin for the indicated times, the cells were washed with ice-cold PBS and harvested using a cell scraper. The cell suspensions were centrifuged at $16{,}000 \times g$ for 5 min, and the cell pellets were lysed in a lysis buffer and incubated on ice for 10 min. The cell lysates were centrifuged at $16{,}000 \times g$ for 10 min, and the supernatant (total protein) was normalized using a Bradford protein assay kit. Aliquots of protein were resolved by sodium dodecyl sulfate-polyacrylamide gel electrophoresis and transferred onto a nitrocellulose membrane. The membrane was blocked with 10% nonfat milk (w/v) in tris-buffered saline with tween (TBST) (0.1 M Tris-HCl, pH 7.5, 1.5 M NaCl, 1% Tween20) for 2 h and incubated for approximately 24 h with TYR primary antibody. The immunoblots were then incubated with appropriate secondary antibodies for 2 h and detected using an enhanced chemiluminescence detection kit.

4.11. Statistical Analysis

One-way ANOVA and a Student's t-test (Systat Inc., Evanston, IL, USA) were used to determine statistical significance. Values of $p < 0.05$, 0.01, 0.001, and 0.0001 were considered significant. All results are presented as the mean ± SD of triplicate experiments.

5. Conclusions

The present study revealed that, among three bromophenols isolated from the marine alga *S. latiuscula*, compound **3** followed by **1** exhibited potent competitive tyrosinase inhibition against L-tyrosine substrate. A molecular docking simulation of the catalytic residue revealed the underlying inhibitory mechanism. In addition, compounds **1** and **3** inhibited cellular tyrosinase activity, decreased tyrosinase protein expression levels, and reduced the melanin content in α-MSH-treated B16F10 melanoma cells in a concentration-dependent manner. These results suggest that the increased number of bromine groups in the compound is associated with significant mushroom tyrosinase inhibitory activity. Overall, the strong tyrosinase inhibitory activity exhibited by the bromophenols isolated from *S. latiuscula* makes the alga a possible source for depigmenting agents in cosmetology.

Author Contributions: P.P. participated in study design, isolation, cell-based assays, and wrote some part and revised the manuscript. A.W. performed enzyme assays and drafted the manuscript. S.H.S. performed the molecular docking studies and wrote part of manuscript. H.J.P. collected plant material. H.A.J. was involved in spectral analysis, statistical analysis and wrote part of the manuscript. J.S.C. conceived the study, coordinated the study and interpreted the data. All authors read and approved the final manuscript.

Acknowledgments: This research was supported by the Basic Science Research Program through the National Research Foundation of Korea (NRF) funded by the Ministry of Science and ICT (2012R1A6A1028677).

Conflicts of Interest: The authors declare no conflict of interest.

References

1. Rajapakse, N.; Kim, S.K. Nutritional and digestive health benefits of seaweed. In *Advances in Food and Nutrition Research*; Kim, S.-K., Ed.; Elsevier: San Diego, CA, USA, 2011; Volume 64, pp. 17–28.
2. Suleria, H.; Osborne, S.; Masci, P.; Gobe, G. Marine-based nutraceuticals: An innovative trend in the food and supplement industries. *Mar. Drugs* **2015**, *13*, 6336–6351. [CrossRef]
3. Wells, M.L.; Potin, P.; Craigie, J.S.; Raven, J.A.; Merchant, S.S.; Helliwell, K.E.; Smith, A.G.; Camire, M.E.; Brawley, S.H. Algae as nutritional and functional food sources: Revisiting our understanding. *J. Appl. Phycol.* **2017**, *29*, 949–982. [CrossRef]
4. Jeon, Y.J.; Samarakoon, K.W.; Elvitigala, D.A. Marine-derived pharmaceuticals and future prospects. In *Springer Handbook of Marine Biotechnology*; Springer-Verlag Berlin Heidelberg: Berlin, Germany, 2015; pp. 957–968.
5. Siahaan, E.A.; Pangestuti, R.; Kim, S.K. Seaweeds: Valuable ingredients for the pharmaceutical industries. In *Grand Challenges in Marine Biotechnology*; Springer International Publishing AG: Cham, Switzerland, 2018; pp. 49–95.
6. Thomas, N.; Kim, S.K. Beneficial effects of marine algal compounds in cosmeceuticals. *Mar. Drugs* **2013**, *11*, 146–164. [CrossRef]
7. Lerner, A.B.; Fitzpatrick, T.B. Treatment of melanin hyperpigmentation. *JAMA* **1953**, *152*, 577–582. [CrossRef]
8. Rigopoulos, D.; Gregoriou, S.; Katsambas, A. Hyperpigmentation and melasma. *J. Cosmet. Dermatol.* **2007**, *6*, 195–202. [CrossRef]
9. Brown, D.A. Skin pigmentation enhancers. In *Comprehensive Series in Photosciences*; Elsevier Science: Amsterdam, The Netherlands, 2001; Volume 3, pp. 637–675.
10. Costin, G.E.; Hearing, V.J. Human skin pigmentation: Melanocytes modulate skin color in response to stress. *FASEB J.* **2007**, *21*, 976–994. [CrossRef]
11. Cichorek, M.; Wachulska, M.; Stasiewicz, A.; Tymińska, A. Skin melanocytes: Biology and development. *Postepy. Dermatol. Alergol.* **2013**, *30*, 30. [CrossRef]
12. Tsatmali, M.; Ancans, J.; Thody, A.J. Melanocyte function and its control by melanocortin peptides. *J. Histochem. Cytochem.* **2002**, *50*, 125–133. [CrossRef]
13. Kobayashi, T.; Urabe, K.; Winder, A.; Jiménez-Cervantes, C.; Imokawa, G.; Brewington, T.; Solano, F.; García-Borrón, J.; Hearing, V. Tyrosinase related protein 1 (TRP1) functions as a DHICA oxidase in melanin biosynthesis. *EMBO J.* **1994**, *13*, 5818–5825. [CrossRef]
14. Körner, A.M.; Pawelek, J. Dopachrome conversion: A possible control point in melanin biosynthesis. *J. Invest. Dermatol.* **1980**, *75*, 192–195. [CrossRef]
15. Steel, K.; Davidson, D.R.; Jackson, I. TRP-2/DT, a new early melanoblast marker, shows that steel growth factor (c-kit ligand) is a survival factor. *Development* **1992**, *115*, 1111–1119. [PubMed]
16. Valencia, J.C.; Watabe, H.; Chi, A.; Rouzaud, F.; Chen, K.G.; Vieira, W.D.; Takahashi, K.; Yamaguchi, Y.; Berens, W.; Nagashima, K. Sorting of Pmel17 to melanosomes through the plasma membrane by AP1 and AP2: Evidence for the polarized nature of melanocytes. *J. Cell Sci.* **2006**, *119*, 1080–1091. [CrossRef]
17. Kawakami, Y.; Robbins, P.F.; Wang, R.F.; Parkhurst, M.; Kang, X.; Rosenberg, S.A. The use of melanosomal proteins in the immunotherapy of melanoma. *J. Immunother.* **1998**, *21*, 237–246. [CrossRef]
18. Bertolotto, C.; Abbe, P.; Hemesath, T.J.; Bille, K.; Fisher, D.E.; Ortonne, J.P.; Ballotti, R. Microphthalmia gene product as a signal transducer in cAMP-induced differentiation of melanocytes. *J. Cell Biol.* **1998**, *142*, 827–835. [CrossRef]
19. Levy, C.; Khaled, M.; Fisher, D.E. MITF: Master regulator of melanocyte development and melanoma oncogene. *Trends Mol. Med.* **2006**, *12*, 406–414. [CrossRef]
20. Shibahara, S.; Yasumoto, K.I.; Amae, S.; Udono, T.; Watanabe, K.I.; Saito, H.; Takeda, K. Regulation of pigment cell-specific gene expression by MITF. *Pigment Cell Res.* **2000**, *13*, 98–102. [CrossRef]
21. Fitzpatrick, T.B.; Becker, S.W.; Lerner, A.B.; Montgomery, H. Tyrosinase in human skin: Demonstration of its presence and of its role in human melanin formation. *Science* **1950**, *112*, 223–225. [CrossRef]
22. Ortonne, J.P. Photoprotective properties of skin melanin. *Br. J. Dermatol.* **2002**, *146*, 7–10. [CrossRef]
23. Pomerantz, S.H.; Warner, M.C. 3,4-Dihydroxy-L-phenylalanine as the tyrosinase cofactor occurrence in melanoma and binding constant. *J. Biol. Chem.* **1967**, *242*, 5308–5314. [PubMed]
24. Riley, P. Melanin. *Int. J. Biochem. Cell Biol.* **1997**, *29*, 1235–1239. [CrossRef]

25. Cha, S.H.; Ko, S.C.; Kim, D.; Jeon, Y.J. Screening of marine algae for potential tyrosinase inhibitor: Those inhibitors reduced tyrosinase activity and melanin synthesis in zebrafish. *J. Dermatol.* **2011**, *38*, 354–363. [CrossRef]
26. Wang, H.M.D.; Chen, C.C.; Huynh, P.; Chang, J.S. Exploring the potential of using algae in cosmetics. *Bioresour. Technol.* **2015**, *184*, 355–362. [CrossRef] [PubMed]
27. Kang, H.S.; Kim, H.R.; Byun, D.S.; Son, B.W.; Nam, T.J.; Choi, J.S. Tyrosinase inhibitors isolated from the edible brown alga *Ecklonia stolonifera*. *Arch. Pharm. Res.* **2004**, *27*, 1226–1232. [CrossRef] [PubMed]
28. Yoon, N.Y.; Eom, T.K.; Kim, M.M.; Kim, S.K. Inhibitory effect of phlorotannins isolated from *Ecklonia cava* on mushroom tyrosinase activity and melanin formation in mouse B16F10 melanoma cells. *J. Agric. Food Chem.* **2009**, *57*, 4124–4129. [CrossRef] [PubMed]
29. Heo, S.J.; Ko, S.C.; Cha, S.H.; Kang, D.H.; Park, H.S.; Choi, Y.U.; Kim, D.; Jung, W.K.; Jeon, Y.J. Effect of phlorotannins isolated from *Ecklonia cava* on melanogenesis and their protective effect against photo-oxidative stress induced by UV-B radiation. *Toxicol. In Vitro* **2009**, *23*, 1123–1130. [CrossRef]
30. Matos, M.J.; Santana, L.; Uriarte, E.; Delogu, G.; Corda, M.; Fadda, M.B.; Era, B.; Fais, A. New halogenated phenylcoumarins as tyrosinase inhibitors. *Bioorg. Med. Chem. Lett.* **2011**, *21*, 3342–3345. [CrossRef]
31. Ismail, T.; Shafi, S.; Srinivas, J.; Sarkar, D.; Qurishi, Y.; Khazir, J.; Alam, M.S.; Kumar, H.M.S. Synthesis and tyrosinase inhibition activity of trans-stilbene derivatives. *Bioorg. Chem.* **2016**, *64*, 97–102. [CrossRef] [PubMed]
32. Onul, N.; Ertik, O.; Mermer, N.; Yanardag, R. Synthesis and biological evaluation of S-substituted perhalo-2-nitrobuta-1,3-dienes as novel xanthine oxidase, tyrosinase, elastase, and neuraminidase inhibitors. *J. Chem.* **2018**, *2018*. [CrossRef]
33. Xu, X.; Yang, H.; Khalil, Z.; Yin, L.; Xiao, X.; Neupane, P.; Bernhardt, P.; Salim, A.; Song, F.; Capon, R. Chemical diversity from a Chinese marine red alga, *Symphyocladia latiuscula*. *Mar. Drugs* **2017**, *15*, 374. [CrossRef] [PubMed]
34. Huang, H.L.; Wang, B.G. Antioxidant capacity and lipophilic content of seaweeds collected from the Qingdao coastline. *J. Agric. Food Chem.* **2004**, *52*, 4993–4997. [CrossRef]
35. Kang, H.S.; Chung, H.Y.; Kim, J.Y.; Son, B.W.; Jung, H.A.; Choi, J.S. Inhibitory phlorotannins from the edible brown alga *Ecklonia stolonifera* on total reactive oxygen species (ROS) generation. *Arch. Pharm. Res.* **2004**, *27*, 194–198. [CrossRef]
36. Choi, J.S.; Park, H.J.; Jung, H.A.; Chung, H.Y.; Jung, J.H.; Choi, W.C. A cyclohexanonyl bromophenol from the red alga *Symphyocladia latiuscula*. *J. Nat. Prod.* **2000**, *63*, 1705–1706. [CrossRef] [PubMed]
37. Duan, X.J.; Li, X.M.; Wang, B.G. Highly brominated mono-and bis-phenols from the marine red alga *Symphyocladia latiuscula* with radical-scavenging activity. *J. Nat. Prod.* **2007**, *70*, 1210–1213. [CrossRef] [PubMed]
38. Xu, X.; Yin, L.; Gao, L.; Gao, J.; Chen, J.; Li, J.; Song, F. Two new bromophenols with radical scavenging activity from marine red alga *Symphyocladia latiuscula*. *Mar. Drugs* **2013**, *11*, 842–847. [CrossRef] [PubMed]
39. Chung, H.Y.; Choi, H.R.; Park, H.J.; Choi, J.S.; Choi, W.C. Peroxynitrite scavenging and cytoprotective activity of 2,3,6 tribromo-4,5-dihydroxybenzyl methyl ether from the marine alga *Symphyocladia latiuscula*. *J. Agric. Food Chem.* **2001**, *49*, 3614–3621. [CrossRef]
40. Choi, J.S.; Bae, H.J.; Kim, S.J.; Choi, I.S. In vitro antibacterial and anti-inflammatory properties of seaweed extracts against acne inducing bacteria, *Propionibacterium acnes*. *J. Environ. Biol.* **2011**, *32*, 313.
41. Xu, X.; Yin, L.; Wang, Y.; Wang, S.; Song, F. A new bromobenzyl methyl sulphoxide from marine red alga *Symphyocladia latiuscula*. *Nat. Prod. Res.* **2013**, *27*, 723–726. [CrossRef]
42. Xu, X.; Yin, L.; Gao, J.; Gao, L.; Song, F. Antifungal bromophenols from marine red alga *Symphyocladia latiuscula*. *Chem. Biodivers.* **2014**, *11*, 807–811. [CrossRef]
43. Park, H.J.; Kurokawa, M.; Shiraki, K.; Nakamura, N.; Choi, J.S.; Hattori, M. Antiviral activity of the marine alga *Symphyocladia latiuscula* against herpes simplex virus (HSV-1) in vitro and its therapeutic efficacy against HSV-1 infection in mice. *Biol. Pharm. Bull.* **2005**, *28*, 2258–2262. [CrossRef]
44. Paudel, P.; Seong, S.H.; Park, H.J.; Jung, H.A.; Choi, J.S. Anti-diabetic activity of 2,3,6-tribromo-4,5-dihydroxybenzyl derivatives from *Symphyocladia latiuscula* through PTP1B downregulation and α-glucosidase inhibition. *Mar. Drugs* **2019**, *17*, 166. [CrossRef]
45. Wang, W.; Okada, Y.; Shi, H.; Wang, Y.; Okuyama, T. Structures and aldose reductase inhibitory effects of bromophenols from the red alga *Symphyocladia latiuscula*. *J. Nat. Prod.* **2005**, *68*, 620–622. [CrossRef]

46. Jin, H.J.; Oh, M.Y.; Jin, D.H.; Hong, Y.K. Identification of a Taq DNA polymerase inhibitor from the red seaweed *Symphyocladia latiuscula*. *J. Environ. Biol.* **2008**, *29*, 475–478.
47. Lee, J.H.; Park, S.E.; Hossain, M.A.; Kim, M.Y.; Kim, M.N.; Chung, H.Y.; Choi, J.S.; Yoo, Y.H.; Kim, N.D. 2,3,6-Tribromo-4,5-dihydroxybenzyl methyl ether induces growth inhibition and apoptosis in MCF-7 human breast cancer cells. *Arch. Pharm. Res.* **2007**, *30*, 1132–1137. [CrossRef] [PubMed]
48. De Vries, D.J.; Beart, P.M. Fishing for drugs from the sea: Status and strategies. *Trends Pharmacol. Sci.* **1995**, *16*, 275–279. [CrossRef]
49. Guillerme, J.B.; Couteau, C.; Coiffard, L. Applications for marine resources in cosmetics. *Cosmetics* **2017**, *4*, 35. [CrossRef]
50. Kim, S.K. Marine cosmeceuticals. *J. Cosmet. Dermatol.* **2014**, *13*, 56–67. [CrossRef] [PubMed]
51. Seo, Y.W.; Yoo, J.S. Screening for antioxidizing and tyrosinase-inhibitory activities of the extracts of marine algae from Busan coastal area. *Ocean Polar Res.* **2003**, *25*, 129–132. [CrossRef]
52. Wagle, A.; Seong, S.H.; Joung, E.J.; Kim, H.R.; Jung, H.A.; Choi, J.S. Discovery of a highly potent tyrosinase inhibitor, luteolin 5-*O*-β-D-glucopyranoside, isolated from *Cirsium japonicum* var. *maackii* (Maxim.) Matsum., Korean thistle: Kinetics and computational molecular docking simulation. *ACS Omega* **2018**, *3*, 17236–17245.
53. Lineweaver, H.; Burk, D. The determination of enzyme dissociation constants. *J. Am. Chem. Soc.* **1934**, *56*, 658–666. [CrossRef]
54. Kim, J.H.; Morgan, A.M.; Tai, B.H.; Van, D.T.; Cuong, N.M.; Kim, Y.H. Inhibition of soluble epoxide hydrolase activity by compounds isolated from the aerial parts of *Glycosmis stenocarpa*. *J. Enzyme Inhib. Med. Chem.* **2016**, *31*, 640–644. [CrossRef]
55. Wagle, A.; Seong, S.H.; Jung, H.A.; Choi, J.S. Identifying an isoflavone from the root of *Pueraria lobata* as a potent tyrosinase inhibitor. *Food Chem.* **2019**, *276*, 383–389. [CrossRef] [PubMed]
56. Azam, M.S.; Kwon, M.; Choi, J.; Kim, H.R. Sargaquinoic acid ameliorates hyperpigmentation through cAMP and ERK-mediated downregulation of MITF in α-MSH-stimulated B16F10 cells. *Biomed. Pharmacother.* **2018**, *104*, 582–589. [CrossRef] [PubMed]
57. Bae, S.J.; Ha, Y.M.; Kim, J.A.; Park, J.Y.; Ha, T.K.; Park, D.; Chun, P.; Park, N.H.; Moon, H.R.; Chung, H.Y. A novel synthesized tyrosinase inhibitor: (E)-2-((2,4-dihydroxyphenyl) diazenyl) phenyl 4-methylbenzenesulfonate as an azo-resveratrol analog. *Biosci. Biotechnol. Biochem.* **2013**, *77*, 65–72. [CrossRef] [PubMed]

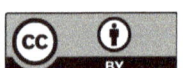

© 2019 by the authors. Licensee MDPI, Basel, Switzerland. This article is an open access article distributed under the terms and conditions of the Creative Commons Attribution (CC BY) license (http://creativecommons.org/licenses/by/4.0/).

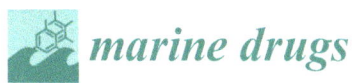

Article

Effects of Fucoidans from Five Different Brown Algae on Oxidative Stress and VEGF Interference in Ocular Cells

Philipp Dörschmann [1], Kaya Saskia Bittkau [2], Sandesh Neupane [2], Johann Roider [1], Susanne Alban [2] and Alexa Klettner [1,*]

1. Department of Ophthalmology, University Medical Center, University of Kiel, Arnold-Heller-Str. 3, Haus 25, 24105 Kiel, Germany; Philipp.Doerschmann@uksh.de (P.D.); johann.roider@uksh.de (J.R.)
2. Department of Pharmaceutical Biology, Pharmaceutical Institute, University of Kiel, Gutenbergstraße 76, 24118 Kiel, Germany; kbittkau@pharmazie.uni-kiel.de (K.S.B.); sneupane@pharmazie.uni-kiel.de (S.N.); salban@pharmazie.uni-kiel.de (S.A.)
* Correspondence: alexakarina.klettner@uksh.de; Tel.: +49-431-500-24283

Received: 20 March 2019; Accepted: 25 April 2019; Published: 30 April 2019

Abstract: Background: Fucoidans are interesting for potential usage in ophthalmology, and especially age-related macular degeneration. However, fucoidans from different species may vary in their effects. Here, we compare fucoidans from five algal species in terms of oxidative stress protection and vascular endothelial growth factor (VEGF) interference in ocular cells. Methods: Brown algae (*Fucus vesiculosus*, *Fucus distichus* subsp. *evanescens*, *Fucus serratus*, *Laminaria digitata*, *Saccharina latissima*) were harvested and fucoidans isolated by hot-water extraction. Fucoidans were tested in several concentrations (1, 10, 50, and 100 µg/mL). Effects were measured on a uveal melanoma cell line (OMM-1) (oxidative stress), retinal pigment epithelium (RPE) cell line ARPE19 (oxidative stress and VEGF), and primary RPE cells (VEGF). Oxidative stress was induced by H_2O_2 or tert-Butyl hydroperoxide (TBHP). Cell viability was investigated with methyl thiazolyl tetrazolium (MTT or MTS) assay, and VEGF secretion with ELISA. Affinity to VEGF was determined by a competitive binding assay. Results: All fucoidans protected OMM-1 from oxidative stress. However, in ARPE19, only fucoidan from *Saccharina latissima* was protective. The affinity to VEGF of all fucoidans was stronger than that of heparin, and all reduced VEGF secretion in ARPE19. In primary RPE, only the fucoidan from *Saccharina latissima* was effective. Conclusion: Among the fucoidans from five different species, *Saccharina latissima* displayed the most promising results concerning oxidative stress protection and reduction of VEGF secretion.

Keywords: fucoidan; age-related macular degeneration; VEGF; oxidative stress; *Saccharina latissima*; *Fucus vesiculosus*; *Fucus distichus* subsp. *evanescens*; *Fucus serratus*; *Laminaria digitata*

1. Introduction

Fucoidans are sulfated polysaccharides found in the cell walls of brown algae. Common to all fucoidans is a high amount of L-fucose, yet their structures are complex and variable among different species [1]. Fucoidans have been described as exerting interesting pharmacological activities including, e.g., anti-inflammatory, antitumorigenic, and anti-angiogenic effects [1,2]. In particular, a fucoidan has been found to be potentially beneficial in age-related macular degeneration (AMD), the most common cause of blindness and severe vision loss in the Western world [3,4]. AMD is a disease of the elderly in which photoreceptors and retinal pigment epithelial cells of the macula, the area of high acuity vision, degenerate, and, in the more severe exudative subtype of the disease (wet AMD), vessels grow from the choroid under and into the retina. These immature vessels are leaky and lead to fluid accumulation and tissue destruction. The pathogenesis of AMD is complex and not fully elucidated. It is a multifactorial disease and several factors are involved in its pathogenesis. The most important ones are oxidative stress and, in wet AMD, the secretion of vascular endothelial growth factor (VEGF) by cells of the retinal pigment epithelium (RPE) [5–7]. Other factors such as impaired complement regulation, lipid dysregulation, and inflammation are also of importance for AMD development [8–10]. Currently, there is no cure for AMD, and the only treatment options are VEGF inhibitors, which need to be regularly injected in the eye [11]. Although these inhibitors have been a great progress in AMD therapy, long-term treatment usually cannot keep up the initial beneficial effects, and may lead to macular atrophy [12,13]. New treatment options would, therefore, be of great benefit.

Fucoidan could be of interest for the development of new AMD therapeutics, since it has been described to be anti-inflammatory, blood lipid-reducing and, most importantly, protective against oxidative stress and VEGF-inhibiting [4].

Our group has previously shown that commercially available fucoidan (from *Fucus vesiculosus*) exhibits interesting effects on RPE cells including reduction of VEGF secretion and reduction of angiogenesis [3]. However, the commercially available fucoidan is poorly defined, with pronounced variability in structural composition and degree of purity between batches [14,15]. Furthermore, fucoidans from different species differ in their composition and may thus exert different biological effects. This renders the search for the most suitable fucoidan for specific applications such as AMD an important quest [4,16].

In the current study, we compared the fucoidans of five species of brown algae (*Saccharina latissima* (SL), *Laminaria digitata* (LD), *Fucus serratus* (FS), *Fucus vesiculosus* (FV), and *Fucus distichus* subsp. *evanescens* (FE) in terms of two important factors for AMD development, i.e., oxidative stress and VEGF secretion in ocular cells, as well as their binding affinity to VEGF. For this comparison, the algal material of all five species were harvested in summer, identically prepared, and then extracted according to the same standardized protocol, leading to the fucoidans SL, LD, FS, FV, and FE.

2. Results

2.1. Oxidative Stress Protection

2.1.1. OMM-1 Cells

The potency of oxidative stress protection of the fucoidan from five different algae species was compared in two different systems. We have previously shown that commercial fucoidan from *Fucus vesiculosus* protected several uveal melanoma cells, including OMM-1, from oxidative stress induced by H_2O_2 [17]. In this study, we used the uveal melanoma cell line OMM-1.

Prior to the experiments with fucoidans, the concentration of H_2O_2 causing about 50% cell death had to be evaluated. While the concentrations of 100 µM (78.67 ± 13.22%), 200 µM (85.67 ± 17.02%) and 400 µM (81.00 ± 15.51%) showed no effect on cell survival, 1000 µM displayed a significant reduction of cell viability compared to the control (1000 µM 58.33 ± 17.98%, $p < 0.05$) (Figure 1a). A concentration of 1000 µM H_2O_2 was therefore chosen for the following experiments.

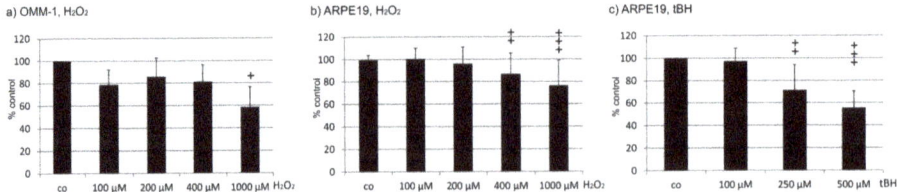

Figure 1. Characterization of the susceptibility of cell lines to oxidative stress. Cell viability was tested in OMM-1 (**a**) and ARPE19 (**b**) exposed to H_2O_2 (**a,b**) and tert-Butyl hydroperoxide (TBHP) (**c**). Significance was evaluated with Friedman's ANOVA and Student's *t*-test, + $p < 0.05$, ++ $p < 0.01$, +++ $p < 0.001$ compared to control ($n > 3$).

In the experiments concerning the fucoidan from *Saccharina latissima*, incubation of OMM-1 treated with 1 mM H_2O_2 and SL fucoidan induced significant changes according to ANOVA testing. Incubation with 1 mM H_2O_2 resulted in a reduction of cell viability to 68.75% (±5.07). Incubation with 1 µg/mL induced no significant protection (72.00 ± 3.04%), while 10 µg/mL, 50 µg/mL, as well as 100 µg/mL all significantly increased cell viability (92.13 ± 3.41%; 93.00 ± 3.57%, and 85.88 ± 7.03%, respectively; all $p < 0.001$) (Figure 2a). In the experiments testing fucoidan from *Laminaria digitata*, incubation with 1 mM H_2O_2 reduced cell viability to 57.50% (±2.29). The differences between the groups treated with LD fucoidan were significant in ANOVA testing. Incubations with any concentration of LD fucoidan tested resulted in a highly significant protection of cell viability (all $p < 0.001$) (1 µg/mL 83.25 ± 3.60%; 10 µg/mL 101.75 ± 4.71%; 50 µg/mL 100.88 ± 5.51%; 100 µg/mL 92.75 ± 7.03%) (Figure 2b). Testing fucoidan from *Fucus serratus*, incubation with 1 mM H_2O_2 resulted in a reduction of cell viability to 39.00% (±3.67). In ANOVA testing, significant differences between the groups could be detected. FS fucoidan increased cell viability significantly, but viability remained considerably low (1 µg/mL 45.25 ± 3.35%, $p < 0.01$; 10 µg/mL 59.88 ± 3.02%, $p < 0.001$; 50 µg/mL 58.63 ± 5.10%, $p < 0.001$; 100 µg/mL 52.38 ± 5.87% $p < 0.001$) (Figure 2c). When testing the fucoidan from *Fucus vesiculosus*, incubation with 1 mM H_2O_2 resulted in a reduction of cell viability to 63.50% (±2.60). In ANOVA testing, significant differences between the groups could be detected. All concentrations of FV fucoidan resulted in a significantly increased viability of cells (1 µg/mL 75.75 ± 10.50%, $p < 0.01$; 10 µg/mL 97.88 ± 14.93%, $p < 0.001$; 50 µg/mL 96.36 ± 13.30%, $p < 0.001$; 100 µg/mL 87.88 ± 11.13%, $p < 0.001$) (Figure 2d). Finally, when testing the fucoidan from *Fucus distichus* subsp. *evanescens*, incubation with 1 mM H_2O_2 resulted in a reduction of cell viability to 36.50% (±8.44). In ANOVA testing, significant differences between the groups could be detected. FE fucoidan significantly increased viability when used at 1–50 µg/mL (1 µg/mL 54.38 ± 18.00%, $p < 0.05$: 10 µg/mL 69.5 ± 17.43%, $p < 0.001$; 50 µg/mL 62.00 ± 18.10%, $p < 0.01$) but not at 100 µg/mL (55.00 ± 22.63%) (Figure 2e).

Taken together, all fucoidans were protective against oxidative stress-induced reduction of viability, and all showed a similar pattern, with the highest viability rates at 10 and 50 µg/mL. However, the fucoidans displayed significant differences when their effects were compared. LD fucoidan clearly showed the strongest protective effect, which was significantly higher than that of SL (for 1 and 10 µg/mL $p < 0.001$; 50 µg/mL $p < 0.001$), significantly higher than that of FE (1 µg/mL $p < 0.01$; 10–100 µg/mL $p < 0.001$), and significantly higher than FS (all $p < 0.001$). FV was significantly more effective than FE (1 µg/mL $p < 0.05$; 10–100 µg/mL $p < 0.01$) and significantly more effective than FS (all $p < 0.001$). Finally, SL was significantly more protective than FE (1 µg/mL $p < 0.05$; 10 µg/mL $p < 0.01$; 50 µg/mL $p < 0.001$; 100 µg/mL $p < 0.01$) and more protective than FS (all $p < 0.001$). FE and FS, however, displayed no statistically significant differences (Table 1). Ranging the protective effect, LD > FV > SL > FE > FS.

Table 1. Comparison of the protective effects of the different fucoidans at different concentrations against oxidative stress cell death in OMM-1 cells induced with 1 mM H_2O_2.

Compared Fucoidans	1 µg/mL	10 µg/mL	50 µg/mL	100 µg/mL
LD vs. FV	not significant (ns)	ns	ns	ns
LD vs. SL	$p < 0.001$	$p < 0.001$	$p < 0.01$	ns
LD vs. FE	$p < 0.05$	$p < 0.001$	$p < 0.001$	$p < 0.001$
LD vs. FS	$p < 0.001$	$p < 0.001$	$p < 0.001$	$p < 0.001$
FV vs. SL	ns	ns	ns	ns
FV vs. FE	$p < 0.05$	$p < 0.01$	$p < 0.01$	$p < 0.01$
FV vs. FS	$p < 0.001$	$p < 0.001$	$p < 0.001$	$p < 0.001$
SL vs. FE	$p < 0.05$	$p < 0.01$	$p < 0.001$	$p < 0.01$
SL vs. FS	$p < 0.001$	$p < 0.001$	$p < 0.001$	$p < 0.001$
FE vs. FS	ns	ns	ns	ns

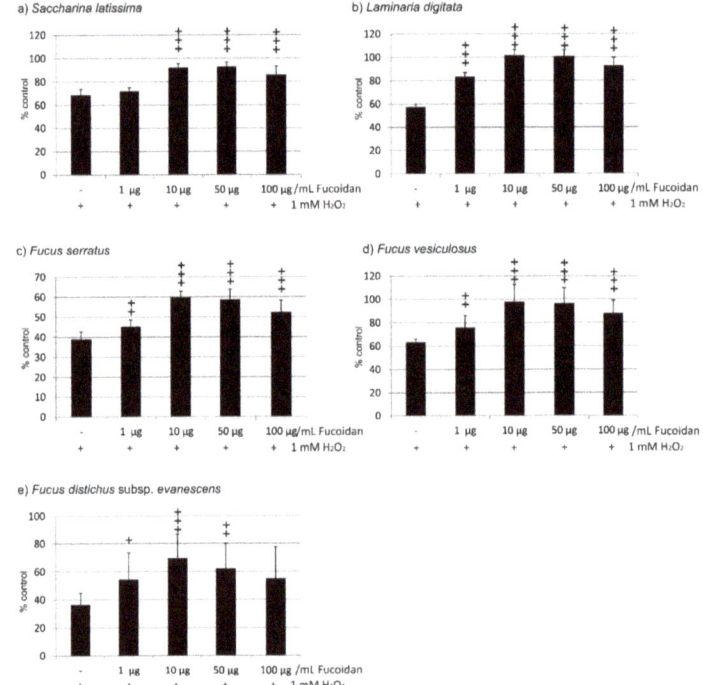

Figure 2. Cell viability of OMM-1 cells challenged with 1 mM H_2O_2 after incubation with fucoidan from (**a**) *Saccharina latissima* (SL), (**b**) *Laminaria digitata* (LD), (**c**) *Fucus serratus* (FS), (**d**) *Fucus vesiculosus* (FV), (**e**) *Fucus distichus* subsp. *evanescens* (FE). Cell viability was measured by MTS assay and is depicted as mean and standard deviation, with the control set as 100%. All fucoidans tested displayed protective effects, with the efficacy of LD > FV > SL > FE > FS. Significance was evaluated with Friedman's ANOVA and subsequent Student's *t*-test, + $p < 0.05$, ++ $p < 0.01$, +++ $p < 0.001$, all versus 1 mM H_2O_2 ($n = 8$).

2.1.2. ARPE19 Cells

ARPE19 cells are an immortal RPE cell line. One important role of RPE cells is protection against oxidative stress [18]. We tested the appropriate concentration of H_2O_2 for the following experiments, but ARPE19 cells turned out to be rather resistant to oxidative stress induced by hydrogen peroxide, which is consistent with the literature [19]. Treatment with H_2O_2 induced a significant reduction in cell viability, detected in ANOVA. While incubation with 100 and 200 µM H_2O_2 did not induce any significant reduction in cell viability compared to the control (100 µM 11.45 ± 9.65%; 200 µM 96.07 ± 14.75%), 400 and 1000 µM H_2O_2 significantly reduced cell survival (400 µM 86.75 ± 18.62%, $p < 0.01$; 1000 µM 76.2 ± 22.74%, $p < 0.001$). However, none of these concentrations reduced cell survival to approximately 50% (Figure 1b). We then tested tert-Butyl hydroperoxide (TBHP) on ARPE19 cells, which induced a significant reduction in cell viability (detected in ANOVA) and showed a concentration-dependent effect with a significant reduction of cell viability at 500 µM (100 µM 97.24 ± 11.56%, 250 µM ± 22.66%; 500 µM 55.33 ± 15.3%) (Figure 1c). Therefore, for the following experiments, a concentration of 500 µM TBHP was chosen.

In the experiments concerning the fucoidan of *Saccharina latissima*, incubation with 500 µg/mL TBHP induced a reduction in cell viability to 48.50 ± 8.44%. ANOVA testing showed significant differences between the groups. Incubation with 1 µg/mL induced no significant protection (55.63 ± 14.48%), while 10 µg/mL, 50 µg/mL, and 100 µg/mL significantly increased cell viability (71.50 ± 13.37%, $p < 0.01$; 73.25 ± 12.59%, $p < 0.001$; 64.00 ± 9.46%, $p < 0.01$) (Figure 3a). In the experiments testing fucoidan from *Laminaria digitata*, incubation with 500 µg/mL TBHP induced a reduction in cell viability to 75.50 ± 8.20%. ANOVA testing showed statistically significant differences between the groups. However, none of the administered concentrations of fucoidan protected the cells against loss of cell viability (1 µg/mL 77.88 ± 10.40%; 10 µg/mL 79.38 ± 11.33%; 50 µg/mL 77.75 ± 12.94%; 100 µg/mL 72.50 ± 16.55%) (Figure 3b). Testing fucoidan from *Fucus serratus*, incubation with 500 µM TBHP resulted in a reduction of cell viability to 58.00% (±3.24). ANOVA testing showed statistically significant differences between the groups. Again, none of the tested concentrations of FS fucoidan conferred any protection. On the contrary, 10–100 µg/mL FS fucoidan significantly reduced the viability of the cells (1 µg/mL 54.50 ± 4.21%; 10 µg/mL 53.13 ± 3.18%, $p < 0.05$; 50 µg/mL 51.75 ± 3.56%, $p < 0.01$; 100 µg/mL 44.88 ± 6.27%. $p < 0.001$) (Figure 3c). When testing for fucoidan from *Fucus vesiculosus*, incubation with 500 mM TBHP resulted in a reduction of cell viability to 62.00% (±15.86). ANOVA testing showed statistically significant differences between groups. However, none of the tested concentrations of FV fucoidan induced a significant change in cell viability (1 µg/mL 70.88 ± 16.80%; 10 µg/mL 75.38 ± 16.43%; 50 µg/mL 77.50 ± 18.4%; 69.75 ± 17.69%) (Figure 3d). Finally, when testing fucoidan from *Fucus distichus* subsp. *evanescens*, incubation with 500 mM TBHP resulted in a reduction of cell viability to 63.50% (±4.33). ANOVA testing showed statistically significant differences between groups. While FE fucoidan in concentrations of 1 µg/mL (61.00 ± 3.08%) and 10 µg/mL (61.50 ± 4.06%) displayed no influence on cell viability, both 50 µg/mL and 100 µg/mL FE fucoidan significantly reduced cell viability (50 µg/mL 49.38 ± 4.99%; 100 µg/mL 45.00 ± 5.15%; both $p < 0.001$) (Figure 3e).

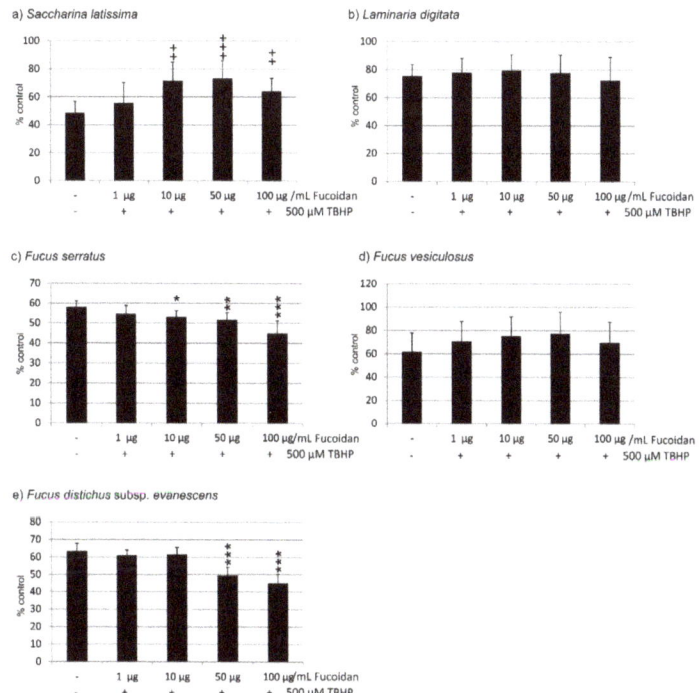

Figure 3. Cell viability of ARPE19 cells challenged with 500 µM TBHP after incubation with fucoidan from (**a**) *Saccharina latissima* (SL), (**b**) *Laminaria digitata* (LD), (**c**) *Fucus serratus* (FS), (**d**) *Fucus vesiculosus* (FV), (**e**) *Fucus distichus* subsp. *evanescens* (FE). Cell viability was measured by MTS assay and is depicted as mean and standard deviation, with the control set as 100%. Only SL fucoidan displayed a protective effect, while FS and FE fucoidans reduced cell viability. Significance was evaluated with Friedman's ANOVA and subsequent Student's *t*-test, ++ $p < 0.01$, +++ $p < 0.001$, for protective effects against 500 µM TBHP, * $p < 0.05$, ** $p < 0.01$ and *** $p < 0.001$ for exacerbating effects against 500 µM TBHP ($n = 8$).

Taken together, the results differ profoundly from those found with OMM-1 cells, with only *Saccharina latissima* showing protection, *Laminaria digitata* and *Fucus vesiculosus* displaying no influence, and *Fucus serratus* and *Fucus distichus* subsp. *evanescens* showing an additional toxic effect on the cells.

In direct comparison, SL fucoidan is significantly different from LD fucoidan (1 µg/mL; $p < 0.01$), from FS fucoidan (10 µg/mL ($p < 0.01$)–100 µg/mL ($p < 0.001$), and from FE fucoidan (50 µg/mL and 100 µg/mL, both $p < 0.001$). The differences between SD fucoidan and FV fucoidan are not significant. Similar results are obtained with LD fucoidan, which does not significantly differ from FV fucoidan, but does differ from FE fucoidan and FS fucoidan in all concentrations tested (FE: 1–10 µg/mL $p < 0.01$, 50–100 µg/mL $p < 0.001$; FS 1–50 µg/mL $p < 0.001$, 100 µg/mL $p < 0.01$). FV fucoidan differs from FE fucoidan at 10–100 µg/mL (10 µg/mL $p < 0.05$; 50–100 µg/mL $p < 0.01$) and from FS fucoidan at all concentrations (1 µg/mL $p < 0.05$, 10–100 µg/mL $p < 0.01$). FE fucoidan differs from FS fucoidan in the lower concentrations (1 µg/mL $p < 0.01$, 10 µg/mL $p < 0.001$) (Table 2).

Table 2. Comparison of the protective effects of the different fucoidans at different concentrations after oxidative stress cell death in ARPE19 cells induced by 500 µM TBHP.

Compared Fucoidans	1 µg/mL	10 µg/mL	50 µg/mL	100 µg/mL
LD vs. FV	ns	ns	ns	ns
LD vs. SL	$p < 0.01$	ns	ns	ns
LD vs. FE	$p < 0.01$	$p < 0.01$	$p < 0.001$	$p < 0.001$
LD vs. FS	$p < 0.001$	$p < 0.001$	$p < 0.001$	$p < 0.01$
FV vs. SL	ns	ns	ns	ns
FV vs. FE	ns	$p < 0.05$	$p < 0.01$	$p < 0.01$
FV vs. FS	$p < 0.05$	$p < 0.01$	$p < 0.01$	$p < 0.01$
SL vs. FE	ns	ns	$p < 0.001$	$p < 0.001$
SL vs. FS	ns	$p < 0.01$	$p < 0.001$	$p < 0.001$
FE vs. FS	$p < 0.01$	$p < 0.001$	ns	ns

2.2. VEGF Secretion

The effect of the five different fucoidans on the secretion of VEGF was compared in two different RPE cell types, the human cell line ARPE19 and primary RPE cells derived from porcine eyes. Untreated ARPE19 cells secreted considerably and significantly less VEGF, with a mean of 416.33 pg/mL (±415.27), in a collection time of 24 h compared to primary porcine RPE cells, which secreted a mean of 2386.88 pg/mL (±824.81) ($p < 0.001$) in a collection time of 4 h, as tested in ANOVA and subsequent *t*-test.

2.2.1. ARPE19

Before testing the five fucoidan extracts, we established the parameters for this test with commercially available fucoidan from *Fucus vesiculosus* (Sigma) with both ARPE19 cells and primary RPE cells (see below). Sigma fucoidan was applied to the cells and supernatant was harvested after 1 day, 3 days, and 7 days. After 7 days, the experiment was terminated and cell viability was measured. Using Sigma fucoidan on ARPE19 cells for one day, no statistical difference could be found in ANOVA (1 µg/mL 82.13 ± 33.16%; 10 µg/mL 79.13 ± 27.21%; 50 µg/mL 72.25 ± 43.1%; 100 µg/mL 89.13 ± 45.02%). After 3 days of incubation, a strong VEGF reduction could be seen, which was significant in ANOVA and was significant at concentrations of 50 µg/mL and 100 µg/mL in further testing (1 µg/mL 110.83 ± 35.94%; 10 µg/mL 71.83 ± 52.07%; 50 µg/mL 63.83 ± 34.62%, $p < 0.05$; 100 µg/mL 50.33 ± 37.33%, $p < 0.05$; day 7: 1 µg/mL 120 ± 79.39%; 10 µg/mL 105.00 ± 83.01%; 50 µg/mL 93.83 ± 69.61%; 100 µg/mL 56.83 ± 50.33%) (Figure 4 a). In addition, we tested the effect of heparin as a known VEGF-binding control compound. At all days, a significant reduction could be detected in ANOVA testing. At the first day, a significant reduction was found for a concentration of 100 µg/mL heparin (1 µg/mL 84.25 ± 37.56%; 10 µg/mL 96.50 ± 40.33%; 50 µg/mL 67.50 ± 58.41%; 100 µg/mL 44.13 ± 20.18%, $p < 0.001$). For day 3 and day 7, both 50 µg/mL and 100 µg/mL displayed a significant reduction of VEGF (day 3: 1 µg/mL 94.17 ± 61.81%; 10 g/ml 59.50 ± 40.01%; 50 µg/mL 43.50 ± 28.39%, $p < 0.01$; 100 µg/mL 24.50 ± 26.30%, $p < 0.001$; day 7: 1 µg/mL 112.33 ± 79.45%; 10 µg/mL 77.67 ± 70.13%; 50 µg/mL 36.83 ± 40.01%,

$p < 0.01$; 100 µg/mL 17.17 ± 34.40%, $p < 0.001$) (Figure 4b). No significant reduction in cell viability could be detected after 7 days (1 µg/mL 148.17 ± 37.12%; 10 µg/mL 127.00 ± 20.98%; 50 µg/mL 101.00 ± 21.93%; 100 µg/mL 78.83 ± 28.11%) (Figure 4c).

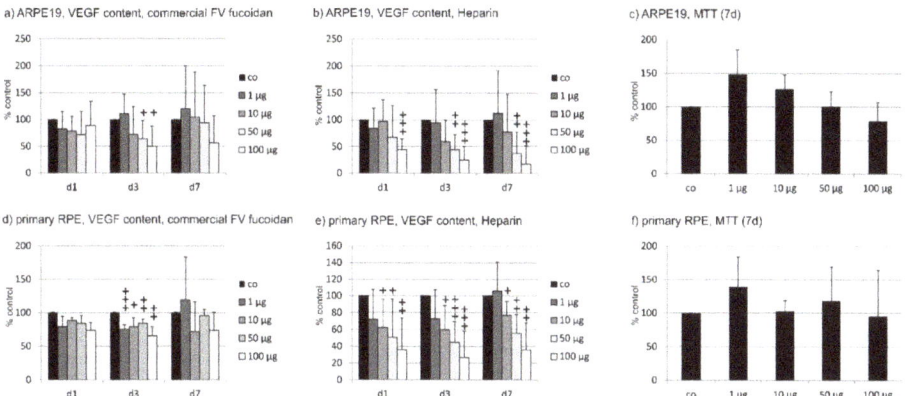

Figure 4. Effect of incubation time for vascular endothelial growth factor (VEGF) experiments. Commercially available fucoidan from *Fucus vesiculosus* was applied for 1 day (d1), 3 days (d3), and 7 days (d7), respectively, at indicated concentrations, to ARPE19 (**a**) or primary porcine retinal pigment epithelium (RPE) (**d**). In addition, heparin was tested on ARPE19 (**b**) and RPE cells (**e**). Cell viability was tested after 7 days (**c**, **f**). VEGF reduction was primarily seen after 3 days of incubation. Heparin showed a dose-dependent effect with similar significant reductions at all tested time points for concentrations of 10–100 µg/mL. No toxic effect was seen after 7 days in either cell type. Significance was evaluated with Friedman's ANOVA and subsequent Student's t-test, + $p < 0.05$ ++ $p < 0.01$, +++ $p < 0.001$ against the control ($n = 4$–6).

Based on these results, we investigated VEGF content after 3 days of incubation with fucoidan for all following experiments. VEGF content was normalized to cell viability and displayed in relation to an untreated control.

After 3 days, fucoidan from all algae tested showed a significant reduction in ANOVA. Fucoidan from *Saccharina latissima* showed a reduction of VEGF when applied in concentrations of 10–100 µg/mL (1 µg/mL 1.07 ± 0.15; 10 µg/mL 0.76 ± 0.11, $p < 0.01$; 50 µg/mL 0.69 ± 0.13, $p < 0.01$; 100 µg/mL 0.46 ± 0.21, $p < 0.001$) (Figure 5a). Fucoidan from *Laminaria digitata* significantly reduced VEGF content in all concentrations tested (1 µg/mL 0.35 ± 0.24; 10 µg/mL 0.18 ± 0.17; 50 µg/mL 0.38 ± 0.28; 100 µg/mL 0.14 ± 0.11; all $p < 0.001$) (Figure 5b). Similarly, all concentrations of fucoidan from *Fucus serratus* showed significant inhibition of VEGF (1 µg/mL 0.45 ± 0.11; 10 µg/mL 0.54 ± 0.28; 50 µg/mL 0.38 ± 0.39; 100 µg/mL 0.05 ± 0.11; all $p < 0.001$) (Figure 5c). Fucoidan from *Fucus vesiculosus* reduced VEGF at concentrations 1 µg/mL (0.50 ± 0.22, $p < 0.001$) and 50–100 µg/mL (50 µg/mL 0.33 ± 0.29; 100 µg/mL 0.16 ± 0.15, both $p < 0.001$), but not 10 µg/mL (0.77 ± 0.60) (Figure 5d). Fucoidan from *Fucus distichus* subsp. *evanescens* reduced VEGF at all concentrations tested (1 µg/mL 0.41 ± 0.22; 10 µg/mL 0.48 ± 0.28; 50 µg/mL 0.50 ± 0.30; 100 µg/mL 0.04 ± 0.05; all $p < 0.001$) (Figure 5e).

In ARPE19 cells, all tested fucoidans reduced the amount of secreted VEGF, with the highest concentration (100 µg/mL) generally displaying the strongest effect. The differences between the different fucoidans are not as profound as those found in protective effects and are generally limited to effects seen at certain concentrations. LD fucoidan differs only slightly from FV or FS fucoidan (both 10 µg/mL, $p < 0.05$) or from FE fucoidan (10 µg/mL and 100 µg/mL both $p < 0.05$), while there were significant differences compared to SL fucoidan in all concentrations tested (1–10 µg/mL $p < 0.001$; 50 µg/mL $p < 0.05$; 100 µg/mL $p < 0.01$). SL fucoidan significantly differed from FV fucoidan in all concentrations but 10 µg/mL (1 µg/mL $p < 0.001$; 50 µg/mL $p < 0.05$; 100 µg/mL $p < 0.01$), while it differed from FE and FS fucoidan at concentrations of 1 µg/mL and 100 µg/mL (both $p < 0.001$). FV fucoidan did not display any significant differences from FS fucoidan, and only at 100 µg/mL when compared to FE fucoidan ($p < 0.05$). Finally, FE and FS fucoidan did not display any significant differences (Table 3). Ranging the effect on VEGF secretion results in LD > FS > FE > FV > SL.

Table 3. Comparison of the effect of the different fucoidans at different concentrations on VEGF secretion in ARPE19 cells.

Compared Fucoidans	1 µg/mL	10 µg/mL	50 µg/mL	100 µg/mL
LD vs. FV	ns	$p < 0.05$	ns	ns
LD vs. SL	$p < 0.001$	$p < 0.001$	$p < 0.05$	$p < 0.01$
LD vs. FE	ns	$p < 0.05$	ns	$p < 0.05$
LD vs. FS	ns	$p < 0.05$	ns	ns
FV vs. SL	$p < 0.001$	ns	$p < 0.05$	$p < 0.01$
FV vs. FE	ns	ns	ns	$p < 0.05$
FV vs. FS	ns	ns	ns	ns
SL vs. FE	$p < 0.001$	ns	ns	$p < 0.001$
SL vs. FS	$p < 0.001$	ns	ns	$p < 0.001$
FE vs. FS	ns	ns	ns	ns

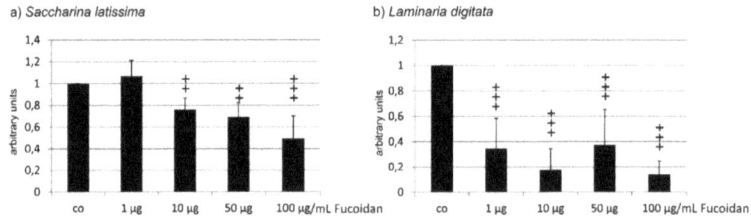

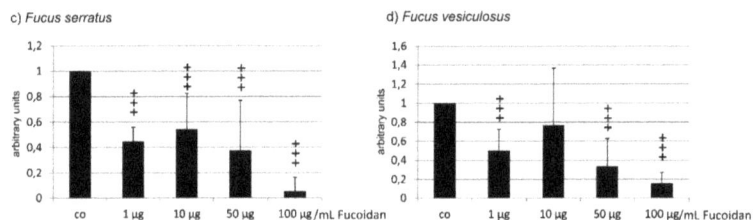

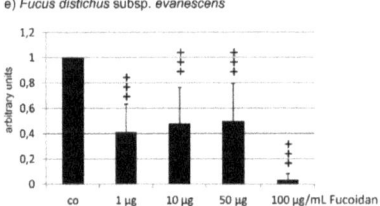

Figure 5. VEGF secretion in ARPE19 cells after incubation with different concentrations of fucoidan. (**a**) *Saccharina latissima* (SL), (**b**) *Laminaria digitata* (LD), (**c**) *Fucus serratus* (FS), (**d**) *Fucus vesiculosus* (FV), (**e**) *Fucus distichus* subsp. *evanescens* (FE). VEGF content was evaluated by ELISA and normalized to cell viability. Control = 1. In ARPE19 cells, all fucoidans reduced VEGF content with the efficacy of LD > FS > FE > FV > SL. Significance was evaluated with Friedman's ANOVA and subsequent Student's t-test, ++ $p < 0.01$, +++ $p < 0.001$ compared to the control ($n = 6$–8).

2.2.2. Primary RPE

The pretesting of Sigma fucoidan on cells for 1 day, 3 days, and 7 days led to the following. In primary porcine RPE cells, we found no significant reduction of VEGF content in the supernatant after 1 day (1 µg/mL 79.25 ± 15.04%; 10 µg/mL 88.00 ± 4.69%; 50 µg/mL 84.25 ± 11.87%; 100 µg/mL 74.25 ± 11.18%). After 3 days, however, a significant reduction could be detected in ANOVA and was found in all concentrations assessed (1 µg/mL 75.50 ± 6.46%, $p < 0.001$; 10 µg/mL 78.75 ± 13.33%, $p < 0.05$; 50 µg/mL 84.00 ± 6.83%; $p < 0.01$; 100 µg/mL 65.5 ± 13.92%, $p < 0.01$). This effect was no longer seen after 7 days (1 µg/mL 119.00 ± 64.18%; 10 µg/mL 71.75 ± 44.70%; 50 µg/mL 95.75 ± 9.07%); 100 µg/mL 73.75 ± 27.21%) (Figure 4d). In addition, we have tested the effect of heparin as a known VEGF binding control compound. At all three tested days, a significant reduction could be detected in ANOVA and concentrations of 10, 50, and 100 µg/mL heparin significantly reduced VEGF in a dose-dependent manner (day 1: 1 µg/mL 72.167 ± 35.32%; 10 µg/mL 62.17 ± 33.44%, $p < 0.05$; 50 µg/mL 50.83 ± 44.91%, $p < 0.05$: 100 µg/mL 36.00 ± 37.70%, $p < 0.01$; day 3: 1 µg/mL 73.17 ± 34.11%; 10 µg/mL 59.60 ± 28.78%, $p < 0.05$; 50 µg/mL 44.50 ± 25.11%, $p < 0.001$; 100 µg/m. 26.33 ± 31.40%, $p < 0.001$; day 7: 1 µg/mL 106.00 ± 34.58%; 10 µg/mL 76.60 ± 16.88%, $p < 0.05$; 50 µg/mL 55.80 ± 22.00%, $p < 0.01$; 100 µg/mL 36.00 ± 31.98%, $p < 0.01$) (Figure 4e). No significant reduction of cell viability could be seen after 7 days (1 µg/mL 139.17 ± 45.20%; 10 µg/mL 103.16 ± 15.38%; 118.00 ± 51.54%; 100 µg/mL 95.50 ± 68.63%) (Figure 4f). Based on these results, we investigated VEGF content after 3 days for all following experiments. VEGF content was normalized to cell viability and displayed in relation to untreated controls.

After 3 days, fucoidan from *Saccharina latissima* reduced the VEGF content of RPE cells at a concentration of 10 µg/mL (0.77 ± 0.17, $p < 0.01$), while the other concentrations showed no significant effect (1 µg/mL 0.97 ± 0.07; 50 µg/mL 1.33 ± 0.66; 100 µg/mL 0.92 ± 0.27) (Figure 6a). None of the other fucoidans reduced VEGF content in RPE cells. Fucoidan from *Laminaria digitata* did not reduce VEGF secretion in primary porcine RPE cells in any concentration tested; however, a significant increase was detected in ANOVA, significantly increasing the VEGF signal at concentrations of 50 µg/mL and 100 µg/mL (1 µg/mL 1.27 ± 0.57; 10 µg/mL 1.44 ± 0.63; 50 µg/mL 1.59 ± 0.43, $p < 0.01$; 1.58 ± 0.24, $p < 0.001$) (Figure 5b). Fucoidan from *Fucus serratus* displayed no significant influence on VEGF secretion in primary porcine RPE at any concentration tested (1 µg/mL 0.96 ± 0.08; 10 µg/mL 1.05 ± 0.28; 50 µg/mL 1.14 ± 0.38; 100 µg/mL 1.40 ± 0.64) (Figure 6c). Fucoidan from *Fucus vesiculosus* did not reduce VEGF in any tested concentration but, similar to LD fucoidan, displayed a significant increase in ANOVA testing, increasing the VEGF signal at concentrations of 50 and 100 µg/mL (1 µg/mL 1.28 ± 0.62; 10 µg/mL 1.97 ± 1.46; 50 µg/mL 1.78 ± 0.44, $p < 0.001$; 100 µg/mL 1.74 ± 0.52, $p < 0.01$) (Figure 6d). Fucoidan from *Fucus distichus* subsp. *evanescens* displayed similar results. While no reduction of VEGF content could be seen at any tested concentration, significant differences could be detected in ANOVA, with 50 µg/mL and 100 µg/mL displaying an increase in VEGF content (1 µg/mL 1.31 ± 0.59; 10 µg/mL 1.81 ± 1.18; 50 µg/mL 2.02 ± 0.98, $p < 0.05$; 100 µg/mL 1.67 ± 0.43, $p < 0.01$) (Figure 6e).

In primary RPE cells, only *Saccharina latissima* showed a reductive effect on VEGF content in the supernatant. When comparing the different fucoidans, significant differences were only found between SL and LD fucoidan (at a concentration of 10 µg/mL) and between FV and FS fucoidan (at a concentration of 50 µg/mL) (Table 4).

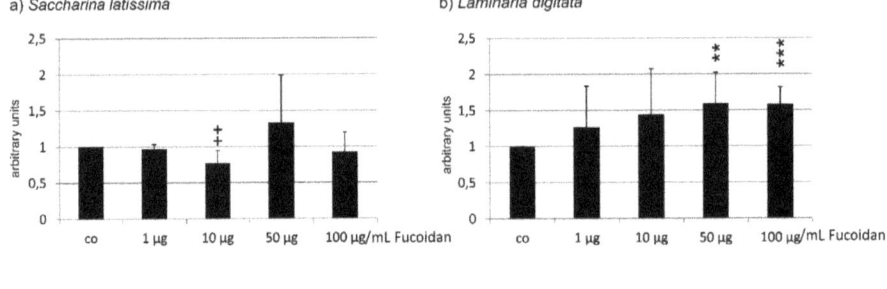

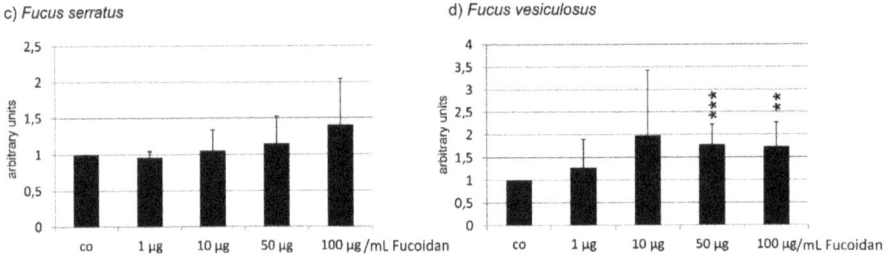

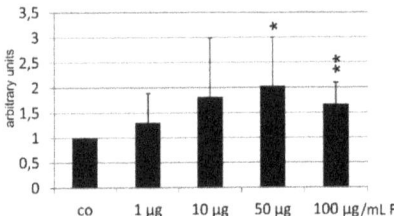

Figure 6. VEGF secretion of primary porcine RPE cells after incubation with different concentrations of fucoidan from (**a**) *Saccharina latissima* (SL), (**b**) *Laminaria digitata* (LD), (**c**) *Fucus serratus* (FS), (**d**) *Fucus vesiculosus* (FV), (**e**) *Fucus distichus* subsp. *evanescens* (FE). VEGF content was evaluated in ELISA and normalized to cell viability. Control = 1. In RPE cells, only SL fucoidan reduced the VEGF content of RPE cells (10 µg/mL), while LD, FV, and FE induced a higher signal at concentrations of 50 and 100 µg/mL. Significance was evaluated with Friedman's ANOVA and subsequent Student's *t*-test, + $p < 0.05$ reduction compared to the control, * $p < 0.05$, ** $p < 0.01$ and *** $p < 0.001$ ($n = 7$).

Table 4. Comparison of the effect of different fucoidans at different concentrations on VEGF secretion in primary porcine RPE cells.

Compared Fucoidans	1 µg/mL	10 µg/mL	50 µg/mL	100 µg/mL
LD vs. FV	ns	ns	ns	ns
LD vs. SL	ns	$p < 0.05$	ns	ns
LD vs. FE	ns	ns	ns	ns
LD vs. FS	ns	ns	ns	ns
FV vs. SL	ns	ns	ns	ns
FV vs. FE	ns	ns	ns	ns
FV vs. FS	ns	ns	$p < 0.05$	ns
SL vs. FE	ns	ns	ns	ns
SL vs. FS	ns	ns	ns	ns
FE vs. FS	ns	ns	ns	ns

2.3. Binding Affinity to VEGF

In the pathogenesis of the exudative form of AMD, VEGF is an important factor [5,6]. VEGF inhibitors are currently used as a therapy standard [11]. As has been known for a long time that heparin and other sulfated polysaccharides have a high affinity for VEGF [20], fucoidans may not only reduce the secretion of VEGF but also directly antagonize its actions. Therefore, we investigated the binding affinity of fucoidans to VEGF in comparison to heparin, and aimed to identify those fucoidans with the strongest binding affinity to VEGF.

In the competitive VEGF binding assay used, the replacement of biotinylated heparin by the test compound was measured. At a concentration of 0.5 µg/mL, maximum binding of biotinylated heparin was achieved (data not shown). By adding increasing concentrations of unlabeled heparin, the detection of biotinylated heparin decreased (data not shown). As expected, incubation with a mixture of 0.5 µg/mL heparin and 0.5 µg/mL biotinylated heparin reduced the signal to 49.96% (±7.28) and thus the binding of biotinylated heparin to VEGF. All five fucoidans showed a significant affinity to VEGF compared to the control, tested in ANOVA and subsequent testing (SL 26.13 ± 13.46%; LD 28.57 ± 13.20%; FS 10.63 ± 6.43%; FV 21.27 ± 4.69% and FE 16.97 ± 9.91%) (Figure 7). Moreover, the three *Fucus* fucoidans bound significantly more strongly to VEGF than heparin ($p < 0.01$) (Table 5). Although FS and FE showed a slightly higher affinity, there were no significant differences between the five fucoidans (Table 5).

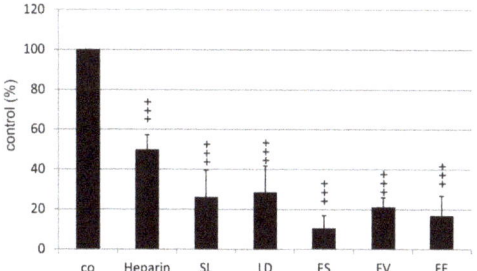

Figure 7. VEGF binding affinity of fucoidans from *Saccharina latissima* (SL), *Laminaria digitata* (LD), *Fucus serratus* (FS), *Fucus vesiculosus* (FV), *Fucus distichus* subsp. *evanescens* (FE), and of heparin. Significance was evaluated with Friedman's ANOVA and subsequent Student's t-test, +++ $p < 0.001$ compared to control (biotinylated heparin).

Table 5. Comparison of the VEGF binding affinity of fucoidans and heparin.

Compared Substances	Significance
Heparin vs. FV	$p < 0.01$
Heparin vs. FS	$p < 0.01$
Heparin vs. FE	$p < 0.01$
Heparin vs. LD	ns
Heparin vs. SL	ns
LD vs. FV	ns
LD vs. SL	ns
LD vs. FE	ns
LD vs. FS	ns
FV vs. SL	ns
FV vs. FE	ns
FV vs. FS	ns
SL vs. FE	ns
SL vs. FS	ns
FE vs. FS	ns

3. Discussion

Fucoidans are of great interest to biomedical research, especially considering their possible application in age-related macular degeneration [4]. However, the effects of fucoidans can profoundly vary depending on their origin and method of extraction. Therefore, generalized statements about their activities should be avoided.

In this study, we have compared fucoidans from five different brown algae species harvested in summer and obtained from the same supplier (Coastal Research & Management, Kiel, Germany). The preparation of the algal material as well as the extraction and purification of the fucoidans were performed in parallel according to a standardized procedure. Therefore, this study is well equipped to reliably examine the effects of fucoidans from different algal species. The aim was to compare the beneficial properties of fucoidans with regard to age-related macular degeneration.

In our study, we focused on two major factors important for the development of age-related macular degeneration, i.e., oxidative stress and VEGF. While interference with these is without doubt of great interest, we are aware that other activities, e.g., anticomplementary, anti-inflammatory effects, or influence on lipid metabolism, are also potentially beneficial for impairing AMD pathogenesis and are of high interest for further testing.

We have previously shown that OMM-1 cells are protected by commercially available fucoidan [17]. In contrast to uveal melanoma cells, RPE cells are intrinsically strongly protected against oxidative stress [18], so we tested oxidative stress protection both in OMM-1 cell lines, which we know could be protected by fucoidans, having demonstrated this for commercial fucoidan from *Fucus vesiculosus* [17], as well as the RPE cell line ARPE19. All five fucoidans protected OMM-1 cells from oxidative stress, confirming our previous results. However, fucoidans can differ in their properties depending on the test system or the cell types due to distinct cellular and molecular pathways. A major task of RPE cells is oxidative stress protection [18] and, as mentioned above, they are naturally highly resistant to oxidative stress. ARPE19 cells, as an RPE cell line, consequently behaved differently from OMM-1 cells, not only concerning their susceptibility to oxidative stress itself, but also their reaction to fucoidans. In contrast to OMM-1 cells, only SL fucoidan displayed a protection of cell viability, while FE and FS fucoidan even exacerbated the effect.

Little is known about oxidative stress pathways in uveal melanoma cells, but an increased susceptibility due to the reduction of superoxide dismutase activity in uveal melanoma cells has been described [21]. There is a debate about the direct reactive oxygen species (ROS) scavenging effect of fucoidans. The ROS scavenging potency of fucoidan has been described in several publications [22–25], but it has recently been demonstrated in cell-free systems that these measured effects are mainly due to co-extracted phenolic and terpenoid compounds in the fucoidan preparations [15,26]. Generally, the scavenging effect of fucoidan against hydrogen peroxide has been described to be rather weak [24,25]. Our results even suggest that the in vitro ROS scavenging activity may be irrelevant as, in contrast to SL and LD, the three *Fucus* fucoidans showed an ROS scavenging effect (manuscript in preparation) but did not protect ARPE19 cells from oxidative stress.

However, independent of all of the results from simple cell-free assays, fucoidans may exhibit antioxidative activity by cellular effects. Accordingly, fucoidan has been shown to increase the expression of superoxide dismutase (SOD) in several experimental models and activate the transcription factor nuclear factor erythroid 2-like 2 (Nrf2), the "master regulator" of the antioxidative stress response [27–32]. Both the overall protective effect of our fucoidans on OMM-1 and the limited protective effect on ARPE19 cells (only found for *Saccharina latissima* fucoidan) could be explained via these pathways. As mentioned above, uveal melanoma cells have been described to have a reduced SOD activity [21]. Hence, the SOD-inducing effect of fucoidans could protect these cells against an oxidative stress insult. In contrast, RPE cells have a high intrinsic stress response level mediated by Nrf2 [18]. Indeed, knock-out of Nrf2 renders RPE cells highly susceptible to oxidative stress insults [33] and Nrf2 knock-out mice develop AMD-like features at an older age [34]. It is feasible that these protective pathways are already at maximum efficacy, so that any further enhancement by fucoidans may be impossible. Therefore, the different effects of fucoidans on the two cell lines are assumed to be due to distinct impacts on the respective cellular pathways. Further research needs to be conducted to elucidate these pathways. It should be noted, however, that oxidative stress protection in AMD is not only needed for (the rather resistant) RPE cells, but also for the rather fragile photoreceptor cells [35]. Therefore, the effect of fucoidans on oxidative stress-induced photoreceptor cell death should also be evaluated in further studies.

A major contributor to the pathology of wet AMD is the growth factor VEGF, and its inhibition is the only current treatment option for AMD patients. We have previously shown that commercially obtained fucoidan from *Fucus vesiculosus* additively reduced VEGF expression when co-applied with the VEGF inhibitor bevacizumab [3]. On the molecular level, the interaction of fucoidan with VEGF differs profoundly from that of the current therapeutic anti-VEGF molecules. VEGF antibody-derived compounds bevacizumab and ranibizumab, as well as the fusion protein aflibecept, interact with specific amino acids in the receptor-binding domain of VEGF, causing a steric inhibition of the binding of VEGF to its receptor [36], with differences in affinities between the compounds [37]. The interaction of fucoidan and other heparin-related compounds is complex, however, depending on features such as sulfation and molecular weight [38,39]. Furthermore, fucoidan has been shown to also have a binding affinity to VEGF receptors and to facilitate the internalization of VEGF receptors, blocking the binding and in-vitro functions of VEGF [38,40,41].

In our current study, we were able to demonstrate antagonization as well as a reduction of VEGF secretion in ARPE19 cells, in which all five fucoidans were effective. In primary porcine RPE cells, however, only SL displayed a significant effect.

Fucoidan was found to influence Stat3-regulated promoters, which includes the promoter of VEGF [42]. But it should be noted that we have previously shown that in unchallenged primary RPE cells, Stat3 is not involved in constitutive VEGF expression [43]. Therefore, this mechanism of fucoidan-mediated VEGF reduction is not feasible. We have also previously shown that VEGF is positively regulated in an autocrine way via the VEGFR-2 [43,44], whereby fucoidan has been shown to bind to VEGF165 and to competitively inhibit the interaction of VEGF with VEGFR2 [39,40]. This pathway has been suggested to be involved in VEGF reduction mediated by fucoidan [3,40]. Such an extracellular mode of action for fucoidans is now supported by the binding of the five fucoidans to VEGF. Their affinity was significantly higher than that of heparin, whereas heparan sulfate was not able to reduce the binding of biotinylated heparin to VEGF. Interaction of VEGF with heparin sulfate on the cell surface was found to be involved in effective VEGFR2 activation [45]. Thus, the fucoidans may competitively prevent this interaction and thus attenuate signaling through VEGFR2, resulting in reduced VEGF expression and secretion. In line with this assumed mode of action are the findings that the intraocular injection of heparan sulfate or heparin in mice eyes with aberrant angiogenesis results in reduced neovascularization [46]. Given the even higher affinity to VEGF of fucoidans, this seems promising.

The amount of VEGF secreted by primary RPE cells in this study was much higher than that of ARPE19 cells (596.72 pg/h for primary RPE vs. 17.35 pg/h for ARPE19; factor 34.4). In the presence of such high VEGF concentrations, the VEGF antagonizing mode of action obviously became ineffective, explaining the discrepant results in ARPE19 cells and RPE cells. Therefore, the effect of SL on VEGF secretion in primary RPE cells is even more remarkable.

Our data clearly show a positive effect of the tested fucoidans in terms of oxidative stress protection and VEGF inhibition, with the most promising fucoidan extracted from *Saccharina latissima*. Among the tested fucoidans, SL had the highest degree of sulfation, the highest molecular weight, and the highest degree of purity (under submission). But these parameters cannot explain its superiority or the ranking of the other fucoidans. Fucoidans from *Saccharina latissima* have been previously shown to be highly biologically active compared to those from other brown algae species [15,16]. Furthermore, in line with our finding concerning VEGF inhibition, fucoidans from *Saccharina latissima* have been shown to inhibit angiogenesis in tumor models [47]. However, it seems too early to decide that the other fucoidans are not worth further investigation. Other activities beneficial for AMD therapy should be regarded as well. Further preclinical and clinical research is warranted, but fucoidans may be a potential treatment option for age-related macular degeneration. To develop potential therapeutics from fucoidan, in addition to finding the most suitable source and a sustainable and reliable harvest and extraction method, bioavailability and application forms need to be tested.

In addition, VEGF secretion and oxidative stress are also involved in the pathomechanisms of diabetic retinopathy [48,49]. Therefore, fucoidans may also be of great interest for diabetic patients, especially considering that fucoidan may also reduce blood glucose levels and ameliorate hypertension [4].

In conclusion, we compared fucoidan from five brown algae species in terms of three activities that are considered promising for the treatment of AMD, i.e., their capacity for oxidative stress protection, inhibition of VEGF secretion, and binding affinity to VEGF. Based on these three basic parameters, the fucoidan from *Saccharina latissima* turned out to be most suitable for further investigations.

4. Material and Methods

4.1. Cell Culture

The uveal melanoma cell line OMM-1 [50] was a kind gift from Dr. Sarah Coupland and was cultivated in an appropriate medium (RPMI, Merck, Darmstadt, Germany, supplemented with 10% fetal calf serum and 1% penicillin/streptomycin). The immortal human RPE cell line ARPE19 was obtained from American Type Culture Collection (ATCC) and cultivated in an appropriate medium (Dulbecco's Modified Eagle's Medium (DMEM), supplemented with penicillin/streptomycin (1%), non-essential amino acids (1%), 4-(2-hydroxyethyl)-1-piperazineethanesulfonic acid (HEPES) (25%), and 10% fetal calf serum).

Primary RPE cells were prepared as previously described [51,52]. In brief, RPE cells were harvested from cleaned porcine eyes by trypsin incubation and cultivated in an appropriate medium (DMEM, HyClone, Thermo Fisher Sc., Bremen, Germany, supplemented with penicillin/streptomysin (1%), HEPES (25%), non-essential amino acids (1%), all Merck, Darmstadt, Germany, and 10% fetal calf serum, Linaris GmbH, Wertheim-Bettingen, Germany). RPE and ARPE19 cells were used at confluence and OMM-1 at 80% confluence for further experimentation.

4.2. Fucoidans

Fucoidans were extracted from dried stocks of the species *Saccharina latissima* (SL; Atlantic, Funningsfjord, Faroe Island), *Fucus vesiculosus* (FV; Baltic, Kiel Bay, Germany), *Laminaria digitata* (LD; Atlantic; Churchbay, Island), *Fucus distichus* subsp. *evanescens* (FE; Baltic, Kiel Cana, Germany), and *Fucus serratus* (FS; Baltic, Kiel Bay, Germany), all harvested in summer and provided by Coastal Research & Management, Kiel, Germany. The fucoidans were extracted as previously described [53]. Briefly, the pulverized algal material was defatted by Soxhlet extraction with 99% (v/v) ethanol, and was then extracted with aqueous 2% calcium chloride for 2 h at 85 °C under reflux conditions. The supernatants of the raw extracts were concentrated and precipitated with ice-cold ethanol in a final concentration of 60% (w/w). After centrifugation, the sediments were dissolved in demineralized water, dialyzed, and lyophilized. In addition, commercially available fucoidan from Sigma (Sigma-Aldrich, Deisenhofen, Germany, F8190) was used. Fucoidan was solved in Ampuwa bidest (Fresenius, Schweinfurt, Germany), and then further diluted with appropriate cell medium for the cell experiments and phosphate buffered saline (PBS) for the VEGF binding assay, filtered through a 0.2 μm filter (Sarstedt, Nümbrecht, Germany), and applied to the cells in final concentrations of 1, 10, 50, and 100 μg/mL.

4.3. Oxidative Stress

4.3.1. OMM-1

OMM-1 cells were treated with hydrogen peroxide (H_2O_2) to induce oxidative stress-related cell death, as previously shown [17]. As OMM-1 is a cancer cell line that may change its characteristics during subculture, we evaluated the appropriate concentrations of H_2O_2 resulting in approximately 50% cell viability. In order to assess this, OMM-1 cells were treated with different concentrations (100, 200, 400, 1000 mM) of H_2O_2 for 24 h and cell viability was investigated by MTS assay (see below). To investigate the potential protective effects of the different fucoidans, a concentration of 1 mM H_2O_2 was chosen. Cells were treated with fucoidan (1, 10, 50, and 100 µg/mL) 30 min prior to the application of H_2O_2.

4.3.2. ARPE19

Corresponding experiments to find the appropriate H_2O_2 concentration for ARPE19 cells revealed that none of the tested concentrations of H_2O_2 (100 µM, 200 µM, 400 µM, 1000 µM) induced a cell death of about 50% after 24 h, as detected by MTS assay. In addition, the cell death rate was highly variable after H_2O_2 incubation (see results). Therefore, we tested tert-Butyl hydroperoxide (TBHP), a more stable inducer of oxidative stress in RPE cells [33], at concentrations of 100 µM, 250 µM, and 500 µM, for 24 h and investigated cell viability by MTS assay, as described below. In order to investigate the potential protective effect of the different fucoidans, a concentration of 500 µM TBHP was chosen. Cells were treated with fucoidan 30 min prior to the insult.

4.4. Methyl Thiazolyl Tetrazolium (MTT) Assay

MTT assay is a common method in cell research [54] and was conducted as previously described [3]. In brief, after treatment with the fucoidans, the cells were washed and incubated with 0.5 mg/mL MTT (dissolved in DMEM without phenol red). After removal and further washing of the cells, cells were lysed with dimethyl sulfoxide (DMSO) and the absorbance was measured at 550 nm with a spectrometer (Elx800, BioTek, Bad Friedrichshall, Germany).

4.5. MTS Assay

The MTS assay is a commercially available viability assay and was used according to the manufacturers' instructions (CellTiter 96® AQueous One Solution Cell Proliferation Assay (Promega, Mannheim, Germany)). The cell viability assay was performed in 96 well plates in phenol red-free medium with the same supplements described above. In each well, 20 µL of MTS solution was added for 1 h.

4.6. VEGF ELISA

VEGF was detected in the supernatants of ARPE19 and primary RPE cells using commercially available ELISA kits (R&D Systems, Wiesbaden, Germany) according to the manufacturer's instructions. To establish the parameters of VEGF ELISA, we investigated time-dependent VEGF secretion in ARPE19 and primary RPE cells in the presence and absence of commercially available fucoidan from *Fucus vesiculosus* (Sigma-Aldrich, F8190) for 1 day, 3 days, and 7 days. A cell viability assay (MTT) was conducted after 7 days. According to these results, an incubation time of 3 days was chosen for experiments with the five different fucoidans. The medium was changed 24 h prior in ARPE19 cells and 4 h prior in primary RPE cells and the supernatant collected. Measured VEGF content was normalized for cell survival and is depicted in relation to that of untreated control cells.

4.7. Competitive VEGF Binding Assay

The affinity to VEGF of the test compounds was investigated with a competitive VEGF-binding assay using biotinylated heparin. In addition to the fucoidans, heparin (EDQM, no. Y0001282, Strasbourg, France) was tested.

The wells of a 96-well Nunc-Immuno MaxiSorp microplate (Sigma-Aldrich, Deisenhofen, Germany) were coated with 0.1 µg recombinant human VEGF 165 (R&D Systems Cat. 293-VE/CF) dissolved in 100 µL PBS overnight at 4 °C. After washing with PBS, the coated wells were blocked for 90 min at 37 °C with 100 µL of 5 mg/mL bovine serum albumin (BSA, dissolved in PBS) and subsequently washed three times with PBS. During the blocking, 65 µL of 1 µg/mL heparin, biotin conjugate (Merck, Darmstadt, Germany) in PBS, and 65 µL of 1 µg/mL test compounds in PBS were preincubated at 4 °C. For the blank and the 100% binding value, 100 µL PBS and 100 µL of 0.5 µg/mL biotinylated heparin in PBS, respectively, were preincubated at 4 °C. Aliquots of 100 µL of these solutions were pipetted into the coated microplate wells and incubated for 2 h at 37 °C with gentle agitation. After three washing steps, 100 µL of streptavidin alkaline phosphate conjugate (Southern Biotech/, Birmingham, AL, USA, stock solution diluted 1:3000 with PBS) was incubated for 1 h at 37 °C with gentle agitation. The next steps involved three washings with PBS and incubation with 100 µL p-nitrophenyl phosphate substrate system (Sigma-Aldrich, Deisenhofen, Germany) for 30 min in the dark. The reaction was stopped by addition of 25 µL 3 N NaOH, and the absorbance was measured at 405 nm. Blank values in the absence of biotinylated heparin were subtracted from the measured values. The reduction of the binding of biotinylated heparin by the test compounds is indicated as a percentage in relation to the binding of the biotinylated heparin alone.

4.8. Statistics

All experiments testing fucoidans were independently repeated at least six times, experiments for establishing oxidative stress response were repeated at least three times, and the VEGF binding experiments were performed in duplicates on three different days. Statistics were calculated using Statistica 7 (Statsoft, Tulsa, OK, USA) and Microsoft Excel (Excel 2010, Microsoft, Redmond, WA, USA). A Friedman's ANOVA was performed, and, if a significant difference between groups was detected, a subsequent Student's *t*-test was conducted. A p value of <0.05 was considered significant. All bars represent mean and standard deviation.

Author Contributions: Conceptualization, A.K. and S.A.; Methodology, A.K., P.D., S.A., K.S.B., S.N.; Software, A.K.; Validation, A.K., P.D., S.A., K.S.B and S.N.; Formal Analysis, P.D., A.K., K.S.B., S.A., S.N.; Investigation, P.D., K.S.B.; Resources, J.R., A.K., S.A.; Data Curation, A.K., S.A.; Writing-Original Draft Preparation, A.K., S.A.; Writing-Review & Editing, A.K., P.D., K.S.B., S.N., J.R., S.A.; Visualization, A.K.; Supervision, A.K., S.A., J.R.; Project Administration, A.K.; Funding Acquisition, A.K., J.R.

Funding: The research was funded by EU InterReg Deutschland–Denmark and the European Regional Development Fund, Project FucoSan, grant number 39-1.0-16. AK was funded by the Hermann–Wacker Foundation.

Acknowledgments: This study is part of the FucoSan–Health from the Sea project and is supported by EU InterReg Deutschland–Denmark and the European Regional Development Fund. We especially thank Coastal Research & Management, Kiel, for the provision of the algae.

Conflicts of Interest: The authors declare no conflict of interest.

References

1. Li, B.; Lu, F.; Wei, X.; Zhao, R. Fucoidan: Structure and bioactivity. *Molecules* **2008**, *13*, 1671–1695. [CrossRef] [PubMed]
2. Fitton, J.H.; Stringer, D.N.; Karpiniec, S.S. Therapies from Fucoidan: An Update. *Mar. Drugs* **2015**, *13*, 5920–5946. [CrossRef] [PubMed]
3. Dithmer, M.; Fuchs, S.; Shi, Y.; Schmidt, H.; Richert, E.; Roider, J.; Klettner, A. Fucoidan reduces secretion and expression of vascular endothelial growth factor in the retinal pigment epithelium and reduces angiogenesis in vitro. *PLoS ONE* **2014**, *9*, e89150. [CrossRef]

4. Klettner, A. Fucoidan as a potential therapeutic for major blinding diseases—A hypothesis. *Mar. Drugs* **2016**, *14*, E31. [CrossRef]
5. Miller, J.W. Age-related macular degeneration revisited–piecing the puzzle: The LXIX Edward Jackson memorial lecture. *Am. J. Ophthalmol.* **2013**, *155*, 1–35. [CrossRef] [PubMed]
6. Klettner, A. Age-related macular degeneration-biology and treatment. *Med. Monatsschr. Pharm.* **2015**, *38*, 258–264. [PubMed]
7. Bellezza, I. Oxidative Stress in Age-Related Macular Degeneration: Nrf2 as Therapeutic Target. *Front. Pharmacol.* **2018**, *9*, 1280. [CrossRef]
8. Copland, D.A.; Theodoropoulou, S.; Liu, J.; Dick, A.D. A Perspective of AMD Through the Eyes of Immunology. *Invest. Ophthalmol. Vis. Sci.* **2018**, *59*, AMD83–AMD92. [CrossRef]
9. Handa, J.T.; Cano, M.; Wang, L.; Datta, S.; Liu, T. Lipids, Oxidized Lipids, Oxidation-specific Epitopes, and Age-related Macular Degeneration. *Biochim. Biophys. Acta* **2017**, *1862*, 430–440. [CrossRef]
10. Toomey, C.B.; Johnson, L.V.; Bowes Rickman, C. Complement factor H in AMD: Bridging genetic associations and pathobiology. *Prog. Retin. Eye Res.* **2018**, *62*, 38–57. [CrossRef]
11. Schmidt-Erfurth, U.; Chong, V.; Loewenstein, A.; Larsen, M.; Souied, E.; Schlingemann, R.; Eldem, B.; Monés, J.; Richard, G.; Bandello, F. European Society of Retina Specialists. Guidelines for the management of neovascular age-related macular degeneration by the European Society of Retina Specialists (EURETINA). *Br. J. Ophthalmol.* **2014**, *98*, 1144–1167. [CrossRef]
12. Rofagha, S.; Bhisitkul, R.B.; Boyer, D.S.; Sadda, S.R.; Zhang, K.; SEVEN-UP Study Group. Seven-year outcomes in ranibizumab-treated patients in ANCHOR, MARINA, and HORIZON: A multicenter cohort study (SEVEN-UP). *Ophthalmology* **2013**, *120*, 2292–2299. [CrossRef]
13. Zarubina, A.V.; Gal-Or, O.; Huisingh, C.E.; Owsley, C.; Freund, K.B. Macular Atrophy Development and Subretinal Drusenoid Deposits in Anti-Vascular Endothelial Growth Factor Treated Age-Related Macular Degeneration. *Invest. Ophthalmol. Vis. Sci.* **2017**, *58*, 6038–6045. [CrossRef]
14. Moryak, V.K.; Kim, J.; Kim, E. Algal fucoidan: Structural and size-dependent bioactivities and their perspectives. *Appl. Microbiol. Biotechnol.* **2012**, *93*, 71–82. [CrossRef]
15. Schneider, T.; Ehrig, K.; Liewert, I.; Alban, S. Interference with the CXCL12/CXCR4 axis as potential antitumor strategy: Superiority of a sulfated galactofucan from the brown alga Saccharina latissima and fucoidan over heparins. *Glycobiology* **2015**, *25*, 812–824. [CrossRef]
16. Cumashi, A.; Ushakova, N.A.; Preobrazhenskaya, M.E.; D'Incecco, A.; Piccoli, A.; Totani, L.; Tinari, N.; Morozevich, G.E.; Berman, A.E.; Bilan, M.I.; et al. A comparative study of the anti-inflammatory, anticoagulant, antiangiogenic, and antiadhesive activities of nine different fucoidans from brown seaweeds. *Glycobiology* **2007**, *17*, 541–552. [CrossRef]
17. Dithmer, M.; Kirsch, A.M.; Richert, E.; Fuchs, S.; Wang, F.; Schmidt, H.; Coupland, S.E.; Roider, J.; Klettner, A. Fucoidan does not exert anti-tumorigenic effects on uveal melanoma cell lines. *Mar. Drugs* **2017**, *15*, 193. [CrossRef]
18. Klettner, A. Oxidative stress induced cellular signaling in RPE cells. *Front. Biosci. (Schol. Ed.)* **2012**, *4*, 392–411. [CrossRef]
19. Karlsson, M.; Kurz, T. Attenuation of iron-binding proteins in ARPE-19 cells reduces their resistance to oxidative stress. *Acta Ophthalmol.* **2016**, *94*, 556–564. [CrossRef]
20. Folkman, J.; Shing, Y. Control of angiogenesis by heparin and other sulfated polysaccharides. *Adv. Exp. Med. Biol.* **1992**, *313*, 355–364.
21. Blasi, M.A.; Maresca, V.; Roccella, M.; Roccella, F.; Sansolini, T.; Grammatico, P.; Balestrazzi, E.; Picardo, M. Antioxidant pattern in uveal melanocytes and melanoma cell cultures. *Invest. Ophthalmol. Vis. Sci.* **1999**, *40*, 3012–3016.
22. Rupérez, P.; Ahrazem, O.; Leal, J.A. Potential antioxidant capacity of sulfated polysaccharides from the edible marine brown seaweed Fucus vesiculosus. *J. Agric. Food Chem.* **2002**, *50*, 840–845. [CrossRef]
23. Wang, J.; Zhang, Q.; Zhang, Z.; Li, Z. Antioxidant activity of sulfated polysaccharide fractions extracted from Laminaria japonica. *Int. J. Biol. Macromol.* **2008**, *42*, 127–132. [CrossRef]
24. Kim, E.A.; Lee, S.H.; Ko, C.I.; Cha, S.H.; Kang, M.C.; Kang, S.M.; Ko, S.C.; Lee, W.W.; Ko, J.Y.; Lee, J.H.; et al. Protective effect of fucoidan against AAPH-induced oxidative stress in zebrafish model. *Carbohydr. Polym.* **2014**, *102*, 185–191. [CrossRef]

25. Abu, R.; Jiang, Z.; Ueno, M.; Okimura, T.; Yamaguchi, K.; Oda, T. In vitro antioxidant activities of sulfated polysaccharide ascophyllan isolated from Ascophyllum nodosum. *Int. J Biol. Macromol.* **2013**, *59*, 305–312. [CrossRef]
26. Lahrsen, E.; Liewert, I.; Alban, S. Gradual degradation of fucoidan from Fucus vesiculosus and its effect on structure, antioxidant and antiproliferative activities. *Carbohydr. Polym.* **2018**, *192*, 208–216. [CrossRef]
27. Wang, Y.Q.; Wei, J.G.; Tu, M.J.; Gu, J.G.; Zhang, W. Fucoidan Alleviates Acetaminophen-Induced Hepatotoxicity via Oxidative Stress Inhibition and Nrf2 Translocation. *Int. J. Mol. Sci.* **2018**, *19*, 4050. [CrossRef]
28. Ryu, M.J.; Chung, H.S. Fucoidan reduces oxidative stress by regulating the gene expression of HO-1 and SOD-1 through the Nrf2/ERK signaling pathway in HaCaT cells. *Mol. Med. Rep.* **2016**, *14*, 3255–3260. [CrossRef]
29. Kim, H.; Ahn, J.H.; Song, M.; Kim, D.W.; Lee, T.K.; Lee, J.C.; Kim, Y.M.; Kim, J.D.; Cho, J.H.; Hwang, I.K.; et al. Pretreated fucoidan confers neuroprotection against transient global cerebral ischemic injury in the gerbil hippocampal CA1 area via reducing of glial cell activation and oxidative stress. *Biomed. Pharmacother.* **2019**, *109*, 1718–1727. [CrossRef]
30. Vomund, S.; Schäfer, A.; Parnham, M.J.; Brüne, B.; von Knethen, A. Nrf2, the Master Regulator of Anti-Oxidative Responses. *Int. J. Mol. Sci.* **2017**, *18*, 2772. [CrossRef]
31. Foresti, R.; Bucolo, C.; Platania, C.M.; Drago, F.; Dubois-Randé, J.L.; Motterlini, R. Nrf2 activators modulate oxidative stress responses and bioenergetic profiles of human retinal epithelial cells cultured in normal or high glucose conditions. *Pharmacol. Res.* **2015**, *99*, 296–307. [CrossRef] [PubMed]
32. Pittalà, V.; Fidilio, A.; Lazzara, F.; Platania, C.B.M.; Salerno, L.; Foresti, R.; Drago, F.; Bucolo, C. Effects of Novel Nitric Oxide-Releasing Molecules against Oxidative Stress on Retinal Pigmented Epithelial Cells. *Oxid. Med. Cell Longev.* **2017**, *2017*, 1420892. [CrossRef] [PubMed]
33. Koinzer, S.; Reinecke, K.; Herdegen, T.; Roider, J.; Klettner, A. Oxidative Stress Induces Biphasic ERK1/2 Activation in the RPE with Distinct Effects on Cell Survival at Early and Late Activation. *Curr. Eye Res.* **2015**, *40*, 853–857. [CrossRef] [PubMed]
34. Tode, J.; Richert, E.; Koinzer, S.; Klettner, A.; von der Burchard, C.; Brinkmann, R.; Lucius, R.; Roider, J. Thermal Stimulation of the Retina Reduces Bruch's Membrane Thickness in Age Related Macular Degeneration Mouse Models. *Transl. Vis. Sci. Technol.* **2018**, *7*, 2. [CrossRef] [PubMed]
35. German, O.L.; Agnolazza, D.L.; Politi, L.E.; Rotstein, N.P. Light, lipids and photoreceptor survival: Live or let die? *Photochem. Photobiol. Sci.* **2015**, *14*, 1737–1753. [CrossRef]
36. Klettner, A.; Roider, J. Treating age-related macular degeneration - interaction of VEGF-antagonists with their target. *Mini Rev. Chem.* **2009**, *9*, 1127–1135. [CrossRef]
37. Platania, C.B.; Di Paola, L.; Leggio, G.M.; Romano, G.L.; Drago, F.; Salomone, S.; Bucolo, C. Molecular features of interaction between VEGFA and anti-angiogenic drugs used in retinal diseases: A computational approach. *Front. Pharmacol.* **2015**, *6*, 248. [CrossRef] [PubMed]
38. Hu, M.; Cui, N.; Bo, Z.; Xiang, F. Structural Determinant and Its Underlying Molecular Mechanism of STPC2 Related to Anti-Angiogenic Activity. *Mar. Drugs* **2017**, *15*, 48. [CrossRef]
39. Koyanagi, S.; Tanigawa, N.; Nakagawa, H.; Soeda, S.; Shimeno, H. Oversulfation of fucoidan enhances its anti-angiogenic and antitumor activities. *Biochem. Pharmacol.* **2003**, *65*, 173–179. [CrossRef]
40. Chen, H.; Cong, Q.; Du, Z.; Liao, W.; Zhang, L.; Yao, Y.; Ding, K. Sulfated fucoidan FP08S2 inhibits lung cancer cell growth in vivo by disrupting angiogenesis via targeting VEGFR2/VEGF and blocking VEGFR2/Erk/VEGF signaling. *Cancer Lett.* **2016**, *382*, 44–52. [CrossRef]
41. Narazaki, M.; Segarra, M.; Tosato, G. Sulfated polysaccharides identified as inducers of neuropilin-1 internalization and functional inhibition of VEGF165 and semaphorin3A. *Blood* **2008**, *111*, 4126. [CrossRef]
42. Rui, X.; Pan, H.F.; Shao, S.L.; Xu, X.M. Anti-tumor and anti-angiogenic effects of Fucoidan on prostate cancer: Possible JAK-STAT3 pathway. *BMC Complement. Altern. Med.* **2017**, *17*, 378. [CrossRef]
43. Klettner, A.; Westhues, D.; Lassen, J.; Bartsch, S.; Roider, J. Regulation of constitutive vascular endothelial growth factor secretion in retinal pigment epithelium/choroid organ cultures: p38, nuclear factor κB, and the vascular endothelial growth factor receptor-2/phosphatidylinositol 3 kinase pathway. *Mol. Vis.* **2013**, *19*, 281–291.
44. Klettner, A.; Kaya, L.; Flach, J.; Lassen, J.; Treumer, F.; Roider, J. Basal and apical regulation of VEGF-A and placenta growth factor in the RPE/choroid and primary RPE. *Mol. Vis.* **2015**, *21*, 736–748.

45. Cébe Suarez, S.; Pieren, M.; Cariolato, L.; Arn, S.; Hoffmann, U.; Bogucki, A.; Manlius, C.; Wood, J.; Ballmer-Hofer, K. A VEGF-A splice variant defective for heparan sulfate and neuropilin-1 binding shows attenuated signaling through VEGFR-2. *Cell. Mol. Life Sci.* **2006**, *63*, 2067–2077. [CrossRef]
46. Nishiguchi, K.M.; Kataoka, K.; Kachi, S.; Komeima, K.; Terasaki, H. Regulation of pathologic retinal angiogenesis in mice and inhibition of VEGF-VEGFR2 binding by soluble heparan sulfate. *PLoS ONE* **2010**, *5*, e13493. [CrossRef]
47. Croci, D.O.; Cumashi, A.; Ushakova, N.A.; Preobrazhenskaya, M.E.; Piccoli, A.; Totani, L.; Ustyuzhanina, N.E.; Bilan, M.I.; Usov, A.I.; Grachev, A.A.; et al. Fucans, but not fucomannoglucuronans, determine the biological activities of sulfated polysaccharides from Laminaria saccharina brown seaweed. *PLoS ONE* **2011**, *6*, e17283. [CrossRef]
48. Platania, C.B.M.; Maisto, R.; Trotta, M.C.; D'Amico, M.; Rossi, S.; Gesualdo, C.; D'Amico, G.; Balta, C.; Herman, H.; Hermenean, A.; et al. Retinal and circulating miRNA expression patterns in diabetic retinopathy: An in silico and in vivo approach. *Br. J. Pharmacol.* **2019**, in press. [CrossRef]
49. Platania, C.B.M.; Leggio, G.M.; Drago, F.; Salomone, S.; Bucolo, C. Computational systems biology approach to identify novel pharmacological targets for diabetic retinopathy. *Biochem. Pharmacol.* **2018**, *158*, 13–26. [CrossRef]
50. Luyten, G.P.; Naus, N.C.; Mooy, C.M.; Hagemeijer, A.; Kan-Mitchell, J.; Van Drunen, E.; Vuzevski, V.; De Jong, P.T.; Luider, T.M. Establishment and characterization of primary and metastatic uveal melanoma cell lines. *Int. J. Cancer* **1996**, *66*, 380–387. [CrossRef]
51. Wiencke, A.K.; Kiilgaard, J.F.; Nicolini, J.; Bundgaard, M.; Röpke, C.; La Cour, M. Growth of cultured porcine retinal pigment epithelial cells. *Acta Ophthalmol. Scand.* **2003**, *81*, 170–176. [CrossRef]
52. Klettner, A.; Roider, J. Comparison of bevacizumab, ranibizumab, and pegaptanib in citro: Efficiency and possible additional pathways. *Invest. Ophthalmol. Vis. Sci.* **2008**, *49*, 4523–4527. [CrossRef]
53. Ehrig, K.; Alban, S. Sulfated galactofucan from the brown alga Saccharina latissima–variability of yield, structural composition and bioactivity. *Mar. Drugs* **2014**, *13*, 76–101. [CrossRef]
54. Riss, T.L.; Moravec, R.A.; Niles, A.L.; Duellman, S.; Benink, H.A.; Worzella, T.J.; Minor, L. Cell Viability Assays. In *Assay Guidance Manual [Internet]*; Sittampalam, G.S., Coussens, N.P., Brimacombe, K., Grossman, A., Arkin, M., Auld, D., Austin, C., Baell, J., Bejcek, B., Caaveiro, J.M.M., et al., Eds.; (MD), Eli Lilly & Company and the National Center for Advancing Translational Sciences: Bethesda, MD, USA, 2013.

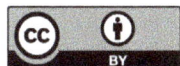

© 2019 by the authors. Licensee MDPI, Basel, Switzerland. This article is an open access article distributed under the terms and conditions of the Creative Commons Attribution (CC BY) license (http://creativecommons.org/licenses/by/4.0/).

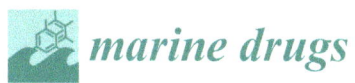

Article

Isolation and Purification of a Neuroprotective Phlorotannin from the Marine Algae *Ecklonia maxima* by Size Exclusion and High-Speed Counter-Current Chromatography

Xuezhen Zhou, Mengqi Yi, Lijian Ding *, Shan He and Xiaojun Yan *

Li Dak Sum Yip Yio Chin Kenneth Li Marine Biopharmaceutical Research Center, College of Food and Pharmaceutical Sciences, Ningbo University, Ningbo 315800, China; zhouxuezhen@nbu.edu.cn (X.Z.); ymqnbu@163.com (M.Y.); heshan@nbu.edu.cn (S.H.)
* Correspondence: dinglijian@nbu.edu.cn (L.D.); yanxiaojun@nbu.edu.cn (X.Y.); Tel.: +86-574-8760-4388 (L.D.)

Received: 28 March 2019; Accepted: 3 April 2019; Published: 4 April 2019

Abstract: Phlorotannins are polyphenolic metabolites of marine brown algae that have been shown to possess health-beneficial biological activities. An efficient approach using a combination of high-speed counter-current chromatography (HSCCC) and size exclusion chromatography with a Sephadex LH-20 has been successfully developed for the isolation and purification of a neuroprotective phlorotannin, eckmaxol, from leaves of the marine brown algae, *Ecklonia maxima*. The phlorotannin of interest, eckmaxol, was isolated with purity >95% by HSCCC using an optimized solvent system composed of *n*-hexane–ethyl acetate–methanol–water (2:8:3:7, v/v/v/v) after Sephadex LH-20 size exclusion chromatography. This compound was successfully purified in the quantity of 5.2 mg from 0.3 kg of the *E. maxima* crude organic extract. The structure of eckmaxol was identified and assigned by NMR spectroscopic and mass spectrometric analyses. The purification method developed for eckmaxol will facilitate the further investigation and development of this neuroprotective agent as a drug lead or pharmacological probe. Furthermore, it is suggested that the combination of HSCCC and size exclusion chromatography could be more widely applied for the isolation and purification of phlorotannins from marine algae.

Keywords: phlorotannin; eckmaxol; high-speed counter-current chromatography; NMR spectroscopy; mass spectrometry; isolation and purification; *Ecklonia maxima*

1. Introduction

Phlorotannins are the major phloroglucinol-derived polyphenols of wide occurrence among marine brown algae, and these have been extensively investigated for various biological activities such as antioxidant, anticancer, anti-inflammatory, anti-allergic, antidiabetic, antihypertensive, and neuroprotective effects [1–4]. *Ecklonia maxima* is a brown seaweed that is distributed along the west coast of South Africa [5]. The leaves of *E. maxima* are frequently used as source materials for producing alginate, animal feed, nutritional supplements, fertilizers, and for preparation of different medications, including alpha-glucosidase inhibitors applied for the treatment of diabetes mellitus [5,6]. Eckmaxol (**1**; Figure 1) is a recently reported phlorotannin obtained from the ethyl acetate extract of *E. maxima* as described in our previous study. This phlorotannin possesses many beneficial properties, including protection against Aβ oligomer induced neurotoxicity in SH-SY5Y cells in vitro [7]. Additional material is required to further investigate the functions of **1** in mammalian systems for the development of this compound as a new pharmacological probe or potential drug lead for treating Alzheimer's disease.

Unfortunately, the reported purification of phlorotannins has typically included repeated column chromatography steps and preparative HPLC, which is time-consuming, leads to the loss of target phlorotannins due to oxidization during the long process, and is not industrially viable due to the cost of solid supports (e.g., resin or gel) for separation. Accordingly, these techniques are not typically suitable for purification of large quantities of material unless no other methods can complete the task [8,9]. Alternatively, high-speed counter-current chromatography (HSCCC) is a liquid-liquid separation chromatography that can reduce the separation time and cost, and offers effectively total sample recovery due to the lack of a solid support matrix that can degrade or permanently retain target molecules [10]. HSCCC has recently been applied to the isolation of various natural products, most typically coming from plants [11–13]. However, no previous report has disclosed the use of HSCCC for the isolation and purification of phlorotannins. The purpose of this study was to develop an efficient method for the preparative isolation and purification of eckmaxol (**1**) using the combined methods HSCCC and Sephadex LH-20, which are both nondestructive and nonabsorptive (e.g., lossless) techniques.

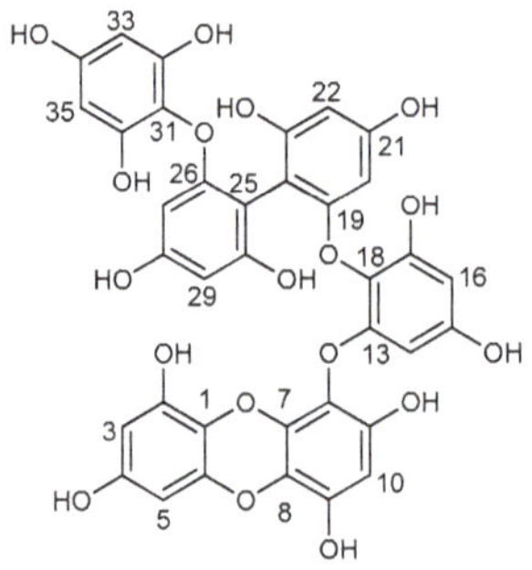

Figure 1. Chemical structure of eckmaxol (**1**).

2. Results and Discussion

2.1. Enrichment of Eckmaxol by Sephadex LH-20 Size Exclusion Chromatography

Due to the large amounts of pigments and other unknown polyphenols contained in the crude ethanolic extract of *E. maxima*, it is difficult to separate and isolate **1** with high purity by HSCCC in one step. In order to effectively enrich the targeted compound, the crude extract was first subjected to size exclusion chromatography on a Sephadex LH-20 gravity column. The LH-20 column was eluted with an isocratic solvent system of dichloromethane–methanol (1:1). A total of six fractions (250 mL each) were successively collected, named Fractions A–F. Fr. C was determined to contain **1** in high quantity, and this sample was concentrated to dryness and stored in a refrigerator (4 °C) for later HSCCC separation.

2.2. Optimization of UPLC Analysis for Eckmaxol

A ultra-performance liquid chromatography (UPLC) method was developed to ensure the baseline separation of the target compound and impurities, and evaluate the size exclusion chromatography fraction C. Different flow rates, elution modes, detection wavelengths and column temperatures were screened. The result indicated that the target compound was baseline separated with methanol-water (methanol: 0–10 min, 10%–90%) as the solvent system, when the flow rate, column temperature and detection wavelength were set at 0.4 mL/min, 25 °C and 254 nm. Preliminary assignment of **1** in the chromatogram was made by comparison of peak retention time and UV spectrum against a previously derived authentic standard. The UPLC chromatogram of fraction C showed the major, but not only peak, as being **1** (Figure 2A).

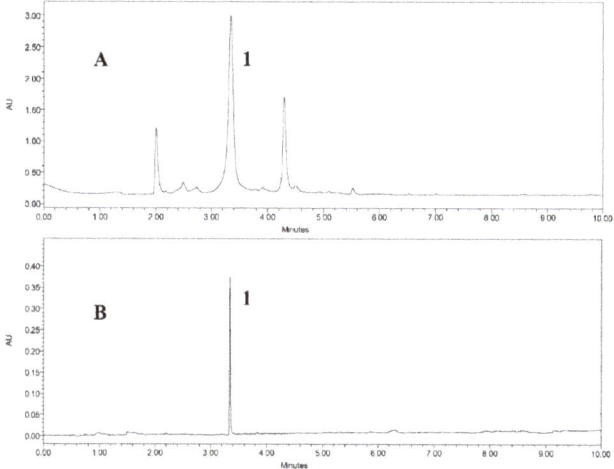

Figure 2. Representative ultra-performance liquid chromatography (UPLC) chromatograms (254 nm) of samples prepared from *E. maxima* (**A**). Fraction C from the size exclusion chromatography of the crude ethyl acetate extract; (**B**) Subfraction of C that contains **1** after preparative separation by high-speed counter-current chromatography (HSCCC).

2.3. Selection of the HSCCC Two-Phase Solvent System

Since HSCCC relies on two immiscible liquids to function as stationary and mobile phases, the selection of a suitable biphasic solvent system plays a vital role in successful separations. It has been suggested that the partition coefficient (K) is the most important parameter in solvent system selection, which should be $0.5 \leq K \leq 2$ (close to 1, best) to get a good separation for HSCCC in a suitable run time [13,14]. As previously reported in the literature [15,16], the two-phase solvent system "HEMWat", comprising *n*-hexane–ethyl acetate–methanol–water, has been widely applied in the separation of natural products by HSCCC. Five sets of different proportional two-phase HEMWat solvent systems were carried out to determine the partition value, K, of the target compound at various volume ratios of n-hexane/ethyl acetate/methanol/water (3:10:3:10, 1:3:1:3, 2:7:3:7, 2:8:3:7, all v/v/v/v) by UPLC analysis of each partition. The results, shown in Table 1, indicated that the two-phase solvent system of 2:8:3:7 *n*-hexane/ethyl acetate/methanol/water, v/v/v/v, provided a suitable partition value for eckmaxol of K = 1.15 with good resolution and short elution time.

Table 1. K values of target compound **1** in different ratios of the HEMWat solvent system.

Solvent System	Ratio (v/v/v/v)	K
n-hexane/ethyl acetate/methanol/water	3:10:3:10	0.32
n-hexane/ethyl acetate/methanol/water	1:3:1:3	0.75
n-hexane/ethyl acetate/methanol/water	2:7:3:7	1.78
n-hexane/ethyl acetate/methanol/water	2:8:3:7	1.15

2.4. HSCCC Separation

The selected fraction C from the size exclusion chromatography of the ethanol extract from *E. maxima* (300 mg) was applied for HSCCC separation with the chosen two-phase solvent system, *n*-hexane-ethyl acetate–methanol–water (2:8:3:7). In order to optimize the resolution and reduce the separation time, different flow rates and rotation speeds were evaluated. It was found that when the flow rate was 2 mL/min and rotation speed was 850 rpm, a good separation was achieved for elution of **1** with a good stationary phase retention of 65.7%. The HSCCC peak fraction corresponding to **1**

(5.2 mg) was collected and determined to have purity of 95.83% by UPLC analysis (Figure 2B). The resulting HSCC chromatogram is shown in Figure 3, demonstrating the good resolution and peak shape of compound **1** at t_R = 140 min.

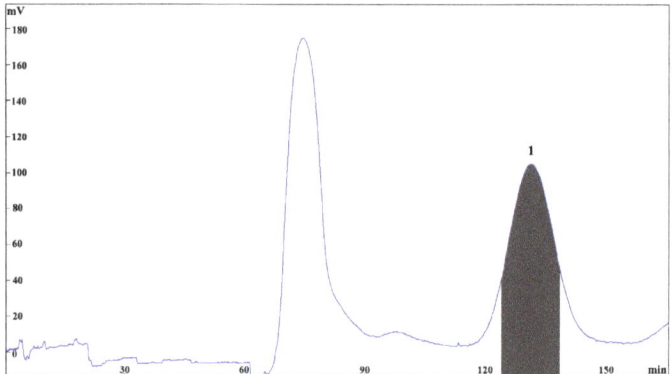

Figure 3. HSCCC chromatogram of the fraction C of the ethanol extract from *E. maxima* using the two-phase solvent system composed of n-hexane–EtOAc–MeOH–water (2:8:3:7, v/v/v/v); stationary phase: upper phase of solvent system; mobile phase: lower aqueous phase of solvent system; column capacity 320 mL; rotation speed 850 rpm; column temperature 25 °C; flow rate 2.0 mL/min; detection, 254 nm; sample injected, 300 mg in 6 mL biphasic solution; retention of the stationary phase, 65.7%; peak identification: eckmaxol (**1**).

2.5. Identification of Chemical Structure

Compound **1** was identified by HR-ESI-MS, ^{1}H-NMR, and ^{13}C-NMR after purification by HSCCC, and its detailed data are shown in Table 2. Its molecular formula $C_{36}H_{24}O_{18}$ was deduced by HR-ESI-MS data at m/z 743.0896 [M − H]$^-$. Compound **1** was identified as a phlorotannin, eckmaxol, with the chemical structure as shown in Figure 1. The structure of eckmaxol was first disclosed in a Japanese patent application (JP 2013-49639), but the assignment of its spectroscopic data was never reported.

Table 2. ^{1}H (500 MHz) and ^{13}C-NMR (125 MHz) spectroscopic data of eckmaxol (**1**) in CDOD_3.

Pos.	δ_H	δ_C	Pos.	δ_H	δ_C
1		124.8	19		157.1
2		151.3	20	5.93 (1H, d, J = 2.4 Hz, H-20)	94.2
3	6.11 (1H, d, J = 2.4 Hz, H-3)	97.6	21		159.2
4		156.4	22	6.32 (1H, d, J = 2.4 Hz, H-22)	98.7
5	5.86 (1H, d, J = 2.4 Hz, H-5)	94.7	23		143.3
6		154.4	24		102.0
7		123.5	25		101.8
8		137.5	26		156.1
9		143.5	27	6.20 (1H, d, J = 2.0 Hz, H-27)	95.2
10	6.20 (1H, s, H-10)	98.9	28		159.3
11		146.3	29	6.28 (1H, d, J = 2.0 Hz, H-29)	98.3
12		124.7	30		158.5
13		153.4	31		124.0
14	6.01 (1H, d, J = 2.4 Hz, H-14)	99.3	32		151.6
15		158.7	33	6.03 (1H, s, H-33)	96.1
16	5.94 (1H, d, J = 2.4 Hz, H-16)	95.2	34		156.1
17		146.7	35	6.03 (1H, s, H-35)	96.1
18		123.8	36		151.6

3. Materials and Methods

3.1. Reagents and Materials

All solvents used for HSCCC were of analytical grade (Huadong Chemicals, Hangzhou, China). Reverse osmosis Milli-Q water (18 M) (Millipore, Bedford, MA, USA) was used for all solutions and dilutions. Methanol used for UPLC analyses was of chromatographic grade and purchased from Anpel Laboratory Technologies (Shanghai, China). The CD_3OD used for NMR analyses was purchased from Tenglong Weibo Technology (Qingdao, China). The sample of *E. maxima* (no. 801) was kindly provided by Shandong Jiejing Group Co., Ltd. in China, collected from the seashore of South Africa.

3.2. Apparatus

HSCCC was carried out using a model TBE-300C high-speed countercurrent chromatograph (Tauto Biotech Co. Ltd., Shanghai, China), containing a self-balancing three-coil centrifuge rotor equipped with three preparative multilayer coils and a total capacity of 320 mL. The internal diameter of PTFE (Polytetrafluoroethylene) tubing was 1.9 mm. The apparatus maximum rotational speed is 1000 rpm and has a 20 mL manual sample loop. The revolution radius was 5 cm and the value of the multilayer coil varied from 0.5 at the internal terminal to 0.8 at the external terminal. An integrated TBP 5002 (Tauto Biotech Co. Ltd.) was used to pump the two-phase HSCCC solvent system, and the UV absorbance of the effluent was measured at 254 nm by a UV 1001 detector (Shanghai Sanotac Scientific Instruments Co. Ltd., Shanghai, China). A DC-0506 constant temperature regulator (Tauto Biotech Co. Ltd.) was used to control the temperature during HSCCC. An N2000 data analysis system (Institute of Automation Engineering, Zhejiang University, Hangzhou, China) was employed for HSCCC data collection and analysis. The UPLC equipment was using a Waters Acquity a UPLC BEH C18 column (100 mm × 2.1 mm, 1.7 µm particle size) equipped with a model 2998 diode array detector and Empower System (Waters Co., Milford, MA, USA). NMR experiments including ^1H, ^{13}C, DEPT, ^1H-^1H COSY, HSQC, and HMBC were carried out using a Varian 500 MHz NMR spectrometer (Palo Alto, CA, USA) spectrometer. HR-ESI-MS data was measured using a Waters Q-TOF Premier LC/MS spectrometer (Waters Co., Milford, MA, USA). Column chromatography (CC) was carried out with Sephadex LH-20 (Amersham Biosciences, Piscataway, NJ, USA).

3.3. Preparation of Crude Sample from E. maxima for HSCCC

The leaves of *E. maxima* were cut into pieces. The fresh pieces (~0.3 kg, wet) were extracted three times with 1 L of 80% ethanol ($EtOH/H_2O$) for 1.5 h by sonication at room temperature (25 °C). The crude extract was concentrated in a rotary vacuum evaporator and partitioned. Then the dried EtOAc extract (1 g) was subjected to column chromatography with Sephadex LH-20 gel for fractionation to furnish fractions A–F, each eluted with a mixed solvent system of dichloromethane–methanol (1:1). Fr. C was concentrated to dryness and stored in a refrigerator (4 °C) for later HSCCC separation.

3.4. Preparation of Two-Phase Solvent System and Sample Solution

The HSCCC experiments were performed using a two-phase solvent system comprising *n*-hexane/ethyl acetate/methanol/water (2:8:3:7, v/v/v/v) solvent. The two phases were separated after thoroughly equilibrating the mixture in a separating funnel at 25 °C. The upper organic phase was used as the stationary phase, and the lower aqueous phase was employed as the mobile phase.

3.5. HSCCC Separation

The HSCCC column was initially filled with the organic stationary phase and rotated at 850 rpm; the mobile phase was pumped into the column in the descending mode at the same flow rate used for separation (2 mL/min). When the mobile phase emerged from the column, it indicated that hydrodynamic equilibrium had been achieved. The concentrated fraction C (300 mg) obtained from the 80% EtOH extract of *E. maxima* was dissolved in 6 mL of a 1:1 (v/v) mixture of the two HSCCC solvent system phases and injected to the sample port. The effluent from the HSCCC was monitored by UV at 254 nm, and 6 mL fractions were collected in 8 mL tubes by a fraction collector.

3.6. Analysis and Identification of the Target Compound

The fraction generated by preparative HSCCC was evaluated by UPLC. The sample was separated with a CH_3OH/H_2O gradient (flow 0.4 mL/min, 10%–90% CH_3OH from 0–10 min). The effluent was continuously monitored by a UV detector at 254 nm. The fraction that showed only one peak in the chromatogram was respectively pooled together to yield the compound (5.2 mg, t_R 3.3 min).

4. Conclusions

In conclusion, an efficient method relying on HSCCC after size exclusion chromatography on Sephadex LH-20 was used to preparative separation of eckmaxol (**1**) from the leaves of *E. maxima* in a lossless two chromatic step procedure. It was important to preliminarily fractionate the crude extract for HSCCC separation to improve the resolution and efficiency. The solvent system of *n*-hexane/ethyl acetate/methanol/water (2:8:3:7, *v/v/v/v*) was used to isolate eckmaxol (**1**). The separation condition was selected as follow: flow rate 2.0 mL/min, rotary speed 850 rpm, column temperature 25 °C. Under the optimized HSCCC condition, 5.2 mg eckmaxol with the high purity of 95.83% was isolated from 300 mg of fraction C of *E. maxima*. This is the first report of the isolation of eckmaxol (**1**) by integrating HSCCC and size exclusion chromatography, and this method could be used for the effective isolation of different phlorotannins. This convenient and economical approach will be applicable for scale-up production of eckmaxol to increase the yield. The purification method developed for eckmaxol will also facilitate the further investigation and development of this neuroprotective agent as a drug lead or pharmacological probe, ideally through future in vivo studies.

Author Contributions: X.Z., L.D. and X.Y. conceived and designed the experiments. X.Z and M.Y. S.H. performed the experiments. X.Z., L.D. and S.H. analyzed the data. X.Z. and L.D. wrote the paper.

Acknowledgments: The authors acknowledge the National Key Research and Development Program of China (2018YFC0310900), the National Natural Science Foundation of China (41776168, 41706167), Ningbo Public Service Platform for High-Value Utilization of Marine Biological Resources (NBHY-2017-P2), the Natural Science Foundation of Ningbo (2018A610303, 2018A610320), Ningbo Sci. & Tech. Projects for Common Wealth (2017C10016), the National 111 Project of China (D16013), the Li Dak Sum Yip Yio Chin Kenneth Li Marine Biopharmaceutical Development Fund, and the K.C. Wong Magna Fund in Ningbo University. We appreciate C. Benjamin Naman (Ningbo University, China and University of California, San Diego, USA) for critical reading and linguistic editing of the manuscript.

Conflicts of Interest: The authors declare no conflict of interest.

References

1. Li, Y.X.; Wijesekara, I.; Li, Y.; Kim, S.K. Phlorotannins as bioactive agents from brown algae. *Process Biochem.* **2011**, *46*, 2219–2224. [CrossRef]
2. Kannan, R.R.R.; Aderogba, M.A.; Ndhlala, A.R.; Stirk, W.A.; Staden, J.V. Acetylcholinesterase inhibitory activity of phlorotannins isolated from the brown alga, *Ecklonia maxima* (Osbeck) Papenfuss. *Food Res. Int.* **2013**, *54*, 1250–1254. [CrossRef]
3. A-Reum, K.; Tai-Sun, S.; Min-Sup, L.; Ji-Young, P.; Kyoung-Eun, P.; Na-Young, Y.; Jong-Soon, K.; Jae-Sue, C.; Byeong-Churl, J.; Dae-Seok, B. Isolation and identification of phlorotannins from *Ecklonia stolonifera* with antioxidant and anti-inflammatory properties. *J. Agr. Food Chem.* **2009**, *57*, 3483–3489.
4. Thomas, N.V.; Kim, S.K. Potential pharmacological applications of polyphenolic derivatives from marine brown algae. *Environ. Toxicol. Phar.* **2011**, *32*, 325–335. [CrossRef] [PubMed]
5. Rengasamy, K.R.R.; Aderogba, M.A.; Amoo, S.O.; Stirk, W.A.; Johannes, V.S. Potential antiradical and alpha-glucosidase inhibitors from *Ecklonia maxima* (Osbeck) Papenfuss. *Food Chem.* **2013**, *141*, 1412–1415. [CrossRef] [PubMed]

6. Rengasamy, K.R.R.; Kulkarni, M.G.; Stirk, W.A.; Staden, J.V. Eckol—A new plant growth stimulant from the brown seaweed *Ecklonia maxima*. *J. Appl. Phycol.* **2015**, *27*, 581–587. [CrossRef]
7. Wang, J.; Zheng, J.; Huang, C.; Zhao, J.; Lin, J.; Zhou, X.; Naman, C.B.; Wang, N.; Gerwick, W.H.; Wang, Q. Eckmaxol, a phlorotannin extracted from *Ecklonia maxima*, produces anti-β-amyloid oligomer neuroprotective effects possibly via directly acting on glycogen synthase kinase 3β. *ACS Chem. Neurosci.* **2018**, *9*, 1349–1356. [CrossRef] [PubMed]
8. Shibata, T.; Ishimaru, K.; Kawaguchi, S.; Yoshikawa, H.; Hama, Y. Antioxidant activities of phlorotannins isolated from Japanese Laminariaceae. *J. Appl. Phycol.* **2008**, *20*, 705–711. [CrossRef]
9. Nakai, M.; Kageyama, N.; Nakahara, K.; Miki, W. Phlorotannins as radical scavengers from the extract of *Sargassum ringgoldianum*. *Mar. Biotechnol.* **2006**, *8*, 409–414. [CrossRef] [PubMed]
10. Duan, W.; Ji, W.; Wei, Y.; Zhao, R.; Chen, Z.; Geng, Y.; Jing, F.; Wang, X. Separation and purification of fructo-oligosaccharide by High-Speed Counter-Current Chromatography coupled with precolumn derivatization. *Molecules* **2018**, *23*, 381. [CrossRef] [PubMed]
11. Yan, R.; Shen, J.; Liu, X.; Zou, Y.; Xu, X. Preparative isolation and purification of hainanmurpanin, meranzin, and phebalosin from leaves of Murraya exotica L. using supercritical fluid extraction combined with consecutive high-speed countercurrent chromatography. *J. Sep. Sci.* **2018**, *41*, 2092. [CrossRef] [PubMed]
12. Guo, W.; Dong, H.; Wang, D.; Yang, B.; Wang, X.; Huang, L. Separation of seven polyphenols from the rhizome of *Smilax glabra* by offline two dimension recycling HSCCC with extrusion mode. *Molecules* **2018**, *23*, 505. [CrossRef] [PubMed]
13. Liu, Y.; Zhou, X.; Naman, C.B.; Lu, Y.; Ding, L.; He, S. Preparative separation and purification of trichothecene mycotoxins from the marine fungus *Fusarium* sp. LS68 by high-speed countercurrent chromatography in stepwise elution mode. *Mar. Drugs* **2018**, *16*, 73. [CrossRef] [PubMed]
14. Wang, J.; Gu, D.; Wang, M.; Guo, X.; Li, H.; Dong, Y.; Guo, H.; Wang, Y.; Fan, M.; Yang, Y. Rational approach to solvent system selection for liquid–liquid extraction–assisted sample pretreatment in counter–current chromatography. *J. Chromatogr. B* **2017**, *1053*, 16–19. [CrossRef] [PubMed]
15. Shaheen, N.; Lu, Y.; Geng, P.; Shao, Q.; Wei, Y. Isolation of four phenolic compounds from *Mangifera indica*. L flowers by using normal phase combined with elution extrusion two-step high speed countercurrent chromatography. *J. Chromatogr. B* **2017**, *1046*, 211–217. [CrossRef] [PubMed]
16. Kong, Q.; Ren, X.; Hu, R.; Yin, X.; Jiang, G.; Pan, Y. Isolation and purification of two antioxidant isomers of resveratrol dimer from the wine grape by counter-current chromatography. *J. Sep. Sci.* **2016**, *39*, 2374–2379. [CrossRef] [PubMed]

 © 2019 by the authors. Licensee MDPI, Basel, Switzerland. This article is an open access article distributed under the terms and conditions of the Creative Commons Attribution (CC BY) license (http://creativecommons.org/licenses/by/4.0/).

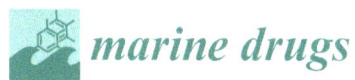

Article

Antitumoral Effect of Laurinterol on 3D Culture of Breast Cancer Explants

Sara García-Davis [1,2], Ezequiel Viveros-Valdez [1], Ana R. Díaz-Marrero [2], José J. Fernández [2], Daniel Valencia-Mercado [3], Olga Esquivel-Hernández [4], Pilar Carranza-Rosales [5], Irma Edith Carranza-Torres [1,5,*] and Nancy Elena Guzmán-Delgado [6,*]

1. Facultad de Ciencias Biológicas (FCB), Universidad Autónoma de Nuevo León (UANL), Av. Pedro de Alba s/n, 66450 San Nicolás de los Garza, Nuevo León, México; sara.garciadv@uanl.edu.mx (S.G.-D.); jose.viverosvld@uanl.edu.mx (E.V.-V.)
2. Instituto Universitario de Bio-Orgánica Antonio González (IUBO AG), Centro de Investigaciones Biomédicas de Canarias (CIBICAN), Universidad de La Laguna (ULL), Avda. Astrofísico F. Sánchez, 2, 38206 La Laguna, Tenerife, Spain; adiazmar@ull.edu.es (A.R.D.-M.); jjfercas@ull.edu.es (J.J.F.)
3. Servicio de Oncología Ginecológica, Unidad Médica de Alta Especialidad, Hospital de Gineco-Obstetricia No. 23, Instituto Mexicano del Seguro Social (IMSS), Avenida Constitución y Félix U. Gómez s/n, Colonia Centro, 64000 Monterrey, Nuevo León, México; davame7@hotmail.com
4. Departamento de Anatomía Patológica, Unidad Médica de Alta Especialidad, Hospital de Gineco-Obstetricia No. 23, Instituto Mexicano del Seguro Social (IMSS), Avenida Constitución y Félix U. Gómez s/n, Colonia Centro, 64000 Monterrey, Nuevo León, México; oesh10@gmail.com
5. Centro de Investigación Biomédica del Noreste (CIBIN), Instituto Mexicano del Seguro Social (IMSS), Calle Jesús Dionisio González # 501, Col. Independencia, 64720 Monterrey, Nuevo León, México; carranza60@yahoo.com.mx
6. División de Investigación en Salud, Unidad Médica de Alta Especialidad, Hospital de Cardiología No. 34, Instituto Mexicano del Seguro Social (IMSS), Av. Lincoln S/N esquina con Enfermera María de Jesús Candia, Col. Valle Verde 2do. Sector, 64360 Monterrey, Nuevo León, México
* Correspondence: mitzba@hotmail.com (I.E.C.-T.); nancyegd@gmail.com (N.E.G.-D.); Tel.: +52-81-8190-4036 (I.E.C.-T.); +52-81-8399-4300 (ext. 40606) (N.E.G.-D.)

Received: 22 February 2019; Accepted: 25 March 2019; Published: 29 March 2019

Abstract: Macroalgae represent an important source of bioactive compounds with a wide range of biotechnological applications. Overall, the discovery of effective cytotoxic compounds with pharmaceutical potential is a significant challenge, mostly because they are scarce in nature or their total synthesis is not efficient, while the bioprospecting models currently used do not predict clinical responses. Given this context, we used three-dimensional (3D) cultures of human breast cancer explants to evaluate the antitumoral effect of laurinterol, the major compound of an ethanolic extract of *Laurencia johnstonii*. To this end, we evaluated the metabolic and histopathological effects of the crude extract of *L. johnstonii* and laurinterol on Vero and MCF-7 cells, in addition to breast cancer explants. We observed a dose-dependent inhibition of the metabolic activity, as well as morphologic and nuclear changes characteristic of apoptosis. On the other hand, a reduced metabolic viability and marked necrosis areas were observed in breast cancer explants incubated with the crude extract, while explants treated with laurinterol exhibited a heterogeneous response which was associated with the individual response of each human tumor sample. This study supports the cytotoxic and antitumoral effects of laurinterol in in vitro cell cultures and in ex vivo organotypic cultures of human breast cancer explants.

Keywords: laurinterol; *Laurencia*; antitumoral; breast cancer explants; organotypic culture; ex vivo

1. Introduction

Marine environments are an interesting source of compounds holding a variety of therapeutic properties as a result of the vast diversity of lifeforms inhabiting the oceans. Among them, algae are one of the most prolific sources of bioactive compounds. Unfortunately, over the last two decades, only nine marine-derived drugs were approved for clinical therapy in spite of more than 18,000 new marine compounds described in that time frame. Additionally, it is interesting to see that six out of these nine approved drugs are currently used in cancer therapies [1].

The genus *Laurencia* is one of the richest sources of novel compounds among red algae. It is widely distributed throughout tropical and temperate zones. In particular, *L. johnstonii* is an endemic species of the Gulf of California in Mexico [2], present throughout the year in regions compatible with its temperate biogeographic affinity [3].

As a consequence of its wide distribution, the biological activity of metabolites isolated from *Laurencia* species were tested. Laurinterol (L1) is a brominated sesquiterpene frequently found in *Laurencia* species and mollusks of genus *Aplysia* [4]. Its antibacterial [5–7], cytotoxic [7,8], antifouling [9], Na/K ATPase inhibition [10], and insecticidal and repellent [11] properties were reported. Recently, our group reported L1 anti-*Acanthamoeba* activity [12].

Breast cancer is the most common cancer worldwide, impacting 2.1 million women each year, and it is the second highest cause of cancer death in women with 627,000 deaths in 2018 [13]. The most common drugs used for breast cancer therapy include anthracyclines, such as doxorubicin and epirubicin, taxanes, such as paclitaxel and docetaxel, 5-fluorouracil (5-FU), cyclophosphamide, and carboplatin. In most cases, combinations of two or three of these drugs are used [14]. However, there is a need for new anti-cancer agents with fewer and/or less significant side effects, and the effectiveness of available option treatments is still limited. In addition, resistance to chemotherapy is an important problem in breast cancer management, and multidrug resistance (MDR) was observed as a result of cross-resistance to other cytotoxic agents to which patients were never exposed [15]. Drug resistance in cancer can be mediated via different mechanisms, such as alterations affecting cell-cycle dynamics, susceptibility of cells undergoing apoptosis, uptake and efflux of drugs, cellular drug metabolism, intracellular compartmentalization of drugs, or repair of drug-induced damage [15].

As a result of the numerous research group efforts to find new targets and novel anticancer compounds, recently, a number of medical advances improved the treatment options against breast cancer, many of which are geared toward the individual characteristics of the patient and the tumoral tissue. The goal of these kinds of treatments is to be as effective as possible, while keeping minimal side effects and treating only the patients who will benefit from a specific therapy [16,17].

After decades of research, experimental models that are able to correlate the compounds' activity with their clinical efficacy in humans, as well as to predict an individual response to treatment, are still needed. In this regard, an organotypic culture of tumor-derived slices is a robust model that retains the tumor microenvironment and allows extrapolating the effect of antineoplastic agents in terms of physiology, metabolism, and pharmacokinetics [18]; it is a promising option between two-dimensional (2D) cell culture and pre-clinical trials, while decreasing the high risk of failure in the drug development pipeline and improving the therapeutic response prediction.

Taking into consideration the cytotoxic activity of *Laurencia*-derived metabolites [4,8,12,19–22], the rapid breast cancer increment, and the need for more effective drugs, we analyzed the antineoplastic effect of L1, the major compound isolated from *L. johnstonii*, using ex vivo organotypic cultures of human breast cancer explants.

2. Results and Discussion

2.1. Extraction and Isolation

The marine environment is an interesting source of bioactive compounds with uncommon chemical features. Among marine organisms, algae are one of the major sources of new compounds after sponges, microorganisms, and phytoplankton [1]. Red algae of the genus *Laurencia* are considered as one of the richest sources of new secondary metabolites with a huge chemical variation influenced by environmental and genetic factors [4]. The study of endemic organisms, such as *L. johnstonii*, adapted to live under particular environmental conditions, is a significant aspect to consider in the search of potential bioactive secondary metabolites. In a previous work, we observed better bioactivity profiles in extracts of *Laurencia* species collected in the Gulf of California compared to those of species inhabiting the Pacific coast from the Baja California peninsula [23].

L1 (Figure 1) was isolated from the ethanolic extract of *L. johnstonii* [24] and represented 70% of the whole crude extract (CE), a relevant fact if we consider that one of the major challenges in the biodiscovery process is the supply problem [1]. L1 is a brominated sesquiterpene with a cyclolaurane skeleton, widely obtained from *Laurencia* species [4] and recently isolated from *L. johnstonii* [12]. L1 belongs to the significant group of marine haloaryl secondary metabolites, molecules of relevance for their interesting biological activity [25].

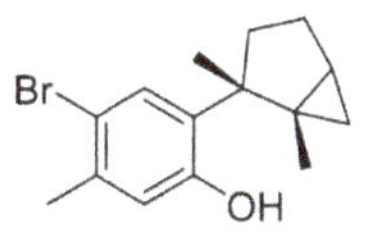

Figure 1. Laurinterol (L1).

2.2. Cytotoxicity Assays

CE and L1 cytotoxic activity were evaluated against Vero and MCF-7 cell lines. Vero cells are used worldwide as a normal cell line control to assess in vitro cytotoxic effects [26,27], due to its susceptibility to various types of microbes, toxins, and chemical compounds. This cell line is often used in natural product screening assays [28–30] and in cancer studies as a normal cell line control group [31]. Cell viability was measured by addition of WST-1 after 24 h of incubation, and it was estimated from the cell population of the control and cell populations after treatments. CE and L1 were assayed at various concentrations and they displayed a dose-dependent inhibition; controls were dimethyl sulfoxide (DMSO), paclitaxel (TX), and cisplatin (CIS). CE showed half maximal inhibitory concentration (IC_{50}) values of 26.18 µg/mL and 28.05 µg/mL for Vero and MCF-7 cell lines, respectively, whereas L1 IC_{50} values were 15.68 µg/mL for Vero and 16.07 µg/mL for MCF-7 cells. Figure 2 shows the percentage of cell viability at two different concentrations of CE and L1, one lower (10 µg/mL) and one higher (30 µg/mL) concentration than the IC_{50} values obtained for both cell lines. Both CE and L1 showed similar viability percentage, due to the great amount of L1 in the CE. The cytotoxic effects of *Laurencia* extracts against different cell lines were reported [23,32,33], showing a wide spectrum of toxicity according to the species, geography, and solvent used for the extraction. L1 was also evaluated in cell lines including MCF-7, with similar results to our findings [8]. Additionally, CE induced a notable or discrete hormetic effect at 10 µg/mL in Vero cells or MCF-7 cells; hormesis is a biphasic dose-dependent response that induces an adaptive effect on the cells characterized by low-dose stimulation and high-dose inhibition [34] (Figure 2).

After a period of 24 h, morphological alterations were observed under the microscope in cells incubated with the treatments. Control subject cells in plain growth medium and cells incubated with 1% DMSO appeared to be healthy, displaying well-defined cell–cell junctions and a normal confluent monolayer, while cells treated with antineoplastics (TX and CIS), CE, and L1 became rounder and shrunken, with cell–cell junctions disrupted and detachment from the surface of the plate, denoting cell death (data not shown).

The cytological effects of L1 in MCF-7 breast cancer cell monolayers were studied using an in situ hematoxylin and eosin (H&E) staining assay (Figure 3). The untreated control cells (Figure 3A) showed the characteristic cell monolayers irregularly shaped, with well-defined junctions and preserved nucleus–cytoplasm ratio, with a prominent nucleus and more than one nucleolus in each cell. Cells incubated with 1% DMSO (Figure 3B) showed a similar morphology to the untreated cells. In the cells treated with CE (Figure 3C), the cytotoxic effect was characterized by the presence of cytoplasmic vacuoles of different sizes in all cells (asterisks), and by the monolayers' partial rupture where cytoplasmic junctions can be observed in empty spaces (ES) instead of cells, while their nucleoli became less prominent. In contrast, the cytotoxic effect of L1 (Figure 3D) is notably different than the CE; in this case, it is possible to observe the cell monolayer's complete rupture, loss of cell morphology, and loss of the nucleus–cytoplasm ratio, as well as cell shrinkage and nuclear pyknosis (arrow). The morphologic and nuclear changes observed in the present study are apoptotic cell death characteristics [35], and they were described in breast cancer cell lines treated with antiproliferative agents [36], extracts [37], and pure compounds, such as curcumin [38]; this also agrees with Kim et al., who reported that a crude extract of *L. okamurai* containing laurinterol can induce apoptosis through a p53-dependent pathway in melanoma cells [22].

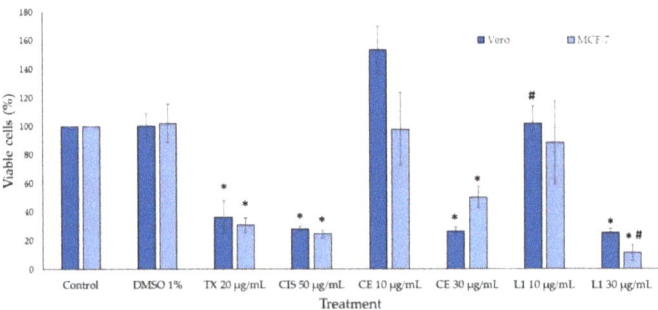

Figure 2. Viability of treated cells. TX: paclitaxel, CIS: cisplatin, CE: crude extract, L1: laurinterol. $n = 3$ ± standard deviation (SD); * $p < 0.01$ compared to the control, # $p < 0.05$ compared to CE.

The CE cytological effects are similar to those induced by TX (Figure 3E), while L1 induces damage similar to CIS (Figure 3F), suggesting different molecular damage mechanisms. At this level, both chemotherapeutic drugs exhibit a greater antiproliferative effect, as they showed a marked inhibition of monolayer formation. Considering that L1 is the major compound in the CE, it could be expected that the observed cytological effect would also be similar. In order to establish the possible relationship between the CE and L1 mechanism of action with the antineoplastics TX and CIS, additional studies are required. On the other hand, it is also possible that the cytological differences induced by the CE and L1 can be attributed to other minor metabolites present in the CE, such as the bromo-sesquiterpene aplysin, which was also found in the CE of *L. johnstonii* [12] and which was reported as a powerful apoptosis inductor [4,39–41]. Other minor compounds isolated from *L. johnstonii* (isolaurinterol, α-bromocuparane, α-isobromocuparane [12], johnstonol [42], and prepacifenol epoxide [43]) also showed cytotoxicity in cell lines [19–21,44,45] and murine macrophages [12], with isolaurinterol showing the highest toxicity. With regard to the apoptosis in MCF-7 cells described in this work, further studies are needed to identify the underlying mechanism.

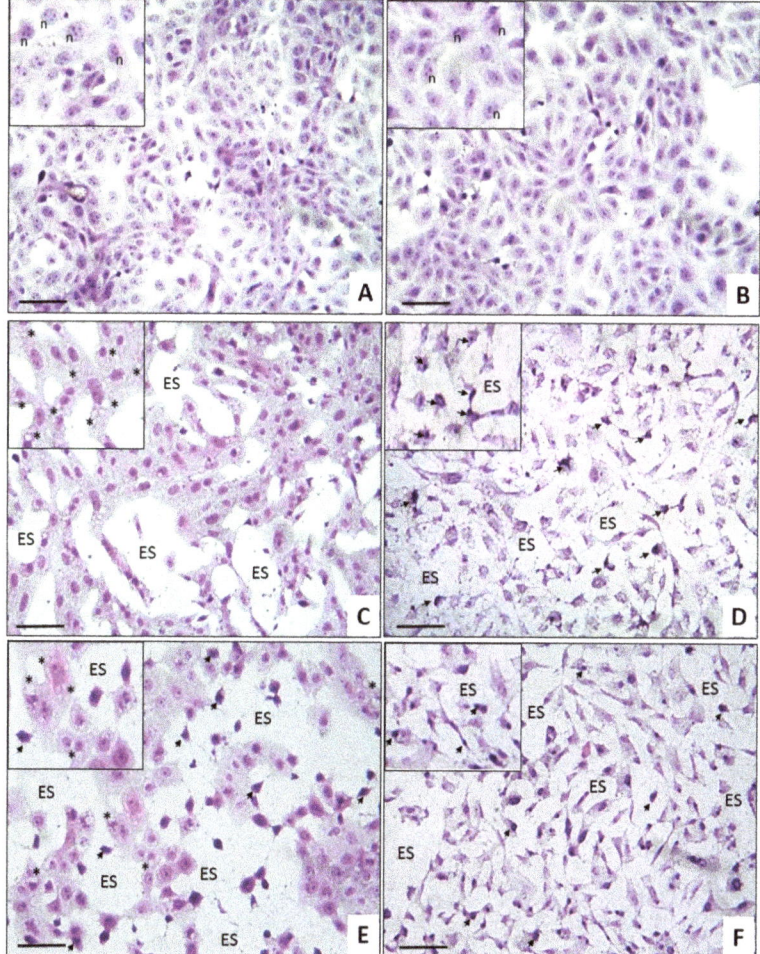

Figure 3. Cytological effects of CE and L1 on MCF-7 cells. Monolayers of MCF-7 human breast cancer cells were incubated with (**A**) cell culture medium, (**B**) 1% dimethyl sulfoxide (DMSO), (**C**) 30 µg/mL CE, (**D**) 30 µg/mL L1, (**E**) 20 µg/mL TX, and (**F**) 50 µg/mL CIS. Inserts in all images show better morphologic details. (Arrows indicate nuclear pyknosis; n, nucleolus; ES, empty space). Hematoxylin and eosin (H&E) in situ staining. Scale bar: 100 µm. Total magnification: 200×.

2.3. Antitumoral Effect on Breast Cancer Explants

In the last few decades, seaweed chemical profiles revealed a significant number of promising cytotoxic compounds against a wide variety of cancer cell lines. However, in vivo studies with these compounds are limited most likely because they are either scarce in nature or they are too structurally complex for their total synthesis. Furthermore, the majority of these in vivo studies were performed in mice with induced carcinogenesis, and human cancer cell line xenografts in immunocompromised mice, guinea-pigs, and zebrafish, which do not reflect the in vivo situation [45]. Despite these models' improvements, it is still not possible to predict clinical results [46].

Considering the results described above, and the necessity for more predictive models to identify cytotoxic compounds with high success rates to proceed toward the clinical trial phase, we decided to evaluate the effect of the CE and L1 in a more robust three-dimensional (3D) model that is able to maintain the tumor environment ex vivo. Precision-cut tissue slices represent an intermediate experimental approach between in vivo and in vitro models, which retain histological and three-dimensional structure, with inter- and extracellular interactions, cell matrix components, and metabolic capacity [47]. There are several studies that report ex vivo tumor responses to anticancer drugs in tissue slices in breast [48–52], liver [53], head and neck [54,55], colorectal [56], gastric, esophagogastric [57], lung [58], pancreatic [59,60], prostate, and bladder [61] cancers. Since different types of tumors display different growth and culture characteristics, the aforementioned studies served to standardize a number of differing tumor-slice culture systems; for example, recently, we used breast tumor explants prepared from precision-cut breast slices to study the antitumoral effect of a number of natural compounds [62].

In order to evaluate the effect of CE and L1, ex vivo cultures of breast cancer explants were obtained after surgery from nine breast cancer patients with histopathological diagnosis of infiltrating ductal/lobular adenocarcinoma. Clinical and histopathological data of the subjects are summarized in Table 1. Four tumor samples were used in four independent assays to evaluate the effect of the CE (Figure 4; Figure 5), while the other five samples were used to test L1 (Figures 6 and 7).

Table 1. Clinical and histopathological subject data.

Patient	Age	[1] CS (grading)	[2] HT	[3] TS	[4] ER	[5] PR	[6] HER2	[7] MC
1	38	T2N1M0 (IIIA)	ID	3	(+)	(+)	(−)	LA
2	54	T4dN1M0 (IIIB)	ID	5	(+)	(+)	(−)	LA
3	46	T3N1M0 (IIIA)	ID	4	(−)	(−)	(+)	HER2
4	63	T2N0M0 (IIA)	ID	3	(−)	(−)	(+)	HER2
5	61	T2N0M0 (IIA)	ID	4	(−)	(−)	(+)	HER2
6	42	T4bN0M0 (IIIB)	ID	4	(−)	(−)	(−)	BL
7	74	T4bN0M0 (IIIB)	IL	4	(+)	(+)	(−)	LA
8	39	T2N2M0 (IIIB)	ID	5	(−)	(−)	(−)	BL
9	57	T3N1M0 (IIIA)	IL	5.5	(+)	(+)	(−)	LA

[1] Clinical stage; [2] histologic type; [3] tumor size (cm); [4] estrogen receptor; [5] progesterone receptor; [6] HER2 status; [7] molecular classification. Patient age in years; ID: infiltrating ductal; IL: infiltrating lobular; LA: luminal A; BL: basal-like.

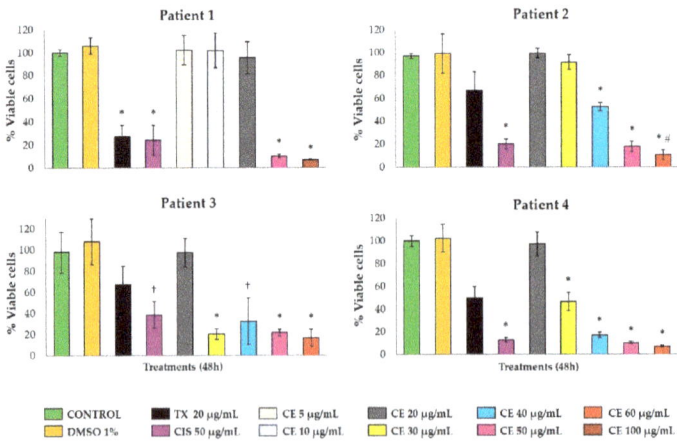

Figure 4. Effect of CE on the metabolic viability of human breast tissue explants. Different concentrations of CE (5–100 μg/mL) were tested in tissue samples from four different patients with breast cancer. CIS (50 μg/mL) was used as a pharmacologic control. Data are expressed as means ± standard deviation (SD). * $p < 0.01$, † $p < 0.05$ compared to the control; # $p < 0.01$ compared to CIS.

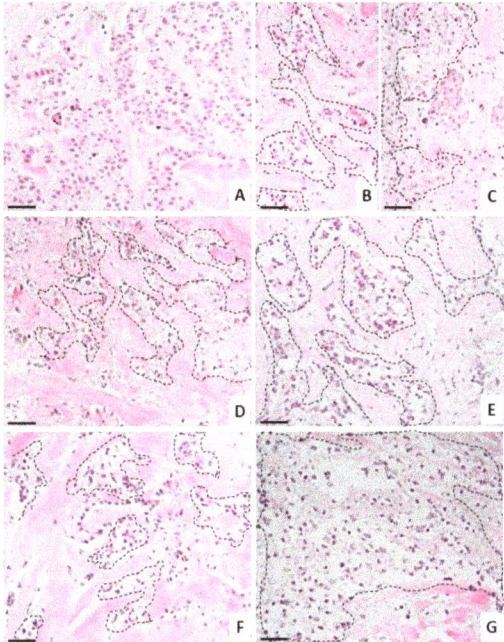

Figure 5. Histopathological analysis of breast tissue explants treated with crude extract (CE). Representative images of CE's effect on human breast tumor tissue explants. (**A**) Tumor explants not subjected to treatment were incubated in culture medium, or incubated in the presence of (**B**) 20 µg/mL TX, (**C**) 50 µg/mL CIS, and different concentrations of CE: (**D**) 30 µg/mL, (**E**) 40 µg/mL, (**F**) 50 µg/mL, and (**G**) 60 µg/mL. H&E staining. Dotted areas indicate necrosis of the tissue. Scale bar: 100 µm. Total magnification: 100×.

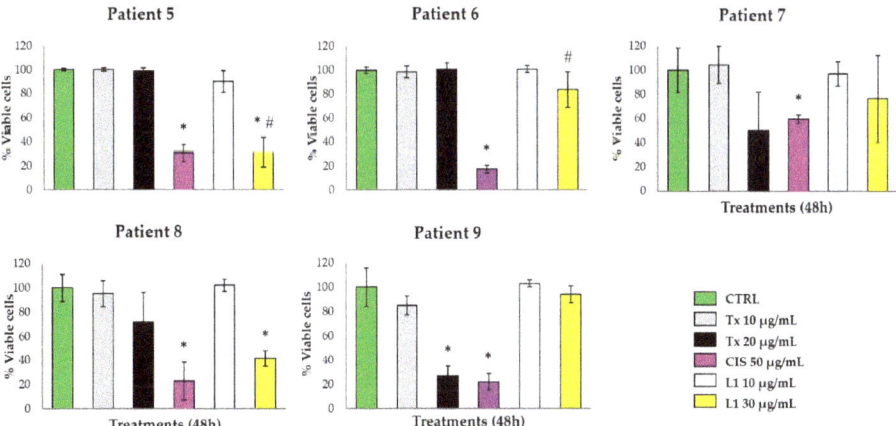

Figure 6. Effect of L1 on the metabolic viability of human breast tissue explants. Tissue explants of human breast tumor from five patients were incubated with DMEM/F12 supplemented medium and treated with L1 at 10 and 30 µg/mL. TX (20 µg/mL) and CIS (50 µg/mL) were used as pharmacological controls. Data are expressed as means ± standard deviation (SD). * $p < 0.05$ compared to the control; # $p < 0.05$ compared to TX (20 µg/mL).

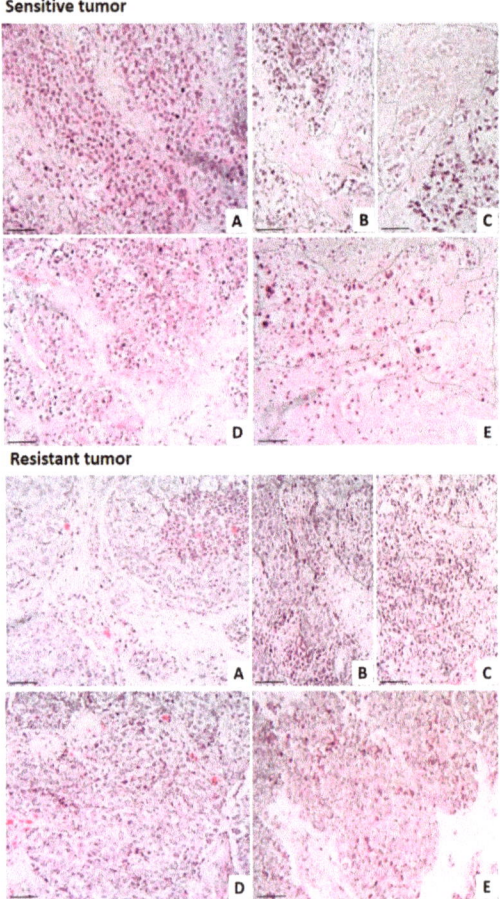

Figure 7. Human breast tumors with different responses to laurinterol (L1). Representative images of human breast tumors that were sensitive (upper panel) and resistant (lower panel) to L1. (**A**) Control tissue explants were grown in culture medium; treated explants were incubated in the presence of (**B**) TX, (**C**) CIS, (**D**) 10 µg/mL L1, and (**E**) 30 µg/mL L1. Dotted areas indicate necrotic tissue. H&E staining. Scale bar: 100 µm. Total magnification: 100×.

A range from 40 to 64 breast cancer explants with a 4-mm diameter and 250–300-µm thickness were obtained from each tumor, and they were incubated for 48 h at 37 °C with different treatments (as referred to in the tumor explant treatment section). Since human tumor tissue is not always available in same quantity/quality to prepare tissue explants, we decided to use a CE dose range from small to higher concentrations (5–100 µg/mL) in explants from Patient 1. On the other hand, because the crude extract did not show activity at small concentrations, we re-adjusted the concentration (20–60 µg/mL) for the next three patients' explants.

The explants' metabolic activity was measured with the Alamar Blue™ assay. CE-treated breast tumor samples showed a considerable reduction in tumor metabolic viability at concentrations greater than 30 µg/mL, similar to the effect of the antineoplastic drug CIS (Figure 4). Patients 2 to 4 showed partial resistance to the metabolic activity reduction with TX. According to the histopathological analysis (Figure 5), untreated tumor tissue was preserved (Figure 5A) and both antineoplastics, TX (Figure 5B) and CIS (Figure 5C), induced marked necrosis areas in the neoplastic cells (dotted areas), although CIS exhibited a more marked necrotic effect. CE also induces necrosis, which increased gradually depending on its concentration (Figure 5D–G).

The metabolic activity of breast tumor explants treated with L1 at 30 µg/mL concentration provoked a marked viability reduction in patients 5 and 8, with a higher effect on the metabolic viability of the tumor tissue compared to TX. Samples from patients 7 and 9 were resistant to the L1 antineoplastic effect, and patient 6 was resistant to TX and L1. All five samples were sensitive to the antineoplastic CIS (Figure 6). The resistance to the antineoplastic drugs used as pharmacologic controls in the present study is possibly due to a reduced intracellular drug concentration of taxol [16], and a reduction of cellular drug uptake of cisplatin by the cancerous cells [17].

As a complement for the in vitro and the metabolic viability assays, histopathological analyses were performed. Histomorphologic findings from the untreated breast tumor explants (control) showed that the tissue typical architecture was preserved under culture conditions (Figure 7A). As expected, the antineoplastic drugs induced necrosis in the neoplastic cell groups to both the sensitive samples and the resistant ones (Figure 7B,C). No tissue damage was observed in the sensitive tumor sample incubated with L1 at 10 µg/mL; however, marked necrotic cell death was induced with the 30 µg/mL concentration. On the other hand, no toxic effects were observed on the resistant tumor samples incubated with 10 µg/mL and 30 µg/mL L1 (Figure 7D,E). Additionally, we evaluated the possible synergistic effect between L1 and TX; however, no effect was detected in either the metabolic activity or the histopathological analysis (data not shown).

The tumor samples used in the present work were classified according to the main breast cancer molecular subtypes as luminal A, luminal B, HER2 non-luminal, and basal-like. As it is known in breast cancer, the overexpression of the estrogen receptor (ER), the progesterone receptor (PR), and oncogenes such as *HER2*, among other biomarkers, are routinely checked with immunohistochemistry, and they are associated with prognosis and prediction of treatment response. The best-characterized breast cancer subtypes are designated as luminal A, luminal B, HER2, and basal-like [63,64].

Our results suggest that there is no predictive relationship between the molecular subtype and the treatment response; the existence of different breast cancer subtypes within a single tumor [65] may account for these results. Despite the samples included in this study belonging to the same histological type, the differential response to the treatments may be due to each patient's complex inherent response, and the heterogeneity inside each tumor sample. Similar results were reported by van der Kuip et al., who found a wide treatment response gamma ranging from strong resistance to intermediate response, sensible to the antineoplastic, when exposing breast cancer slices from 10 patients diagnosed with invasive ductal type to different taxol doses [48].

In addition to intratumoral heterogeneity, our results exhibit how patient response to treatment varies on a case by case basis. Therefore, assays aimed toward predicting whether or not an individual tumor responds to cancer treatments are needed, and we believe that tumor-derived organotypic cultures provide a suitable approach to deal with said requirement [50,54,56,57,60,62], since they comprise various cells that are collectively important for tissue homeostasis, as well as tumor response [66]. As it was proven in the present study, cell cultures are a helpful approach as a first screening option due to their simplicity. Nevertheless, overcoming the unrealistic monolayer culture's growth conditions remains a necessity and an interesting opportunity for future studies.

3. Materials and Methods

3.1. General Experimental Procedures

Optical rotations were measured in CH_2Cl_2 on a PerkinElmer 241 polarimeter (Waltham, MA, USA) using an Na lamp. NMR spectra were recorded on a Bruker AVANCE 500 MHz (Bruker Biospin, Fällanden, Switzerland). NMR spectra were obtained dissolving samples in $CDCl_3$ (99.9%) and chemical shifts are reported relative to solvent (δ_H 7.26 and δ_C 77.0 ppm) and TMS as an internal pattern. HR-ESI-MS data were obtained on an LCT Premier XE Micromass spectrometer (Waters,

Milford, CT, USA). Thin-layer chromatography (TLC; Merck, Darmstadt, Germany) was visualized by spraying with cobalt chloride reagent 2% (10% sulfuric acid) and heating.

Paclitaxel, cisplatin, DMEM/F12 medium, fetal bovine serum, gentamicin, penicillin–streptomycin, and Alamar Blue™ were obtained from Invitrogen (Gran Island, NY, USA). The reagents for general use were purchased from Sigma-Aldrich (St. Louis, MO, USA).

3.2. Biological Material

L. johnstonii was collected by hand during the summer off the coast of Baja California Sur, Mexico (24°21′10.8″ north (N), 110°16′58.8″ west (W)). A voucher specimen (code 13-003) was deposited at the Herbarium of the Laboratory of Marine Algae of the Interdisciplinary Center of Marine Science (CICIMAR) and it was identified by Dr. Rafael Riosmena Rodríguez from the Autonomous University of Baja California Sur (UABCS, La Paz, B.C.S., México).

3.3. Extraction and Isolation

Washed and dried specimens of *L. johnstonii* were crushed and extracted with EtOH for three days at 25 °C under gentle agitation. The dissolvent was replaced three times and the ethanol was combined and filtered through a Whatman no. 4 filter paper. Solvent was removed using a rotatory vacuum evaporator. Then, 10 g of the resulting extract was chromatographed in Sephadex LH-20 (500 × 70 mm, CH$_3$OH 100%) to obtain five fractions. Fraction 4 (1 g) was separated in a Silicagel open column (25 × 5 cm) using a stepwise gradient of *n*-hexane–ethyl acetate to yield pure L1 (*n*-hexane 100%, 707.9 mg).

Laurinterol (**L1**): C$_{15}$H$_{19}$BrO, HR-ESI-MS *m/z* 293.0531 [M − H]$^-$ (calculated C$_{15}$H$_{18}$O^{79}Br, 293.0541), 295.0518 [M − H]$^-$ (calculated C$_{15}$H$_{18}$O^{81}Br, 295.0521) $[\alpha]_D^{25}$ + 17 (*c* 0.15, CH$_2$Cl$_2$) ^{1}H NMR (CDCl$_3$) δ 0.55 (1H, dd, *J* = 7.9, 4.8 Hz, H-12), 0.58 (1H, t, *J* = 4.6 Hz, H-12), 1.15 (1H, dt, *J* = 8.1, 4.3 Hz, H-3), 1.28 (1H, m, H-5), 1.32 (3H, s, H-13), 1.41 (3H, s, H-14), 1.66 (1H, dd, *J* = 12.3, 8.0 Hz, H-4), 1.95 (1H, tdd, *J* = 12.3, 8.1, 4.4, H-4), 2.09 (1H, dd, *J* = 13.2, 8.1 Hz, H-5), 2.29 (3H, s, H-15), 5.26 (1H, br, s, 7-OH), 6,61 (1H, s, H-8), 7.61 (1H, s, H-11); ^{13}C NMR (CDCl$_3$) δ 16.2 (C-12), 18.6 (C-13), 22.2 (C-14), 23.5 (C-15), 24.4 (C-3), 25.3 (C-4), 29.6 (C-2), 35.9 (C-5), 114.9 (C-10), 118.8 (C-8), 132.3 (C-11), 134.0 (C-6), 135.9 (C-9), 153.3 (C-7).

3.4. Cell Culture

Vero (kidney normal epithelial cell line, ATTC® number CCL-81™, Manassas, VA, USA) and MCF-7 (mammary adenocarcinoma cell line, ATCC® number CCL-2™) cells were grown in MEM and DMEM/F12 medium (1:1 mixture containing 2.5 mM L-glutamine, 15 mM HEPES, 0.5 mM sodium pyruvate, 17.5 mM D-Glucose, and 1.2 g/L sodium bicarbonate) supplemented with 10% (*v/v*) FBS and penicillin–streptomycin, respectively. Cultures were routinely maintained at 37°C in a humidified 5% CO$_2$ atmosphere.

3.5. Cytotoxicity Activity

The assays were performed in 96-well microplates, containing 15,625 cells/cm^2 (5 × 10^3 cells/well) and exposed to different concentrations of the extract and the pure compound for 24 h. Cell viability was measured by WST-1 addition and 90 min of incubation. The absorbance was measured at 450 nm, and the concentration of the samples that inhibited 50% of the cell growth (IC$_{50}$) was calculated. Three experiments were performed in triplicate. DMSO (1%), CIS (50 μg/mL), and TX (20 μg/mL) were used as controls. TX concentration was chosen on basis of our previous work [62]. Cisplatin concentration was selected by testing several doses in MCF-7 cells and breast cancer explants.

3.6. In Situ H&E Staining of MCF-7 Cells

To elucidate partially the damage mechanism induced by both CE and L1, we performed an in situ staining that allowed observing, at a cellular level and in greater detail, the toxic effects induced by different compounds. The MCF-7 breast cancer cell line (52,632 cells/cm^2 = 5 × 10^5 cells/well) was cultured on sterile glass coverslips contained in six-well microplates and incubated at 37 °C with 5% CO_2 for 24 h. Afterward, the cultures were incubated for additional 24 h in the presence of culture medium (untreated control), 1% DMSO (solvent control), 30 µg/mL CE, and 30 µg/mL L1. The antineoplastic drugs TX and CIS (20 and 50 µg/mL, respectively) were used as pharmacological control references. After the incubation time with the treatments, the cells were fixed and stained in situ by H&E staining, and permanent preparations were made, and they were observed with a Zeiss Axiostar Plus brightfield microscope (Jena, Germany). Representative photographs of all treatments were obtained with a 5.0 MP Moticam camera (Richmond, BC, Canada).

3.7. Tumor Samples

The approval to work with human tissues was obtained from the Institutional Review Board (Instituto Mexicano del Seguro Social, Coordinación de Investigación en Salud. R-2014-785-022,). With previous informed consent, infiltrating ductal/lobular adenocarcinoma samples were obtained from nine patients undergoing mastectomy or excisional biopsy for the carcinoma remaining removed as surgical waste once sufficient tissue was assured for clinical diagnosis at the Hospital de Ginecología y Obstetricia (UMAE # 23, Monterrey, Nuevo León, México) from the Instituto Mexicano del Seguro Social (clinical and histopathological data are described in Table 1). Tissues were collected in cold serum-free DMEM/F12 medium and transported at 4 °C to the laboratory for immediate processing.

3.8. Preparation of Slices and Explants from Breast Cancer

Breast cancer human tissue slices of 4 mm diameter and 250–300 µm thickness were obtained using the Krumdieck tissue slicer (Alabama Research & Development, Munford, AL, USA) with constant flow of KB buffer at 4 °C gassed with carbogen gas as described previously [62]. In total, 40 to 64 breast tumor explants were prepared and placed in 24-well microplates containing DMEM/F12 supplemented medium with 10% (v/v) FBS, 25 mM D-glucose, 1% ITS (insulin-transferrin-selenium), 1 mM sodium pyruvate, plus penicillin–streptomycin, and incubated for 1 h at 37 °C, 5% CO_2, with agitation at 30 rpm. The interval between the tumor resection and the explant incubation was no more than 2 h.

3.9. Treatment of Tumor Explants

After pre-incubation, in order to confirm the tumor samples' viability, control explants (0 h) were placed in 24-well microplates containing 1 mL of DMEM/F12 supplemented medium and incubated for 4 h at 37 °C, 5% CO_2/95% air, with agitation at 30 rpm. Depending on the explants' availability, 40 to 64 explants were cultured per assay, with four to six explants per treatment or experimental condition. Treated explants were incubated for 48 h at 37°C, 5% CO_2, with agitation at 30 rpm with the following compounds: 20 µg/mL TX, 50 µg/mL CIS, 5–100 µg/mL CE, 10 and 30 µg/mL L1, and 10 µg/mL L1 + 10 µg/mL TX. Controls were medium and 1% DMSO.

3.10. Alamar Blue™ Viability Assay

After 48 h of incubation with the compounds, as well as the culture medium (control), the explants were incubated for an additional 4 h with 10% Alamar Blue™ in 500 µL of DMEM/F12 supplemented medium at 37 °C in the conditions described earlier. Afterward, 100 µL was collected from each sample and transferred to a 96-well microplate to read fluorescence at 530-nm excitation/590-nm emission wavelengths. The percentage of viability relative to control was obtained by calculating the percentage of Alamar Blue™ reduction per explant [62].

3.11. Histopatological Analysis

After incubation with the treatments, the breast cancer explants were fixed in 10% neutral formalin and embedded in paraffin using conventional histological techniques. Tissue sections of 4 μm were prepared on a microtome and mounted on glass slides. Afterward, the slides were deparaffinized and stained with hematoxylin and eosin (H&E). The stained preparations were observed by a pathologist using a Zeiss Axiostar Plus Brightfield microscope, and photographs were obtained with a 5.0 Moticam camera. Histopathological analysis was performed by two independent pathologists, and the morphological parameters analyzed included necrosis, viable/damaged tumor cells, and inflammation.

3.12. Statistical Analysis

Statistical analysis was performed with SPSS version 20.0 software. Quantitative data were expressed as means and standard deviation. Differences in continuous variables with normal distribution were analyzed with Student's *t*-test or the Mann–Whitney *U* test for non-normal distributions.

4. Conclusions

To our knowledge, this is the first study of a marine natural product in human breast tumor-derived organotypic culture, which supports the known in vitro cytotoxic activity of laurinterol in a more complex system. Our results show a dose-dependent inhibition of the metabolic activity and morphological changes characteristic of apoptotic cell death in cells treated with the crude extract and laurinterol. Meanwhile, breast cancer explants treated with the extract showed reduced metabolic viability and necrosis areas, while explants treated with laurinterol exhibited a heterogeneous response associated with the individual response of each tumor sample. This study emphasizes the importance of the 3D culture of human cancer tissue slices or tissue explants to improve the selection of new therapeutic options from different sources before preclinical studies, as well as a functional drug testing in personalized oncology, enabling the prediction of the interpersonal tumor response.

Author Contributions: N.E.G.D. and I.E.C.T. conceived and designed the experiments; S.G.D. and E.V.V. collected the algae, prepared the extracts, and determined the cytotoxic activity; S.G.D. performed isolation and purification experiments, and wrote the paper; A.R.D.M. and J.J.F. analyzed the chemical data; D.V.M. selected and provided the tumor samples; N.E.G.G. also performed the histopathological analysis; O.E.H. performed histopathological analysis; I.E.C.T. determined the antitumoral activity; P.C.R. contributed to the ex vivo antitumoral assays, and reviewed the manuscript. All authors reviewed and commented on the manuscript.

Funding: The authors thank funds from CONACYT fellowships 290666 (S.G.D) and 209488 (I.E.C.T.); CTQ2014-55888-C03-01/R (Ministerio de Economía y Competitividad, J.J.F.); FIS/IMSS/PROT/G14/1298 (Coordinación de Investigación en Salud del Instituto Mexicano del Seguro Social, P.C.R.).

Acknowledgments: The authors also thank Rafael Riosmena Rodríguez (UABCS) for taxonomic classification of specimens of *Laurencia johnstonii* and QBP Consuelo Coronado Martínez for the excellent technical assistance.

Conflicts of Interest: The authors declare no conflicts of interest.

References

1. Alves, C.; Silva, J.; Pinteus, S.; Gaspar, H.; Alpoim, M.C.; Botana, L.M.; Pedrosa, R. From marine origin to therapeutics: The antitumor potential of marine algae-derived compounds. *Front. Pharmacol.* **2018**, *9*, 777. [CrossRef] [PubMed]
2. Guiry, M.D.; Guiry, M.D. AlgaBase. World-wide electronic publication, National University of Irland, Galway. Available online: www.algaebase.org (accessed on 12 May 2018).
3. Vázquez-Borja, R. *Análisis Comparativo de la Ficoflora de Baja California Sur*; Maestría en Ciencias, Instituto Politécnico Nacional: Mexico City, Mexico, 1999.
4. Harizani, M.; Ioannou, E.; Roussis, V. The *Laurencia* paradox: An endless source of chemodiversity. *Prog. Chem. Org. Nat. Prod.* **2016**, *102*, 91–252. [CrossRef]

5. Vairappan, C.S.; Suzuki, M.; Abe, T.; Masuda, M. Halogenated metabolites with antibacterial activity from the Okinawan *Laurencia* species. *Phytochemistry* **2001**, *58*, 517–523. [CrossRef]
6. Vairappan, C.S.; Kawamoto, T.; Miwa, H.; Suzuki, M. Potent antibacterial activity of halogenated compounds against antibiotic-resistant bacteria. *Planta Med.* **2004**, *70*, 1087–1090. [CrossRef] [PubMed]
7. Tsukamoto, S.; Yamashita, Y.; Ohta, T. New cytotoxic and antibacterial compounds isolated from sea hare, *Aplysia kurodai*. *Mar Drugs* **2005**, *3*, 22–28. [CrossRef]
8. Kladi, M.; Xenaki, H.; Vagias, C.; Papazafiri, P.; Roussis, V. New cytotoxic sesquiterpenes from the red algae *Laurencia obtusa* and *Laurencia microcladia*. *Tetrahedron* **2006**, *62*, 182–189. [CrossRef]
9. Oguri, Y.; Watanabe, M.; Ishikawa, T.; Kamada, T.; Vairappan, C.; Matsuura, H.; Kaneko, K.; Ishii, T.; Suzuki, M.; Yoshimura, E.; Nogata, Y. New marine antifouling compounds from the red alga *Laurencia* sp. *Mar. Drugs* **2017**, *15*, 267. [CrossRef] [PubMed]
10. Okamoto, Y.; Nitanda, N.; Ojika, M.; Sakagami, Y. Aplysiallene, a new bromoallene as an Na, K-ATPase inhibitor from the sea hare, *Aplysia kurodai*. *Biosci. Biotechnol. Biochem.* **2001**, *65*, 474–476. [CrossRef] [PubMed]
11. Ishii, T.; Nagamine, T.; Nguyen, B.C.; Tawata, S. Insecticidal and repellent activities of laurinterol from the Okinawan red alga *Laurencia nidifica*. *Rec. Nat. Prod.* **2017**, *11*, 63–68.
12. García-Davis, S.; Sifaoui, I.; Reyes-Batlle, M.; Viveros-Valdez, E.; Piñero, J.E.; Lorenzo-Morales, J.; Fernández, J.J.; Díaz-Marrero, A.R. Anti-Acanthamoeba activity of brominated sesquiterpenes from *Laurencia johnstonii*. *Mar. Drugs* **2018**, *16*, 443. [CrossRef] [PubMed]
13. WHO. Cancer Fact Sheet. Available online: www.who.int/cancer/prevention/diagnosis-screening/breast-cancer/en/ (accessed on 22 January 2019).
14. Perez, E.A. Impact, mechanisms, and novel chemotherapy strategies for overcoming resistance to anthracyclines and taxanes in metastatic breast cancer. *Breast. Cancer Res. Treat.* **2009**, *114*, 195–201. [CrossRef]
15. Ambudkar, S.V.; Dey, S.; Hrycyna, C.A.; Ramachandra, M.; Pastan, I.; Gottesman, M.M. Biochemical, cellular, and pharmacological aspects of the multidrug transporter. *Annu. Rev. Pharmacol Toxicol.* **1999**, *39*, 361–398. [CrossRef]
16. Maass, N.; Schütz, F.; Fasching, P.A.; Fehm, T.; Janni, W.; Kümmel, S.; Lüfner, D.; Wallwiener, M.; Lux, M.P. Breast cancer update 2014—Focus on the patient and the tumor. *Geburtshile Frauenheilkd.* **2015**, *75*, 170–182. [CrossRef]
17. Taran, F.A.; Schneeweiss, A.; Lux, M.P.; Janni, W.; Hartkopf, A.D.; Nabieva, N.; Overkamp, F.; Kolberg, H.C.; Hadji, P.; Tesch, H.; Wöckel, A. Update breast cancer 2018 (Part 1)—Primary breast cancer and biomarkers. *Geburtshile Frauenheilkd.* **2018**, *78*, 235–245. [CrossRef] [PubMed]
18. Carranza-Rosales, P.; Guzmán-Delgado, N.E.; Carranza-Torres, I.E.; Viveros-Valdez, E.; Morán-Martínez, J. Breast organotypic cancer models. *Curr. Top. Microbiol. Immunol.* **2018**, 1–25. [CrossRef]
19. Sun, J.; Shi, D.; Ma, M.; Wang, S.; Han, L.; Yang, Y.; Fan, X.; Shi, J.; He, L. Sesquiterpenes from the red alga *Laurencia tristicha*. *J. Nat. Prod.* **2005**, *68*, 915–919. [CrossRef] [PubMed]
20. Zaleta-Pinet, D.A.; Holland, I.P.; Muñoz-Ochoa, M.; Murillo-Alvarez, J.I.; Sakoff, J.A.; van Altena, I.A.; McCluskey, A. Cytotoxic compounds from *Laurencia pacifica*. *Org. Med. Chem. Lett.* **2014**, *4*, 8. [CrossRef] [PubMed]
21. Zhang, X.; Zhuang, T.; Liang, Z.; Li, L.; Xue, M.; Liu, J.; Liang, H. Breast cancer suppression by aplysin is associated with inhibition of PI3K/AK/FOXO3a pathway. *Oncotarget* **2017**, *8*, 63923–63934. [CrossRef] [PubMed]
22. Kim, M.M.; Mendis, E.; Kim, S.K. *Laurencia okamurai* extract containing laurinterol induces apoptosis in melanoma cells. *J. Med. Food* **2008**, *11*, 260–266. [CrossRef] [PubMed]
23. García-Davis, S.; Murillo-Alvarez, I.; Muñoz-Ochoa, M.; Carranza-Torres, E.; Garza-Padrón, R.; Morales-Rubio, E.; Viveros-Valdez, E. Bactericide, antioxidant and cytotoxic activities from marine algae of genus *Laurencia* collected in Baja California Sur. *Int. J. Pharmacol.* **2018**, *14*, 391–396. [CrossRef]
24. Irie, T.; Suzuki, M.; Masamune, T. Laurinterol and debromolaurinterol constituents from Laurencia intermedia. *Tetraheron Lett.* **1966**, *7*, 1837–1840. [CrossRef]
25. Jesus, A.; Correia-da-Silva, M.; Alfonso, C.; Pinto, M.; Cidade, H. Isolation and potential biological applications of haloaryl secondary metabolites from macroalgae. *Mar. Drugs* **2019**, *17*, 73. [CrossRef]

26. Fernández Freire, P.; Peropadre, A.; Pérez Martín, J.M.; Herrero, O.; Hazen, M.J. An integrated cellular model to evaluate cytotoxic effects in mammalian cell lines. *Toxicol. In Vitro* **2009**, *23*, 1553–1558. [CrossRef] [PubMed]
27. Sombatsri, A.; Thummanant, Y.; Sribuhom, T.; Wongphakham, P.; Senawong, T.; Yenjai, C. Atalantums H-K from the peels of *Atalantia monophylla* and their cytotoxicity. *Nat. Prod Res.* **2019**. [CrossRef] [PubMed]
28. Kumarihamy, M.; Ferreira, D.; Croom, E.M., Jr.; Sahu, R.; Tekwani, B.L.; Duke, S.O.; Khan, S.; Techen, N.; Nanayakkara, N.P.D. Antiplasmodial and cytotoxic cytochalasins from an endophytic fungus, *Nemania* sp. UM10M, isolated from a diseased *Torreya taxifolia* Leaf. *Molecules* **2019**, *24*, 777. [CrossRef] [PubMed]
29. Mashjoor, S.; Yousefzadi, M.; Esmaeili, M.A.; Rafiee, R. Cytotoxicity and antimicrobial activity of marine macro algae (Dictyotaceae and Ulvaceae) from the Persian Gulf. *Cytotechnology* **2016**, *68*, 1717–1726. [CrossRef]
30. Sit, N.W.; Chan, Y.S.; Lai, S.C.; Lim, L.N.; Looi, G.T.; Tay, P.L.; Tee, Y.T.; Woon, Y.Y.; Khoo, K.S.; Ong, H.C. In vitro antidermatophytic activity and cytotoxicity of extracts derived from medicinal plants and marine algae. *J. Mycol. Med.* **2018**, *28*, 561–567. [CrossRef]
31. Siddiqui, S.; Ahmad, R.; Khan, M.A.; Upadhyay, S.; Husain, I.; Srivastava, A.N. Cytostatic and anti-tumor potential of Ajwa date pulp against human hepatocellular carcinoma HepG2 cells. *Sci. Rep.* **2019**, *9*, 245. [CrossRef]
32. Stein, E.M.; Andreguetti, D.X.; Rocha, C.S.; Fujii, M.T.; Baptista, M.S.; Colepicolo, P.; Indig, G.L. Search for cytotoxic agents in multiple *Laurencia* complex seaweed species (Ceramiales, Rhodophyta) harvested from the Atlantic Ocean with emphasis on the Brazilian State of Espírito Santo. *Rev. Bras. Farmacogn.* **2011**, *21*, 239–243. [CrossRef]
33. Esselin, H.; Sutour, S.; Liberal, J.; Cruz, M.T.; Salgueiro, L.; Siegler, B.; Freuze, I.; Castola, V.; Paoli, M.; Bighelli, A.; et al. Chemical composition of *Laurencia obtuse* extract and isolation of a New C_{15} acetogenin. *Molecules* **2017**, *22*. [CrossRef]
34. Garzon, C.D.; Flores, F.J. Hormesis: Biphasic dose-responses to fungicides in plant pathogens and their potential threat to agriculture. In *Fungicides—Showcases of Integrated Plant Disease Management from Around the World*; Mizuho, N., Ed.; InTech: Rijeka, Croatia, 2013; pp. 311–328. [CrossRef]
35. Afford, S.; Randhawa, S. Apoptosis. *Mol. Pathol.* **2000**, *53*, 55–63. [CrossRef] [PubMed]
36. Mgbonyebi, O.P.; Russo, J.; Russo, I.H. Roscovitine induces cell death and morphological changes indicative of apoptosis in MDA-MB-231 breast cancer cells. *Cancer Res.* **1999**, *59*, 1903–1910. [PubMed]
37. Mahassni, S.H.; Al-Reemi, R.M. Apoptosis and necrosis of human breast cancer cells by an aqueous extract of garden cress (*Lepidium sativum*) seeds. *Saudi J. Biol. Sci.* **2013**, *20*, 131–139. [CrossRef]
38. Lv, Z.D.; Liu, X.P.; Zhao, W.J.; Dong, Q.; Li, F.N.; Wang, H.B.; Kong, B. Curcumin induces apoptosis in breast cancer cells and inhibits tumor growth in vitro and *in vivo*. *Int. J. Clin. Exp. Pathol.* **2014**, *7*, 2818.
39. Gong, A.J.; Gong, L.L.; Yao, W.C.; Ge, N.; Lu, L.X.; Liang, H. Aplysin induces apoptosis in glioma cells through HSP90/AKT pathway. *Exp. Biol. Med.* **2015**, *240*, 639–644. [CrossRef]
40. Shakeel, E.; Akhtar, S.; Khan, M.K.A.; Lohani, M.; Arif, J.M.; Siddiqui, M.H. Molecular docking analysis of aplysin analogs targeting survivin protein. *Bioinformation* **2017**, *13*, 293–300. [CrossRef]
41. Shakeel, E.; Sharma, N.; Akhtar, S.; Khan, M.K.A.; Lohani, M.; Siddiqui, M.H. Decoding the antineoplastic efficacy of aplysin targeting Bcl-2: A de novo perspective. *Comput. Biol. Chem.* **2018**, *77*, 390–401. [CrossRef]
42. Sims, J.J.; Fenical, W.; Wing, R.M.; Radlick, P. Marine natural products III. Johnstonnol, an unusual halogenated epoxide from the red alga *Laurencia johnstonii*. *Tetrahedron Lett.* **1972**, *13*, 195–198. [CrossRef]
43. Faulkner, J.D.; Stallard, M.O.; Ireland, C. Prepacifenol epoxide, a halogenated sesquiterpene diepoxide. *Tetrahedron Lett.* **1974**, *15*, 3571–3574. [CrossRef]
44. Liu, J.; Ma, N.; Liu, G.; Zheng, L.; Lin, X. Aplysin sensitizes cancer cells to TRAIL by suppressing P38 MAPK/survivin pathway. *Mar. Drugs* **2014**, *12*, 5072–5088. [CrossRef]
45. Rocha, D.H.A.; Seca, A.M.L.; Pinto, D.C.G.A. Seaweed secondary metabolites in vitro and in vivo anticancer activity. *Mar. Drugs* **2018**, *16*, 410. [CrossRef]
46. Hait, W.N. Anticancer drug development: The grand challenges. *Nat. Rev. Drug Discov.* **2010**, *9*, 253–254. [CrossRef]

47. De Graaf, I.A.; Olinga, P.; de Jager, M.H.; Merema, M.T.; de Kanter, R.; Van de Kerkhof, E.G.; Groothuis, G.M. Preparation and incubation of precisión-cut liver and intestinal slice for application in drug metabolism and toxicity studies. *Nat. Protoc.* **2010**, *5*, 1540–1551. [CrossRef]
48. Van der Kuip, H.; Mürdter, T.E.; Sonnenberg, M.; McClenllan, M.; Gutzeit, S.; Gerteis, A.; Simon, W.; Fritz, P.; Aulitzky, W.E. Short term culture of breast cancer tissues to study the activity of the anticancer drug taxol in an intact tumor environment. *BMC Cancer* **2006**, *6*, 86. [CrossRef] [PubMed]
49. Mestres, P.; Morguet, A.; Schmidt, W.; Kob, A.; Thedinga, E. A new method to assess drug sensitivity on breast tumor acute slices preparation. *Ann. N. Y. Acad. Sci.* **2006**, *1091*, 460–469. [CrossRef]
50. Holliday, D.L.; Moss, M.A.; Pollock, S.; Lane, S.; Shaaban, A.M.; Millican-Slater, R.; Nash, C.; Hanby, A.M.; Speirs, V. The practicalities of using tissue slices as preclinical organotypics breast cancer models. *J. Clin. Pathol.* **2013**, *66*, 253–255. [CrossRef] [PubMed]
51. Naipal, K.A.T.; Verkaik, N.S.; Sánchez, H.; van Deurzen, C.H.M.; den Bakker, M.A.; Hoeijmakers, J.H.J.; Kanaar, R.; Vreeswijk, M.P.G.; Jager, A.; van Gent, D.C. Tumor slice culture system to assess drug response of primary breast cancer. *BMC Cancer* **2016**, *16*, 78. [CrossRef]
52. Garcia-Chagollan, M.; Carranza-Torres, I.E.; Carranza-Rosales, P.; Guzmán-Delgado, N.E.; Ramírez-Montoya, H.; Martínez-Silva, M.G.; Mariscal-Ramirez, I.; Barrón-Gallardo, C.A.; Pereira-Suárez, A.L.; Aguilar-Lemarroy, A. Expression of NK cell Surface receptors in breast cancer tissue as predictors of resistance to antineoplastic treatment. *Technol. Cancer Res. Treat.* **2018**, *17*. [CrossRef] [PubMed]
53. Kern, M.A.; Haugg, A.M.; Eiteneuer, E.; Konze, E.; Drebber, U.; Dienes, H.P.; Breuhahn, K.; Schirmacher, P.; Kasper, H.U. Ex vivo analysis of antineoplastic agents in precision-cut tissue slices of human origin: Effects of cyclooxygenase-2 inhibition in hepatocellular carcinoma. *Liver Int.* **2006**, *26*, 604–612. [CrossRef]
54. Gerlach, M.M.; Merz, F.; Kubick, C.; Wittekind, C.; Lordick, F.; Dietz, A.; Bechmann, I. Slice cultures from head and neck squamous cell carcinoma: A novel test system for drug susceptibility and mechanisms of resistance. *Br. J. Cancer* **2014**, *110*, 479–488. [CrossRef] [PubMed]
55. Peria, M.; Donnadieu, J.; Racz, C.; Ikoli, J.F.; Galmiche, A.; Chauffert, B.; Page, C. Evaluation of individual sensitivity of head and neck squamous cell carcinoma to cetuximab by short-term culture of tumor slices. *Head Neck* **2016**, *38* (Suppl. 1), E911–E915. [CrossRef] [PubMed]
56. Unger, F.T.; Bentz, S.; Krüger, J.; Rosenbrock, C.; Schaller, J.; Pursche, K.; Sprüssel, A.; Juhl, H.; David, K.A. Precision cut cancer tissue slices in anticancer drug testing. *J. Mol. Pathophysiol.* **2015**, *4*, 108–121. [CrossRef]
57. Koefer, J.; Kallendrusch, S.; Merz, F.; Kubick, C.; Kassahun, W.T.; Schumacher, G.; Moebius, C.; Gäßler, N.; Schopow, N.; Geister, D.; Wiechmann, V.; et al. Organotypic slice cultures of human gastric and esophagogastric junction cancer. *Cancer Med.* **2016**, *5*, 1444–1453. [CrossRef]
58. Peranzoni, E.; Bougherara, H.; Barrin, S.; Mansuet-Lupo, A.; Alifano, M.; Damotte, D.; Donnadieu, E. Ex vivo imaging of resident CD8 T lymphocytes in human lung tumor slices using confocal microscopy. *J. Vis. Exp.* **2017**, *130*. [CrossRef]
59. Dayot, S.; Speisky, D.; Couvelard, A.; Bourgoin, P.; Gratio, V.; Cros, J.; Rebours, V.; Sauvanet, A.; Bedossa, P.; Paradis, V.; et al. In vitro, in vivo and ex vivo demonstration of the antitumoral role of hypocretin-1/orexin-A and almorexant in pancreatic ductal adenocarcinoma. *Oncotarget* **2018**, *9*, 6952–6967. [CrossRef] [PubMed]
60. Lim, C.Y.; Chang, J.H.; Lee, K.M.; Yoon, Y.C.; Kim, J.; Park, I.Y. Organotypic slice cultures of pancreatic ductal adenocarcinoma preserve the tumor microenvironment and provide a plataform for drugs response. *Pancreatology* **2018**, *18*, 913–927. [CrossRef] [PubMed]
61. Van de Merbel, A.F.; van der Horst, G.; van der Mark, M.H.; van Uhm, J.I.M.; van Gennep, E.J.; Kloen, P.; Beimers, L.; Pelger, R.C.M.; van der Plujim, G. An ex vivo tissue culture model for the assessment of individualized drug responses in prostate and bladder cancer. *Front. Oncol.* **2018**, *8*, 400. [CrossRef] [PubMed]
62. Carranza-Torres, I.E.; Guzmán-Delgado, N.E.; Coronado-Martínez, C.; Bañuelos-García, J.I.; Viveros-Valdez, E.; Morán-Martínez, J.; Carranza-Rosales, P. Organotypic culture of breast tumor explants as a multicellular system for the screening of natural compounds with antineoplastic potential. *Biomed. Res. Int.* **2015**, *2015*, 618021. [CrossRef]
63. Ross, J.S.; Linette, G.P.; Stec, J.; Clark, E.; Ayers, M.; Leschly, N.; Symmans, W.F.; Hortobagyi, G.N.; Pusztai, L. Breast cancer biomarkers an molecular medicine. *Expert Rev. Mol. Diagn.* **2003**, *3*, 573–585. [CrossRef]

64. Brenton, J.D.; Carey, L.A.; Ahmed, A.A.; Caldas, C. Molecular classification and molecular forecasting of breast cancer: Ready for clinical application? *J. Clin. Oncol.* **2005**, *23*, 7350–7360. [CrossRef]
65. Yeo, S.K.; Guan, J.L. Breast cancer: Multiples subtypes within a tumor? *Trends Cancer* **2017**, *3*, 753–760. [CrossRef] [PubMed]
66. Hoarau-Véchot, J.; Rafii, A.; Touboul, C.; Pasquier, J. Halfway between 2D and animal models: Are 3D cultures the ideal tool to study cancer-microenvironment interactions? *Int. J. Mol. Sci.* **2018**, *19*, 181. [CrossRef] [PubMed]

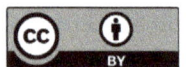

© 2019 by the authors. Licensee MDPI, Basel, Switzerland. This article is an open access article distributed under the terms and conditions of the Creative Commons Attribution (CC BY) license (http://creativecommons.org/licenses/by/4.0/).

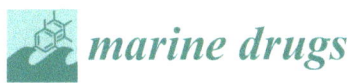

Review

Seaweed Secondary Metabolites with Beneficial Health Effects: An Overview of Successes in In Vivo Studies and Clinical Trials

Gonçalo P. Rosa [1], Wilson R. Tavares [2], Pedro M. C. Sousa [2], Aida K. Pagès [2], Ana M. L. Seca [1,3,*] and Diana C. G. A. Pinto [3,*]

1. cE3c—Centre for Ecology, Evolution and Environmental Changes/Azorean Biodiversity Group & University of Azores, Rua Mãe de Deus, 9501-801 Ponta Delgada, Portugal; goncalo.p.rosa@uac.pt
2. Faculty of Sciences and Technology, University of Azores, 9501-801 Ponta Delgada, Portugal; wrt-94@hotmail.com (W.R.T.); sdoffich@gmail.com (P.M.C.S.); aidakane.1@hotmail.com (A.K.P.)
3. QOPNA & LAQV-REQUIMTE, Department of Chemistry, University of Aveiro, 3810-193 Aveiro, Portugal
* Correspondence: ana.ml.seca@uac.pt (A.M.L.S.); diana@ua.pt (D.C.G.A.P.); Tel.: +351-296-650-174 (A.M.L.S.); +351-234-363-401-407 (D.C.G.A.P.)

Received: 25 November 2019; Accepted: 18 December 2019; Published: 20 December 2019

Abstract: Macroalgae are increasingly viewed as a source of secondary metabolites with great potential for the development of new drugs. In this development, in vitro studies are only the first step in a long process, while in vivo studies and clinical trials are the most revealing stages of the true potential and limitations that a given metabolite may have as a new drug. This literature review aims to give a critical overview of the secondary metabolites that reveal the most interesting results in these two steps. Phlorotannins show great pharmaceutical potential in in vivo models and, among the several examples, the anti-dyslipidemia activity of dieckol must be highlighted because it was more effective than lovastatin in an in vivo model. The IRLIIVLMPILMA tridecapeptide that exhibits an in vivo level of activity similar to the hypotensive clinical drug captopril should still be stressed, as well as griffithsin which showed such stunning results over a variety of animal models and which will probably move onto clinical trials soon. Regarding clinical trials, studies with pure algal metabolites are scarce, limited to those carried out with kahalalide F and fucoxanthin. The majority of clinical trials currently aim to ascertain the effect of algae consumption, as extracts or fractions, on obesity and diabetes.

Keywords: seaweeds; secondary metabolites; in vivo studies; clinical trials; health effects; dieckol; eckol; fucoxanthin; kahalalide F

1. Introduction

In the last few years, macroalgae attracted increasing attention from many industries of diverse branches such as fuel, plastics, cosmetics, pharmaceuticals, and food [1,2]. In fact, the chemical diversity within red (Rhodophyta), green (Chlorophyta), and brown (Phaeophyta) macroalgae offers the possibility of finding a wide variety of primary and secondary metabolites, with interesting properties and applications [1,3–7]. Primary metabolites are directly involved in physiological functions, under normal growth conditions, such as reproduction, while secondary metabolites are mainly excretory products produced under different stress conditions, such as exposure to ultraviolet (UV) radiation, changes in temperature and salinity, or environmental pollutants. Primary algal metabolites are the normal ones, such as proteins, polysaccharides, and lipids, whereas the main secondary metabolites produced in algae tissues are phenolic compounds, halogenated compounds, sterols, terpenes, and small peptides, among other bioactive compounds [8–11].

Studies focusing on the preparation of macroalgae extracts and their chemical characterization revealed a large range of seaweed compounds with very interesting biological activities including antitumor, anti-inflammatory, antimicrobial, antidiabetic, antivirus, antihypertensive, fat-lowering, and neuroprotective activities [12–15].

The large volume of studies proving the seaweed compound activities in in vitro systems [16–19] hints the need for further advancements in the knowledge about macroalgae compound efficiency in living systems (in vivo) and their use in the development of pharmaceuticals. In vitro studies are very relevant and yield very important information, but they only represent the first step of a long process, and the results obtained rarely reveal anything about the effects of a compound in vivo, because the responses observed in vitro can be magnified, diminished, or totally different in a more complex and integrated system. In fact, in vivo studies and clinical trials are those which contribute most to truly understanding the real potential of compounds as future pharmaceuticals.

In this regard, the present work intends to present insight into the results obtained in the last few years regarding secondary metabolites, such as phlorotannins, halogenated compounds, fucoxanthin, and fucosterol isolated from macroalgae, involved in in vivo studies and clinical trials, identifying the research opportunities and knowledge gaps, to valorize these compounds and their natural resources. The intention is not to present an exhaustive survey of all published works, but rather a selection of authors based on the following criteria: in-depth studies involving pure compounds most characteristic from seaweeds, and studies in which the applied dose was less than 100 mg/kg, with a few exceptions justified in the discussion of these studies.

2. In Vivo Studies

Several compounds isolated from macroalgae reached the in vivo stage of investigation into their biological effects, which means that researchers recognize their potential and are willing to prove their full pharmacological value. In this regard, the paragraphs below review and discuss the most significant results obtained in these in vivo studies.

2.1. Phlorotannins

Phlorotannins are a class of inimitable complex polyphenol compounds produced by brown seaweed as secondary metabolites and biosynthesized via the acetate malonate pathway [20,21]. They are basically constituted by phloroglucinol (1,3,5-trihydroxybenzene) base units with different degrees of polymerization. Phlorotannin classification is based on the types of linkages between the phloroglucinol units, and there are four subclasses, namely, phlorotannins with ether linkages (fuhalols and phlorethols), those with phenyl linkages (fucols), those with both ether and phenyl linkages (fucophlorethols), and those with a dibenzodioxin linkage (eckols) [22] (Figure 1).

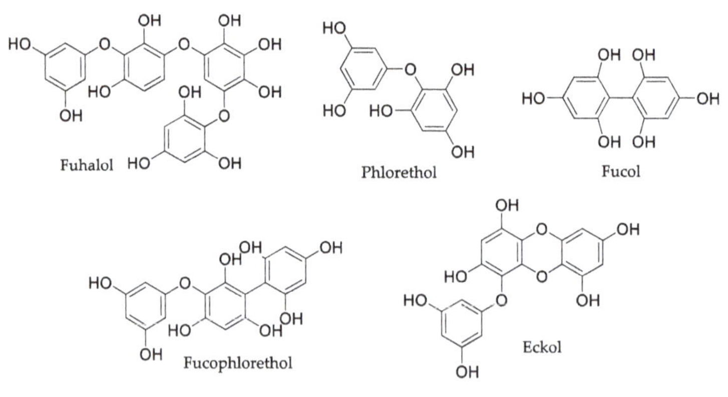

Figure 1. Examples of different subclasses of phlorotannins.

Phlorotannin presence, either in free form or forming complexes with different components of the cell walls, like alginic acid [23], is essential to the physiological integrity of algae and to numerous important other roles such as chemical defense against bacteria, epiphytes, and hydroids, protection against oxidative damage that occurs in response to interactions with other organisms or the abiotic environment such as UV radiation, and changes in nutrient availability [24,25].

Due to their important roles in the physiology of brown algae, these compounds attracted a lot of research interest, with many studies addressing their isolation [26–29]. Moreover, as reviewed by Imbs and Zvyagintseva [30], there were a high number of studies describing the important in vitro activities of phlorotannins including anti-inflammatory, antitumor, and antibacterial activities, among others, which led researchers to advance the study of these compounds, trying to prove their biological activities in vivo. The main results of those studies are summarized in Table 1, and the most relevant aspects are discussed below, while the compounds' chemical structures are presented in Figure 2.

Table 1. Summary of in vivo activity of phlorotannins.

Compound	Source	Model	Dose	Activity
Phloroglucinol 1	*Eisenia bicyclis* (Kjellman) Setchell [31], *Ecklonia cava* Kjellman [32–34]	ICR mice	20 µM	Suppression of acetic acid-induced vessel hyperpermeability (20%) and CMC-induced leucocyte migration (36.4%) [31].
		Balb/c mice	50 and 100 mg/kg (b.w.)	Protects against γ-radiation damage increasing survival rate (70% and 90% against 40% in the control group, observed 30 days after exposure to lethal doses of ionizing radiation) [32].
		Balb/c mice	25 mg/kg (b.w.)	Reduction of breast tumor growth by 82% compared to untreated group [35].
		NOD scid gamma mice	25 mg/kg (b.w.)	33.3% less metastasis of breast cancer cells and extended survival rate (40% after 10 weeks against 0% untreated group) [36].
		C57BL/6J mice	100 mg/kg (b.w.)	13% improvement in glucose tolerance compared to untreated group. 60% inhibition of glucose synthesis in primary mouse hepatocytes [37].
		ICR mice	20 mg/kg (b.w.)	Enhanced jejunal crypt survival (26.4%) and reduction of apoptotic cells (32.5%) in jejunal crypts after γ-ray exposure [33].
		HR-1 hairless mice	100 mg/kg (b.w.)	High reduction of UV-B-induced wrinkle formation (25%), epidermal thickness (62%), and elastic fiber degeneration (75%) when compared with control group [38].
		Balb/c mice	10 mg/mouse * (topical application)	Protection against UV-B-induced DNA damage by induction of NER pathway: Increase of 50% in XPC expression and of 66% in ERCC1 expression [39].
		Zebrafish embryos	50 µM	Reduction of H_2O_2 induced oxidative stress damage, with survival rate of 90% against 60% in untreated group [34].

Table 1. Cont.

Compound	Source	Model	Dose	Activity
Octaphlorethol A 2	Ishige sinicola (Setchell and N.L. Gardner) Chihara [40], Ishige foliacea Okamura [41–43]	SHR rats	10 mg/kg (b.w.)	Reduction of 21.9 mmHg in systolic blood pressure against 26.3 mmHg obtained with captopril [40].
		Zebrafish embryos	50 µM	Decrease glucose-induced ROS generation (10%) and lipid peroxidation (20%). Increase survival rate (50%) [41].
		Zebrafish embryos	12.6 µM *	Decrease of AAPH-induced ROS formation (30%) and lipid peroxidation (25%) when compared with the untreated group. Toxic at concentration higher than 50.4 µM [42].
		Zebrafish embryos	25 µM	Inhibition of melanin synthesis (27.8%) and tyrosinase activity (32.8%) Inhibitory activity higher than arbutin at 500 µM [43].
Diphlorethohydroxycarmalol 3	Ishige okamurae Yendo [44,45]	HR-1 hairless mice	2 mM	Inhibition of $PM_{2.5}$ exposure-induced lipid peroxidation (25%), protein carbonylation (37.5), and epidermal height (12%) [44].
		Balb/c mice	100 mg/kg (b.w.)	Protection against radiation-induced cell damage and increase by 30% in number of crypt cells compared with untreated group. Maintained villi height. Reduction of 50% of lipid peroxidation in liver. Bone marrow cell viability increased (40%) [46].
		Zebrafish embryos	48.8 µM *	Decrease of fine-dust particle-induced NO (50%) and ROS production (32%). Decrease inflammation-induced cell death (40%) [47].
		Zebrafish embryos	2 µM	Suppression of high glucose-induced dilation in the retinal vessel diameter (64.9%) and vessel formation (35.6%) [48].
Eckol 4	Ecklonia sp. and Eisenia sp. [49,50]	ICR mice	75 nmol/mouse	Inhibition of ear edema induced by AA (12.7%), by TPA (40.0%), and by OXA (19.3%) [51].
		Kunming mice	0.5 mg/kg (b.w.)	Hepatoprotection by reduction of ALT (41.6%) and AST (26%) on CCl_4-induced liver injury; decrease in expression of caspase-3 (77%), TNF-α (23%), IL-1β (%), IL-6 (26%), and lipid peroxidation (21%); increase in expression of Bcl-2 (33.3%) and IL-10 (33%). Increase in GSH (31%) and SOD (19.5%) [52].
		ICR mice	50 mg/kg (b.w.)	Anticoagulant action by increasing tail bleeding time (135%). Less active than heparin [53].
		ICR mice	20 mg/kg (b.w.)	Enhanced jejunal crypt survival (17.7%) and reduction of apoptotic cells (37.5%) in jejunal crypts after γ-ray exposure [33].

Table 1. Cont.

Compound	Source	Model	Dose	Activity
Eckol 4	Ecklonia sp. and Eisenia sp. [49,50]	C57BL/6 mice	10 mg/kg (b.w.)	Radioprotection increasing survival rate (58%), hematopoietic recovery (50%), reduction of DNA damage in lymphocytes (27.8%), and increase in CD3$^+$ T cell (44.3%) and CD45R/B220+ pan B cell (27.6%) populations after γ-ray exposure [54].
		C57BL/6 mice	10 mg/kg (b.w.)	Inhibition of γ-radiation-induced lymphocyte apoptosis (33.33%), and intestinal cell apoptosis (16.63%) [55].
		Sprague-Dawley rats	20 mg/kg (b.w.)	Anti-hyperlipidemic effect by reduction of TG (27.2%), TC (38.6%), AI (49%), and LDL (56.5%) level and increased level of HDL (10.5%). Activity level similar to lovastatin [56].
		ICR mice	20 μM	Suppression of acetic acid-induced vessel hyperpermeability (50%) and leucocyte migration (50%) [31].
		Zebrafish	50 μM	Photoprotection by reduction of UV-B induced ROS formation (43%), NO levels (33%), cell death (78%), and hyperpigmentation (50%) [57].
Dieckol 5	Ecklonia sp. and Eisenia sp. [49,58]	IgE/antigen-sensitized mice	20 mg/kg (b.w.) *	Administration prior to IgE sensitization, reduced mast cell degranulation, and edema formation (80%) [59].
		Sprague-Dawley rats	20 mg/kg (b.w.)	Reduction of TG (31%), TC (43.4%), AI (72.6%), and LDL (75.5%) level and increased level of HDL (35.4%). More active than lovastatin [56].
		ICR mice	20 μM	Suppression of acetic acid-induced vessel hyperpermeability (70%) and CMC-induced leucocyte migration (55%) [31].
		C57BL/KsJ-db/db mice	20 mg/kg (b.w.)	Antidiabetic effect by reduction of lipid peroxidation (87%) body weight (7%), blood glucose (40%), and blood insulin (50%). Increased the activity of SOD (8.5%), CAT (0.5%), and GSH-px (0.1%), and over-expression of AMPK (60%) and Akt (100%) [58].
		ICR mice	50 mg/kg (b.w.)	Anticoagulant effect by increasing tail bleeding time (173.8%). Less active than heparin [53].
		Zebrafish embryos	20 μM	Reduction of heart rate (13%), ROS formation (35%), NO level (18%), lipid peroxidation (10%), and cell death (10%) in high glucose-induced oxidative stress. Reduction of over-expression of iNOS (20%) and COX-2 (15%) [60].
		Zebrafish embryos	20 μM	Reduction of ROS formation (80%), lipid peroxidation (5%), and cell death (15%) on ethanol-induced damage [61].

Table 1. Cont.

Compound	Source	Model	Dose	Activity
Phlorofucofuroeckol A 6	Eisenia arborea Areschouga [a] [51,62]; Ecklonia stolonifera Okamura [63]	Zebrafish embryos	41.5 µM	Decreased AAPH-induced ROS levels (40%), lipid peroxidation (48%), and cell death (70%) [64].
		ICR mice	75 nmol/mouse	Inhibition of ear edema induced by AA (30.5%), by TPA (31.7%), and by OXA (23.4%). EGCG inhibits 12.9%, 13.8%, and 5.7% of ear edema induced by AA, TPA, and OXA, respectively [51].
Phlorofucofuroeckol B 7	Eisenia arborea Areschoug [a] [51,62]; Ecklonia stolonifera Okamura [63]	ICR mice	75 nmol/mouse	Inhibition of ear edema induced by AA (42.2%), by TPA (38.4%), and by OXA (41.0%). EGCG inhibits 12.9%, 13.8%, and 5.7% of ear edema induced by AA, TPA, and OXA, respectively [51].
6,6'-Bieckol 8	Eisenia arborea Areschoug [a] [51,65]; Ecklonia stolonifera Okamura [63]	SHR rats	20 mg/kg (b.w.)	Reduction of 28.6 mmHg in systolic blood pressure, against 31.3 mmHg obtained with captopril [66].
		ICR mice	75 nmol/mouse	Inhibition of ear edema induced by AA (41.9%), by TPA (34.2%), and by OXA (17.8%). EGCG inhibits 12.9%, 13.8%, and 5.7% of ear edema induced by AA, TPA, and OXA, respectively [51].
6,8'-Bieckol 9	Eisenia arborea Areschoug [a] [51,62]	ICR mice	75 nmol/mouse	Inhibition of ear edema induced by AA (39.8%), by TPA (49.4%), and by OXA (77.8%). EGCG inhibits 12.9%, 13.8%, and 5.7% of ear edema induced by AA, TPA, and OXA, respectively [51].
8,8'-Bieckol 10	Eisenia arborea Areschoug [a] [51]	ICR mice	75 nmol/mouse	Inhibition of ear edema induced by AA (21.0%), by TPA (31.7%), and by OXA (32.3%). EGCG inhibits 12.9%, 13.8%, and 5.7% of ear edema induced by AA, TPA, and OXA, respectively [51].
Eckstolonol 11	Ecklonia cava Kjellman [67], Ecklonia stolonifera Okamura [68]	C57BL/6N mice	50 mg/kg (b.w.)	Decrease in sleep latency and increase (1.4×) in the amount of NREMS [67].

* Unit converted for comparison purposes. [a] The current accepted name is Ecklonia arborea (Areschoug) M. D. Rothman, Mattio and J. J. Bolton.

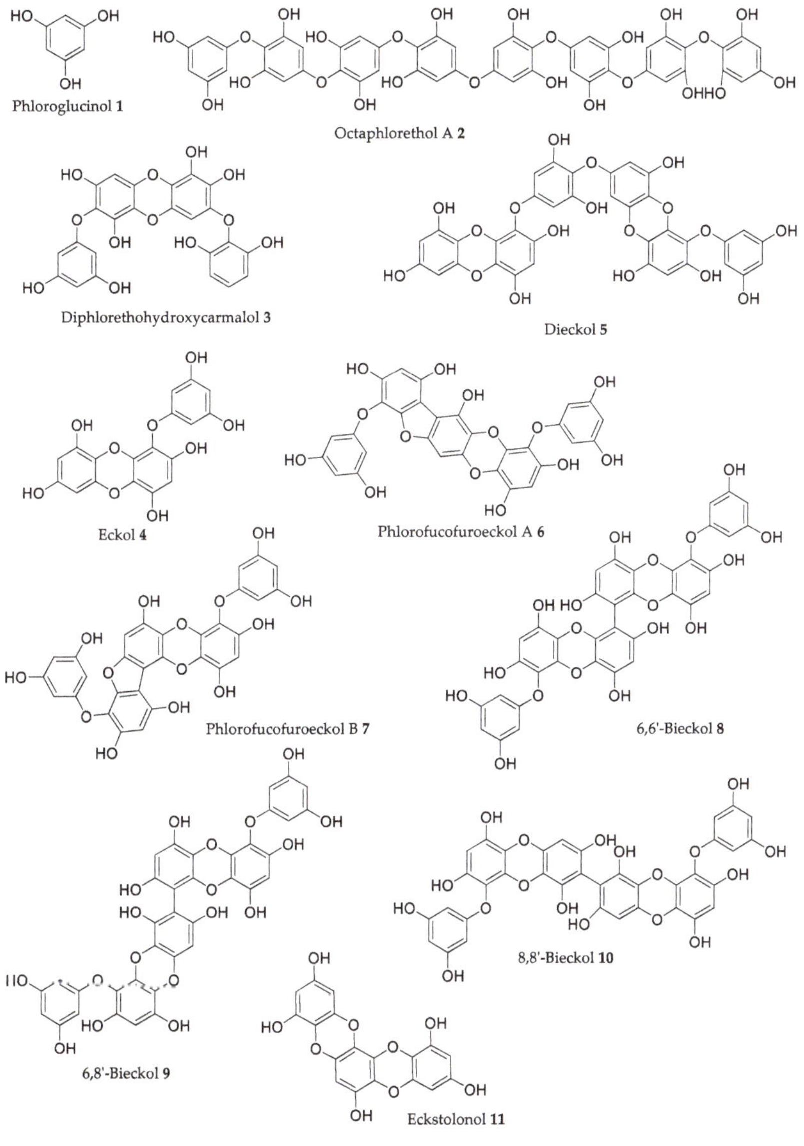

Figure 2. Chemical structures of phlorotannins referred to in Table 1 with relevant in vivo activities.

2.1.1. Phloroglucinol

Phloroglucinol **1** (Figure 2), the basic unit of phlorotannins, was found to reduce H_2O_2-induced toxicity in zebrafish, with the treated group (50 µM of **1**) presenting a survival rate of 90% against only 60% in the control group [34]. The augmented survival rate was correlated with a reduction of H_2O_2-induced cell death, lipid peroxidation, and ROS formation. Moreover, this compound accelerates liver regeneration after metronidazole (MNZ)-induced apoptosis at a concentration of 400 µM [34].

The effects of **1** on the blood glucose level and the regulation of glucose synthesis in the liver were also investigated. As shown in Table 1, phloroglucinol **1** (100 mg/kg b.w.) significantly improved glucose tolerance in C57BL/6J male mice whose diet was high in fat and inhibited glucose synthesis in primary mouse hepatocytes [37]. This phlorotannin also exerts efficient cell protection against ionizing radiation and extends the survival of mice exposed to a lethal dose of γ-radiation. Thirty days after exposure, there was a survival rate of 90% in the group treated with 100 mg/kg (b.w) of **1** and 70% in the group treated with 50 mg/kg (b.w.), while, in the control group, only 40% of the mice survived [32]. It was proposed that the protection against γ-radiation is mainly due to the antioxidant effects of **1**, namely, the inhibition of ROS formation, leading to the inhibition of mitogen-activated protein kinase kinase-4 (MKK4/SEK1), c-Jun NH_2-terminal kinase (JNK), and activator protein-1 (AP-1) cascades [32,69]. Moon et al. [33] found that administration of **1** (20 mg/kg b.w.) could enhance the jejunal crypt survival by 26.4% and decreased the number of apoptotic cells in the jejunal crypts by 32.5% when compared with the untreated irradiated group (Table 1).

Phloroglucinol **1** (100 mg/kg b.w.) protects hairless mice against UV-B-induced photodamage in the skin, by significantly reducing (25%–75%) wrinkle formation, epidermal thickness, and elastic fiber degeneration [38]. The levels of UV-B-induced DNA damage are also decreased by **1** since the topical application of 10 mg/mouse was found to increase the expression levels of xeroderma pigmentosum complementation group C (XPC) and excision repair cross-complementation 1 (ERCC1). These components are essential for the activation of the nucleotide excision repair (NER) pathway, which is the mechanism responsible for DNA repairing [39]. Phloroglucinol **1** also exhibits breast anticancer activity at 25 mg/kg (b.w.), either by decreasing tumor growth or by suppressing the metastatic ability of breast cancer cells that spread to the lungs, contributing in both cases to an increase of survival time in mice (Table 1) [35,36]. Since there is still no suitable therapeutic agent that blocks the progression of breast cancer, these results can be of clinical importance for the treatment of metastatic breast cancer.

2.1.2. Octaphlorethol A

Octaphlorethol A **2**, a rare phlorotannin, decreased oxidative stress induced either by 2,2′-azobis (2-amidinopropane) (AAPH) [42] or by high levels of glucose [41] in zebrafish embryos (Table 1). This phlorotannin is toxic for the embryos at concentrations above 50.4 μM; however, at concentrations lower than 25.2 μM, a strong antioxidant effect was noted without traces of toxicity [42]. These toxicity values against zebrafish are supported by the data obtained by Kim et al. [43], which found that more than 90% of subject embryos survived upon exposure to **2** at concentrations below 25 μM, which was not significantly different from the findings in the control group. Moreover, the same authors reported that this compound significantly inhibited melanin synthesis (27.8%) and tyrosinase activity (32.8%) at a concentration of 25 μM, which is higher than the 15% and 17.3% of inhibition obtained with the reference compound, arbutin, at 500 μM, for melanin synthesis and tyrosinase activity, respectively. These results indicate that **2** has a potential for application in skin-whitening formulations [43].

A dose of 10 mg/kg (b.w.) of **2** led to a reduction of 21.9 mmHg in the systolic blood pressure (SBP) in spontaneously hypertensive rats (SHR), against the 26.3 mmHg reduction obtained using the same dosage of the reference drug captopril. The anti-hypertensive effect was maintained for 6 h, and the authors suggested this effect was due to the induction of NO production, which is a vasodilator [40].

2.1.3. Diphlorethohydroxycarmalol

Diphlorethohydroxycarmalol **3**, which was only isolated from *Ishige okamurae* Yendo, has a protective effect against radiation exposure. Ahn et al. [46] reported that treatment with **3** (100 mg/kg b.w.) in mice before γ-ray irradiation significantly protected the intestinal crypt cells in the jejunum and maintained villi height, compared with those of the control-treated irradiated group. Mice pretreated with **3** also exhibited dose-dependent increases in the bone marrow cell viability up to a maximum of 40% at 100 mg/kg (b.w.) [46].

Diphlorethohydroxycarmalol **3** decreased the oxidative stress caused to the skin tissue of HR-1 hairless mice by fine particulate matter with a diameter ≤2.5 μm ($PM_{2.5}$), a major pollutant present in the atmosphere [44] (Table 1). Exposure to $PM_{2.5}$ caused lipid peroxidation and protein carbonylation, and increased epidermal height, which were inhibited by **3**. Moreover, $PM_{2.5}$ induced apoptosis and mitogen-activated protein kinase (MAPK) protein expression; however, these changes were attenuated by **3** [44].

Fernando et al. [47] reported for the first time the use of a zebrafish embryo model for evaluating the inflammatory effects of fine dust (FD) particles, which are a major aggressive agent in air pollution. The authors determined that a concentration of 48.8 µM of **3** significantly decreased NO and ROS production and prevented fine dust inflammation-induced cell death [47]. The effect of **3** against high glucose-induced angiogenesis in zebrafish embryos was studied, and it was found that the treatment of embryos with a concentration of 2 µM of **3** suppressed high glucose-induced dilation in the retinal vessel diameter and vessel formation (Table 1). Moreover, **3** exhibits the ability to inhibit high glucose-induced vascular endothelial growth factor receptor 2 (VEGFR-2) expression and its downstream signaling cascade [48]. Hence, **3** seems to be a potential agent for the development of drugs against angiogenesis induced by diabetes.

2.1.4. Eckol

Eckol **4** presented anti-inflammatory activity in various in vivo studies. Kim et al. [31] found that a concentration of 20 µM of **4** significantly suppressed acetic acid-induced hyperpermeability and carboxy-methylcellulose-induced leucocyte migration in mice at a much higher level than **1** (Table 1). A dosage of 75 nmol of **4** per mouse decreased mouse ear edema induced by different sensitizers, such as arachidonic acid (AA), 12-O-tetradecanoylphorbol-13-acetate (TPA), and oxazolone (OXA), by 12.7%, 40.0%, and 19.3%, respectively (Table 1) [51]. This shows that **4** can modulate various targets of the inflammatory cascade.

On the other hand, **4** at a very low dosage (0.5 mg/kg b.w.) has an hepatoprotective effect on mice by modulating anti-apoptotic and antioxidant mechanisms and suppressing the expression of pro-inflammatory cytokines, like tumor necrosis factor (TNF), interleukin (IL)-1, and IL-6, and by upregulating the expression of IL-10, an anti-inflammatory interleukin [52].

Kim et al. [53] reported that **4** presented anticoagulant activity in a mouse model. A dosage of 50 mg/kg (b.w.) increased the in vivo tail bleeding time from 51.5 to 121 s, which is an increase of more than 100%. However, this result was lower than that obtained with heparin, the commercial anticoagulant (165 s).

Eckol **4** (20 mg/kg b.w.) also significantly reduced the level of triglycerides (TG), total cholesterol (TC), atherogenic index (AI), and low-density lipoprotein cholesterol (LDL) and increased level of the high-density lipoprotein cholesterol (HDL), in SD rats, by similar values to those presented by lovastatin (Table 1), a therapeutic agent used in the treatment of hypercholesterolemia [56].

Park et al. [54] found that the administration of 10 mg/kg (b.w.) of **4** to γ-ray irradiated C57BL/6 mice led to an improvement in hematopoietic recovery and in the repair of damaged DNA in immune cells and an enhancement of their proliferation, which was severely suppressed by ionizing radiation (Table 1). It was also found that the same dose decreased lymphocyte apoptosis by 33.33% and intestinal cell apoptosis by 16.63%, which was correlated with a decrease in the amount of pro-apoptotic p53 and Bax proteins and an increase in the level of Bcl-2, an anti-apoptotic protein, indicating that its over-expression, which leads to resistance to DNA damage, is involved in protection of gastrointestinal cells after irradiation [55]. Furthermore, Moon et al. [33] found that **4** at a higher dose (20 mg/kg b.w.) enhanced jejunal crypt survival and protected against apoptosis induced by radiation in ICR mice jejunal crypts, albeit to a lesser extent than the values obtained for **1** (Table 1). These findings indicate that **4** should be a candidate for adjuvant therapy to alleviate radiation-induced injuries to cancer patients; however, as far as we were able to assess, there were no further advancements in this regard.

Pre-treatment with **4** (50 µM) reduced ROS and NO formation by about 43% and 33%, respectively, in zebrafish embryos following UV-B irradiation. It also reduced UV-B-induced cell death by 78% and hyperpigmentation by about 50%, when compared to the untreated control group, showing the photoprotection effectiveness of **4**. The compound presented low toxicity at the tested concentration [57].

2.1.5. Dieckol

Dieckol 5 was able to impair the oxidative stress effects induced by ethanol in zebrafish embryos [61]. A concentration of 20 µM decreased ROS formation by 80% and lipid peroxidation by 5%. The attenuation of oxidative stress led to a 15% decrease in ethanol-induced liver cell death, showing that dieckol possesses a hepatoprotective effect [61]. Dieckol at the same dose also decreased the oxidative effects caused by high glucose, by significantly reducing heart rate, ROS, lipid peroxidation, and cell death in zebrafish (Table 1) [60]. Furthermore, high glucose levels induced the over-expression of inducible nitric oxide synthase (iNOS) and cyclooxygenase-2 (COX-2), whereas 5 treatment reduced it [60].

Additionally, the antioxidant effects of 5 also play an important role in the attenuation of type II diabetes. C57BL/KsJ-db/db diabetic mice, when injected with 20 mg/kg (b.w.) of 5, showed a significant reduction of blood glucose level, serum insulin level, and body weight, when compared to the untreated group [58]. Nonetheless, 5 also promoted the increase of the activity of antioxidant enzymes, including superoxide dismutase (SOD), catalase (CAT), and glutathione peroxidase (GSH-px) in liver tissues, and it increased levels of the phosphorylation of AMPK and Akt in muscle tissues (Table 1), suggesting that 5 can be developed as a therapeutic agent for type II diabetes [58].

Like phlorotannin 4, 5 also suppressed acetic acid-induced hyperpermeability and carboxy-methylcellulose-induced leucocyte migration in mice [31], albeit to a higher level than 4, leading to the conclusion that the number of OH groups in the 5 structure increases its anti-inflammatory activity. The authors proved the influence of the OH groups of 5 on its activity by protecting those groups with a methyl substituent, and the activity obtained for methyl-dieckol was reduced by about 35% [31].

The comparison between 5 and 4 was also verified for anticoagulant activity. Kim et al. [53] found that 5 increased the in vivo tail bleeding time by 173.8%, from 51.5 to 141 s, whereas 4 only increased this time to 121 s, and heparin increased tail bleeding time to 165 s.

Dieckol also presented a better potential for treating dyslipidemia than 4 since it reduced all the parameters measured by Yoon et al. [56] at a higher level than that obtained with 4 and even lovastatin (Table 1). As an example of the efficiency of 5 in the treatment of dyslipidemia, a dose of 20 mg/kg (b.w.) of 5 decreased total cholesterol by 43.4% when compared with the untreated group, whereas lovastatin (25 mg/kg (b.w.)) only decreased this parameter by 15.3% [56].

Dieckol 5 also presents anti-allergy effects since oral administration of 5 and 20 mg/kg (b.w.), before IgE sensitization, markedly abrogated mast cell degranulation and edematous changes in vivo [59]. However, the authors also suggested that the inhibition of the passive cutaneous anaphylaxis could be mainly attributed to the anti-inflammatory effects of 5.

2.1.6. Other Phlorotannins

In the literature revision performed for the present work, phlorotannins other than those already known were found with in vitro activities reported, while they only had one or two studies addressing their in vivo activities, unlike the compounds discussed above. However, some of these activities are interesting; thus, the studies addressing the less studied phlorotannins are discussed to demonstrate the interest of future studies on these phlorotannins.

Phlorofucofuroeckol B 7 suppressed 42.2%, 38.4%, and 41.0% of ear swelling in mice induced by AA, TPA, and OXA, respectively (Table 1), whereas the suppression of ear edema induced by those three sensitizers showed was significantly lower for isomer 6 (23.4%–31.7%) [51]. This indicates that the change of the 3″,5″-dihydroxybenzyl group from C-8 in 6 to C-11 in 7 increases the compound's anti-inflammatory capacity. The results presented by 7 were also better than those obtained for 4 (Table 1). The interesting activities shown in vivo by this phlorotannin 7 justify the realization of further studies, including more deep SAR studies to establish its action mechanism.

Administration of 6,6′-bieckol 8 (Figure 2) to mouse (75 nmol per mouse) caused the reduction of ear swelling after sensitization with AA and TPA by 41.9% and 34.2%, respectively, which is an anti-inflammatory effect similar to phlorofucofuroeckol B **7**, although **8** had a much smaller anti-inflammatory effect on the OXA-induced mouse model (17.8%) [51]. On the other hand, the administration of 6,8'-bieckol **9** was able to inhibit 77.8% of mouse ear swelling when the sensitizer was OXA, which was the highest value obtained by Sugiura et al. [51], while the administration of **10** yielded an inhibition of 32.3%. These results show clearly that the position of the linkage has a great influence on the anti-inflammatory activity of phlorotannins. Compounds **4** and **6–10** exhibited anti-inflammatory effects identical to or higher than epigallocatechin gallate (EGCG), the compound used as a positive control.

Ko et al. [66] found that a dose of 20 mg/kg (b.w.) of **8** led to a reduction of 28.6 mmHg in the SBP in SHR, whereas the same dosage of the reference drug captopril decreased SBP by 31.3 mmHg. This phlorotannin **8** is less active than octaphlorethol **2** [40] since the dose of **8** used was two times higher than the dose of **2** (Table 1). Thus, the latter seems to be more promising for anti-hypertensive applications.

The phlorotannin eckstolonol **11** significantly decreased sleep latency in a concentration-dependent manner and increased the amount of non-rapid eye movements (NREMS) in C57BL/6N mice by 1.4-fold at 50 mg/kg (b.w.) [67]. At this dose, **11** administered in conjunction with pentobarbital was also capable of increasing sleep duration when compared to the control (only pentobarbital), showing that this phlorotannin can also potentiate the effects of other hypnotic drugs. It was found that **11** acts as a partial agonist to the GABAA–BZD receptors [67], similar to the action mode of benzodiazepines, showing its potential as a hypnotic drug.

In addition to the good results presented by phlorotannins in in vivo studies, which showed their high pharmaceutical potential, there were some studies [31,44] where there was no information about the actual amount of compound administered, which hindered their comparison with other studies, as well as the reproducibility of the results. Also, the majority of the referenced studies, particularly those using a murine model, had a small group of individuals per study group (4–6), which may not be very representative of the real effect of the compounds. Future studies should increase the number of test subjects to increase the statistical power of the findings.

2.2. Peptides

2.2.1. Griffithsin

One of the most biologically interesting families of peptides extracted from macroalgae is the lectins. They are a structurally diverse group of highly specific and reversibly carbohydrate-binding proteins [70]. The three groups of macroalgae (Rhodophyta, Phaeophyta, and Chlorophyta) can produce lectins [71], and these lectins present great potential for the development of new drugs [72–76]. In fact, because of the highly specific way lectins bind to sugars outside cell surfaces inhibiting cell proliferation [77,78], lectins primarily show antiviral, antibacterial, and antifungal activities [73,79–81]. The most interesting lectin and also the one with the most in vivo studies is griffithsin **12** (Figure 3) (Table 2).

Table 2. Summary of in vivo activity of seaweed peptides.

Compound	Algae	Model	Activity	Dose
Griffithsin 12	Griffithsia sp. [82]	Balb/c mice	100% of mice survival from a high dose of SARS-CoV (compared to 30% survival in control group) [83].	10 mg/kg (b.w.)/day
		Balb/c mice	Protected 100% of mice from a lethal JEV dose (compared to 0% survival in control) [84].	5 mg/kg (b.w.)/day
		Chimeric uPA$^+$/$^+$-SCID mice	Protected mice from hepatitis C infection (viral load below detection limit in treated mice) [85].	5 mg/kg (b.w.)/day
		Balb/c mice	Significantly protected mice from HSV-2 vaginal infection (0/5 treated mice were infected compared to 3/5 infected in control group, after 7 days) [86].	20μL of 0.1% griffithsin gel
		New Zealand rabbits	Caused no mucosal damage or inflammatory responses with intravaginal administration [87].	0.1% griffithsin gel
		Balb/c mice	Significantly protected mice from HSV-2 vaginal infection and HPV16 pseudovirus challenge [88].	20 μL gel of griffithsin–carrageenan combination (0.1% 12 and 3% CG)
		Rhesus macaques	Did not negatively impact the mucosal proteome or microbiome [89].	0.1% griffithsin gel
Tridecapeptide 13	Palmaria palmata (Linnaeus) F. Weber and D. Mohr [90]	SHR mice	After 2 h, significant 33 mmHg SBP reduction; captopril at same dose caused 29 mmHg SBP reduction [90].	3 mg/kg (b.w.)
Dipeptide 14	Undaria pinnatifida (Harvey) Suringar [91]	SHR mice	16 mmHg SBP reduction after 3 h; captopril at same dose caused 17 mmHg SBP reduction [91].	1 mg/kg (b.w.)
Phycoerythrin 15	Porphyra haitanensis T.J. Chang and B.F. Zheng [a], Grateloupia turuturu Yamada, Gracilaria lemaneiformis (Bory) Greville [b] [92–94]	S180 tumor-bearing mice	Reduced tumor growth by 41.3%. Increase TNF-α level, lymphocyte proliferation, and SOD activity [92].	300 mg/kg (b.w.)
		N2 Caenorhabditis elegans	Increased Caenorhabditis elegans lifespan (15 ± 0.1 to 19.9 ± 0.3 days), increased thermal stress resistance (22.2% ± 2.5% to 41.6% ± 2.5% mean survival) and oxidative stress resistance (30.1% ± 3.2% to 63.1% ± 6.4% mean survival) [95].	100 μg/mL
		CL4176 Caenorhabitis elegans	Significant reduction of senile plaque formation (2-fold reduction in grayscale values [96].	100 μg/mL
Kahalalide F 16	Bryopsis sp. [97]	Athymic mice with xenografted tumors	Reduced prostate tumor growth by 50% and 35% [98].	0.245 and 0.123 mg/kg (b.w.)

[a] The current accepted name is *Pyropia haitanensis* (T. J. Chang and B. F. Zheng) N. Kikuchi and M. Miyata). [b] The current accepted name is *Gracilariopsis lemaneiformis* (Bory de Saint-Vincent) E. Y. Dawson, Acleto and Foldvik.

Griffithsin was first isolated from aqueous extracts of *Griffithsia* sp., and it exhibits antiviral activity [82]. This 121-amino-acid peptide **12** showed no significant homology (>30%) with other known proteins and exhibited potent in vitro antiviral activity (EC_{50} values ranging from 0.043 to 0.63 nM) [82], which enticed researchers to perform several subsequent in vivo studies.

Ser-Leu-Thr-His-Arg-Lys-Phe-Gly-Gly-Ser-Pro-Phe-Ser-Gly-Ile-Ser-Ser-Ile-Ala-Val-Arg-Ser-Gly-Ser-
Tyr-Leu-Asp-X-Ile-Ile-Ile-Asp-Gly-Val-His-His-Gly-Gly-Ser-Gly-Gly-Asn-Leu-Ser-Pro-Thr-Phe-Thr-
Phe-Gly-Ser-Gly-Glu-Tyr-Ile-Ser-Asn-Met-Thr-Ile-Arg-Ser-Gly-Asp-Tyr-Ile-Asp-Asn-Ile-Ser-Phe-Glu-
Thr-Asn-Met-Gly-Arg-Arg-Phe-Gly-Pro-Tyr-Gly-Gly-Ser-Gly-Gly-Ser-Ala-Asn-Thr-Leu-Ser-Asn-Val-
Lys-Val-Ile-Gln-Ile-Asn-Gly-Ser-Ala-Gly-Asp-Tyr-Leu-Asp-Ser-Leu-Asp-Ile-Tyr-Tyr-Glu-Gln-Tyr

Griffithsin 12

Ile-Arg-Leu-Ile-Ile-Val-Leu-Met-Pro-Ile-Leu-Met-Ala

Tridecapeptide 13

Dipeptide 14

Met-Leu-Asp-Ala-Phe-Ser-Arg-Val-Ile-Ser-Asn-
Ala-Asp-Ala-Lys-Ala-Ala-Tyr-Val-Gly-Gly-Ser-
Asp-Leu-Gln-Ala-Leu-Arg-Thr-Phe-Ile-Ser-
Asp-Gly-Asn-Lys-Arg-Leu-Asp-Ala-Val-Asn-
Tyr-Ile-Val-Ser-Asn-Ser-Ser-Cys-Ile-Val-Ser-
Asp-Ala-Ile-Ser-Gly-Met-Ile-Cys-Glu-Asn-Pro-
Gly-Gly-Asn-Cys-Tyr-Thr-Asn-Arg-Arg-Met-
Ala-Ala-Cys-Leu-Arg-Asp-Gly-Glu-Ile-Ile-Leu-
Arg-Tyr-Ile-Ser-Tyr-Ala-Leu-Leu-Ala-Gly-Asp-
Ser-Ser-Val-Leu-Glu-Asp-Arg-Cys-Leu-Asn-
Gly-Leu-Lys-Glu-Thr-Tyr-Ile-Ala-Leu-Gly-Val-
Pro-Thr-Asn-Ser-Thr-Val-Arg-Ala-Val-Ser-Ile-
Met-Lys-Ala-Ala-Val-Gly-Ala-Phe-Ile-Ser-Asn-
Thr-Ala-Ser-Gln-Arg-Lys-Gly-Glu-Val-Ile-Glu-
Gly-Asp-Cys-Ser-Ala-Leu-Ala-Ala-Glu-Ile-Ala-
Ser-Tyr-Cys-Asp-Arg-Ile-Ser-Ala-Ala-Val-Ser

Phycoerythrin 15

Kahalalide F 16

Figure 3. Amino-acid sequence of seaweed peptides with relevant in vivo activities.

O'Keefe et al. [83] reported the antiviral effect of griffithsin **12** (Figure 3, Table 2) on mouse models infected with an adapted SARS-CoV virus. After injection with a viral dose known to cause at least 75% mouse mortality, mice treated with griffithsin **12** (5 mg/kg b.w. dose intranasally delivered 4 h before infection) showed 100% survival rates, no weight loss, and decreased pulmonary pathology during infection. The compound reduced mice pulmonary viral load and inhibited the deleterious inflammatory response to the virus. In 2013, Ishag et al. [84] once again proved griffithsin's life-saving in vivo efficacy with mice models infected with lethal doses of Japanese encephalitis virus (JEV). Similar to the results obtained by O'Keefe et al. [83], treated mice showed 100% survival rates, as well as reduced viral antigen load in brain tissue. The griffithsin **12** treatment of mice consisted of 5 mg/kg b.w. intraperitoneal injection of the encephalitis virus. The fact that the same 5 mg/kg b.w. dose was so effective against both the SARS-CoV and JEV virus highlights griffithsin's potential as an antiviral agent. Subsequently, Meuleman et al. [85] also used a 5 mg/kg b.w. griffithsin treatment (subcutaneously injected in chimeric uPA-SCID mice) to mitigate hepatitis C liver infection. After one week of virus injection, the results showed significantly lower viral loads (below the limit of detection, <750 IU/mL) in four of the six treated mice, as opposed to easily detectable loads in the control mice. In the following two weeks of the study, while the treated mice started slowly exhibiting signs of infection, the control mice experienced full-blown viremia. Surprisingly, one of the treated mice managed to stay completely below the detection limit throughout the entire study period. These results once again point to the extent and versatility of griffithsin's antiviral activity against taxonomically distinct viruses. Although very interesting, these results feel particularly limited in scope due to the small sample size ($n = 6$ treated and $n = 5$ control mice), a fact that was acknowledged by the authors. Nevertheless, griffithsin's broad-spectrum antiviral action was still very "alluring" to researchers and begged further study. Nixon et al. [86] used murine models to see if a 0.1% griffithsin gel would protect mice from intravaginally applied genital herpes. Results showed that the gel significantly prevented herpes simplex virus 2 infection and proliferation after mucosal surface challenge and subsequent viral introduction in seminal plasma. These results complemented those obtained by O'Keefe et al. [87], which used the rabbit vaginal irritation model to prove griffithsin's safety as a topical microbicide component. Results showed that griffithsin caused no mucosal damage or inflammatory responses. Another study, by Levendosky et al. [88], used a very similar intravaginal challenge methodology to assess topically applied antiviral activity of a griffithsin–carrageenan (**12**-CG) combination against herpes simplex (HSV-2) and human papillomavirus (HPV16). A 20-µL dose of the combination (0.1% **12** and 3% CG) was shown to scientifically reduce HSV-2 vaginal infection (when applied before challenge) and HPV16 (when dosed during and after challenge). The discrepancy between HSV-2 and HPV16 efficacy timeframes is believed to be due to a several-hour "lag" period in HPV's replication cycle. Notwithstanding, these results are in line with previous works and prove griffithsin's action as a broad-spectrum antiviral. To conclude, we present a more recent study by Girard et al. in 2018 [89], who produced and rectally applied griffithsin gels in rhesus monkeys. The study confirmed the safety of griffithsin as an anti-HIV agent, with minimum disturbance of the monkey's rectal proteome and microbiota.

In summary, griffithsin **12** shows tremendous promise as a topical antiviral agent, with great potential concerning the prevention of sexually transmitted infections. The compound's repeatedly proven efficacy, along with the safety studies of O'Keefe et al. [87] and Girard et al. [89], appears to be leading up to a pre-clinical stage of testing, which should happen soon and eventually pave the way for future clinical trials.

2.2.2. ACE and Renin Inhibitory Peptides IRLIIVLMPILMA Tridecapeptide and Phe–Tyr Dipeptide

The search for angiotensin-converting enzyme (ACE) inhibitors is of great biological value due to their inherent hypotensive effects and subsequent applications. Macroalgae were proven to be an especially rich source of compounds with ACE inhibition activity [18,99–104]. Regarding seaweed ACE or renin inhibitors, this review chooses to focus on the IRLIIVLMPILMA tridecapeptide **13** and the Phe–Tyr dipeptide **14** (Figure 3) shown in Table 2, mainly due to their potent hypotensive activity compared to a current pharmaceutical option (captopril), as well as being of more recent relevance and interest.

Fitzgerald et al. [90] studied the hypotensive effect of the renin inhibitor tridecapeptide IRLIIVLMPILMA **13** (Figure 3), previously extracted and purified from *Palmaria palmata* (Linnaeus) F. Weber and D. Mohr hydrolysate [105], using the SHR model. The research group reported that a dose of 3 mg/kg b.w. of tridecapeptide **13** resulted in a decrease in SBP by 33 mmHg after 2 h. This is especially interesting when compared to the positive control (the clinical hypotensive drug captopril), which showed an SBP decrease by 29 mmHg with the same dose. Also noteworthy is that a 34-mmHg SBP decrease was achieved with *Palmaria palmata* (Linnaeus) F. Weber and D. Mohr protein hydrolysate but with a dose of 50 mg/kg b.w.

The SHR model was also used in a somewhat similar study by Sato et al. [91] to test ACE inhibitory peptides purified from *Undaria pinnatifida* (Harvey) Suringar hydrolysate. Seven dipeptides were identified and tested in vivo, of which the Phe–Tyr dipeptide **14** stood out, revealing a statistically significant 16-mmHg SBP decrease after 3 h with a 1 mg/kg b.w. dose and a 26-mmHg SBP decrease after 9 h with only a 0.1 mg/kg b.w. dose. These results were compared to captopril, which showed 17-mmHg and 14-mmHg SBP decreases after 3 and 9 h, respectively, with a 1 mg/kg b.w. dose. In more recent work, Kecel-Gündüz et al. [106] studied poly(lactic-*co*-glycolic acid) nanoparticles as a delivery system for the Phe–Tyr dipeptide **14**, which highlights the continued interest and relevance of this seaweed peptide with great antihypertensive potential.

As previously mentioned, of all the analyzed literature, the IRLIIVLMPILMA tridecapeptide **13** and Phe–Tyr dipeptide **14** (Figure 3, Table 2) are the most promising in vivo hypotensive seaweed compounds identified so far, with a similar effect to clinical drugs.

2.2.3. Phycoerythrin

Phycoerythrin **15** (Figure 3), a red protein pigment complex abundant in Rhodophyta (although many studies use cyanobacteria as a more readily available natural source for this compound), is another polypeptide very interesting, not as a hypotensive agent but rather as an antitumor and anti-aging agent.

After extensive in vitro studies which demonstrated the cytotoxic activity of phycoerythrin **15** (Figure 3) [94,107], Pan et al. [92] demonstrated its activity in vivo using the S180 tumor-bearing mice model (Table 2). Results showed that phycoerythrin injection, at a dose of 300 mg/kg b.w., reduced S180 tumor growth by up to 41.3% in treated mice. These mice also revealed a significant serum increase in the TNF-α level, NK cell kill activity, and lymphocyte proliferation. The antitumor activity obtained is believed to be related to phycoerythrin's antioxidant activity, as shown by the significant increase in superoxide dismutase activity in the serum of treated mice, as well as the significant decrease in mouse liver malondialdehyde level.

Shortly after, Sonani et al. [95] used the *Caenorhabitis elegans* model to test the in vivo antioxidant and anti-aging effects of phycoerythrin. Doses of 100 µg/mL of the compound were found to significantly increase *Caenorhabitis elegans* lifespan both in normal and in oxidative stress conditions. This is indicative of phycoerythrin having a strong anti-aging effect, possibly related to its antioxidant properties.

In more recent work, Chaubey et al. [96] tested the effect of phycoerythrin in a mutant *Caenorhabitis elegans* Alzheimer's disease model. Results showed that a dose of 100 µg/mL of phycoerythrin led to a significant reduction in senile plaque formation when compared to untreated nematodes. This indicates that phycoerythrin might have great potential as a therapeutic agent in neurodegenerative diseases, but more tests are required to confirm this.

2.2.4. Kahalalide F

Kahalalide F **16** (Figure 3) is a cyclic depsipeptide that belongs to the kahalalide protein family. It was first described by Hamann and Scheuer [97], isolated from *Bryopsis* sp. green alga, as well as from the *Elysia rufescens* mollusk, which feeds on *Bryopsis* and bio-accumulates **16** (which is why most studies used the mollusk as a source of this compound). In vitro studies [108] revealed the great cytotoxic potential of **16** against several tumor cell lines, particularly prostate and breast cancer lines, with IC_{50} values ranging from 0.07 to 0.28 µM [109]. In vivo studies carried out by Faircloth and Cuevas [98] showed the tumor response to injected **16** (Figure 3, Table 2) in human breast, prostate, colon, and lung tumor cells xenografted into athymic mice. Treatment with a 0.245 mg/kg (b.w.) dose led to ~50% smaller chemotherapy-resistant DU-145 prostate tumor, while the PC-3 human prostate tumor was reduced by nearly 35% with a 0.123 mg/kg (b.w.) dose. These highly promising results led kahalalide F **16** to the clinical trial phase, which is discussed later.

2.3. Halogenated Secondary Metabolites

Halogenated compounds are also an interesting set of bioactive macroalgae secondary metabolites [17,110–113]. Among these, halogenated terpenes and bromophenols are those whose in vivo studies revealed the greatest potential for new drug development, as discussed below.

Pentahalogenated monoterpene 6*R*-bromo-3*S*-(bromomethyl)-7-methyl-2,3,7-trichloro-1-octene, known by trivial name halomon **17** (Figure 4, Table 3), showed the most promise in in vitro cytotoxic studies (sub-micromolar IC_{50} values) [17], going so far as to be selected by the National Cancer Institute within the NCI60 human tumor cell line anticancer drug screen program, for preclinical studies for drug development. Although this testing never went beyond a preliminary phase, the first results were very promising, showing 40% of "apparent cures" of a very aggressive U251 brain tumor in mouse ip/ip xenograft models [114].

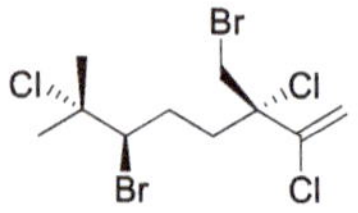

Halomon **17**

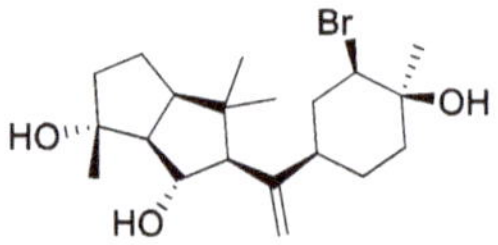

Neorogioltriol **18**

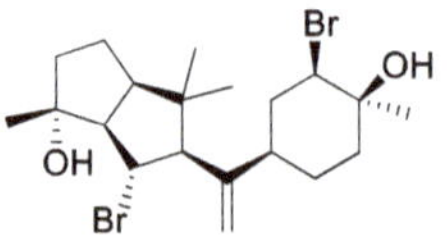

Neorogioldiol **19**

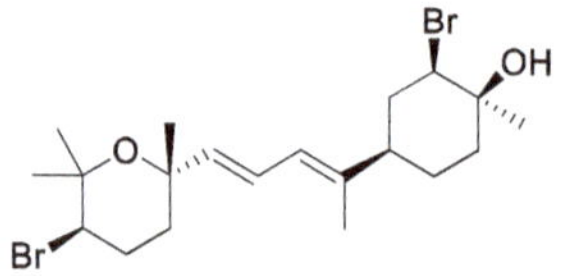

O^{11},15-Cyclo-14-bromo-14,15-dihydrorogiol-3,11-diol **20**

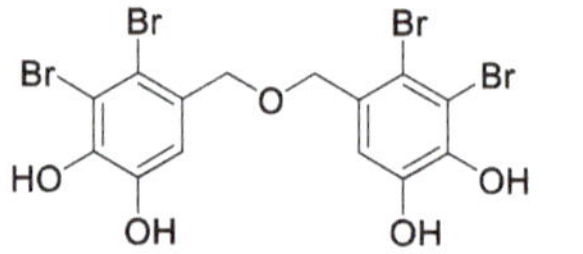

bis (2,3-dibromo-4,5-dihydroxybenzyl) ether (BDDE) **21**

Figure 4. Chemical structure of some halogenated compounds.

Table 3. Summary of in vivo activity of halogenated terpenoids and bromophenols seaweed compounds.

Compound	Source	Model	Activity	Dose
Halomon **17**	*Portieria hornemanii* (Lyngbye) P.C. Silva [114]	U251 brain tumor ip/ip xenograft mouse model	40% "apparent cures" of mouse brain cancer [114].	5 × 50 mg/kg (b.w.)
Neorogioltriol **18**	*Laurencia glandulifera* (Kützing) Kützing [115]	Swiss mice and rats	Reduce writhing response by 88.9% and reduced pain response behavior by 48% [115].	1 mg/kg (b.w.)
		Rats	Reduced paw swelling by 58% after 3 h. 300 mg/kg (b.w.) of acetylsalicylic acid was required to obtain the same effect [116].	1 mg/kg (b.w.)
Neorogioldiol **19**	*Laurencia glandulifera* (Kützing) Kützing, *Laurencia microcladia* Kützing [117,118]	C57BL/6 mice	Reduced inflammatory colon damage and cytokine expression (reduced IL-1β by 6-fold and IL-6 by 40-fold) [117].	0.25 mg/kg (b.w.)
O^{11},15-cyclo-14-bromo-14,15-dihydrorogiol-3,11-diol **20**	*Laurencia glandulifera* (Kützing) Kützing [117]	C57BL/6 mice	Reduced inflammatory colon damage and cytokine expression (reduced IL-1β by 7-fold and IL-6 by 40-fold) [117].	0.25 mg/kg (b.w.)
BDDE **21**	*Odonthalia corymbifera* (S.G. Gmelin) Greville [119], *Leathesia nana* Setchell and N.L. Gardner [a] [120], *Rhodomela confervoides* (Hudson) P.C. Silva [121].	Zebrafish embryos	Reduced SIV growth by 17.7%, 40.4%, and 49.5% [121].	6.25, 12.5, and 25 mM
		Db/db mice	Reduction of blood glucose levels (12.3%) (metformin caused a 10.1% decrease). Decreased glycated hemoglobin, triglycerides and body weight [122].	40 mg/kg (b.w.)

[a] The current accepted name is *Leathesia marina* (Lyngbye) Decaisne.

The latest published results regarding this preclinical trial process were related to halomon **17** tested in CD_2F_1 mice regarding bioavailability, pharmacokinetics, and tissue distribution [123]. The results showed that halomon bioavailability is higher after intraperitoneal injection and subcutaneous injection

(45% and 47%, respectively), while its urinary excretion is minimal. Halomon **17** is distributed in all tissues but with a higher concentration in adipose tissue. The concentration of halomon measured in the brain is comparable to that detected in plasma and most other tissues. Even though preclinical testing never progressed beyond preliminary stages, this never deterred the scientific community's interest in **17** over time, and a more recent study about the action mechanism of **17** proposed that it acts as a DNA methyl transferase-1 inhibitor [124]. However, more deep mechanism studies should be performed.

In addition to these studies, a real obstacle to overcome with halomon **17** is always to obtain enough quantity of the compound. Fuller et al. [114] described this struggle by stating that "slight geographic and/or temporal change" would dramatically affect the terpene content of *Portieria hornemanii*, and that alternative approaches should be considered. Naturally, this problem led to chemists trying to synthesize halomon, with the first success occurring in 1998 by Schlama et al. [125], who reported a 13% overall yield. A result was obtained by Sotokawa et al. [126], reducing the previous 13-step process into three steps, reporting a 25% overall yield but with poor selectivity. Only in 2015 was the first efficient and high-selectivity method described by Bucher et al. [127], a process which was since further optimized by Landry and Burns [128]. Having finally overcome this obstacle after over 25 years, halomon **17** in vivo studies should be restarted as to finally confirm its potential.

Another highly interesting compound is neorogioltriol **18** (Figure 4, Table 3), a tricyclic brominated diterpenoid first isolated from *Laurencia glandulifera* by Chatter et al. [115]. This research group showed that neorogioltriol had analgesic properties. In the writhing test, neorogiotriol produced a dose-dependent response, and a dose of 1 mg/kg (b.w.) was enough to reduce the mouse acetic acid-induced writhing response by 88.9% (Table 3). With the rat model, the formalin test was used to determine if the compound affected neurogenic and/or inflammatory pain. Results showed that neorogiotriol **18** reduced licking time by 48%, but only in the second phase of the formalin test, indicating that the compound has a peripheral analgesic effect, acting on inflammatory pain in a way typical of cyclooxygenase inhibitors. Chatter et al. [115] supplemented their previous work with neorogioltriol **18** by testing its in vivo anti-inflammatory effect on induced rat paw swelling. Results showed that an injected dose of 1 mg/kg (b.w.) of the compound reduced paw swelling by 28% after the first hour and 58% after three hours. To achieve the same anti-inflammatory result with a reference compound, acetylsalicylic acid would require a dose of 300 mg/kg (b.w.) [115].

A more recent paper published by Daskalaki et al. [117] studied two diterpenes, neorogioldiol **19** and O^{11},15-cyclo-14-bromo-14,15-dihydrorogiol-3,11-diol **20** (Figure 4 Table 3). These compounds were used to treat C57BL/6 mice with DSS-induced inflammatory bowel disease (colitis). A 0.25 mg/mouse dose of each compound was intraperitoneally injected every 48 h, in two different groups. The results showed that treated mice demonstrated reduced inflammatory colonic tissue damage, as well as a very significant decreased of pro-inflammatory cytokine messenger RNA (mRNA) (more than 40-fold decrease in the case of interleukin-6). Neorogioldiol **19** and O^{11},15-cyclo-14-bromo-14,15-dihydrorogiol-3,11-diol **20** showed similar activity levels and revealed their great potential for bowel disease inflammatory treatment. More studies should be pursued, particularly to assess the neorogiotriol **18** activity in the previously mentioned colitis model once it is structurally related to compounds **19** and **20**.

Bromophenols are another class of very interesting macroalgae metabolites. Although most studies of this family of compounds only showed in vitro effects so far, a few of them reached the level of being evaluated in an in vivo model. One of the most biologically relevant of such compounds is BDDE **21** (Figure 4, Table 3).

First isolated by Kurihara et al. in 1999 from Rhodophyta *Odonthalia corymbifera*, these researchers showed BDDE **21** as an α-glucosidase inhibitor [119]. After this, some very promising in vitro studies confirmed **21**'s α-glucosidase interaction [129] and showed **21**'s anticancer [120,130] and antifungal activities [131]. A recently published study [122] showed that **21** had in vivo antidiabetic activity. The research group showed that a dose of 40 mg/kg (b.w.), orally administered, was more effective at lowering blood glucose levels in db/db mice than metformin (a clinical antidiabetic drug). The study also showed that **21** significantly reduced glycated hemoglobin, triglyceride levels, and body weight without influencing the mice's food or water intake. This shows that **21** might constitute a powerful antidiabetic drug in the future, but more testing is required to ascertain this possibility. Another interesting in vivo study, using a different animal model, was also published in 2015 by Qi et al. [121], revealing a different effect. In this work, BDDE **21** exhibited potent angiogenesis inhibition activity in zebrafish embryo models [121]. In this work, researchers monitored the embryonic development of the zebrafish sub-intestinal vessel (SIV) when incubated in the presence of **21**. Results showed a statistically significant and dose-dependent response, with 6.25, 12.5, and 25 mM reducing SIV growth by 17.7%, 40.4%, and 49.5%, respectively. This unequivocally proves **21**'s effect as an anti-angiogenesis agent and points to its great potential for cancer therapeutic applications; however, more in vivo antitumor studies are necessary. In summary, there is a considerable diversity of algae halogenated secondary metabolites with very interesting and promising bioactivities, which might lead to future drug developments; however, more testing is required.

2.4. Fucoxanthin

Concerning algal lipids, fucoxanthin **22** (Figure 5), a xanthophyll-like carotenoid, is one of the most studied metabolites because of its beneficial health effects [18,103,132]. Indeed, there are many published reviews and research articles demonstrating and extolling, among others, the nutraceutical, antioxidant, anticancer, anti-obesity, antidiabetic, antimicrobial, and cardiovascular protective effects of fucoxanthin **22** [103,132–139].

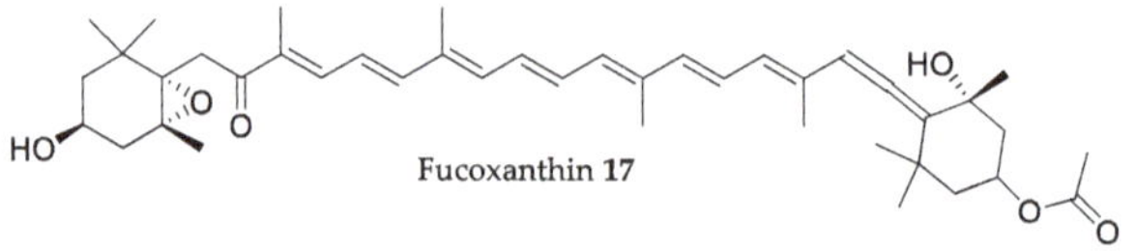

Figure 5. Chemical structure of fucoxanthin.

It is intended here to review the most relevant in vivo studies with pure fucoxanthin, highlighting the impact that each one had on the process of development of fucoxanthin as a drug with many potential therapeutic uses.

Fucoxanthin **22** (Figure 5) seems to have a neuroprotective effect, as evidenced by Hu et al. [140] using the middle cerebral artery occlusion rat model (MCAO) [141]. To assess a neuroprotective effect, the rats were intragastrical administered different doses (30, 60, and 90 mg/kg b.w.) of pure fucoxanthin 1 h before cerebral ischemia was induced. Results showed significant and dose-dependent reductions of neurological deficit scores and percentages of infarcted area in the brain, as well as an attenuation of brain edema. One criticism that could be made of the researchers' work pertains to how they presented the objective results of their essays; the results were presented only in graph form with no supporting table listing the values. This makes it hard to properly and objectively assess the degree to which the neurological parameters tested showed an improvement or not. Nonetheless, the published work did serve to firmly support fucoxanthin as a potential neuroprotective supplement of interest.

Another highly interesting potential pharmaceutical application for fucoxanthin was illustrated in the recently published work by Wang et al. [142], which reports fucoxanthin antitumor activity in a novel lymphangiogenesis inhibition perspective. In this work, the MDA-MB-231 breast cancer xenograft model was used on Balb/c nude mice treated with 6.58 and 32.9 µg doses of **22**. Fucoxanthin was injected daily on the tumor periphery, and tumors were excised after 26 days. Results revealed significant decreases in micro-lymphatic vascular density, from an average of 14.0 ± 2.94 lymphatic vessels to 6.0 ± 0.81 (with 6.58 µg fucoxanthin treatment) and 3.66 ± 1.25 (with 32.9 µg treatment) per tumor. Tumor weight and volume also decreased by more than half in a dose-dependent manner, although, once again, it is difficult to assess this reduction precisely due to the lack of a values table accompanying the results graph. However, these results adequately highlight **22**'s potential in cancer treatment. In another 2019 study by Terasaki et al. [143], this anti-tumor activity was again tested, this time with a colorectal cancer mouse model. In this work, AOM/DSS mice were injected with a 30 mg/kg (b.w.) daily dose of fucoxanthin oil for seven weeks, with subsequent bowel excision and analysis post sacrifice. Results showed that **22** significantly reduced the number of colonic polyps by close to half compared to non-treated mice, with polyp size also significantly reduced to about one-third of the control mice. Objective histological examination showed a reduction in the prevalence of tumors, ulcers, and crypt dysplasia. The authors suggested that this may be linked to **22** promoting anoikis-like cell death, and they supported this hypothesis by showing increased expression (2–5-fold) of key molecular hallmarks for anoikis in treated mice colon cells. These results reinforce **22** as a good candidate for possible anti-cancer drugs. In addition to this bioactivity, a 2019 paper by Jiang et al. [144] highlighted **22**'s potential as an antidepressant. In this work, a lipopolysaccharide-induced depressive-like behavior mouse model was used, to evaluate if **22** treatments would reduce depressive or anxiety associated behaviors. Results showed that treated mice had significantly higher body weight and food intake than control mice, as well as significantly reduced depressive-like behavior and anxiety-like behavior. These behaviors were assessed by presenting the mice with stressful conditions/obstacles and then evaluating their activity. It is important to note that the lower doses of **22** used in this work showed a very marginal depressive behavioral reduction, but the highest dose tested (200 mg/kg b.w.) managed to reduce depressive and anxiety-like behaviors to almost baseline values of non-depressed mice. In other words, a 200 mg/kg (b.w.) dose of **22** significantly reduced depressive behavioral traits to the point where the induced depression was practically "cured". While this dosage is considerably higher than that used in previously mentioned studies, we chose to highlight this neuroprotective bioactivity here due to its novelty and relative relevance.

To finalize, another 2019 study by Su et al. [145] revealed that **22** has great potential as an anti-inflammatory in a mouse sepsis model. In this work, lipopolysaccharides were once again used (albeit at a much higher dose than in the previous study) to induce sepsis, eventually leading to death in the mouse models. The results showed that, while a 10 mg/kg (b.w.) dose of LPS caused a 20% survival rate in the mice, the same dose in mice treated with 1 mg/kg (b.w.) of **22** had a 40% survival rate. A single very small dose of **22** injected 30 min prior to challenge effectively doubled the survival rate of the sepsis mouse model. In addition, treated mice also showed significantly reduced levels of pro-inflammatory cytokines TNF-α (~30% reduction) and IL-6 (~90% reduction) when compared to non-treated mice, as well as significantly inhibiting the NF-κB inflammatory pathway (as shown by the ~50% reduction in p-IκBα, and p-NF-κB). This shows that **22** exhibits a potent anti-inflammatory effect and can effectively have a strong protective effect in an acute inflammatory disease model. In summary, **22** exhibits a multitude of very interesting and diverse potent bioactivities, with studies very recently published. The scientific community appears to have a great interest in this compound, and we hope to see more high-quality in vivo publications in the near future.

2.5. Fucosterol

Fucosterol **23** (Figure 6) is a phytosterol, mostly isolated from brown algae, and it is relatively abundant in this particular algal class. It was widely studied regarding its in vitro health effects [146]; however, in vivo evaluations of fucosterol's health effects are very scarce. In this regard, the present work reviews the existing in vivo studies, and the main observations and conclusions are discussed in the paragraphs below.

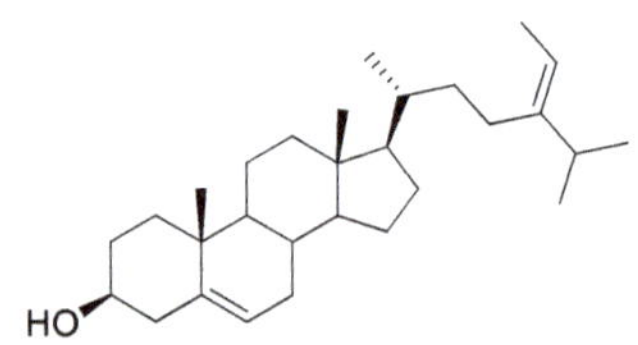

Fucosterol 23

Figure 6. Chemical structure of fucosterol.

One of the first evaluations of the in vivo effects of fucosterol 23 was regarding its anti-diabetic effects, and it was found that, when administered orally at 30 mg/kg in streptozotocin-induced diabetic rats, fucosterol caused a significant decrease of 14.8% in serum glucose concentrations, and exhibited an inhibition of sorbitol accumulations in the lenses of 22.4% when compared to the untreated group [147].

This phytosterol presents antitumor activity in vivo, with a dosage of 40 mg/kg (b.w.), reducing about 75% of tumor weight and 50% of tumor volume after six weeks in lung cancer xenografted C57 BL/6 mice model [148]. In addition, fucosterol 23 (40 mg/kg b.w.) reduced Ki-67 expression, an indicator of cell proliferation, by 60%, and increased cleaved caspase-3 levels by more than 100%, which indicates that 23 acts in the tumor cells by simultaneously decreasing their proliferation and enhancing their apoptosis [148].

Fucosterol 23 also exhibits a protective effect on LPS-induced acute lung injury (ALI), by modulating the expression of pro-inflammatory factors [149]. A dosage of 30 mg/kg (b.w.) of 23 attenuated lung histopathologic changes and the wet-to-dry ratio of lungs in LPS-induced ALI in mice. Furthermore, fucosterol significantly inhibited TNF-a, IL-1ß, and IL-6 levels in both the broncho-alveolar lavage fluid (BALF) and the LPS-stimulated alveolar macrophages, reducing their expression by about 50%, when compared to the untreated group [149]. The fact that 23 is able to inhibit the production of pro-inflammatory molecules suggests that it could be used for the treatment of other inflammatory diseases. This suggestion was confirmed by the findings of Mo et al. [150], where it was observed that fucosterol 23 attenuated serum liver enzyme levels, hepatic necrosis, and apoptosis induced by TNF-α, IL-6, and IL-1β. In fact, a dosage of 50 mg/kg (b.w.) of fucosterol reduced the serum levels of these three pro-inflammatory molecules by 37.5%, 31.3%, and 33.3%, respectively, after 8 h of exposure to concanavalin-A, the inducer of acute liver injury. The authors also found that 23 (50 mg/kg b.w.) also inhibited apoptosis and autophagy by upregulating Bcl-2 (12-fold increase), which decreased levels of functional Bax (50%) and Beclin-1 (46%). Furthermore, reduced P38 MAPK and NF-κB signaling were accompanied by PPARγ activation, showing that fucosterol acts by inhibiting P38 MAPK/PPARγ/NF-κB signaling [150].

Fucosterol 23 is able to reduce the effects of postmenopausal osteoporosis. A study performed with ovariectomized rats found that the bone mineral density of femoral bones was significantly higher in 23 (50 mg/kg b.w.) treated groups than in the untreated group [151]. Additionally, body weight after six weeks of treatment was 6% lower in the fucosterol 23 treated groups, when compared to the untreated group. In terms of serum biomarkers of bone formation and resorption, 23 (100 mg/kg b.w.) tripled the level of serum osteocalcin relative to the untreated group and reduced the serum level of CTx by 60%, which suggests that fucosterol 23 has the potential to activate osteoblasts, stimulate bone formation, suppress differentiation of osteoclasts, and reduce bone resorption [151].

In terms of neurological effects of fucosterol 23, this compound was found to attenuate sAβ_{1-42}-induced cognitive impairment in aging rats [152]. In fact, aged rats treated with only sAβ_{1-42} performed poorly in acquisition training and memory tests, whereas co-infusion of 10 μmol/h of 23 for the four weeks of assay restored the rats' performance to the level of the healthy control. Fucosterol 23 action was via downregulation of GRP78 expression and upregulation of mature brain-derived neurotrophic factor (BDNF) expression in the dentate gyrus, which means it is able to suppress aging-induced endoplasmic reticulum (ER) stress [152].

Fucosterol-induced upregulation of BDNF levels is also linked to other neurological actions, like antidepressant activity. In fact, **23** (20 mg/kg b.w.) administration to Balb/e mice reduced immobility time in the forced swim test, which is a measure of depression, by 82.2 s, a value very similar to that obtained with the positive control, fluoxetine, at the same concentration (85.1 s) [153]. The same effect was observed in the tail suspension test, where both fucosterol **23** and fluoxetine (20 mg/kg b.w.) significantly shortened immobility time in the forced tail suspension test by approximately 80 s, when compared with the untreated group. Fucosterol **23** (20 mg/kg b.w.) significantly increased serotonin, norepinephrine, and the metabolite 5-hydroxyindole acetic acid in the mouse brain, with levels very close to that observed in the brain of mice not subjected to the stress of the tail suspension and forced swimming tests. This suggests that the effects of fucosterol **23** may be mediated through these neurotransmitters [153]. Also, a significant increase in hippocampal brain-derived neurotrophic factor (BDNF) levels was found in the fucosterol 20 mg/kg (b.w.) group, which suggests that the antidepressant effect may be mediated by increasing central BDNF levels [153].

The findings presented show that **23** could be an efficient therapeutic agent for a wide array of health conditions. Regardless, the number of in vivo tests existing with this algal metabolite is still very scarce; thus, we suggest that future works should invest in assessing the full in vivo potential of fucosterol **23**.

3. Clinical Trials

The above-mentioned information regarding the performance of seaweed compounds and derivatives in the in vivo assays shows that these types of compounds have great pharmaceutical potential with some of them already being in clinical trial phases.

Fucoxanthin **22** (Figure 4) is one of them, with two studies scheduled to begin at the end of 2019, one a phase II study that aims at fucoxanthin's effects on metabolic syndrome (ClinicalTrials.gov identifier: NCT03613740) and the other that will test an oral dietary supplement rich with fucoxanthin for improving liver health (ClinicalTrials.gov identifier: NCT03625284).

Additionally, some trials already reached the end and presented their results. Hitoe and Shimoda [154] reported that a month of treatment with 3 mg of **22** per day had weight loss effects in mildly obese Japanese adults (BMI > 25 kg/m^2) since it reduced abdominal fat, body weight, and overall BMI compared to the placebo group. These results are in accordance with those described by Abidov et al. [155] who performed a 16-week clinical trial in 151 women using a dietary supplement named Xanthigen composed of pomegranate seed oil and brown seaweed extract containing 2.4 mg of **22**, which increased resting energy expenditure, and induced body fat reduction and weight loss in obese women (BMI > 30 kg/m^2).

Kahalalide F **16** (Figure 3), as already mentioned in Section 2.2.4, is a promising peptide that is being tested in clinical trials, particularly for its antitumor properties. Martín-Algarra and colleagues [156] investigated the response of patients with advanced malignant melanoma to **16**, through weekly intravenous administration of 650 µg/m^2 until patient refusal, unacceptable toxicity, or disease progression was observed. The results indicated that, contrary to the majority of other chemotherapeutic agents, **16** did not induce severe cardiac, renal, or bone marrow toxicity, alopecia, diarrhea, or mucositis, and it was able to stabilize the disease for more than three months in five of 21 patients (23.8%) who completed the study.

A more recent study [157] evaluated the **16** weekly intravenous administration maximum tolerated dose and infusion times to recommend appropriate doses and treatment times for further phase II clinical studies in patients with advanced solid tumors. Based on the results, the authors recommended a dose of 1000 µg/m^2 of **16** with three hours of treatment per week; however, prolonged infusion times (i.e., 24-h treatment) are also feasible.

Unfortunately, only these two compounds from all those mentioned in Section 2 reached clinical trials, which could be due to diverse complications like obtaining the necessary approvals required to start the study, obtaining volunteers, or isolating the compound of interest in sufficient quantities to allow the studies to unfold.

On the other hand, since seaweeds represent a good source of compounds with pharmaceutical potential and since seaweeds are attaining more interest in Western countries' diets, the majority of clinical trials are currently carried out to ascertain to what extent the consumption of algae improves human health. Thus, the clinical trials discussed below focused on testing the effects of consuming one type of seaweed (or a mixture of them) or its various rich fractions/extracts.

With a quick search on ClinicalTrials.gov, it is possible to find 25 clinical trials that were seaweed-relevant. From those 25 clinical trials, two are active and ongoing, and six are scheduled to start shortly, which shows the current interest and relevance of this topic. Unfortunately, from the 17 already completed clinical trials, only eight had their results published. Additionally, it was possible to find other clinical trials that were not listed on this database, and which contributed also to an overview of this topic with growing interest.

Several clinical studies aimed at evaluating the effect of polysaccharide fractions, extracts, and even whole seaweed on the treatment and prevention of diabetes and obesity. These important aspects that are beyond the scope of this review topic, but we refer our readers to interesting publications about this subject [158–163].

A recent study conducted by Murray et al. [164] found that a single dose up to 2000 mg of a polyphenol-rich *Fucus vesiculosus* Linnaeus extract had no additional lowering effect compared to placebo on postprandial blood glucose or plasma insulin in healthy adults. The authors suggested that future studies with polyphenol-rich marine algal extracts should aim to investigate the glycemic modulating effects in at-risk populations, such as pre-diabetics, since the results may be different.

Another clinical trial from the same year [165] examined, in 60 healthy adults, the effect of brown seaweed extract InSea2® consumption on their postprandial cognitive function. A dose of brown seaweed extract (500 mg), containing 20% phlorotannins, was consumed 30 min before lunch. Attention, episodic memory, and subjective state were the parameters analyzed five times over a 3-h period following lunch with 40-min intervals between measures. The results demonstrated an improvement in cognitive performance following the ingestion of the seaweed extract when compared to the placebo group since accuracy was increased in the choice reaction time and on the digit vigilance tasks. The authors [165] pointed out that, since the brown seaweed extract was a supplement equivalent of 10 g of dried seaweed, the cognitive benefits presented in this work could be obtained from dietary intake of seaweed consumption.

Regarding seaweed consumption, another study [166] investigated the acceptability of *Ascophyllum nodosum* (Linnaeus) Le Jolis-enriched bread as part of a meal by overweight healthy males, to see if it could modulate cholesterolemic and glycemic responses and reduce energy intake. Four hours after the enriched bread consumption at breakfast (using a test meal), the energy intake suffered a significant reduction (16.4%). According to the study results, it is acceptable to incorporate this seaweed into a basic food such as bread, at least at concentrations of up to 4% wholemeal loaf. Considering the interesting results of this acute feeding trial, the authors accentuated that a long-term study regarding the addition of seaweed-enriched bread to diets of participants would help to clarify its potential for the reduction of energy intake, potentially positively affecting their body mass index (BMI).

Higher oxidant status increases the oxidative damage of macromolecules, which, associated with obesity, increases the probability of chronic disease development [167], with obese individuals as a risk group. Baldrick et al. [168] investigated the bioavailability and effect of an *Ascophyllum nodosum* (Linnaeus) Le Jolis polyphenol-rich extract on DNA damage, oxidative stress, and inflammation level. Eighty participants, of which 36 were obese, consumed daily, for eight weeks, a capsule containing 100 mg of *Ascophyllum nodosum* (Linnaeus) Le Jolis polyphenol-rich extract. After the trial period, only the obese individuals presented results significantly distinct from placebo, with a 23% decrease in lymphocyte DNA damage. Thus, this work suggests that long-term consumption of *Ascophyllum nodosum* (Linnaeus) Le Jolis polyphenols rich extract could be beneficial since it could potentially decrease the risk of chronic disease development in obese individuals.

In other lines of research, Allaert et al. [169] found that, when compared with a placebo, a daily intake of a water-soluble extract of *Ulva lactuca* Linnaeus (6.45 mg per kg body weight) for three months significantly improved the depression state of subjects presenting anhedonia (a loss of sensitivity when it comes to feeling pleasure). In the placebo group, 72.5% of participants said they felt an improvement in mood versus 90.1% of the participants in the *Ulva lactuca* Linnaeus extract group (a statistically significant difference). Similarly, 70.8% of doctors judged the subjects in the placebo group to have improved versus 90.9% of the participants in the *Ulva lactuca* Linnaeus extract group. As the authors pointed out, identifying the compound in the seaweed extract responsible for the witnessed effect in this work opens up perspectives for its potential use in depression therapy.

Teas and Irhimeh [170] showed a synergistic effect between the daily consumption of brown seaweed (*Undaria pinnatifida* (Harvey) Suringar) (2.5 g) and spirulina (*Arthrospira platensis* Gomont) (3 g), since it was able to increase immune response and decrease HIV viral fusion/entry and replication in a three-month period. Furthermore, one subject continued in the trial for 13 months and reported decreased HIV viral load (from 3.3 to 2.8 $\log_{10}$) and clinically significant improvement in CD4 (>100 cells/mL). Despite the promising results, it should be noted that the sample size in this work was too small ($n = 11$) to make any generalizations about the efficacy, and further research is imperative.

Since higher levels of serum estradiol (E2) are associated with an increased risk of breast cancer development [171], Teas et al. [172] reported that a daily dose of 5 g of *Alaria esculenta* (Linnaeus) Greville for seven weeks had the ability to modulate serum hormone levels and urinary excretion of estrogen metabolites and phytoestrogens, diminishing breast cancer risk in women. Again, the conclusion of this study was limited by the small number of participants ($n = 15$), which limited the statistical power of the results.

The results of the various clinical trials mentioned above point out that the consumption of algae, particularly brown algae, can be beneficial to human health. However, in our opinion, it is also necessary to perform the identification of the chemical compounds responsible for the observed effects. There are several studies where the authors did not relate the observed effect to any constituent of the seaweed/extract evaluated, and having studies with fractions rich in a given class of compounds does not substitute for the identification of the bioactive metabolites and their health effects. Nevertheless, these studies are also important because they established that some seaweeds can be used for human consumption.

4. Critical Opinion

In the last few years, secondary metabolites isolated from macroalgae gained growing interest, as shown by the numerous articles reporting in vivo studies, with some compounds reaching clinical trial phases. Although many studies presented their results with quality, there were some points that deserve to be highlighted regarding the majority of the consulted papers.

Future in vivo studies, especially those with murine models, should increase the number of individuals for each test group to increase the statistical power of the findings. Also, a reference compound should always be used, to assess the real efficacy of the tested compounds. The frequent lack of clarity in result presentation in several publications was also a downside in interesting and promising studies.

Clinical trial studies with isolated compounds, unfortunately, are scarce. This could be due to diverse complications like obtaining the necessary approvals required to start the study, obtaining volunteers, or obtaining the compound in enough quantities. Additionally, most of the clinical trials aimed at ascertaining to what extent the consumption of algae, as a whole or as extracts or fractions, affects human health, particularly the effects regarding obesity and diabetes. Nonetheless, it is unfortunate that many of the mentioned studies were carried out with such small population samples, which deprives them of statistical power. Another serious flaw in the numerous studies addressing algae extracts is the fact that their chemical composition was not mentioned or is unknown, and extrapolation of the effects of extracts or algae on their secondary metabolites is in no way guaranteed and/or valid. The knowledge of the bioactive metabolites and their activity is important but does not validate the algae's consumption.

Despite the indicated limitations, these extract clinical trials are relevant for qualitative and safety evaluations. In our opinion, these studies will also contribute to the scientific community's interest, resulting in a deeper analysis that will uncover the most active metabolites.

Regardless of that, in most cases, these studies represent the first steps on the way to enhancing algae's potential as a pharmaceutical source of new compounds with promising properties.

5. Conclusions

Phlorotannins show great pharmaceutical potential in vivo. Most of the studies indicated that the main sources of bioactive phlorotannins are algae from the *Eisenia*, *Ecklonia*, and *Ishige* genera. However, this observation can be the result of the studies' geographical distribution. The studies reviewed herein showed that phlorotannins' mechanisms of action are mainly related to the modulation of oxidative stress and the inflammatory cascade. Phloroglucinol **1**, eckol **4**, and dieckol **5** are compounds with a wide range of applications. The dieckol **5** anti-dyslipidemia activity must be highlighted because it is more effective than lovastatin, the clinically used drug. The hepatoprotective activity of eckol **4** should also be emphasized, since a very low dose (0.5 mg/kg b.w.) is needed.

Concerning other non-phlorotannin groups of compounds, it is clear that there is a great variety of very interesting compounds, with many of them in dire need of further testing. Out of these, the bioactive effects of the peptides griffithsin **12**, tridecapeptide IRLIIVLMPILMA **13**, and kahalalide F **16** should be highlighted, as they are arguably the most promising of all non-phlorotannins. Kahalalide F already moved beyond the in vivo stage to clinical trials, whereas tridecapeptide **13**, with a level of activity similar to the clinical drug captopril, and griffithsin **12**, which showed such stunning results over a variety of animal models, will probably move into the clinical trial stage soon. In contrast, there are promising compounds such as halomon **17** and neorogioltriol **18**, which exhibited potent and very relevant bioactivities and were not subjected to clinical trials. Hopefully, the discussion presented in this paper about their activities will interest the scientific community, and further studies will be conducted.

Regarding the fact that clinical trials with isolated compounds are scarce, only those carried out with kahalalide F **16** and fucoxanthin **22** were found, whereas we also analyzed a few clinical trials involving seaweed extracts. It can be concluded that the consumption of brown algae can be beneficial to human health, with *Ascophyllum nodosum* (Linnaeus) Le Jolis as the leading seaweed in clinical trials.

Author Contributions: A.M.L.S. and D.C.G.A.P. conceptualized and revised the paper; G.P.R., P.M.C.S., and W.R.T. conducted the research and wrote the first draft together with A.K.P. All authors have read and agreed to the published version of the manuscript.

Funding: This research was funded by project MACBIOBLUE (MAC/1.1b/086), program Interreg MAC 2014–2020 co-financed by DRCT (Azores Regional Government), supporting G.P. Rosa's grant, as well as by FCT—Fundação para a Ciência e a Tecnologia, the European Union, QREN, FEDER, and COMPETE, through funding the cE3c center (FCT UID/BIA/00329/2013, 2015–2018 and UID/BIA/00329/2019) and the QOPNA research unit (FCT UID/QUI/00062/2019).

Acknowledgments: Thanks are due to the University of Azores and the University of Aveiro.

Conflicts of Interest: The authors declare no conflicts of interest.

Abbreviations

AA	Arachidonic acid
AAPH	2,2′-azobis (2-amidinopropane)
ACE	Angiotensin-converting-enzyme
AI	Atherogenic index
ALI	Acute lung injury
AMPK	Adenosine monophosphate-activated protein kinase
AOM	Azoxymethane
AP-1	Activator protein-1
BALB/c	Strain of laboratory mouse
BALF	Broncho-alveolar lavage fluid
Bax	Bcl-2-associated X
Bcl-2	B-cell lymphoma 2
BDDE	Bis(2,3-dibromo-4,5-dihydroxybenzyl) ether
BDNF	Brain-derived neurotrophic factor
BMI	Body mass index
b.w.	Body weight
C57BL/6	Strain of laboratory mouse
C57BL/6J	Strain of laboratory mouse
C57BL/KsJ-db/db	Strain of laboratory diabetic mouse
CAT	Catalase
CD_2F_1	Strain of laboratory mouse
CD4	Cluster of differentiation 4 cells
CG	Carragenan
CMC-	Carboxy-methylcellulose
COX-2	Cyclooxygenase-2
CTx	C-terminal telopeptide of type-1 collagen
DNA	Deoxyribonucleic acid
DSS	Dextran sodium sulfate
DU-145	Human prostate cancer cell line
E2	Estradiol
EC_{50}	Half maximal effective concentration
EGCG	Epigallocatechin gallate
ER	Endoplasmic reticulum
ERCC1	Excision repair cross-complementation
FD	Fine dust
GABAA-BZD	Gamma-aminobutyric acid A-benzodiazepine
GRP78	Glucose-regulated protein 78
GSH-px	Glutathione peroxidase
HDL	High-density lipoprotein
HIV	Human immunodeficiency virus
HPV16	Human papillomavirus type 16
HSV-2	Herpes simplex virus type 2
IC_{50}	Half maximal inhibitory concentration
ICR	Strain of laboratory mouse
IgE	Immunoglobulin E
IL-1	Interleukin-1
IL-6	Interleukin-6
IL-10	Interleukin-10
iNOS	Inducible nitric oxide synthase
IU	International unit
JEV	Japanese encephalitis virus
JNK	c-Jun NH2-terminal kinase
Ki-67	Proliferation marker protein

LDL	Low-density lipoprotein
LPS	Lipopolysaccharides
MAPK	Mitogen-activated protein kinase
MCAO	Middle cerebral artery occlusion rat model
MDA-MB-231	Human breast adenocarcinoma
MKK4/SEK1	Mitogen-activated protein kinase kinase-4
MNZ	Metronidazole
mRNA	Messenger ribonucleic acid
NCI	National Cancer Institute
NER	Nucleotide excision repair
NF-κB	Nuclear factor kappa B
NK	Natural killer cells
NO	Nitric oxide
NREMS	Non-rapid eye movements
OXA	Oxazolone
PC-3	Human prostate cancer cell line
PM2.5	Particulate matter $\leq$2.5 µm
PPARγ	Peroxisome proliferator-activated receptor gamma
ROS	Reactive oxygen species
S180	Murine sarcoma cancer cell line
sAβ1-42	Soluble amyloid beta peptide (1-42)
SAR	Structure–activity relationship
SARS-CoV	Severe acute respiratory syndrome-related coronavirus
SBP	Systolic blood pressure
SD	Sprague-Dawley rats
SHR	Spontaneously hypertensive rats
SIV	Sub-intestinal vessel
SOD	Superoxide dismutase
TC	Total cholesterol
TG	Triglycerides
TNF	Tumor necrosis factor
TNF-α	Tumor necrosis factor α
TPA	12-O-tetradecanoylphorbol-13-acetate
U251	Human glioblastoma
uPA-SCID	Urokinase-type plasminogen activator severe combined immunodeficient mice
UV	Ultraviolet
VEGFR-2	Vascular endothelial growth factor receptor 2
XPC	Xeroderma pigmentosum complementation group C

References

1. Kiuru, P.; D'Auria, M.V.; Muller, C.D.; Tammela, P.; Vuorela, H.; Yli-Kauhaluoma, J. Exploring marine resources for bioactive compounds. *Planta Med.* **2014**, *80*, 1234–1246. [CrossRef] [PubMed]
2. Loureiro, C.; Medema, M.H.; van der Oost, J.; Sipkema, D. Exploration and exploitation of the environment for novel specialized metabolites. *Curr. Opin. Biotechnol.* **2018**, *50*, 206–213. [CrossRef] [PubMed]
3. Ariede, M.B.; Candido, T.M.; Jacome, A.L.M.; Velasco, M.V.R.; Carvalho, J.C.M.; Baby, A.R. Cosmetic attributes of algae—A review. *Algal Res.* **2017**, *25*, 483–487. [CrossRef]
4. Wang, H.-M.D.; Li, X.-C.; Lee, D.-J.; Chang, J.-S. Potential biomedical applications of marine algae. *Bioresour. Technol.* **2017**, *244*, 1407–1415. [CrossRef]
5. Zhao, C.; Yang, C.; Liu, B.; Lin, L.; Sarker, S.D.; Nahar, L.; Yu, H.; Cao, H.; Xiao, J. Bioactive compounds from marine macroalgae and their hypoglycemic benefits. *Trends Food Sci. Technol.* **2018**, *72*, 1–12. [CrossRef]
6. Tanna, B.; Mishra, A. Nutraceutical potential of seaweed polysaccharides: Structure, bioactivity, safety, and toxicity. *Compr. Rev. Food Sci. Food Saf.* **2019**, *18*, 817–831. [CrossRef]

7. Hsu, H.-Y.; Hwang, P.-A. Clinical applications of fucoidan in translational medicine for adjuvant cancer therapy. *Clin. Trans. Med.* **2019**, *8*, 15. [CrossRef]
8. Pereira, L. *Therapeutic and Nutritional Uses of Algae*, 1st ed.; CRC Press: Boca Raton, FL, USA, 2018; p. 264. ISBN 9781498755382.
9. Thomas, N.V.; Kim, S.-K. Beneficial effects of marine algal compounds in cosmeceuticals. *Mar. Drugs* **2013**, *11*, 146–164. [CrossRef]
10. Stengel, D.B.; Connan, S.; Popper, Z.A. Algal chemodiversity and bioactivity: Sources of natural variability and implications for commercial application. *Biotechnol. Adv.* **2011**, *29*, 483–501. [CrossRef]
11. Holdt, S.L.; Kraan, S. Bioactive compounds in seaweed: Functional food applications and legislation. *J. Appl. Phycol.* **2011**, *23*, 543–597. [CrossRef]
12. Khalid, S.; Abbas, M.; Saeed, F.; Bader-Ul-Ain, H.; Suleira, H.A.R. Therapeutic potential of seaweed bioactive compounds. In *Seaweed Biomaterials*, 1st ed.; Maiti, S., Ed.; IntechOpen: London, UK, 2018; Volume 1, pp. 7–26. [CrossRef]
13. Martins, R.M.; Nedel, F.; Guimarães, V.B.S.; da Silva, A.F.; Colepicolo, P.; de Pereira, C.M.P.; Lund, R.G. Macroalgae extracts from Antarctica have antimicrobial and anticancer potential. *Front. Microbiol.* **2018**, *9*, 412. [CrossRef]
14. Pereira, L. Seaweeds as source of bioactive substances and skin care therapy—cosmeceuticals, algotheraphy, and thalassotherapy. *Cosmetics* **2018**, *5*, 68. [CrossRef]
15. Michalak, I.; Chojnacka, K. Algae as production systems of bioactive compounds. *Eng. Life Sci.* **2015**, *15*, 160–176. [CrossRef]
16. Hussain, E.; Wang, L.-J.; Jiang, B.; Riaz, S.; Butt, G.Y.; Shi, D.-Y. A review of the components of brown seaweeds as potential candidates in cancer therapy. *RSC Adv.* **2016**, *6*, 12592–12610. [CrossRef]
17. Rocha, D.H.A.; Seca, A.M.L.; Pinto, D.C.G.A. Seaweed secondary metabolites in vitro and in vivo anticancer activity. *Mar. Drugs* **2018**, *16*, 410. [CrossRef]
18. Seca, A.M.L.; Pinto, D.C.G.A. Overview on the antihypertensive and anti-obesity effects of secondary metabolites from seaweeds. *Mar. Drugs* **2018**, *16*, 237. [CrossRef]
19. Lefranc, F.; Koutsaviti, A.; Ioannou, E.; Kornienko, A.; Roussis, V.; Kiss, R.; Newman, D. Algae metabolites: From in vitro growth inhibitory effects to promising anticancer activity. *Nat. Prod. Rep.* **2019**, *36*, 810–841. [CrossRef]
20. Wang, T.; Jonsdottir, R.; Liu, H.; Gu, L.; Kristinsson, H.G.; Raghavan, S.; Olafsdottir, G. Antioxidant capacities of phlorotannins extracted from the brown algae *Fucus vesiculosus*. *J. Agric. Food Chem.* **2012**, *60*, 5874–5883. [CrossRef]
21. Meslet-Cladière, L.; Delage, L.; Leroux, C.J.-J.; Goulitquer, S.; Leblanc, C.; Creis, E.; Gall, E.A.; Stiger-Pouvreau, V.; Czjzek, M.; Potin, P. Structure/function analysis of a type iii polyketide synthase in the brown alga *Ectocarpus siliculosus* reveals a biochemical pathway in phlorotannin monomer biosynthesis. *Plant Cell.* **2013**, *25*, 3089–3103. [CrossRef]
22. Singh, I.P.; Sidana, J. Phlorotannins. In *Functional Ingredients from Algae for Foods and Nutraceuticals*, 1st ed.; Domínguez, H., Ed.; Woodhead Publishing: Cambridge, UK, 2013; pp. 181–204. [CrossRef]
23. Leyton, A.; Pezoa-Conte, R.; Barriga, A.; Buschmann, A.H.; Mäki-Arvela, P.; Mikkola, J.-P.; Lienqueo, M.E. Identification and efficient extraction method of phlorotannins from the brown seaweed *Macrocystis pyrifera* using an orthogonal experimental design. *Algal Res.* **2016**, *16*, 201–208. [CrossRef]
24. Gupta, S.; Abu-Ghannam, N. Bioactive potential and possible health effects of edible brown seaweeds. *Trends Food Sci. Technol.* **2011**, *22*, 315–326. [CrossRef]
25. Li, Y.-X.; Wijesekara, I.; Li, Y.; Kim, S.-K. Phlorotannins as bioactive agents from brown algae. *Proc. Biochem.* **2011**, *46*, 2219–2224. [CrossRef]
26. Lee, M.-S.; Shin, T.; Utsuki, T.; Choi, J.-S.; Byun, D.-S.; Kim, H.-R. Isolation and identification of phlorotannins from *Ecklonia stolonifera* with antioxidant and hepatoprotective properties in tacrine-treated HepG2 cells. *J. Agric. Food Chem.* **2012**, *60*, 5340–5349. [CrossRef]
27. Dong, X.; Bai, Y.; Xu, Z.; Shi, Y.; Sun, Y.; Janaswamy, S.; Yu, C.; Qi, H. Phlorotannins from *Undaria pinnatifida* Sporophyll: Extraction, antioxidant, and anti-inflammatory activities. *Mar. Drugs* **2019**, *17*, 434. [CrossRef]

28. Zenthoefer, M.; Geisen, U.; Hofmann-Peiker, K.; Fuhrmann, M.; Kerber, J.; Kirchhofer, R.; Hennig, S.; Peipp, M.; Geyer, R.; Piker, L.; et al. Isolation of polyphenols with anticancer activity from the Baltic Sea brown seaweed *Fucus vesiculosus* using bioassay-guided fractionation. *J. Appl. Phycol.* **2017**, *29*, 2021–2037. [CrossRef]
29. Zhou, X.; Yi, M.; Ding, L.; He, S.; Yan, X. Isolation and purification of a neuroprotective phlorotannin from the marine algae *Ecklonia maxima* by size exclusion and high-speed counter-current chromatography. *Mar. Drugs* **2019**, *17*, 212. [CrossRef]
30. Imbs, T.I.; Zvyagintseva, T.N. Phlorotannins are polyphenolic metabolites of brown algae. *Russ. J. Mar. Biol.* **2018**, *44*, 263–273. [CrossRef]
31. Kim, T.H.; Lee, T.; Ku, S.K.; Bae, J.S. Vascular barrier protective effects of eckol and its derivatives. *Bioorg. Med. Chem. Let.* **2012**, *22*, 3710–3712. [CrossRef]
32. Kang, K.A.; Zhang, R.; Chae, S.; Lee, S.J.; Kim, J.; Kim, J.; Jeong, J.; Lee, J.; Shin, T.; Lee, N.H.; et al. Phloroglucinol (1, 3, 5-trihydroxybenzene) protects against ionizing radiation-induced cell damage through inhibition of oxidative stress in vitro and in vivo. *Chem. Biol. Interact.* **2010**, *185*, 215–226. [CrossRef]
33. Moon, C.; Kim, S.-H.; Kim, J.-C.; Hyun, J.W.; Lee, N.H.; Park, J.W.; Shin, T. Protective effect of phlorotannin components phloroglucinol and eckol on radiation-induced intestinal injury in mice. *Phytother. Res.* **2008**, *22*, 238–242. [CrossRef]
34. Cha, S.-H.; Lee, J.-H.; Kim, E.-A.; Shin, C.H.; Jun, H.-S.; Jeon, Y.-J. Phloroglucinol accelerates the regeneration of liver damaged by H_2O_2 or MNZ treatment in zebrafish. *RSC Adv.* **2017**, *7*, 46164–46170. [CrossRef]
35. Kim, R.-K.; Uddin, N.; Hyun, J.-W.; Kim, C.; Suh, Y.; Lee, S.-J. Novel anticancer activity of phloroglucinol against breast cancer stem-like cells. *Toxicol. Appl. Pharmacol.* **2015**, *286*, 143–150. [CrossRef] [PubMed]
36. Kim, R.-K.; Suh, Y.; Yoo, K.-C.; Cui, Y.-H.; Hwang, E.; Kim, H.-J.; Kang, J.-S.; Kim, M.-J.; Lee, Y.Y.; Lee, S.-J. Phloroglucinol suppresses metastatic ability of breast cancer cells by inhibition of epithelial-mesenchymal cell transition. *Cancer Sci.* **2015**, *106*, 94–101. [CrossRef] [PubMed]
37. Yoon, J.-Y.; Choi, H.; Jun, H.-S. The effect of phloroglucinol, a component of *Ecklonia cava* extract, on hepatic glucose production. *Mar. Drugs* **2017**, *15*, 106. [CrossRef] [PubMed]
38. Im, A.-R.; Nam, K.-W.; Hyun, J.W.; Chae, S. Phloroglucinol reduces photodamage in hairless mice via matrix metalloproteinase activity through MAPK pathway. *Photochem. Photobiol.* **2016**, *92*, 173–179. [CrossRef]
39. Piao, M.J.; Ahn, M.J.; Kang, K.A.; Kim, K.C.; Cha, J.W.; Lee, N.H.; Hyun, J.W. Phloroglucinol enhances the repair of UVB radiation-induced DNA damage via promotion of the nucleotide excision repair system in vitro and in vivo. *DNA Repair* **2015**, *28*, 131–138. [CrossRef]
40. Ko, S.-C.; Jung, W.-K.; Kang, S.-M.; Lee, S.-H.; Kang, M.C.; Heo, S.-J.; Kang, K.-H.; Kim, Y.-T.; Park, S.-J.; Jeong, Y.; et al. Angiotensin I-converting enzyme (ACE) inhibition and nitric oxide (NO)-mediated antihypertensive effect of octaphlorethol A isolated from *Ishige sinicola*: In vitro molecular mechanism and in vivo SHR model. *J. Funct. Foods* **2015**, *18*, 289–299. [CrossRef]
41. Kang, M.-C.; Kim, K.-N.; Lakmal, H.H.C.; Kim, E.-A.; Wijesinghe, W.A.J.P.; Yang, X.; Heo, S.-J.; Jeon, Y.J. Octaphlorethol A isolated from *Ishige foliacea* prevents and protects against high glucose-induced oxidative damage in vitro and in vivo. *Environ. Toxicol. Pharmacol.* **2014**, *38*, 607–615. [CrossRef]
42. Lee, J.-H.; Ko, J.-Y.; Kim, H.-H.; Kim, C.-Y.; Jang, J.-H.; Nah, J.-W.; Jeon, Y.-J. Efficient approach to purification of octaphlorethol A from brown seaweed, *Ishige foliacea* by centrifugal partition chromatography. *Algal Res.* **2017**, *22*, 87–92. [CrossRef]
43. Kim, K.-N.; Yang, H.-M.; Kang, S.-M.; Ahn, G.; Roh, S.W.; Lee, W.; Kim, D.; Jeon, Y.-J. Whitening effect of octaphlorethol A isolated from *Ishige foliacea* in an in vivo zebrafish model. *J. Microbiol. Biotechnol.* **2015**, *25*, 448–451. [CrossRef]
44. Zhen, A.X.; Piao, M.J.; Hyun, Y.J.; Kang, K.A.; Fernando, P.D.S.M.; Cho, S.J.; Ahn, M.J.; Hyun, J.W. Diphlorethohydroxycarmalol attenuates fine particulate matter-induced subcellular skin dysfunction. *Mar. Drugs* **2019**, *17*, 95. [CrossRef] [PubMed]
45. Sanjeewa, K.K.A.; Lee, W.W.; Kim, J.-I.; Jeon, Y.-J. Exploiting biological activities of brown seaweed *Ishige okamurae* Yendo for potential industrial applications: A review. *J. Appl. Phycol.* **2017**, *29*, 3109–3119. [CrossRef]
46. Ahn, M.; Moon, C.; Yang, W.; Ko, E.J.; Hyun, J.W.; Joo, H.G.; Jee, Y.; Lee, N.H.; Park, J.W.; Ko, R.K.; et al. Diphlorethohydroxycarmalol, isolated from the brown algae *Ishige okamurae*, protects against radiation-induced cell damage in mice. *Food Chem. Toxicol.* **2011**, *49*, 864–870. [CrossRef] [PubMed]

47. Fernando, I.P.S.; Kim, H.-S.; Sanjeewa, K.K.A.; Oh, J.-Y.; Jeon, Y.-J.; Lee, W.W. Inhibition of inflammatory responses elicited by urban fine dust particles in keratinocytes and macrophages by diphlorethohydroxycarmalol isolated from a brown alga *Ishige okamurae*. *Algae* **2017**, *32*, 261–273. [CrossRef]
48. Fernando, K.H.N.; Yang, H.-W.; Jiang, Y.; Jeon, Y.-J.; Ryu, B. Diphlorethohydroxycarmalol isolated from *Ishige okamurae* represses high glucose-induced angiogenesis in vitro and in vivo. *Mar. Drugs* **2018**, *16*, 375. [CrossRef]
49. Barbosa, M.; Lopes, G.; Andrade, P.B.; Valentão, P. Bioprospecting of brown seaweeds for biotechnological applications. *Trends Food Sci. Technol.* **2019**, *86*, 153–171. [CrossRef]
50. Manandhar, B.; Paudel, P.; Seong, S.H.; Jung, H.A.; Choi, J.S. Characterizing eckol as a therapeutic aid: A systematic review. *Mar. Drugs* **2019**, *17*, 361. [CrossRef]
51. Sugiura, Y.; Usui, M.; Katsuzaki, H.; Imai, K.; Kakinuma, M.; Amano, H.; Myata, M. Orally administered phlorotannins from *Eisenia arborea* suppress chemical mediator release and cyclooxygenase-2 signaling to alleviate mouse ear swelling. *Mar. Drugs* **2018**, *16*, 267. [CrossRef]
52. Li, S.; Liu, J.; Zhang, M.; Chen, Y.; Zhu, T.; Wang, J. Protective effect of eckol against acute hepatic injury induced by carbon tetrachloride in mice. *Mar. Drugs* **2018**, *16*, 300. [CrossRef]
53. Kim, T.H.; Ku, S.-K.; Bae, J.-S. Antithrombotic and profibrinolytic activities of eckol and dieckol. *J. Cell. Biol.* **2012**, *113*, 2877–2883. [CrossRef]
54. Park, E.; Ahn, G.-N.; Lee, N.H.; Kim, J.M.; Yun, J.S.; Hyun, J.W.; Jeon, Y.-J.; Wie, M.B.; Lee, Y.J.; Park, J.W.; et al. Radioprotective properties of eckol against ionizing radiation in mice. *FEBS Lett.* **2008**, *582*, 925–930. [CrossRef] [PubMed]
55. Park, E.; Lee, N.H.; Joo, H.-G.; Jee, Y. Modulation of apoptosis of eckol against ionizing radiation in mice. *Biochem. Biophys. Res. Commun.* **2008**, *372*, 792–797. [CrossRef] [PubMed]
56. Yoon, N.Y.; Kim, H.R.; Chung, H.Y.; Choi, J.S. Anti-hyperlipidemic effect of an edible brown algae, *Ecklonia stolonifera*, and its constituents on poloxamer 407-induced hyperlipidemic and cholesterol-fed rats. *Arch. Pharm. Res.* **2008**, *31*, 1564–1571. [CrossRef] [PubMed]
57. Cha, S.-H.; Ko, C.-I.; Kim, D.; Jeon, Y.-J. Protective effects of phlorotannins against ultraviolet B radiation in zebrafish (*Danio rerio*). *Vet. Dermatol.* **2012**, *23*, 51–56. [CrossRef] [PubMed]
58. Kang, M.-C.; Wijesinghe, W.A.J.P.; Lee, S.-H.; Kang, S.-M.; Ko, S.-C.; Yang, X.; Kang, N.; Jeon, B.-T.; Kim, J.; Lee, D.-H.; et al. Dieckol isolated from brown seaweed *Ecklonia cava* attenuates type II diabetis in db/db mouse model. *Food Chem. Toxicol.* **2013**, *53*, 294–298. [CrossRef]
59. Ahn, G.; Amagai, Y.; Matsuda, A.; Kang, S.-M.; Lee, W.; Jung, K.; Oida, K.; Jang, H.; Ishizaka, S.; Matsuda, K.; et al. Dieckol, a phlorotannin of *Ecklonia cava*, suppresses IgE-mediated mast cell activation and passive cutaneous anaphylactic reaction. *Exp. Derm.* **2015**, *24*, 968–970. [CrossRef]
60. Kim, E.-A.; Kang, M.-C.; Lee, J.-H.; Kang, N.; Lee, W.; Oh, J.-Y.; Yang, H.-W.; Lee, J.-S.; Jeon, Y.-J. Protective effect of marine brown algal polyphenols against oxidative stressed zebrafish with high glucose. *RSC Adv.* **2015**, *5*, 25738–25746. [CrossRef]
61. Kang, M.-C.; Kim, K.-N.; Kang, S. M.; Yang, X.; Kim, E.-A.; Song, C.B.; Nah, J.-W.; Jang, M.-K.; Lee, J.-S.; Jung, W.-K.; et al. Protective effect of dieckol isolated from *Ecklonia cava* against ethanol caused damage in vitro and in zebrafish model. *Environ. Toxicol. Pharmacol.* **2013**, *36*, 1217–1226. [CrossRef]
62. Sugiura, Y.; Tanaka, R.; Katsuzaki, H.; Imai, K.; Matsushita, T. The anti-inflammatory effects of phlorotannins from *Eisenia arborea* on mouse ear edema by inflammatory inducers. *J. Funct. Foods* **2013**, *5*, 2019–2023. [CrossRef]
63. Wei, R.; Lee, M.-S.; Lee, B.; Oh, C.-W.; Choi, C.-G.; Kim, H.-R. Isolation and identification of anti-inflammatory compounds from ethyl acetate fraction of *Ecklonia stolonifera* and their anti-inflammatory action. *J. Appl. Phycol.* **2016**, *28*, 3535–3545. [CrossRef]
64. Lee, J.-H.; Ko, J.-Y.; Oh, J.-Y.; Kim, E.-A.; Kim, C.-Y.; Jeon, Y.-J. Evaluation of phlorofucofuroeckol-A isolated from *Ecklonia cava* (Phaeophyta) on anti-lipid peroxidation in vitro and in vivo. *Algae* **2015**, *30*, 313–323. [CrossRef]
65. Sugiura, Y.; Usui, M.; Hirotaka, K.; Imai, K.; Miyata, M. Anti-inflammatory effects of 6, 6'-bieckol and 6, 8'-bieckol from *Eisenia arborea* on mouse ear swelling. *J. Food Sci. Technol.* **2017**, *23*, 475–480. [CrossRef]

66. Ko, S.-C.; Kang, M.C.; Kang, N.; Kim, H.-S.; Lee, S.-H.; Ahn, G.; Jung, W.-K.; Jeon, Y.-J. Effect of angiotensin I-converting enzyme (ACE) inhibition and nitric oxide (NO) production of 6, 6-bieckol, a marine algal polyphenol and its antihypertensive effect in spontaneously hypertensive rats. *Proc. Biochem.* **2017**, *58*, 326–332. [CrossRef]
67. Cho, S.; Yoon, M.; Pae, A.N.; Ji, Y.-H.; Cho, N.-C.; Takata, Y.; Urade, Y.; Kim, S.; Yang, H.; Kim, J.; et al. Marine polyphenol phlorotannins promote non-rapid eye movement sleep in mice via the benzodiazepine site of the GABAA receptor. *Psychopharmacology* **2014**, *231*, 2825–2837. [CrossRef]
68. Kang, H.S.; Chung, H.Y.; Jung, J.H.; Son, B.W.; Choi, J.S. A new phlorotannin from the brown alga *Ecklonia stolonifera*. *Chem. Pharm. Bull.* **2003**, *51*, 1012–1014. [CrossRef]
69. Shin, T.; Ahn, M.; Hyun, J.W.; Kim, S.H.; Moon, C. Antioxidant marine algae phlorotannins and radioprotection: A review of experimental evidence. *Acta Histochem.* **2014**, *116*, 669–674. [CrossRef]
70. Hori, K.; Matsubara, K.; Miyazawa, K. Primary structures of two hemagglutinins from the marine red alga, *Hypnea japonica*. *Biochim. Biophys. Acta* **2000**, *1474*, 226–236. [CrossRef]
71. Singh, R.S.; Walia, A.K.; Khattar, J.S.; Singh, D.P.; Kennedy, J.F. Cyanobacterial lectins characteristics and their role as antiviral agents. *Int. J. Biol. Macromol.* **2017**, *102*, 475–496. [CrossRef]
72. Vanderlei, E.S.O.; Patoilo, K.K.N.R.; Lima, N.A.; Lima, A.P.S.; Rodrigues, J.A.G.; Silva, L.M.C.M.; Lima, M.E.P.; Lima, V.; Benevides, N.M.B. Antinociceptive and anti-inflammatory activities of lectin from the marine green alga *Caulerpa cupressoides*. *Int. Immunopharmacol.* **2010**, *10*, 1113–1118. [CrossRef]
73. Akkouh, O.; Ng, T.B.; Singh, S.S.; Yin, C.; Dan, X.; Chan, Y.S.; Pan, W.; Cheung, R.C.F. Lectins with anti-HIV activity: A review. *Molecules* **2015**, *20*, 648–668. [CrossRef]
74. Mu, J.; Hirayama, M.; Sato, Y.; Morimoto, K.; Hori, K. A novel high-mannose specific lectin from the green alga *Halimeda renschii* exhibits a potent anti-influenza virus activity through high-affinity binding to the viral hemagglutinin. *Mar. Drugs* **2017**, *15*, 255. [CrossRef]
75. Fontenelle, T.P.C.; Lima, G.C.; Mesquita, J.X.; Lopes, J.L.S.; de Brito, T.V.; Júnior, F.D.C.V.; Sales, A.B.; Aragão, K.S.; Souza, M.H.L.P.; Barbosa, A.L.D.R.; et al. Lectin obtained from the red seaweed *Bryothamnion triquetrum*: Secondary structure and anti-inflammatory activity in mice. *Int. J. Biol. Macromol.* **2018**, *112*, 1122–1130. [CrossRef]
76. Barre, A.; Simplicien, M.; Benoist, H.; Van Damme, E.J.M.; Rougé, P. Mannose-specific lectins from marine algae: Diverse structural scaffolds associated to common virucidal and anti-cancer properties. *Mar. Drugs* **2019**, *17*, 440. [CrossRef]
77. Gauto, D.F.; Di Lella, S.; Estrin, D.A.; Monaco, H.L.; Martí, M.A. Structural basis for ligand recognition in a mushroom lectin: Solvent structure as specificity predictor. *Carbohydr. Res.* **2011**, *346*, 939–948. [CrossRef]
78. Manning, J.C.; Romero, A.; Habermann, F.A.; Caballero, G.G.; Kaltner, H.; Gabius, H.-J. Lectins: A primer for histochemists and cell biologists. *Histochem. Cell Biol.* **2017**, *147*, 199–222. [CrossRef]
79. Sato, Y.; Morimoto, K.; Hirayama, M.; Hori, K. High mannose-specific lectin (KAA-2) from the red alga *Kappaphycus alvarezii* potently inhibits influenza virus infection in a strain-independent manner. *Biochem. Biophys. Res. Commun.* **2011**, *405*, 291–296. [CrossRef]
80. Pérez, M.J.; Falqué, E.; Domínguez, H. Antimicrobial action of compounds from marine seaweed. *Mar. Drugs* **2016**, *14*, 52. [CrossRef]
81. Kang, H.K.; Lee, H.H.; Seo, C.H.; Park, Y. Antimicrobial and immunomodulatory properties and applications of marine-derived proteins and peptides. *Mar. Drugs* **2019**, *17*, 350. [CrossRef]
82. Mori, T.; O'Keefe, B.R.; Sowder, R.C.; Bringans, S.; Gardella, R.; Berg, S.; Cochran, P.; Turpin, J.A.; Buckheit, R.W.; McMahon, J.B.; et al. Isolation and characterization of griffithsin, a novel HIV-inactivating protein, from the red alga *Griffithsia* sp. *J. Biol. Chem.* **2005**, *280*, 9345–9353. [CrossRef]
83. O'Keefe, B.R.; Giomarelli, B.; Barnard, D.L.; Shenoy, S.R.; Chan, P.K.S.; McMahon, J.B.; Palmer, K.E.; Barnett, B.W.; Meyerholz, D.K.; Wohlford-Lenane, C.L.; et al. Broad-spectrum in vitro activity and in vivo efficacy of the antiviral protein griffithsin against emerging viruses of the family *Coronaviridae*. *J. Virol.* **2010**, *84*, 2511–2521. [CrossRef]
84. Ishag, H.Z.A.; Li, C.; Huang, L.; Sun, M.-X.; Wang, F.; Ni, B.; Malik, T.; Chen, P.-Y.; Mao, X. Griffithsin inhibits japanese encephalitis virus infection in vitro and in vivo. *Arch. Virol.* **2013**, *158*, 349–358. [CrossRef] [PubMed]

85. Meuleman, P.; Albecka, A.; Belouzard, S.; Vercauteren, K.; Verhoye, L.; Wychowski, C.; Leroux-Roels, G.; Palmer, K.E.; Dubuisson, J. Griffithsin has antiviral activity against hepatitis C virus. *Antimicrob. Agents Chemother.* **2011**, *55*, 5159–5167. [CrossRef] [PubMed]
86. Nixon, B.; Stefanidou, M.; Mesquita, P.M.M.; Fakioglu, E.; Segarra, T.; Rohan, L.; Halford, W.; Palmer, K.E.; Herold, B.C. Griffithsin protects mice from genital herpes by preventing cell-to-cell spread. *J. Virol.* **2013**, *87*, 6257–6269. [CrossRef]
87. O'Keefe, B.R.; Vojdani, F.; Buffa, V.; Shattock, R.J.; Montefiori, D.C.; Bakke, J.; Mirsalis, J.; d'Andrea, A.-L.; Hume, S.D.; Bratcher, B.; et al. Scaleable manufacture of HIV-1 entry inhibitor griffithsin and validation of its safety and efficacy as a topical microbicide component. *Proc. Natl. Acad. Sci. USA* **2009**, *106*, 6099–6104. [CrossRef]
88. Levendosky, K.; Mizenina, O.; Martinelli, E.; Jean-Pierre, N.; Kizima, L.; Rodriguez, A.; Kleinbeck, K.; Bonnaire, T.; Robbiani, M.; Zydowsky, T.M.; et al. Griffithsin and carrageenan combination to target herpes simplex virus 2 and human papillomavirus. *Antimicrob. Agents Chemother.* **2015**, *59*, 7290–7298. [CrossRef]
89. Girard, L.; Birse, K.; Holm, J.B.; Gajer, P.; Humphrys, M.S.; Garber, D.; Guenthner, P.; Noël-Romas, L.; Abou, M.; McCorrister, S.; et al. Impact of the griffithsin anti-HIV microbicide and placebo gels on the rectal mucosal proteome and microbiome in non-human primates. *Sci. Rep.* **2018**, *8*, 8059. [CrossRef]
90. Fitzgerald, C.; Aluko, R.E.; Hossain, M.; Rai, D.K.; Hayes, M. Potential of a renin inhibitory peptide from the red seaweed *Palmaria palmata* as a functional food ingredient following confirmation and characterization of a hypotensive effect in spontaneously hypertensive rats. *J. Agric. Food Chem.* **2014**, *62*, 8352–8356. [CrossRef]
91. Sato, M.; Hosokawa, T.; Yamaguchi, T.; Nakano, T.; Muramoto, K.; Kahara, T.; Funayama, K.; Kobayashi, A.; Nakano, T. Angiotensin I-Converting enzyme inhibitory peptides derived from Wakame (*Undaria pinnatifida*) and their antihypertensive effect in spontaneously hypertensive rats. *J. Agric. Food Chem.* **2002**, *50*, 6245–6252. [CrossRef]
92. Pan, Q.; Chen, M.; Li, J.; Wu, Y.; Zhen, C.; Liang, B. Antitumor function and mechanism of phycoerythrin from *Porphyra haitanensis*. *Biol. Res.* **2013**, *46*, 87–95. [CrossRef]
93. Munier, M.; Morançais, M.; Dumay, J.; Jaouen, P.; Fleurence, J. One-step purification of R-phycoerythrin from the red edible seaweed *Grateloupia turuturu*. *J. Chromatogr. B* **2015**, *992*, 23–29. [CrossRef]
94. Li, P.; Ying, J.; Chang, Q.; Zhu, W.; Yang, G.; Xu, T.; Yi, H.; Pan, R.; Zhang, E.; Zeng, X.; et al. Effects of phycoerythrin from *Gracilaria lemaneiformis* in proliferation and apoptosis of SW480 cells. *Oncol. Rep.* **2016**, *36*, 3536–3544. [CrossRef]
95. Sonani, R.R.; Singh, N.K.; Awasthi, A.; Prasad, B.; Kumar, J.; Madamwar, D. Phycoerythrin extends life span and health span of *Caenorhabditis elegans*. *AGE* **2014**, *36*, 9717. [CrossRef]
96. Chaubey, M.G.; Patel, S.N.; Rastogi, R.P.; Srivastava, P.L.; Singh, A.K.; Madamwar, D.; Singh, N.K. Therapeutic potential of cyanobacterial pigment protein phycoerythrin: In silico and in vitro study of BACE1 interaction and in vivo Aβ reduction. *Int. J. Biol. Macromol.* **2019**, *134*, 368–378. [CrossRef]
97. Hamann, M.T.; Scheuer, P.J. Kahalalide F: A bioactive depsipeptide from the sacoglossan mollusk *Elysia rufescens* and the green alga *Bryopsis* sp. *J. Am. Chem. Soc.* **1993**, *115*, 5825–5826. [CrossRef]
98. Faircloth, G.; Cuevas, C. Kahalalide F and ES285: Potent anticancer agents from marine molluscs. In *Progress in Molecular and Subcellular Biology*; Springer: Berlin/Heidelberg, Germany, 2006; Volume 43, pp. 363–379. [PubMed]
99. Suetsuna, K. Purification and identification of angiotensin I-converting enzyme inhibitors from the red alga *Porphyra yezoensis*. *J. Mar. Biotechnol.* **1998**, *6*, 163–167. [PubMed]
100. Suetsuna, K. Separation and identification of angiotensin I-converting enzyme inhibitory peptides from peptic digest of *Hizikia fusiformis* protein. *Bull. Japan. Soc. Sci. Fish.* **1998**, *64*, 862–866. [CrossRef]
101. Suetsuna, K.; Nakano, T. Identification of an antihypertensive peptide from peptic digest of wakame (*Undaria pinnatifida*). *J. Nutr. Biochem.* **2000**, *11*, 450–454. [CrossRef]
102. Suetsuna, K.; Maekawa, K.; Chen, J.-R. Antihypertensive effects of *Undaria pinnatifida* (wakame) peptide on blood pressure in spontaneously hypertensive rats. *J. Nutr. Biochem.* **2004**, *15*, 267–272. [CrossRef]
103. Cardoso, S.M.; Pereira, O.R.; Seca, A.M.L.; Pinto, D.C.G.A.; Silva, A.M.S. Seaweeds as preventive agents for cardiovascular diseases: From nutrients to functional foods. *Mar. Drugs* **2015**, *13*, 6838–6865. [CrossRef]
104. Vijayan, R.; Chitra, L.; Penislusshiyan, S.; Palvannan, T. Exploring bioactive fraction of *Sargassum wightii*: In vitro elucidation of angiotensin-I-converting enzyme inhibition and antioxidant potential. *Int. J. Food Prop.* **2018**, *21*, 674–684. [CrossRef]

105. Fitzgerald, C.; Mora-Soler, L.; Gallagher, E.; O'Connor, P.; Prieto, J.; Soler-Vila, A.; Hayes, M. Isolation and characterization of bioactive pro-peptides with in vitro renin inhibitory activities from the macroalga *Palmaria palmata*. *J. Agric. Food Chem.* **2012**, *60*, 7421–7427. [CrossRef]
106. Kecel-Gündüz, S.; Budama-Kilinc, Y.; Cakir Koc, R.; Kökcü, Y.; Bicak, B.; Aslan, B.; Özel, A.E. Computational design of Phe-Tyr dipeptide and preparation, characterization, cytotoxicity studies of Phe-Tyr dipeptide loaded PLGA nanoparticles for the treatment of hypertension. *J. Biomol. Struct. Dyn.* **2018**, *36*, 2893–2907. [CrossRef]
107. Tan, H.; Gao, S.; Zhuang, Y.; Dong, Y.; Guan, W.; Zhang, K.; Xu, J.; Cui, J. R-Phycoerythrin induces SGC-7901 apoptosis by arresting cell cycle at S-phase. *Mar. Drugs* **2016**, *14*, 166. [CrossRef]
108. Hamann, M.T.; Otto, C.S.; Scheuer, P.J.; Dunbar, D.C. Kahalalides: Bioactive peptides from a marine Mollusk *Elysia rufescens* and its algal diet *Bryopsis* sp. *J. Org. Chem.* **1996**, *61*, 6594–6600. [CrossRef]
109. Suárez, Y.; González, L.; Cuadrado, A.; Berciano, M.; Lafarga, M.; Muñoz, A. Kahalalide F, a new marine-derived compound, induces oncosis in human prostate and breast cancer cells. *Mol. Cancer Ther.* **2003**, *2*, 863–872.
110. Cabrita, M.T.; Vale, C.; Rauter, A.P. Halogenated compounds from marine algae. *Mar. Drugs* **2010**, *8*, 2301–2317. [CrossRef]
111. Soares, A.C. Extraction, isolation, and identification of sesquiterpenes from *Laurencia* species. *Methods Mol. Biol.* **2015**, *1308*, 225–240. [CrossRef]
112. Woolner, V.H.; Gordon, R.M.A.; Miller, J.H.; Lein, M.; Northcote, P.T.; Keyzers, R.A. Halogenated meroditerpenoids from a South Pacific collection of the red alga *Callophycus serratus*. *J. Nat. Prod.* **2018**, *81*, 2446–2454. [CrossRef]
113. Jesus, A.; Correia-da-Silva, M.; Afonso, C.; Pinto, M.; Cidade, H. Isolation and potential biological applications of haloaryl secondary metabolites from macroalgae. *Mar. Drugs* **2019**, *17*, 73. [CrossRef]
114. Fuller, R.W.; Cardellina, J.H.; Jurek, J.; Scheuer, P.J.; Alvarado-Lindner, B.; McGuire, M.; Gray, G.N.; Steiner, J.R.; Clardy, J.; Menez, E.; et al. Isolation and structure/activity features of halomon-related antitumor monoterpenes from the red alga *Portieria hornemannii*. *J. Med. Chem.* **1994**, *37*, 4407–4411. [CrossRef]
115. Chatter, R.; Kladi, M.; Tarhouni, S.; Maatoug, R.; Kharrat, R.; Vagias, C.; Roussis, V. Neorogioltriol: A brominated diterpene with analgesic activity from *Laurencia glandulifera*. *Phytochem. Lett.* **2009**, *2*, 25–28. [CrossRef]
116. Chatter, R.; Othman, R.B.; Rabhi, S.; Kladi, M.; Tarhouni, S.; Vagias, C.; Roussis, V.; Guizani-Tabbane, L.; Kharrat, R. In vivo and in vitro anti-inflammatory activity of neorogioltriol, a new diterpene extracted from the red algae *Laurencia glandulifera*. *Mar. Drugs* **2011**, *9*, 1293–1306. [CrossRef]
117. Daskalaki, M.G.; Vyrla, D.; Harizani, M.; Doxaki, C.; Eliopoulos, A.G.; Roussis, V.; Ioannou, E.; Tsatsanis, C.; Kampranis, S.C. Neorogioltriol and related diterpenes from the red alga *Laurencia* inhibit inflammatory bowel disease in mice by suppressing M1 and promoting M2-like macrophage responses. *Mar. Drugs* **2019**, *17*, 97. [CrossRef]
118. Guella, G.; Pietra, F. A new-skeleton diterpenoid, new prenylbisabolanes, and their putative biogenetic precursor, from the red seaweed *Laurencia microcladia* from II Rogiolo: Assigning the absolute configuration when two chiral halves are connected by single bonds. *Helv. Chim. Acta* **2000**, *83*, 2946–2952. [CrossRef]
119. Kurihara, H.; Mitani, T.; Kawabata, J.; Takahashi, T. Two new bromophenols from the red alga *Odonthalia corymbifera*. *J. Nat. Prod.* **1999**, *62*, 882–884. [CrossRef]
120. Shi, D.; Li, J.; Guo, S.; Su, H.; Fan, X. The antitumor effect of bromophenol derivatives in vitro and *Leathesia nana* extract in vivo. *Chin. J. Ocean. Limnol.* **2009**, *27*, 277–282. [CrossRef]
121. Qi, X.; Liu, G.; Qiu, L.; Lin, X.; Liu, M. Marine bromophenol bis (2, 3-dibromo-4, 5-dihydroxybenzyl) ether, represses angiogenesis in HUVEC cells and in zebrafish embryos via inhibiting the VEGF signal systems. *Biomed. Pharmacother.* **2015**, *75*, 58–66. [CrossRef]
122. Xu, F.; Wang, F.; Wang, Z.; Lv, W.; Wang, W.; Wang, Y. Glucose uptake activities of bis (2,3-dibromo-4,5-dihydroxybenzyl) ether, a novel marine natural product from red alga *Odonthalia corymbifera* with protein tyrosine phosphatase 1B inhibition, in vitro and in vivo. *PLoS ONE* **2016**, *11*, e0147748. [CrossRef]
123. Egorin, M.J.; Sentz, D.L.; Rosen, D.M.; Ballesteros, M.F.; Kearns, C.M.; Callery, P.S.; Eiseman, J.L. Plasma pharmacokinetics, bioavailability, and tissue distribution in CD2F1 mice of halomon, an antitumor halogenated monoterpene isolated from the red algae *Portieria hornemannii*. *Cancer Chemother. Pharmacol.* **1996**, *39*, 51–60. [CrossRef]

124. Andrianasolo, E.H.; France, D.; Cornell-Kennon, S.; Gerwick, W.H. DNA Methyl transferase inhibiting halogenated monoterpenes from the Madagascar red marine alga *Portieria hornemannii*. *J. Nat. Prod.* **2006**, *69*, 576–579. [CrossRef]
125. Schlama, T.; Baati, R.; Gouverneur, V.; Valleix, A.; Falck, J.R.; Mioskowski, C. Total synthesis of (±)-halomon by a Johnson-Claisen rearrangement. *Angew. Chem. Int. Ed. Engl.* **1998**, *37*, 2085–2087. [CrossRef]
126. Sotokawa, T.; Noda, T.; Pi, S.; Hirama, M. A three-step synthesis of halomon. *Angew. Chem. Int. Ed. Engl.* **2000**, *39*, 3430–3432. [CrossRef]
127. Bucher, C.; Deans, R.M.; Burns, N.Z. Highly selective synthesis of halomon, plocamenone, and isoplocamenone. *J. Am. Chem. Soc.* **2015**, *137*, 12784–12787. [CrossRef] [PubMed]
128. Landry, M.L.; Burns, N.Z. Catalytic enantioselective dihalogenation in total synthesis. *Acc. Chem. Res.* **2018**, *51*, 1260–1271. [CrossRef] [PubMed]
129. Liu, M.; Zhang, W.; Wei, J.; Lin, X. Synthesis and α-glucosidase inhibitory mechanisms of bis (2, 3-dibromo-4, 5-dihydroxybenzyl) ether, a potential marine bromophenol α-glucosidase inhibitor. *Mar. Drugs* **2011**, *9*, 1554–1565. [CrossRef]
130. Liu, M.; Zhang, W.; Wei, J.; Qiu, L.; Lin, X. Marine bromophenol bis (2, 3-dibromo-4, 5-dihydroxybenzyl) ether, induces mitochondrial apoptosis in K562 cells and inhibits topoisomerase I in vitro. *Toxicol. Lett.* **2012**, *211*, 126–134. [CrossRef]
131. Liu, M.; Wang, G.; Xiao, L.; Xu, A.; Liu, X.; Xu, P.; Lin, X. Bis (2,3-dibromo-4,5-dihydroxybenzyl) ether, a marine algae derived bromophenol, inhibits the growth of *Botrytis cinerea* and interacts with DNA molecules. *Mar. Drugs* **2014**, *12*, 3838–3851. [CrossRef]
132. Irvani, N.; Hajiaghaee, R.; Zarekarizi, A.R. A review on biosynthesis, health benefits and extraction methods of fucoxanthin, particular marine carotenoids in algae. *J. Med. Plants* **2018**, *17*, 6–30.
133. Zhang, H.; Tang, Y.; Zhang, Y.; Zhang, S.; Qu, J.; Wang, X.; Kong, R.; Han, C.; Liu, Z. Fucoxanthin: A promising medicinal and nutritional ingredient. *Evid. Based Complement. Altern. Med.* **2015**, *2015*, 723515. [CrossRef]
134. Peng, J.; Deng, X.-Q.; Ao, Y.-S.; Yuan, J.-P. Anti-obesity and anti-diabetic effects of fucoxanthin. *Mod. Food Sci. Technol.* **2015**, *31*, 313–325. [CrossRef]
135. Miyashita, K.; Hosokawa, M. Fucoxanthin in the management of obesity and its related disorders. *J. Funct. Foods* **2017**, *36*, 195–202. [CrossRef]
136. Satomi, Y. Antitumor and cancer-preventative function of fucoxanthin: A marine carotenoid. *Anticancer Res.* **2017**, *37*, 1557–1562. [CrossRef] [PubMed]
137. Wang, Z.; Li, H.; Dong, M.; Zhu, P.; Cai, Y. The anticancer effects and mechanisms of fucoxanthin combined with other drugs. *J. Cancer Res. Clin. Oncol.* **2019**, *145*, 293–301. [CrossRef] [PubMed]
138. Karpiński, T.M.; Adamczak, A. Fucoxanthin—An antibacterial carotenoid. *Antioxidants* **2019**, *8*, 239. [CrossRef]
139. Neumann, U.; Derwenskus, F.; Flister, V.F.; Schmid-Staiger, U.; Hirth, T.; Bischoff, S.C. Fucoxanthin, a carotenoid derived from *Phaeodactylum tricornutum* exerts antiproliferative and antioxidant activities in vitro. *Antioxidants* **2019**, *8*, 183. [CrossRef]
140. Hu, L.; Chen, W.; Tian, F.; Yuan, C.; Wang, H.; Yue, H. Neuroprotective role of fucoxanthin against cerebral ischemic/reperfusion injury through activation of Nrf2/HO-1 signaling. *Biomed. Pharmacother.* **2018**, *106*, 1484–1489. [CrossRef]
141. Longa, E.Z.; Weinstein, P.R.; Carlson, S.; Cummins, R. Reversible middle cerebral artery occlusion without craniectomy in rats. *Stroke* **1989**, *20*, 84–91. [CrossRef]
142. Wang, J.; Ma, Y.; Yang, J.; Jin, L.; Gao, Z.; Xue, L.; Hou, L.; Sui, L.; Liu, J.; Zou, X. Fucoxanthin inhibits tumour-related lymphangiogenesis and growth of breast cancer. *J. Cell. Mol. Med.* **2019**, *23*, 2219–2229. [CrossRef]
143. Terasaki, M.; Iida, T.; Kikuchi, F.; Tamura, K.; Endo, T.; Kuramitsu, Y.; Tanaka, T.; Maeda, H.; Miyashita, K.; Mutoh, M. Fucoxanthin potentiates anoikis in colon mucosa and prevents carcinogenesis in AOM/DSS model mice. *J. Nutr. Biochem.* **2019**, *64*, 198–205. [CrossRef]
144. Jiang, X.; Wang, G.; Lin, Q.; Tang, Z.; Yan, Q.; Yu, X. Fucoxanthin prevents lipopolysaccharide-induced depressive-like behavior in mice via AMPK- NF-κB pathway. *Metab. Brain Dis.* **2019**, *34*, 431–442. [CrossRef]

145. Su, J.; Guo, K.; Huang, M.; Liu, Y.; Zhang, J.; Sun, L.; Li, D.; Pang, K.-L.; Wang, G.; Chen, L.; et al. Fucoxanthin, a marine xanthophyll isolated from *Conticribra weissflogii* ND-8: Preventive anti-inflammatory effect in a mouse model of sepsis. *Front. Pharmacol.* **2019**, *10*, 906. [CrossRef] [PubMed]
146. Abdul, Q.A.; Choi, R.J.; Jung, H.A.; Choi, J.S. Health benefit of fucosterol from marine algae: A review. *J. Sci. Food Agric.* **2016**, *96*, 1856–1866. [CrossRef] [PubMed]
147. Lee, Y.S.; Shin, K.H.; Kim, B.-K.; Lee, S. Anti-diabetic activities of fucosterol from *Pelvetia siliquosa*. *Arch. Pharm. Res.* **2004**, *11*, 1120–1122. [CrossRef] [PubMed]
148. Zhangfan, M.; Xiaoling, S.; Ping, D.; Gaoli, L.; Shize, P.; Xiangran, S.; Haifeng, H.; Li, P.; Jie, H. Fucosterol exerts antiproliferative effects on human lung cancer cells by inducing apoptosis, cel cycle arrest and targeting of Raf/MEK/ERK signaling pathway. *Phytomedicine* **2019**, *61*, 152809. [CrossRef]
149. Li, Y.; Li, X.; Liu, G.; Sun, R.; Wang, L.; Wang, J.; Wang, H. Fucosterol attenuates lipopolysaccharide-induced acute lung injury in mice. *J. Surg. Res.* **2015**, *195*, 515–521. [CrossRef]
150. Mo, W.; Wang, C.; Li, J.; Chen, K.; Xia, Y.; Li, S.; Xu, L.; Lu, X.; Wang, W.; Guo, C. Fucosterol protects against concanavalin A-induced acute liver injury: Focus on P38 MAPK/NF-κB pathway activity. *Gastroenterol. Res. Pract.* **2018**, *2018*, 2824139. [CrossRef]
151. Lee, D.-G.; Park, S.-Y.; Chung, W.-S.; Park, J.-H.; Shin, H.-S.; Hwang, E.; Kim, I.-H.; Yi, T.-H. The bone regenerative effects of fucosterol in in vitro and in vivo models of postmenopausal osteoporosis. *Mol. Nutr. Food Res.* **2014**, *58*, 1249–1257. [CrossRef]
152. Oh, J.H.; Choi, J.S.; Nam, T.J. Fucosterol from an edible brown alga *Ecklonia stolonifera* prevents soluble amyloid beta-induced cognitive dysfunction in aging rats. *Mar. Drugs* **2018**, *16*, 368. [CrossRef]
153. Zhen, X.-H.; Quan, Y.-C.; Jiang, H.-Y.; Wen, Z.-S.; Qu, Y.-L.; Guan, L.-P. Fucosterol, a sterol extracted from *Sargassum fusiforme*, shows antidepressant and anticonvulsant effects. *Eur. J. Pharmacol.* **2015**, *768*, 131–138. [CrossRef]
154. Hitoe, S.; Shimoda, H. Seaweed fucoxanthin supplementation improves obesity parameters in mildly obese Japanese subjects. *Funct. Food Health Dis.* **2017**, *7*, 246–262. [CrossRef]
155. Abidov, M.; Ramazanov, Z.; Seifulla, R.; Grachev, S. The effects of xanthigen in the weight management of obese premenopausal women with non-alcoholic fatty liver disease and normal liver fat. *Diabetes Obes. Metab.* **2010**, *12*, 72–81. [CrossRef] [PubMed]
156. Martín-Algarra, S.; Espinosa, E.; Rubió, J.; López, J.J.L.; Manzano, J.L.; Carrión, L.A.; Plazaola, A.; Tanovic, A.; Paz-Ares, L. Phase II study of weekly Kahalalide F in patients with advanced malignant melanoma. *Eur. J. Cancer* **2009**, *45*, 732–735. [CrossRef] [PubMed]
157. Salazar, R.; Cortés-Funes, H.; Casado, E.; Pardo, B.; López-Martín, A.; Cuadra, C.; Tabernero, J.; Coronado, C.; García, M.; Matos-Pita, A.S.; et al. Phase I study of weekly kahalalide F as prolonged infusion in patients with advanced solid tumors. *Cancer Chemother. Pharmacol.* **2013**, *72*, 75–83. [CrossRef] [PubMed]
158. Gómez-Ordóñez, E.; Jiménez-Escrig, A.; Rupérez, P. Dietary fibre and physicochemical properties of several edible seaweeds from the northwestern Spanish coast. *Food Res. Int.* **2010**, *43*, 2289–2294. [CrossRef]
159. Wang, H.; Hong, T.; Li, N.; Zang, B.; Wu, X. Soluble dietary fiber improves energy homeostasis in obese mice by remodeling the gut microbiota. *Biochem. Biophys. Res. Commun.* **2018**, *498*, 146–151. [CrossRef] [PubMed]
160. Ottrey, E.; Jong, J.; Porter, J. Ethnography in nutrition and dietetics research: A systematic review. *J. Acad. Nutr. Diet.* **2018**, *118*, 1903–1942. [CrossRef]
161. Forouhi, N.G.; Misra, A.; Mohan, V.; Taylor, R.; Yancy, W. Dietary and nutritional approaches for prevention and management of type 2 diabetes. *BMJ* **2018**, *361*, k2234. [CrossRef]
162. Sakai, C.; Abe, S.; Kouzuki, M.; Shimohiro, H.; Ota, Y.; Sakinada, H.; Takeuchi, T.; Okura, T.; Kasagi, T.; Hanaki, K. A randomized placebo-controlled trial of an oral preparation of high molecular weight fucoidan in patients with type 2 diabetes with evaluation of taste sensitivity. *Yonago Acta Med.* **2019**, *62*, 14–23. [CrossRef]
163. Paradis, M.-E.; Couture, P.; Lamarche, B. A randomised crossover placebo-controlled trial investigating the effect of brown seaweed (*Ascophyllum nodosum* and *Fucus vesiculosus*) on post challenge plasma glucose and insulin levels in men and women. *Appl. Physiol. Nutr. Metab.* **2011**, *36*, 913–919. [CrossRef]
164. Murray, M.; Dordevic, A.L.; Ryan, L.; Bonham, M.P. The impact of a single dose of a polyphenol-rich seaweed extract on postprandial glycaemic control in healthy adults: A randomised cross-over trial. *Nutrients* **2018**, *10*, 270. [CrossRef]

165. Haskell-Ramsay, C.F.; Jackson, P.A.; Dodd, F.L.; Forster, J.S.; Bérubé, J.; Levinton, C.; Kennedy, D.O. Acute post-prandial cognitive effects of brown seaweed extract in humans. *Nutrients* **2018**, *10*, 85. [CrossRef] [PubMed]
166. Hall, A.C.; Fairclough, A.C.; Mahadevan, K.; Paxman, J.R. *Ascophyllum nodosum* enriched bread reduces subsequent energy intake with no effect on post-prandial glucose and cholesterol in healthy, overweight males. A pilot study. *Appetite* **2012**, *58*, 379–386. [CrossRef] [PubMed]
167. Bray, G.A.; Kim, K.K.; Wilding, J.P.H. Obesity: A chronic relapsing progressive disease process. A position statement of the World Obesity Federation. *Obes. Rev.* **2017**, *18*, 715–723. [CrossRef] [PubMed]
168. Baldrick, F.R.; McFadden, K.; Ibars, M.; Sung, C.; Moffatt, T.; Megarry, K.; Thomas, K.; Mitchell, P.; Wallace, J.M.W.; Pourshahidi, L.K.; et al. Impact of a (poly)phenol-rich extract from the brown algae *Ascophyllum nodosum* on DNA damage and antioxidant activity in an overweight or obese population: A randomized controlled trial. *Am. J. Clin. Nutr.* **2018**, *108*, 688–700. [CrossRef]
169. Allaert, F.-A.; Demais, H.; Collén, P.N. A randomized controlled double-blind clinical trial comparing versus placebo the effect of an edible algal extract (*Ulva lactuca*) on the component of depression in healthy volunteers with anhedonia. *BMC Psychiatry* **2018**, *18*, 215. [CrossRef]
170. Teas, J.; Irhimeh, M.R. Dietary algae and HIV/AIDS: Proof of concept clinical data. *J. Appl. Phycol.* **2012**, *24*, 575–582. [CrossRef]
171. Tian, J.-M.; Ran, B.; Zhang, C.-L.; Yan, D.-M.; Li, X.-H. Estrogen and progesterone promote breast cancer cell proliferation by inducing cyclin G1 expression. *Braz. J. Med. Biol. Res.* **2018**, *51*, 1–7. [CrossRef]
172. Teas, J.; Hurley, T.G.; Hebert, J.R.; Franke, A.A.; Sepkovic, D.W.; Kurzer, M.S. Dietary seaweed modifies estrogen and phytoestrogen metabolism in healthy postmenopausal women. *J. Nutr.* **2009**, *139*, 939–944. [CrossRef]

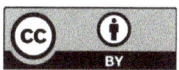

© 2019 by the authors. Licensee MDPI, Basel, Switzerland. This article is an open access article distributed under the terms and conditions of the Creative Commons Attribution (CC BY) license (http://creativecommons.org/licenses/by/4.0/).

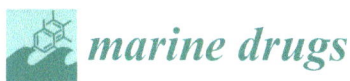

Review

Potential Use of Seaweed Bioactive Compounds in Skincare—A Review

Valentina Jesumani [1], Hong Du [1,*], Muhammad Aslam [1,2], Pengbing Pei [1] and Nan Huang [1]

1. Guangdong Provincial Key Laboratory of Marine Biotechnology College of Sciences, Shantou University, Shantou 515063, China; tina@stu.edu.cn (V.J.); drmaslam@hotmail.com (M.A.); peipengbing1990@126.com (P.P.); 18nhuang@stu.edu.cn (N.H.)
2. Faculty of Marine Sciences, Lasbela University, Uthal 90950, Pakistan
* Correspondence: hdu@stu.edu.cn; Tel.: +86-0754-86502083

Received: 20 September 2019; Accepted: 2 December 2019; Published: 6 December 2019

Abstract: Modern lifestyles have developed new attention on appearance and personal care which attract a huge number of consumers towards cosmetic products. The demand for a skincare product with natural ingredients is rapidly increasing. Seaweeds are major resources for in-demand active compounds with a wide variety of applications. The use of seaweed-derived ingredients in cosmetic products has increased in recent years as many scientific studies have proved the potential skincare properties of seaweed bioactive compounds. This review emphasizes possible skincare properties of seaweed bioactive compounds. The review outlines the mechanism involved in skin problems including hyperpigmentation, premature skin aging, and acne in the first part while the second part focuses on the promising application of seaweeds in skin protection by highlighting the bioactive compound responsible for their bioactivity.

Keywords: seaweeds; hyperpigmentation; skin aging; skincare; photo-protection

---

1. Introduction

Cosmetics are the materials used to enhance or alter the function and appearance of the skin and hair [1]. Kligman created the term "cosmeceutical" to hightlight cosmetic products that can combine the use of both cosmetic and pharmaceutical uses [2]. Cosmeceuticals are often used in dermatology to enhance the skin tone, skin glow, and provide anti-aging benefits [3]. The cosmeceutical industries are most fascinating, profitable, and constantly growing in the world economy. According to reports, an average woman spends $15,000 on beauty products in her lifetime [4]. The cosmetics industry has predicted an annual gross revenue of US $170 billion according to the financial exploration stated by a French-based company, Eurostaf [5]. In 2016, the European cosmetics market was top in the world, esteemed at €77 billion in a wholesale rate, trailed by the US and Brazil [4]. The global beauty market stated that the cosmetic industry will continue to develop due to the growth of the middle class in many developing countries [6]. Based on this encouraging future of the cosmetics industry, many cosmetic products without any side effects have been developed to satisfy the customers' needs. Currently, many synthetic chemicals have been used in cosmetic products, many of them did not get synthetic customer satisfaction due to high cost and unsafe nature in terms of side effects. For example, chemicals like hydroquinone, arbutin, and kojic acid are being used as a skin whitening agent, but they are reported to be unstable and they also cause dermatitis and induce cancer [7–9]. Thus, in recent years, the demand for cosmetic products that containing natural ingredients is rapidly expanding. The advantages of natural ingredients are environmentally friendliness, fewer side effects, and safe use [1,10]. Hence, Cosmeceutical industries are persistently seeking active compounds from natural sources. From this perspective, the marine environment provides numerous marine organisms, including seaweeds with potential bioactive compounds. Seaweeds are rich in bioactive compounds that could be exploited as functional ingredients for cosmetic applications [11]. This review focusses on the cosmetic properties of seaweed bioactive compounds and provides an overview of skin problems and the potential of seaweed bioactive compounds against skin problems.

2. Structure of Skin

The skin is the major organ in the human body. Generally, the skin can be divided into epidermis, dermis, and subcutaneous tissue. The epidermis is the uppermost layer of the skin. It has three types of cells—namely keratinocytes, melanocytes, and Langerhans cells. Keratinocytes are made up of keratin, which on maturation lose water and move up to the uppermost layer of the epidermis called the 'stratum corneum' [12]. The next collection of cells present in the epidermis are melanocytes, the cells that produce melanin, the pigment accountable for skin tone and color. Langerhans cells inhibit the penetration of unwanted foreign materials into the skin. The condition of the epidermis defines the freshness and youthfulness of your skin. The middle layer of the skin is the dermis [13]. Collagen and elastin are the main components of the extracellular matrix (ECM), covering about 90% of the dermis, which are cross-linked and provide support for the skin. Hence, the dermis is responsible for the structural support and elasticity of the skin. Collagen is found in the extracellular matrix of all animal bodies [14]. Hyaluronic acid (HA) is also a main constituent of the dermis. HA plays an important role in moisture absorption and moisture retention [12]. Subcutaneous tissue, which is the third layer located under the dermis, is comprised of connective tissue and fat. The loss of subcutaneous tissue due to age will also lead to facial sagging and wrinkles.

3. UV Induced Skin Damage

The ultraviolet (UV) radiation from the sun extends the earth in a significant amount. UV-C (100–290 nm) is mostly filtered by the atmosphere, but UVA (320–400 nm) and UVB (290–320 nm) rays extend the skin and cause suntan, wrinkles, etc. [15]. UV radiation induces the production of reactive oxygen species (ROS) and also depletes the antioxidant enzymes [16]. These ROS can lead to skin disorders such as hyperpigmentation (dark spots), premature aging, dryness, etc. [17,18].

3.1. Hyperpigmentation

Hyperpigmentation is usually an inoffensive form in which spots of the skin become darker in color than the regular surrounding skin. The overproduction and accumulation of melanin pigment resulted in a change in skin color. Melanogenesis is controlled by an enzyme such as tyrosinase, a glycoprotein [19] present in the membrane of the melanosome which catalyzes the conversion of l-tyrosine to melanin [20]. Melanogenesis is regulated by maturation and translocation of tyrosinase. The translocation of tyrosinases is regulated by the presence of specific carbohydrate moieties [21].

Two types of melanin are synthesized within melanosomes: eumelanin and pheomelanin. The pathway in which melanogenesis occurs is presented in Figure 1. The enzymes such as tyrosinase and tyrosinase related protein (TRP-1 and 2) are produced by the phosphorylation of MITF, which is activated by several signaling pathways such as cAMP, ERK, and Wnt pathways. These signaling pathways are upregulated by the upstream of the receptor such as KIT (ligand SCF) and MC1R (ligand α-MSH, ACTH, and ASP). The KIT receptor activates the cAMP pathway and MC1R activates both cAMP and ERK pathway which further phosphorylates the MITF. This leads to the expression of tyrosinase-related enzymes which further mediates the production of melanin [22–26]. The skin under UV generates the reactive oxygen species (ROS) that activate the α-MSH and MC1R and enhances the production of tyrosinase that leads to the excess generation of melanin [27,28].

3.2. Skin Aging

Skin aging is a complex process that occurs in all living beings that caused by two factors. One is intrinsic in which aging is caused by genetics [29]. The latter one is an extrinsic factor, in which aging occurs due to the exposure of skin to the ultraviolet rays. This type of aging is called photo-aging or premature aging [30]. Reactive oxygen species (ROS) play a key role in skin aging. ROS triggers the various growth factors and cytokine receptors which further stimulate mitogen-activated protein kinase (MAPK) signal transduction and P13/AKT pathway. The AKT pathway inactivates the FoxO which suppresses the expression of antioxidant enzymes in the cell. MAPK upregulates activator protein-1 (AP-1) and NF-κB in the nucleus. The induction of AP-1 gives rise to the MMP expressions [31,32] (Figure 2). MMPs are a collection of zinc-containing extracellular proteinases that degrade the extracellular components, such as collagen and elastic fibers, inducing wrinkle formation [31–33]. ROS also activates the expression of the hyaluronidase enzyme that degrades hyaluronic acid. Hyaluronic acid is present in extracellular matrix, absorbing and retaining water molecules and helping to keep the skin smooth, moist, and lubricated [34–36].

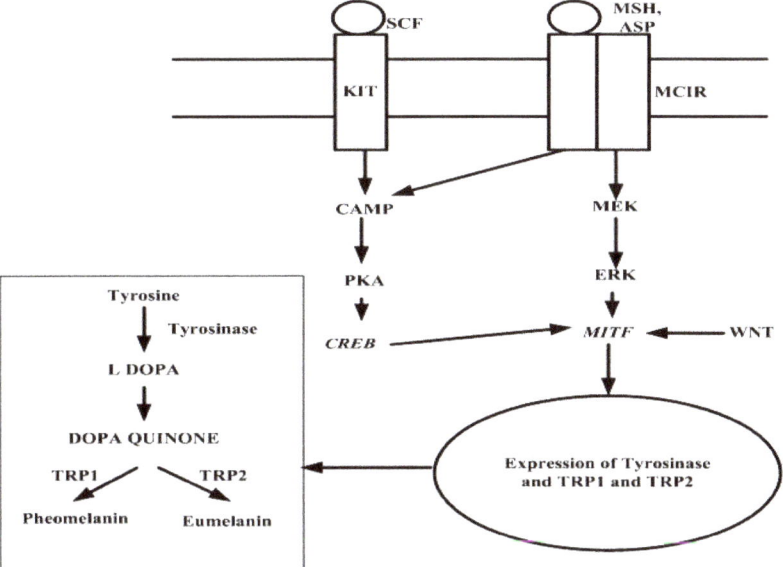

Figure 1. Signaling pathways involved in melanin synthesis. Tyrosinase-related protein (TRP), microphthalmia-associated transcription factor (MITF), adenosine 3′,5′-cyclic monophosphate (cyclic AMP) (cAMP), cAMP response element-binding (CREB), extracellular receptor kinase (ERK), melanocortin 1 receptor (MC1R), wingless-related integration site (Wnt), α-melanocyte-stimulating hormone (MSH), agonist stimulating protein (ASP), and stem cell factor (SCF).

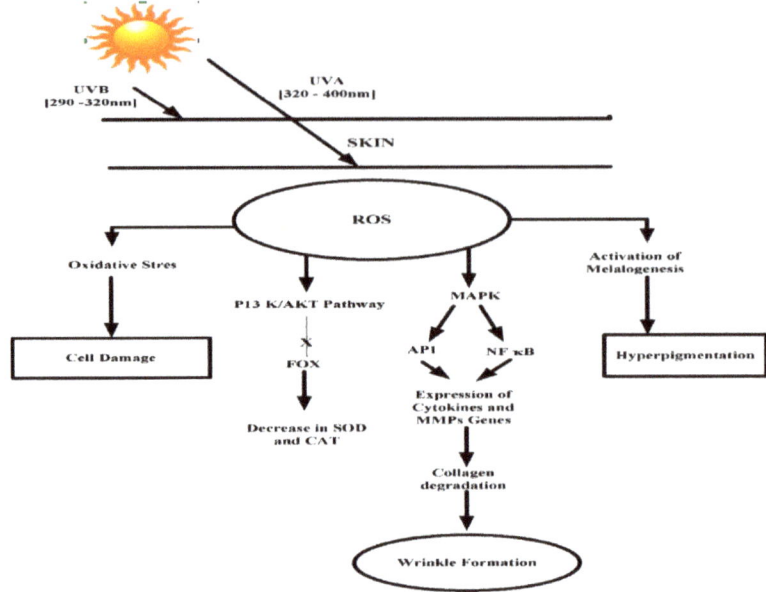

Figure 2. UV induced signaling pathway involved in premature skin aging. Mitogen-activated protein kinase (MAPK), matrix metalloproteinase (MMP), nuclear factor kappa-light-chain-enhancer of activated B cells (NF-κB), activator protein 1 (AP-1).

4. Bacteria-Induced Skin Damage-Acne Vulgaris

Acne vulgaris is a prevalent, chronic skin disorder which affects most of the adult and leads to scar marks. Acne vulgaris is a formation of lesions and prevalently caused by *Propionibacterium acnes*. Acne is spread by enzymes such as lipase, protease, hyaluronidase, and acid phosphatase produced by *P. acnes* [37]. The infection of *P. acne* triggers the immune response by the release of cytokine (IL-12 and IL-8) and the antimicrobial peptide (β-defensins) expression [38]. IL-8 stimulates neutrophils movement which leads to the formation of acne lesions and pus. Neutrophils consequently produce free radicals for killing the bacteria. This excess production of free radicals leads to the development of the inflammatory responses [39]. *Staphylococcus aureus* and *Staphylococcus epidermidis* are also the normal flora of human skin may also cause acne inflammatory response but are less significant than *P. acnes* in this process [40].

5. Seaweeds a Potential Source in the Cosmetic Industry

Nowadays People prefer cosmetic products that have natural ingredients than chemical ones. As the products with natural ingredients are safe to use without any side effects, many consumers go in search of natural products to keep themselves look young with healthy skin. Due to this, the cosmetic industry has also focussed on the ingredients that are derived from natural resources like plant, algae, microbes, and their metabolites. The marine world is extremely demanding for a wide variety of species with multiple bioactive compounds. Macroalgae are major resources for the active compound with a wide variety of applications in many fields (Figure 3) [16].

Macroalgae or seaweeds are the aquatic, photosynthetic organisms taxonomically categorized as algae, and they divided into three groups based on their pigment, the Rhodophyceae (red algae), Phaeophyceae (brown algae), and Chlorophyceae (green algae). Marine algae are considered as sea vegetables which are also used for consumption. Since ancient times seaweeds are also used as an alternative medicine for skin-related diseases. Many studies revealed the potentiality of seaweeds and their major role in antioxidant, antitumor, anti-inflammatory, anti-lipedemic, anti-microbial, and also their anti-allergic properties. Wide applications of seaweeds are based on the valuable bioactive compounds and potent bioactivity. In addition, the compounds derived from marine algae have been given considerable importance in developing a cosmeceutical product [41]. Seaweed compounds—including phenolic compounds, polysaccharides, pigments, PUFA, sterols, proteins, peptides, and mycosporine-like amino acid (MAA)—exhibited a wide range of bioactivity that can be used as active ingredients in cosmetic products (Figure 3) [7,42]. Phenolic compounds are the water-soluble secondary metabolites that have numerous biological activities [43]. It is a diverse group of compounds and the common structural features shared by all the phenol groups. Based on the number of substituents, phenolic compounds can be divided into simple phenols or polyphenols. Flavonoids and gallic acid are the building blocks of polyphenols. Phenolic compounds from seaweeds, like *Ecklonia cava* Kjellman and *Ishige okamurae* Yendo, are proven to have many bioactivities—including anti-oxidant, anti-microbial, anti-inflammatory, anti-cancer, etc. Antioxidant activity of seaweeds is mainly due to the presence of phenolic compounds [43,44]. Among the many phenolic compounds extracted from seaweeds, phlorotannins from brown seaweed are the most important secondary metabolites, with a wide range of functional bioactivity [45]. Phlorotannins are phloroglucinol-based polyphenols found in Marine brown algae. Phloroglucinol units linked to each other in various ways to form phlorotannins [46]. Marine brown algae such as *Ecklonia cava* Kjellman, *E. stolonifera* Okamura, *E. kurome* Okamura, *Ishige okamurae* Yendo, *Hizikia fusiformis* (Harvey) Okamura, *Eisenia bicyclis* (Kjellman) Setchell *Undaria pinnatifida* (Harvey) Suringar, *Sargassum thunbergii* (Mertens ex Roth) Kuntze, and *Laminaria japonica*. Areschoug have been studied the biological activity of phlorotannins [47,48]. Phlorotannins are well known for their wide-ranging applications which include anti-melanogenesis, anti-aging, and antioxidant [49–52]. As a result of the bioactivities, the application of phlorotannins on pharmaceutical, nutraceutical, and cosmeceutical advances [43,53,54].

Polysaccharides are the most important compounds present in seaweeds and are well documented for its biological activity. The green seaweed-like Ulva has the high content of polysaccharide comprises of 65% of dry weight. The other seaweeds that have a large amount of polysaccharide are Ascophyllum, Porphyra, and Palmaria species. The important polysaccharides are ulvan from green seaweeds, fucoidan, alginate, and laminarin from brown seaweeds, agar, and carrageenan from red seaweeds. In this, agar and alginate are used widely in the food industry as thickening and gelling agents. Fucoidan, ulvan, and carrageenan are sulfated polysaccharides that have wide application in many fields. Among these polysaccharides, the fucoidan from brown seaweed has been studied enormously for their bioactivity including antioxidant, anticancer, antimicrobial, hyperlipedemic, anti-inflammatory, etc. [4]. In recent days, many studies recommend the use of polysaccharide as an active ingredient in cosmetic formulations. Polysaccharides have a huge number of cosmetic roles such as hair conditioners, moisturizers, emulsifiers, wound-healing agents, and as a thickening agent [55,56].

Proteins are macromolecules made up of one or more amino acids. Seaweeds are a good source of amino acid. Amino acids are one of the important constitutes of natural moisturizing factor which prevents the water loss in the skin [57]. Seaweeds have amino acids, such as alanine, proline, arginine, serine, histidine, and tyrosine. Palmaria and Porphyra have the maximum amount of arginine, which is considered a natural moisturizing factor that can be used in cosmetic products. Mycosporine-like amino acids are water-soluble low molecular weight molecules. They are categorized by cyclohexane joined with nitrogen as a substitute for amino acid, amino alcohol, or amino group [57]. For seaweeds exposed to extreme stress including UV radiation, Mycosporine-like amino acids defend seaweed from UV radiation and act as a potent photo protector candidate. It also involved in radical scavenging and DNA repair systems. Hence, they have received more attention as UV protection and antioxidant agents in the cosmetic industry [3,16,58]. Furthermore, in recent years, peptides have drawn attention in the field of skincare due to their binding specificity to the target cells and their ability to change the physiological functions in the skin. Bioactivity depends on the composition of amino acids.

Macroalgae contain a large variety of pigments which absorb the light for photosynthesis. The green algae contain the pigment similar to the plants namely chlorophylls a, b, and carotenoids. The red algae have photosynthetic pigments such as chlorophyll a and the phycobilins such as R-phycocyanin and R-phycoerythrin and carotenoids, mostly β-carotene, lutein, and zeaxanthin. The brown algae pigments include the chlorophylls a and c, fucoxanthin, and carotenoids. The pigment act as a shield to the cells from UV irradiation [59]. Seaweeds are an important source of vitamin A, vitamin B, vitamin C, vitamin D, and vitamin E which are widely used in skincare.

The lipid content of seaweeds is generally low and less than 4% of the dried mass, whereas *Sargassum kjellmaniamum* Yendo contains more than 6% [60]. Lipids such as essential fatty acid, glycolipids, sterols, triglycerides, and phospholipids are found in seaweeds. Polyunsaturated fatty acid (PUFA) present in seaweeds is higher than in terrestrial plants. Seaweed fatty acids have anti-allergic and anti-inflammatory activities and also act as an emollient that protects the skin from water loss [61].

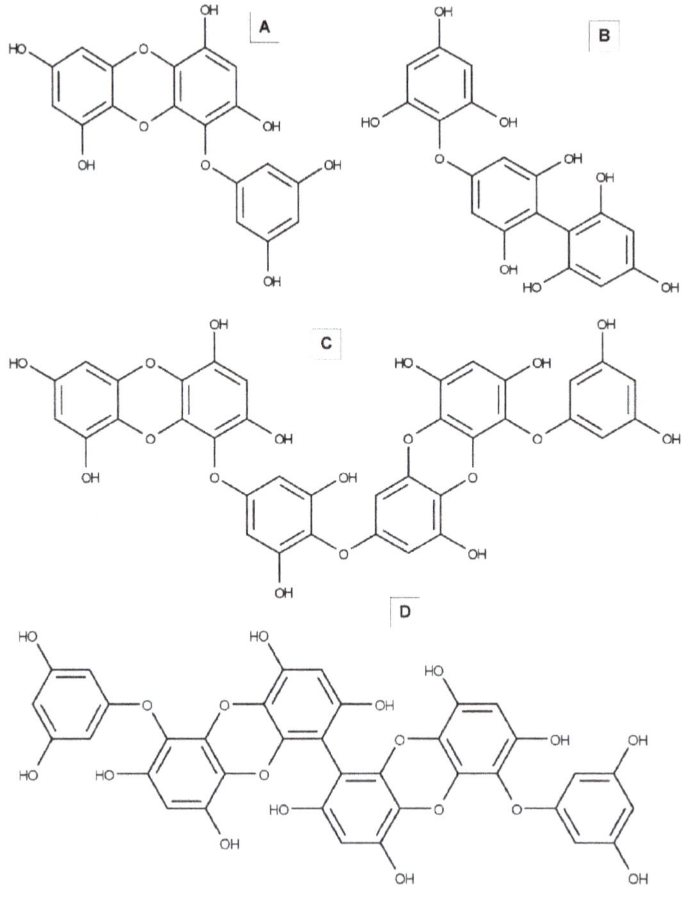

Figure 3. Cont.

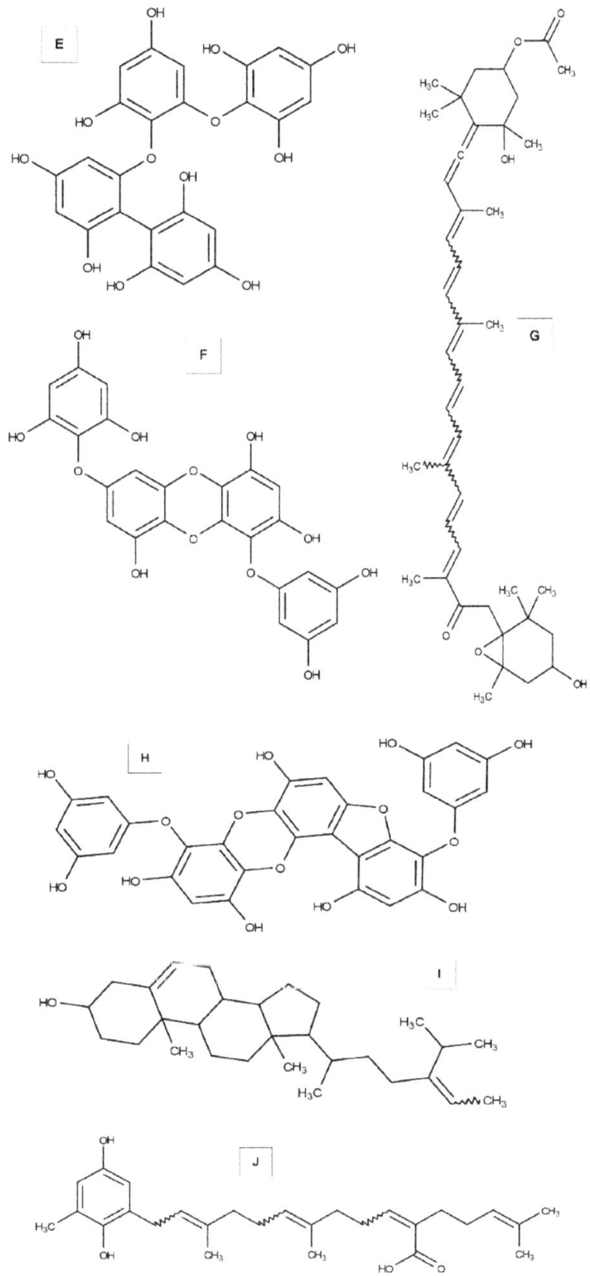

Figure 3. *Cont.*

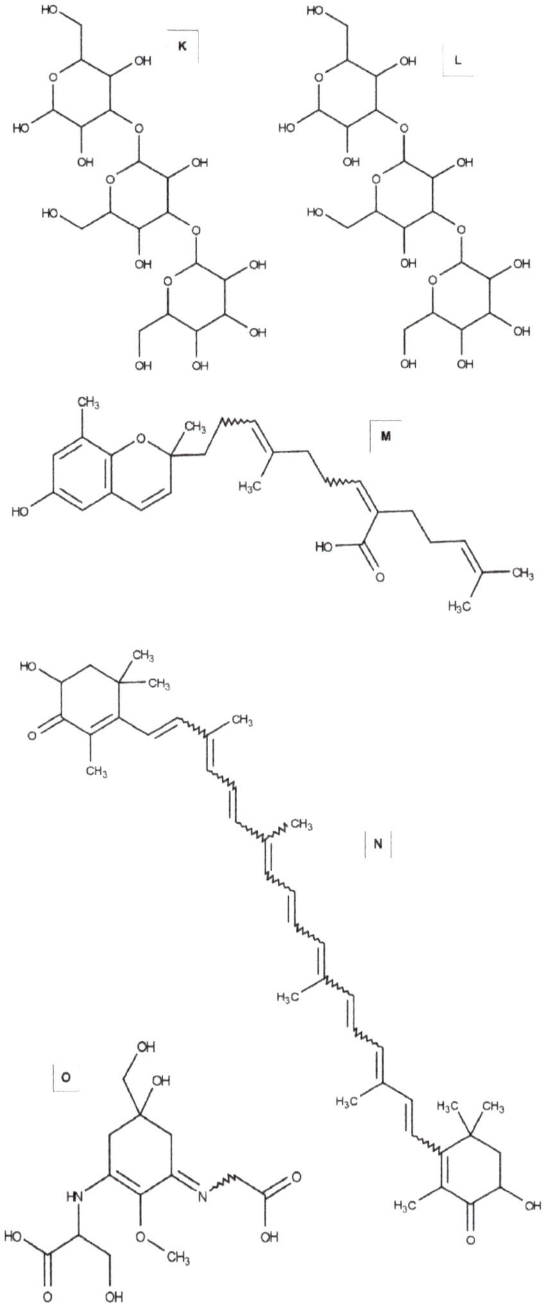

Figure 3. Seaweed bioactive compounds with skincare potentials. (**A**) Eckol; (**B**) Fucophloroethol; (**C**) Dieckol; (**D**) 6,6 Bieckol; (**E**) Fucodiphloroethol G; (**F**) 7-phloroeckol; (**G**) Fucoxanthin; (**H**) phlorofucofuroeckol; (**I**) Fucosterol; (**J**) Sargahydroquinoic acid; (**K**) Laminarin; (**L**) Porphyra 334, (**M**) Sargachromenol; (**N**) Astaxanthin; (**O**) Shinorine [3,22,42,47,57].

6. Skincare Application of Seaweeds

In recent years, seaweeds have been most desirable source of research for their bioactivity and bioactive compounds like polyphenols, fucoidan, phlorotannins, carotenoids, etc. Beauty care products have been focused on compounds with potential antioxidant activity, MMPs, and tyrosinase inhibitory activity in order to reduce ROS caused by UV radiation and also to delay skin aging.

6.1. Tyrosinase Inhibition Activity of Seaweed

Tyrosinase is the enzyme that catalyzes the synthesis of melanin, a pigment that is responsible for skin color. Hyperpigmentation is caused due to the abnormal accumulation of melanin pigments in the skin. Overexposure to UV rays induces abnormal melanin synthesis which results in skin pigmentation. Tyrosinase inhibitors may act as a candidate for the control of hyperpigmentation or skin whitening as the tyrosinase catalyzes the melanogenesis [62]. The search for natural tyrosinase inhibitors becomes a great interest for non-toxic and active skin whitening ingredients. Hence, skin whitening agents derived from seaweeds could be advantageous for the cosmetic industry. Researchers screened various seaweed extracts for tyrosinase inhibition activity and found that *Ishige okamurae* Yendo, *Endarachne binghamiae* J.Agardh, *Schizymenia dubyi* (Chauvin ex Duby) J.Agardh, *Ecklonia cava, E. stolonifera* Okamura, and *Sargassum silquastrum* (Mertens ex Turner) C.Agardh showed profound tyrosinase activity and significantly reduced the content of the melanin [63–65]. *S. polycystum* hexane extract had no inhibitory activity on mushroom tyrosinase. However, it showed potential activity on cellular tyrosinase inhibition when examined on cellular tyrosinase [66]. Dieckol is a phlorotannin derivative isolated from *E. stolonifera* showed the tyrosinase inhibition activity with the IC50 of 2.16 µg/mL [67,68]. Fucoxanthin is a carotenoid present in the seaweed exhibits tyrosinase inhibition activity when treated orally and also applied topically in UVB-induced guinea pig [69]. Many studies proved that sulfated polysaccharide, fucoidan extracted from Fucus sp., Sargassum sp., and Laminaria sp. can also be used as a promising tyrosinase inhibitor [70–72]. Fucoidan, the polysaccharide extracted from the brown seaweed such as *Chnoospora minima* (Hering) Papenfuss and *Sargassum polycystum* C.Agardh inhibit the activity of collagenase, elastase and also tyrosinase [70]. Tyrosinase activity was increased by the low molecular weight fucoidan extracted from *Sargassum fusiforme* (Harvey) Setchell [73]. Park et al. [74] were also demonstrated the increased inhibitory activity in low molecular weight fucoidan in a melanoma cell.

Several signaling pathways involved in melanin synthesis. The cAMP pathway is one of the prime regulatory mechanism which increases the expression of microphthalmia-associated transcription factor -MITF. MITF regulates the expression of tyrosinase, tyrosinase-related protein 1,2 which is required for melanogenesis. Ethyl acetate fraction of *Leathesia difformis* Areschoug showed the effect on melanin synthesis and cellular tyrosinase activity by downregulating the CREB, PKA, and cAMP pathways [75]. ERK pathway involves in anti-melanogenesis. The phosphorylation of ERK degrades the MITF which leads to the suppression of melanin synthesis [23]. Fucoidan plays a major role in the anti-melanogenesis by ERK phosphorylation [76]. Another study showed the inhibitory activity of fucoidan on cellular melanin and tyrosinase but in contrast, it lacks the inhibitory activity on the expression of TRP1, TRP2, and MITF [71]. Sargahydroquinoic acid, sargachromenol, and sargaquinoic acid from *S. serratifolium* (C.Agardh) C.Agardh decreased the α-MSH-activated melanogenesis in melanoma cells through the inhibition of CREB signaling pathways without affecting ERK pathway [77]. Sulfated galactans, the polysaccharide from *G. fisheri*, showed no potential inhibition on tyrosinase activity and it proved to be suppressed the activity of tyrosinase by downregulating the MITF, TRP1,2, and tyrosinase mRNA expression, which was concluded by RT-PCR and ELISA [78].

6.2. Collagenase and Elastase Inhibition Activity of Seaweed

The MMPs are a family of degradative enzymes particularly collagenase which is responsible for the degradation of skin matrix especially collagen due to which occurs the skin sagging. The same way enzyme elastase degrades the elastin. This process leads to wrinkles. The compound that inhibits collagenase and elastase activity might act as an active ingredient in an anti-aging product. Overexposure of UV produces ROS which activates the mitogen-activated protein kinases followed by the phosphorylation of transcription factor activator protein1 results in the upregulation of MMPs.

Seaweed polysaccharides play a major role in inhibiting collagenase and elastase activity. Sulfated polysaccharides from *Sargassum fusiforme* (Harvey). Setchell potentially inhibited the activity of intracellular collagenase and elastase by regulating the NF-κB, AP-1, and MAPKs pathways in HDF cells radiated by UVB [79]. Fucoidans isolated from the *Chnoospora minima* (Hering) Papenfuss and *Sargassum polycystum* C.Agardh showed elastase and collagenase inhibition in a dose-dependent manner [70]. Fucoidan inhibited the expression of MMP 1 in UVB-induced dermal fibroblast cells in a dose-dependent manner. It suppressed the expression of MMP by inhibiting the ERK pathway and reduced the expression of MMP1 mRNA. Furthermore, Fucoidan also inhibited the activity of the MMP1 promoter and increased the expression of Type 1 procollagen synthesis [80,81].

Ryu et al. [82] proved that methanol extracts of *Corallina pilulifera* J.V.Lamouroux that are rich in phenolic content inhibited the MMP 2,9 expressions in a dose-dependent manner in UV-induced dermal fibroblast cells. Phlorotannin extracted from *Eisenia bicyclis* (Kjellman) Setchell, *Ecklonia cava* Kjellman, and *E. stolonifera* Okamura strongly inhibit the MMP1 expression. Similarly, phlorotannin from *E. cava* inhibit the expression of MMP 2,9 and also reduced the activity of MMPs at 10 μg/mL. Eckol, dieckol, dioxinodehydroeckol, and bieckol are responsible for the inhibition of MMPs in human dermal fibroblast cells. This previous study also suggested that these phlorotannin derivatives inhibited the expression of NF-kappa B and AP-1 reporter resulting in the suppression of MMP expression [51,83]. The results of all these studies suggest that phlorotannin may act as an active ingredient in preventing photoaging of the skin.

The peptides, namely PYP1-5 and Porphyra 334 from *Porphyra yezoensis* f. coreana Ueda, increased the production of elastin and collagen and decrease the expression of MMP protein [84]. PYP1-5 induced the collagen synthesis by initiate the TGF-b/Smad signaling pathway by increasing the expression of TIMP-1,2 and TGF-b1 protein expression [85]. Likewise, Sargachromanol extracted from *S. horneri* (Turner) C.Agardh also activated the TIMP1,2 and downregulate the expression of MMP [86]. The sterol compound, fucosterol from marine brown algae also enhanced the production of type I procollagen and suppressed the expression of MMPs in human keratinocytes cell by deactivating the MAPK pathway [59]. All these studies revealed the potential protection of seaweed bio compounds towards UVA-induced collagen degradation.

6.3. Hyaluronidase Inhibition

Hyaluronidase is an enzyme that degrades the hyaluronic acid present in the extracellular matrix which results in the skin aging process. Very few studies have been focused on Hyaluronidase inhibition. Phlorotannins derivatives—such as fucophloroethol, fucodiphloroethol, fucotriphloroethol, 7-phloroeckol, phlorofucofuroeckol, and bieckol/dieckol extracted from *Cystoseira nodicaulis* (Withering) M.Roberts exhibited the hyaluronidase activity with the IC50 of 0.73 mg/mL and also proved that the higher molecular weight displayed the strongest activity [87]. Phlorotannins derivatives—such as dieckol, eckol, bieckol, and phlorofucofuroeckol A—extracted from *Eisenia bicyclis* (Kjellman) Setchell and *Ecklonia kurome* Okamura exhibited potent inhibition towards hyaluronidase. Among these phlorotannin derivatives, bieckol exhibited the strongest inhibition with an IC50 value of 40 μM [88].

6.4. Photoprotection Ability

When the skin is exposed to UV radiation, UV rays penetrate into dermis and epidermis and induce the production of ROS which cause damage to DNA. This results in hyperpigmentation, premature aging, sunburn, skin cancer, etc. The extensive use of photoprotection products will help to get rid of the effect caused by the sun UV rays. The macroalgae are exposed to extreme conditions such as UV radiation and it produces the ROS. The seaweeds produce many secondary metabolites that play as an antioxidant that helps to combat those ROS. These antioxidant substances included pigments like fucoxanthin, carotenoids, mycosporine-like amino acids (MAA), and phenols such as phlorotannins and scytonemins [89,90]. These bioactive components are capable of absorbing the UV radiation and keep the human fibroblast cells from UV-induced aging. These secondary metabolites that act as UV filters/sunscreen with antioxidant activity can be extensively used in cosmetic products. Polysaccharides such as fucoidan, laminarin, and alginate extracted from brown algae like *Fucus vesiculosus var. alternans* C.Agardh, *Sargassum sp*, *Turbinaria conoides f. laticuspidata* W.R.Taylor, possessed potent anti-oxidative activity [89].

Cardozo et al. [91] studied the MAA from the red algae, *Gracilaria birdiae* E.M.Plastino & E.C.Oliveira, *G. domingensis* (Kützing) Sonder ex Dickie, and *G. tenuistipitata* C.F.Chang & B.-M.Xia which exhibited the photoprotection activity. Heo et al. [92] studied the photoprotection ability of fucoxanthin on UV induced human fibroblast cells and showed to significantly inhibit the cell damage at 61.24% at 250 µM. Fucoxanthin successfully suppressed the cell damage and apoptotic stimulation induced by UV-B. Fucoxanthin extracted from *Sargassum fusiforme* (Harvey) Setchell and *S.saliquastrum* (Mertens ex Turner) C.Agardh exhibited strong antioxidant activity against DPPH and hydrogen peroxide. Urikura et al. [93] reported that fucoxanthin reduced UV induced ROS in the hairless mice and also suppress the MMP expression.

A red pigment, astaxanthin, exhibited strong antioxidant activity and protects from peroxidation by scavenging the radicals. The activity may be due to the presence of conjugated polyene and terminal ring moieties of astaxanthin help to trap the radicals and therefore exhibit potent antioxidative and photoprotective agents. It also blocked cytokine production. The topical application also demonstrated the photoprotection effect against the cell damage caused by UVB radiation [94]. Lyons et al. [95] studied the photoprotection exhibited by the algal extract that contains astaxanthin by reducing DNA damage and also conserve the cellular antioxidant enzymes in human cells irradiated by UVA. Tetraprenyltoluquinol chromane meroterpenoid extracted from *Sargassum muticum* (Yendo) Fensholt showed potent photoprotection against UV-A radiation and also inhibit the accumulation of intracellular ROS in human dermal fibroblast cells [96].

Phlorotannins extracted from *E. cava* and *E. stolonifera* also provided photoprotection towards UVB rays by reducing the cell damage caused by UVB radiation which is measured by comet assay. It also showed the inhibition against UVB induced oxidative damage with antioxidant activities and also upgrading in cell viability [63,68]. Phlorotannins extracted from *Halidrys siliquosa* (Linnaeus) Lyngbye proved the sunscreen ability based on the sun protection factor and UV-A protection factor. It also was shown to exhibit strong antioxidant activity and proved to have the ability to kill bacteria [97]. Vo et al. [98] isolated fucofuroeckol-A, which exhibited the photoprotection activity against damage caused by UVB radiation. The aqueous extracts of *Hydropuntia cornea* (J.Agardh) M.J.Wynne and *Gracilariopsis longissima* (S.G.Gmelin) Steentoft, L.M.Irvine & Farnham exhibited a photo-protective activity with the sun protection factor of 7.5 and 4.8. The MAA Porphyra-334 and Shinorine were extracted from *Porphyra rosengurttii* J.Coll & J.Cox tested for their photo-protective activity and photo-stability without producing any free radicals. The formulated product of these two demonstrated wide-ranging protection against UV. MAA can also absorb UV light and also act as a sunscreen [99,100]. Porphyra-334 from the *Porphyra umbilicalis* Kützing reduced the intracellular ROS induced by UV-A radiation and also suppressed the expression of MMPs. It also acts as a better UV filter compared to synthetic sunscreens [84,101].

6.5. Moisture Retention Ability

Maintaining moisture in the skin is important to skincare and it improves the skin texture and state, i.e., young and healthy. Extract from *Undaria pinnatifida* (Harvey) Suringar, *Codium tomentosum* Stackhouse, *Durvillea antarctica* (Chamisso) Hariot, *Cladosiphon okamuranus* Tokida, *A. nodosum* (Linnaeus) Le Jolis, *Pediastrum duplex* Meyen, and *Polysiphonia lanosa* (Linnaeus). Tandy exhibited skin hydrating properties and protects the skin from dryness. Polysaccharides have maximum water holding capacity which can act as a humectant and moisturizer in cosmetic industry. Polysaccharides from *Laminaria japonica* Areschoug were shown to have greater hydrating and moisturizing effects than hyaluronic acid. The formulation prepared by incorporating *Laminaria japonica* extract shown to improve the skin moisture [3,4,6]. Shao et al. [102] isolated sulfated polysaccharide from the green algae *Ulva fasciata* Delile displayed a higher capability both in the moisture-absorption and moisture retention for 96 h when compared with glycerol. Wang et al. [103] extracted the polysaccharide from *Saccharina japonica* (Areschoug) C.E.Lane, C.Mayes, Druehl & G.W.Saunders; *Porphyra haitanensis* T.J.Chang & B.F.Zheng; *Codium fragile* (Suringar) Hariot; *Enteromorpha linza* (Linnaeus) J.Agardh and *Bryopsis plumose* (Hudson) C.Agardh and studied for the moisture absorption and retention. The authors also proved that the sulfate content and molecular weight plays a major role in the moisture-holding capacity [103].

6.6. Antimicrobial Activity

Antimicrobial property of the seaweeds can be used in cosmetic products as a preservative that could delay the shelf life of the cosmetic product by killing the microorganisms especially fungi that could spoil the product. Seaweeds exhibited antifungal activity for possible use in substituting chemical preservations. Seaweeds such as *Sargassum vulgare* C.Agardh, *Colpomenia sinuosa* (Mertens ex Roth) Derbès & Solier, *Dictyopteris membranacea* Batters, *Cystoseira barbata* (Stackhouse) C.Agardh, and *Dictyota* dichotoma (Hudson) J.V.Lamouroux, showed the strongest antifungal effect against *Cladosporium cladosporioides, Alternaria alternata, Fusarium oxysporum, Aspergillus niger, Epicoccum nigrum, A.ochraceus, Penicillium citrinum*, and *A. flavus* [104]. Extract from *Halimeda tuna* (J.Ellis & Solander) J.V.Lamouroux also showed the antifungal activity against *Candida albicans, Aspergillus niger, A. flavus, Alternaria, Trichophyton rubrum, Epidermophyton floccossum, T. mentagrophytes*, and *Penicillium sp.* [44]. Saidani et al. [105] studied the antifungal activity of seaweed, in which the seaweed, *Rhodomela confervoides* (Hudson) P.C.Silva reported for the strongest inhibition against *Candida albicans* and *Mucor ramaniannus* and the seaweed, *Padina pavonica* (Linnaeus) Thivy against the *Candida albicans*. Phlorotannin derivative, Dieckol from *E.cava* showed the antifungal activity with the MIC of 200 μM against *Trichophyton rubrum* [106]. Alghazeer et al. [107] screened the 19 seaweed extracts and tested them for their antibacterial activity. Their data revealed that all the extracts showed inhibition against gram-positive and gram-negative bacteria including *E. coli, Staphylococcus aureus*, and *S. epidermis*. Among the 19 species the brown algae *Cystoseira crinita* Duby showed the strongest antibacterial activity. *Ulva rigidis* also showed the strongest inhibition against *S. aureus* and *Escherichia coli* [108]. These studies confirmed the role of seaweeds and their extract as a preservative.

The skin may also be contaminated by some microorganisms which could create skin problems that can be overcome by the antimicrobial potential of the seaweeds derived biological compounds. *Propionibacterium acnes, Staphylococcus aureus*, and *S. epidermis* are some of the normal microflora present in the skin. *P. acnes* is the main inducers of acne. *S. aureus* and *S. epidermis* are harmless microflora, but it can enter the skin epidermis through the wound and cause infection by secreting the toxins [109]. This leads to pimples, abscesses, and also blisters. Therefore, the antimicrobial potential of seaweed could be used effectively in cosmetic formulations in the prevention of skin acne [4,109]. Ruxton and Jenkins [110] discussed the anti-acne activity of seaweed oligosaccharide-zinc complex extracted from *Laminaria digitata* (Hudson) J.V.Lamouroux which also reduces the signs of acne by reducing the sebum production. Ethyl acetate extraction of *Fucus evanescens* C.Agardh showed antibacterial ability against methicillin-resistant *S. aureus* and *P. acnes* [111]. Choi et al. [112] screened 57 seaweed species for the antimicrobial activity against *P. acnes* in which 15 species exhibited the antiacne activity. The methanol extract of *E. cava, E. kurome, Ishige sinicola* (Setchell & N.L.Gardner) Chihara, and *Symphyocladia latiuscula* (Harvey) Yamada showed potent activity with the maximum MIC of 0.31 mg/mL. Phlorotannins isolated from *E. bicyclis* showed effective inhibitory activity against human acne producing bacteria such as *P. acnes, Staphylococcus aureus*, and *S. epidermidis* [113]. Carrageenan extracted from red algae of the genus Corallina inhibited the bacteria *S. epidermidis* with a MIC of 0.325 mg/mL, whereas sulfated galactan from Corallina showed the bactericidal activity against *Enterococcus faecalis* and *S. epidermidis* [114]. These studies defined that the seaweed compound can act as an ingredient for the anti-acne product due to its inhibitory activity against *P. acnes*, *S. aureus*, and *S. epidermidis*.

7. Conclusions

Due to the overexposure of human skin to several environmental stress—such as UV and pollution—it increases the production of ROS that leads to many skin related problems such as hyperpigmentation, premature aging, etc. The seaweeds in the marine environment have the biosynthesis of secondary metabolites for its survival under stress conditions. These biologically active components present in the seaweeds paves the way to be used as an active ingredient in the cosmetic industries due to their potent skin protection ability. The active components from the seaweeds could be used as an antioxidant, antibacterial whitening agent, anti-aging, and anti-acne, and also for moisturization in cosmetic industries.

8. Future Perspectives

This review examines the potentiality of seaweed-derived compounds in applications to combat skin whitening and aging in cosmetic industries. Though most of the seaweeds are studied for its cosmetic properties, still many species are not explored. Hence, the standardization of cost-effective and efficient methods to extract the bioactive compounds with higher productivity and activity is in demand. In addition to efficiency, the molecular mechanism of their activity and safety concerns of these compounds are very significant for future challenges in the cosmetics industry.

Author Contributions: V.J. conceived, organized, and wrote the manuscript. P.P., N.H., and M.A. analyzed the information from the references. H.D. and M.A. revised the manuscript and H.D. contributed to the final version of the manuscript.

Funding: This research was supported by the China Agriculture Research System (CARS-50), Start-Up Funding of Shantou University (NTF18004), and Department of Education of Guangdong Province (2017KQNCX076).

Conflicts of Interest: The authors declare no conflict of interest.

Abbreviations

ECM	Extracellular matrix
HA	Hyaluronic acid
ROS	Reactive oxygen species
TRP	Tyrosinase related protein
MITF	Microphthalmia-associated transcription factor
cAMP	Adenosine 3′,5′-cyclic monophosphate (cyclic AMP)
CREB	cAMP response element-binding
ERK	Extracellular receptor kinase
ASP	Agonist stimulating protein
SCF	Stem cell factor
Wnt	Wingless-related integration site
MC1R	Melanocortin 1 receptor
α-MSH	α-Melanocyte-stimulating hormone
MAPK	Mitogen-activated protein kinase
MMP	Matrix metalloproteinase
NF-κB	Nuclear factor kappa-light-chain-enhancer of activated B cells
AP-1	Activator protein 1
IL-12 and IL-8	Interleukin 12
TLR2	Toll-like receptor 2
MAA	Mycosporine-like amino acid
PUFA	Polyunsaturated fatty acid

References

1. Siahaan, E.A.; Pangestuti, R.; Munandar, H.; Kim, S.-K. Cosmeceuticals properties of Sea Cucumbers: Prospects and trends. *Cosmetics* **2017**, *4*, 26. [CrossRef]
2. Kligman, A.M. Cosmetics A dermatologists looks to the future: Promises and problems. *Dermatol. Clin.* **2000**, *18*, 699–709. [CrossRef]
3. Pimentel, F.; Alves, R.; Rodrigues, F.; Oliveira, M. Macroalgae-Derived Ingredients for Cosmetic Industry—An Update. *Cosmetics* **2017**, *5*, 2. [CrossRef]
4. Wang, H.M.D.; Chen, C.C.; Huynh, P.; Chang, J.S. Exploring the potential of using algae in cosmetics. *Bioresour. Technol.* **2015**, *184*, 355–362. [CrossRef]
5. Arora, N.; Agarwal, S.; Murthy, R.S.R. Latest technology advances in cosmeceuticals. *Int. J. Pharm. Sci. Drug Res.* **2012**, *4*, 168–182.
6. Łopaciuk, A.; Łoboda, M. Global beauty industry trends in the 21st century. In *Management, Knowledge and Learning International Conference, Zadar, Croatia, 19–21 June 2013*; ToKnowPress: Celje, Slovenia, 2013; pp. 19–21.
7. Priyan, S.F.; Kim, K.N.; Kim, D.; Jeon, Y.J. Algal polysaccharides: Potential bioactive substances for cosmeceutical applications. *Crit. Rev. Biotechnol.* **2019**, *39*, 99–113. [CrossRef]
8. Gao, X.H.; Zhang, L.; Wei, H.; Chen, H.D. Efficacy and safety of innovative cosmeceuticals. *Clin. Dermatol.* **2008**, *26*, 367–374. [CrossRef]
9. Takizawa, T.; Imai, T.; Onose, J.; Ueda, M.; Tamura, T.; Mitsumori, K.; Izumi, K.; Hirose, M. Enhancement of hepatocarcinogenesis by kojic acid in rat two-stage models after initiation with N-bis (2-hydroxypropyl) nitrosamine or N-diethylnitrosamine. *Toxicol. Sci.* **2004**, *81*, 43–49. [CrossRef]
10. Ahmed, A.B.; Adel, M.; Karimi, P.; Peidayesh, M. Pharmaceutical, cosmeceutical, and traditional applications of marine carbohydrates. *Adv. Food Nutr. Res.* **2014**, *73*, 197–220.
11. Sudhakar, K.; Mamat, R.; Samykano, M.; Azmi, W.H.; Ishak, W.F.W.; Yusaf, T. An overview of marine macroalgae as bioresource. *Renew. Sustain. Energy Rev.* **2018**, *91*, 165–179. [CrossRef]
12. Farage, M.A.; Miller, K.W.; Elsner, P.; Maibach, H.I. Structural characteristics of the aging skin: A review. *Cutan. Ocul. Toxicol.* **2007**, *26*, 343–357. [CrossRef] [PubMed]
13. Meyer, W.; Seegers, U. Basics of skin structure and function in elasmobranchs: A review. *J. Fish Biol.* **2012**, *80*, 1940–1967. [CrossRef] [PubMed]
14. Rahman, M.A. Collagen of extracellular matrix from marine invertebrates and its medical applications. *Mar. Drugs* **2019**, *17*, 118. [CrossRef] [PubMed]
15. Ebrahimzadeh, M.A.; Enayatifard, R.; Khalili, M.; Ghaffarloo, M.; Saeedi, M.; Charati, J.Y. Correlation between sun protection factor and antioxidant activity, phenol and flavonoid contents of some medicinal plants. *Iran. J. Pharm. Res.* **2014**, *13*, 1041–1047.
16. Berthon, J.Y.; Nachat-Kappes, R.; Bey, M.; Cadoret, J.P.; Renimel, I.; Filaire, E. Marine algae as attractive source to skin care. *Free Radic. Res.* **2017**, *51*, 555–567. [CrossRef]
17. González, S.; Fernández-Lorente, M.; Gilaberte-Calzada, Y. The latest on skin photoprotection. *Clin. Dermatol.* **2008**, *26*, 614–626. [CrossRef]
18. Roy, A.; Sahu, R.K.; Matlam, M.; Deshmukh, V.K.; Dwivedi, J.; Jha, A.K. In vitro techniques to assess the proficiency of skin care cosmetic formulations. *Pharmacogn. Rev.* **2013**, *7*, 97–106.
19. Parvez, S.; Kang, M.; Chung, H.S.; Cho, C.; Hong, M.C.; Shin, M.K.; Bae, H. Survey and mechanism of skin depigmenting and lightening agents. *Phytother. Res.* **2006**, *20*, 921–934. [CrossRef]
20. Chang, T.S. Natural melanogenesis inhibitors acting through the down-regulation of tyrosinase activity. *Materials* **2012**, *5*, 1661–1685. [CrossRef]
21. Imokawa, G.; Mishima, Y. Importance of glycoproteins in the initiation of melanogenesis: An electron microscopic study of B-16 melanoma cells after release from inhibition of glycosylation. *J. Investig. Dermatol.* **1986**, *87*, 319–325. [CrossRef]
22. Azam, M.; Choi, J.; Lee, M.S.; Kim, H.R. Hypopigmenting effects of brown algae-derived phytochemicals: A review on molecular mechanisms. *Mar. Drugs* **2017**, *15*, 297. [CrossRef] [PubMed]
23. D'Mello, S.; Finlay, G.; Baguley, B.; Askarian-Amiri, M. Signaling pathways in melanogenesis. *Int. J. Mol. Sci.* **2016**, *17*, 1144. [CrossRef] [PubMed]

24. Shin, H.; Hong, S.D.; Roh, E.; Jung, S.-H.; Cho, W.-J.; Hong Park, S.; Yoon, D.Y.; Ko, S.M.; Hwang, B.Y.; Hong, J.T. cAMP-dependent activation of protein kinase A as a therapeutic target of skin hyperpigmentation by diphenylmethylene hydrazinecarbothioamide. *Br. J. Pharmacol.* **2015**, *172*, 3434–3445. [CrossRef] [PubMed]
25. Wu, L.C.; Lin, Y.Y.; Yang, S.Y.; Weng, Y.T.; Tsai, Y.T. Antimelanogenic effect of c-phycocyanin through modulation of tyrosinase expression by upregulation of ERK and downregulation of p38 MAPK signaling pathways. *J. Biomed. Sci.* **2011**, *18*, 74. [CrossRef]
26. Chandra, M.; Levitt, J.; Pensabene, C.A. Hydroquinone therapy for post-inflammatory hyperpigmentation secondary to acne: Not just prescribable by dermatologists. *Acta Dermto Venereol.* **2012**, *92*, 232–235. [CrossRef]
27. Chou, T.H.; Ding, H.Y.; Hung, W.J.; Liang, C.H. Antioxidative characteristics and inhibition of α-melanocyte-stimulating hormone-stimulated melanogenesis of vanillin and vanillic acid from *Origanum vulgare*. *Exp. Dermatol.* **2010**, *19*, 742–750. [CrossRef]
28. Pilawa, B.; Buszman, E.; Latocha, M.; Wilczok, T. Free radicals in DOPA-melanin-chloroquine complexes. *Pol. J. Med. Phys. Eng.* **2007**, *10*, 35–42.
29. Makrantonaki, E.; Adjaye, J.; Herwig, R.; Brink, T.C.; Groth, D.; Hultschig, C. Age-specific hormonal decline is accompanied by transcriptional changes in human sebocytes in vitro. *Aging Cell* **2006**, *5*, 331–344. [CrossRef]
30. Pientaweeratch, S.; Panapisal, V.; Tansirikongkol, A. Antioxidant, anti-collagenase and anti-elastase activities of *Phyllanthus emblica*, *Manilkara zapota* and silymarin: An in vitro comparative study for anti-aging applications. *Pharm. Biol.* **2016**, *54*, 1865–1872. [CrossRef]
31. Kim, Y.H.; Chung, C.B.; Kim, J.G.; Ko, K.I.; Park, S.H.; Kim, J.H.; Kim, K.H. Anti-wrinkle activity of ziyuglycoside I isolated from a *Sanguisorba officinalis* root extract and its application as a cosmeceutical ingredient. *Biosci. Biotechnol. Biochem.* **2008**, *72*, 303–311. [CrossRef]
32. Leem, K.H. Effects of Olibanum extracts on the collagenase activity and procollagen synthesis in Hs68 human fibroblasts and tyrosinase activity. *Adv. Sci. Technol. Lett.* **2015**, *88*, 172–175.
33. Ndlovu, G.; Fouche, G.; Tselanyane, M.; Cordier, W.; Steenkamp, V. In vitro determination of the anti-aging potential of four southern African medicinal plants. *BMC Complement. Altern. Med.* **2013**, *13*, 304–311. [CrossRef] [PubMed]
34. Papakonstantinou, E.; Roth, M.; Karakiulakis, G. Hyaluronic acid: A key molecule in skin aging. *Dermato Endocrinol.* **2012**, *4*, 253–258. [CrossRef] [PubMed]
35. Stern, R.; Maibach, H.I. Hyaluronan in skin: Aspects of aging and its pharmacologic modulation. *Clin. Dermatol.* **2008**, *26*, 106–122. [CrossRef] [PubMed]
36. Girish, K.S.; Kemparaju, K. The magic glue hyaluronan and its eraser hyaluronidase: A biological overview. *Life Sci.* **2007**, *80*, 1921–1943. [CrossRef] [PubMed]
37. Patil, V.; Bandivadekar, A.; Debjani, D. Inhibition of *Propionibacterium acnes* lipase by extracts of Indian medicinal plants. *Int. J. Cosmet. Sci.* **2012**, *34*, 234–239. [CrossRef]
38. Tanghetti, E.A. The role of inflammation in the pathology of acne. *J. Clin. Aesthetic Dermatol.* **2013**, *6*, 27–35.
39. Poomanee, W.; Chaiyana, W.; Mueller, M.; Viernstein, H.; Khunkitti, W.; Leelapornpisid, P. In-vitro investigation of anti-acne properties of *Mangifera indica* L. kernel extract and its mechanism of action against *Propionibacterium acnes*. *Anaerobe* **2018**, *52*, 64–74.
40. Chomnawang, M.T.; Surassmo, S.; Nukoolkarn, V.S.; Gritsanapan, W. Antimicrobial effects of Thai medicinal plants against acne-inducing bacteria. *J. Ethnopharmacol.* **2005**, *10*, 330–333. [CrossRef]
41. Brunt, E.G.; Burgess, J.G. The promise of marine molecules as cosmetic active ingredients. *J. Cosmet. Sci.* **2018**, *40*, 1–15. [CrossRef]
42. Pallela, R.; Na-Young, Y.; Kim, S.K. Anti-photoaging and photoprotective compounds derived from marine organisms. *Mar. Drugs* **2010**, *8*, 1189–1202. [CrossRef]
43. Fernando, I.S.; Kim, M.; Son, K.T.; Jeong, Y.; Jeon, Y.J. Antioxidant activity of marine algal polyphenolic compounds: A mechanistic approach. *J. Med. Food* **2016**, *19*, 615–628. [CrossRef]
44. Indira, K.; Balakrishnan, S.; Srinivasan, M.; Bragadeeswaran, S.; Balasubramanian, T. Evaluation of in vitro antimicrobial property of seaweed (*Halimeda tuna*) from Tuticorin coast, Tamil Nadu, Southeast coast of India. *Afr. J. Biotechnol.* **2013**, *12*, 284–289.

45. Liu, N.; Fu, X.; Duan, D.; Xu, J.; Gao, X.; Zhao, L. Evaluation of bioactivity of phenolic compounds from the brown seaweed of *Sargassum fusiforme* and development of their stable emulsion. *J. Appl. Phycol.* **2018**, *30*, 1955–1970. [CrossRef]
46. Pérez, M.J.; Falqué, E.; Domínguez, H. Antimicrobial action of compounds from marine seaweed. *Mar. Drugs* **2016**, *14*, 52. [CrossRef]
47. Li, Y.X.; Wijesekara, I.; Li, Y.; Kim, S.K. Phlorotannins as bioactive agents from brown algae. *Process Biochem.* **2011**, *46*, 2219–2224. [CrossRef]
48. Zou, Y.; Qian, Z.-J.; Li, Y.; Kim, M.-M.; Lee, S.-H.; Kim, S.K. Antioxidant effects of phlorotannins isolated from *Ishige okamurae* in free radical mediated oxidative systems. *J. Agric. Food Chem.* **2008**, *56*, 7001–7009. [CrossRef]
49. Lee, M.S.; Yoon, H.D.; Kim, J.I.; Choi, J.S.; Byun, D.S.; Kim, H.R. Dioxinodehydroeckol inhibits melanin synthesis through PI3K/Akt signalling pathway in alpha-melanocyte-stimulating hormone-treated B16F10 cells. *Exp. Dermatol.* **2012**, *21*, 471–473. [CrossRef]
50. Kim, K.N.; Yang, H.M.; Kang, S.M.; Ahn, G.N.; Roh, S.W.; Lee, W.; Kim, D.K.; Jeon, Y.J. Whitening effect of octaphlorethol A isolated from *Ishige foliacea* in an in vivo zebrafish model. *J. Microbiol. Biotechnol.* **2015**, *25*, 448–451. [CrossRef]
51. Joe, M.J.; Kim, S.N.; Choi, H.Y.; Shin, W.S.; Park, G.M.; Kang, D.W.; Kim, Y.K. The inhibitory effects of eckol and dieckol from *Ecklonia stolonifera* on the expression of matrix metalloproteinase-1 in human dermal fibroblasts. *Biol. Pharm. Bull.* **2006**, *29*, 1735–1739. [CrossRef]
52. Jun, Y.J.; Lee, M.; Shin, T.; Yoon, N.; Kim, J.H.; Kim, H.R. Eckol enhances heme oxygenase-1 expression through activation of Nrf2/JNK pathway in HepG2 cells. *Molecules* **2014**, *19*, 15638–15652. [CrossRef] [PubMed]
53. Wijesekara, I.; Yoon, N.Y.; Kim, S.K. Phlorotannins from *Ecklonia cava* (Phaeophyceae): Biological activities and potential health benefits. *Biofactors* **2010**, *36*, 408–414. [CrossRef] [PubMed]
54. Saraf, S.; Kaur, C.D. Phytoconstituents as photoprotective novel cosmetic formulations. *Pharmacogn. Rev.* **2010**, *4*, 1–11. [CrossRef] [PubMed]
55. Venkatesan, J.; Anil, S.; Kim, S.K. Introduction to Seaweed Polysaccharides. In *Seaweed Polysaccharides*; Elseiver: Amsterdam, The Netherlands, 2017; pp. 1–9.
56. Percival, E. The polysaccharides of green, red and brown seaweeds: Their basic structure, biosynthesis and function. *Br. Phycol. J.* **1979**, *14*, 103–117. [CrossRef]
57. Pereira, L. Seaweeds as source of bioactive substances and skin care therapy—Cosmeceuticals, algotheraphy, and thalassotherapy. *Cosmetics* **2018**, *5*, 68. [CrossRef]
58. Pangestuti, R.; Siahaan, E.; Kim, S.K. Photoprotective substances derived from marine algae. *Mar. Drugs* **2018**, *16*, 399. [CrossRef]
59. Kim, M.S.; Oh, G.H.; Kim, M.J.; Hwang, J.K. Fucosterol inhibits matrix metalloproteinase expression and promotes type-1 procollagen production in UVB-induced HaCaT cells. *Photochem. Photobiol.* **2013**, *89*, 911–918. [CrossRef]
60. Sánchez-Machado, D.I.; López-Cervantes, J.; López-Hernández, J.; Paseiro-Losada, P. Fatty acids, total lipid, protein and ash contents of processed edible seaweeds. *Food Chem.* **2004**, *85*, 439–444. [CrossRef]
61. Dawczynski, C.; Schubert, R.; Jahreis, G. Amino acids, fatty acids, and dietary fibre in edible seaweed products. *Food Chem.* **2007**, *103*, 891–899. [CrossRef]
62. Liang, C.; Lim, J.H.; Kim, S.H.; Kim, D.S. Dioscin: A synergistic tyrosinase inhibitor from the roots of Smilax china. *Food Chem.* **2012**, *134*, 1146–1148. [CrossRef]
63. Heo, S.J.; Ko, S.C.; Kang, S.M.; Cha, S.H.; Lee, S.H. Inhibitory effect of diphlorethohydroxycarmalol on melanogenesis and its protective effect against UV-B radiation-induced cell damage. *Food Chem. Toxicol.* **2010**, *48*, 1355–1361. [CrossRef] [PubMed]
64. Cha, S.H.; Ko, S.C.; Kim, D.; Jeon, Y.J. Screening of marine algae for potential tyrosinase inhibitor: Those inhibitors reduced tyrosinase activity and melanin synthesis in zebrafish. *J. Dermatol.* **2011**, *38*, 354–363. [CrossRef] [PubMed]
65. Kang, H.S.; Kim, H.R.; Byun, D.S.; Son, B.W.; Nam, T.J.; Choi, J.S. Tyrosinase inhibitors isolated from the edible brown alga *Ecklonia stolonifera*. *Arch. Pharm. Res.* **2004**, *27*, 1226. [CrossRef] [PubMed]

66. Chan, Y.Y.; Kim, K.H.; Cheah, S.H. Inhibitory effects of *Sargassum polycystum* on tyrosinase activity and melanin formation in B16F10 murine melanoma cells. *J. Ethnopharmacol.* **2011**, *137*, 1183–1188. [CrossRef] [PubMed]
67. Babitha, S.; Kim, E.K. Effect of marine cosmeceuticals on the pigmentation of skin. In *Marine Cosmeceuticals: Trends and Prospect*; CRC Press: Boca Raton, FL, USA, 2011; pp. 63–66.
68. Heo, S.J.; Ko, S.C.; Cha, S.H.; Kang, D.H.; Park, H.S.; Choi, Y.U.; Jeon, Y.J. Effect of phlorotannins isolated from *Ecklonia cava* on melanogenesis and their protective effect against photo-oxidative stress induced by UV-B radiation. *Toxicol. In Vitro* **2009**, *23*, 1123–1130. [CrossRef]
69. Shimoda, H.; Tanaka, J.; Shan, S.J.; Maoka, T. Anti-pigmentary activity of fucoxanthin and its influence on skin mRNA expression of melanogenic molecules. *J. Pharm. Pharmacol.* **2010**, *62*, 1137–1145. [CrossRef]
70. Fernando, I.S.; Sanjeewa, K.A.; Samarakoon, K.W.; Kim, H.S.; Gunasekara, U.K.D.S.S.; Park, Y.J.; Jeon, Y.J. The potential of fucoidans from *Chnoospora minima* and *Sargassum polycystum* in cosmetics: Antioxidant, anti-inflammatory, skin-whitening, and antiwrinkle activities. *J. Appl. Phycol.* **2018**, *30*, 3223–3232. [CrossRef]
71. Wang, Z.J.; Xu, W.; Liang, J.W.; Wang, C.S.; Kang, Y. Effect of fucoidan on b16 murine melanoma cell melanin formation and apoptosis. *Afr. J. Tradit. Complement. Altern. Med.* **2017**, *14*, 149–155. [CrossRef]
72. Yu, P.; Sun, H. Purification of a fucoidan from kelp polysaccharide and its inhibitory kinetics for tyrosinase. *Carbohydr. Polym.* **2014**, *99*, 278–283. [CrossRef]
73. Chen, B.J.; Shi, M.J.; Cui, S.; Hao, S.X.; Hider, R.C.; Zhou, T. Improved antioxidant and anti-tyrosinase activity of polysaccharide from *Sargassum fusiforme* by degradation. *Int. J. Biol. Macromol.* **2016**, *92*, 715–722. [CrossRef]
74. Park, E.J.; Choi, J.I. Melanogenesis inhibitory effect of low molecular weight fucoidan from *Undaria pinnatifida*. *J. Appl. Phycol.* **2017**, *29*, 2213–2217. [CrossRef]
75. Seo, G.Y.; Ha, Y.; Park, A.H.; Kwon, O.W.; Kim, Y.J. *Leathesia difformis* Extract Inhibits α-MSH-Induced Melanogenesis in B16F10 Cells via Down-Regulation of CREB Signaling Pathway. *Int. J. Mol. Sci.* **2019**, *20*, 536.
76. Song, Y.S.; Balcos, M.C.; Yun, H.Y.; Baek, K.J.; Kwon, N.S.; Kim, M.K.; Kim, D.S. ERK activation by fucoidan leads to inhibition of melanogenesis in Mel-Ab cells. *Korean J. Physiol. Pharmacol.* **2015**, *19*, 29–34. [CrossRef] [PubMed]
77. Azam, M.S.; Joung, E.J.; Choi, J.; Kim, H.R. Ethanolic extract from *Sargassum serratifolium* attenuates hyperpigmentation through CREB/ERK signaling pathways in α-MSH-stimulated B16F10 melanoma cells. *J. Appl. Phycol.* **2017**, *29*, 2089–2096. [CrossRef]
78. Pratoomthai, B.; Songtavisin, T.; Gangnonngiw, W.; Wongprasert, K. In vitro inhibitory effect of sulfated galactans isolated from red alga *Gracilaria fisheri* on melanogenesis in B16F10 melanoma cells. *J. Appl. Phycol.* **2018**, *30*, 2611–2618. [CrossRef]
79. Wang, L.; Lee, W.; Oh, J.; Cui, Y.; Ryu, B.; Jeon, Y.J. Protective Effect of Sulfated Polysaccharides from Celluclast-Assisted Extract of *Hizikia fusiforme* Against Ultraviolet B-Induced Skin Damage by Regulating NF-κB, AP-1, and MAPKs Signaling Pathways In Vitro in Human Dermal Fibroblasts. *Mar. Drugs* **2018**, *16*, 239. [CrossRef]
80. Moon, H.J.; Lee, S.R.; Shim, S.N.; Jeong, S.H.; Stonik, V.A.; Rasskazov, V.A.; Lee, Y.H. Fucoidan inhibits UVB-induced MMP-1 expression in human skin fibroblasts. *Biol. Pharm. Bull.* **2008**, *31*, 284–289. [CrossRef]
81. Moon, H.J.; Lee, S.H.; Ku, M.J.; Yu, B.C.; Jeon, M.J.; Jeong, S.H.; Lee, Y.H. Fucoidan inhibits UVB-induced MMP-1 promoter expression and down regulation of type I procollagen synthesis in human skin fibroblasts. *Eur. J. Dermatol.* **2009**, *19*, 129–134. [CrossRef]
82. Ryu, B.; Qian, Z.J.; Kim, M.M.; Nam, K.W.; Kim, S.K. Anti-photoaging activity and inhibition of matrix metalloproteinase (MMP) by marine red alga, *Corallina pilulifera* methanol extract. *Radiat. Phys. Chem.* **2009**, *78*, 98–105. [CrossRef]
83. Kong, C.S.; Kim, J.A.; Ahn, B.N.; Kim, S.K. Potential effect of phloroglucinol derivatives from *Ecklonia cava* on matrix metalloproteinase expression and the inflammatory profile in lipopolysaccharide-stimulated human THP-1 macrophages. *Fish. Sci.* **2011**, *77*, 867–873. [CrossRef]
84. Ryu, J.; Park, S.J.; Kim, I.H.; Choi, Y.H.; Nam, T.J. Protective effect of porphyra-334 on UVA-induced photoaging in human skin fibroblasts. *Int. J. Mol. Med.* **2014**, *34*, 796–803. [CrossRef] [PubMed]

85. Kim, C.R.; Kim, Y.M.; Lee, M.K.; Kim, I.H.; Choi, Y.H.; Nam, T.J. Pyropia yezoensis peptide promotes collagen synthesis by activating the TGF-β/Smad signaling pathway in the human dermal fibroblast cell line Hs27. *Int. J. Mol. Med.* **2017**, *39*, 31–38. [CrossRef] [PubMed]
86. Kim, J.A.; Ahn, B.N.; Kong, C.S.; Kim, S.K. The chromene sargachromanol E inhibits ultraviolet A-induced ageing of skin in human dermal fibroblasts. *Br. J. Dermatol.* **2013**, *168*, 968–976. [CrossRef] [PubMed]
87. Ferreres, F.; Lopes, G.; Gil-Izquierdo, A.; Andrade, P.B.; Sousa, C.; Mouga, T.; Valentão, P. Phlorotannin extracts from fucales characterized by HPLC-DAD-ESI-MSn: Approaches to hyaluronidase inhibitory capacity and antioxidant properties. *Mar. Drugs* **2012**, *10*, 2766–2781. [CrossRef]
88. Shibata, T.; Fujimoto, K.; Nagayama, K.; Yamaguchi, K.; Nakamura, T. Inhibitory activity of brown algal phlorotannins against hyaluronidase. *Int. J. Food Sci. Technol.* **2002**, *37*, 703–709. [CrossRef]
89. Wang, H.M.D.; Li, X.C.; Lee, D.J.; Chang, J.S. Potential biomedical applications of marine algae. *Bioresour. Technol.* **2017**, *244*, 1407–1415. [CrossRef]
90. Cruces, E.; Flores-Molina, M.R.; Díaz, M.J.; Huovinen, P.; Gómez, I. Phenolics as photoprotective mechanism against combined action of UV radiation and temperature in the red alga *Gracilaria chilensis*? *J. Appl. Phycol.* **2018**, *30*, 1247–1257. [CrossRef]
91. Cardozo, K.H.; Marques, L.G.; Carvalho, V.M.; Carignan, M.O.; Pinto, E.; Marinho-Soriano, E.; Colepicolo, P. Analyses of photoprotective compounds in red algae from the Brazilian coast. *Rev. Bras. Farmacogn.* **2011**, *21*, 202–208. [CrossRef]
92. Heo, S.J.; Jeon, Y.J. Protective effect of fucoxanthin isolated from *Sargassum siliquastrum* on UV-B induced cell damage. *J. Photochem. Photobiol. B Biol.* **2009**, *95*, 101–107. [CrossRef]
93. Urikura, I.; Sugawara, T.; Hirata, T. Protective effect of fucoxanthin against UVB-induced skin photoaging in hairless mice. *Biosci. Biotechnol. Biochem.* **2011**, *75*, 757–760. [CrossRef]
94. Hama, S.; Takahashi, K.; Inai, Y.; Shiota, K.; Sakamoto, R.; Yamada, A.; Kogure, K. Protective effects of topical application of a poorly soluble antioxidant astaxanthin liposomal formulation on ultraviolet-induced skin damage. *J. Pharm. Sci.* **2012**, *101*, 2909–2916. [CrossRef] [PubMed]
95. Lyons, N.M.; O'Brien, N.M. Modulatory effects of an algal extract containing astaxanthin on UVA-irradiated cells in culture. *J. Dermatol. Sci.* **2002**, *30*, 73–84. [CrossRef]
96. Balboa, E.M.; Li, Y.X.; Ahn, B.N.; Eom, S.H.; Domínguez, H.; Jiménez, C.; Rodríguez, J. Photodamage attenuation effect by a tetraprenyltoluquinol chromane meroterpenoid isolated from *Sargassum muticum*. *J. Photochem. Photobiol. B* **2015**, *148*, 51–58. [CrossRef] [PubMed]
97. Le Lann, K.; Surget, G.; Couteau, C.; Coiffard, L.; Cérantola, S.; Gaillard, F.; Stiger-Pouvreau, V. Sunscreen, antioxidant, and bactericide capacities of phlorotannins from the brown macroalga *Halidrys siliquosa*. *J. Appl. Phycol.* **2016**, *28*, 3547–3559. [CrossRef]
98. Vo, T.S.; Kim, S.-K.; Ryu, B.; Ngo, D.H.; Yoon, N.-Y.; Bach, L.G.; Hang, N.T.N.; Ngo, D.N. The Suppressive Activity of Fucofuroeckol-A Derived from Brown Algal *Ecklonia stolonifera* Okamura on UVB-Induced Mast Cell Degranulation. *Mar. Drugs* **2018**, *16*, 1. [CrossRef]
99. Álvarez-Gómez, F.; Korbee, N.; Casas-Arrojo, V.; Abdala-Díaz, R.T.; Figueroa, F.L. UV Photoprotection, Cytotoxicity and Immunology Capacity of Red Algae Extracts. *Molecules* **2019**, *24*, 341. [CrossRef]
100. Oren, A.; Gunde-Cimerman, N. Mycosporines and mycosporine-like amino acids: UV protectants or multipurpose secondary metabolites? *FEMS Microbiol. Lett.* **2007**, *269*, 1–10. [CrossRef]
101. Daniel, S.; Cornelia, S.; Fred, Z. UV-A sunscreen from red algae for protection against premature skin aging. *Cosmet. Toilet. Manuf. Worldw.* **2004**, *129*, 139–143.
102. Shao, P.; Shao, J.; Han, L.; Lv, R.; Sun, P. Separation, preliminary characterization, and moisture-preserving activity of polysaccharides from *Ulva fasciata*. *Int. J. Biol. Macromol.* **2015**, *72*, 924–930. [CrossRef]
103. Wang, J.; Jin, W.; Hou, Y.; Niu, X.; Zhang, H.; Zhang, Q. Chemical composition and moisture-absorption/retention ability of polysaccharides extracted from five algae. *Int. J. Biol. Macromol.* **2013**, *57*, 26–29. [CrossRef]
104. Khallil, A.M.; Daghman, I.M.; Fady, A.A. Antifungal Potential in Crude Extracts of Five Selected Brown Seaweeds Collected from the Western Libya Coast. *J. Micro. Creat.* **2015**, *1*, 103. [CrossRef]
105. Saidani, K.; Bedjou, F.; Benabdesselam, F.; Touati, N. Antifungal activity of methanolic extracts of four Algerian marine algae species. *Afr. J. Biotechnol.* **2012**, *11*, 9496–9500. [CrossRef]
106. Lee, M.H.; Lee, K.B.; Oh, S.M.; Lee, B.H.; Chee, H.Y. Antifungal activities of dieckol isolated from the marine brown alga *Ecklonia cava* against *Trichophyton rubrum*. *J. Korean Soc. Appl. Biol.* **2010**, *53*, 504–507. [CrossRef]

107. Alghazeer, R.; Whida, F.; Abduelrhman, E.; Gammoudi, F.; Azwai, S. Screening of antibacterial activity in marine green, red and brown macroalgae from the western coast of Libya. *Nat. Sci.* **2013**, *5*, 7. [CrossRef]
108. Sahnouni, F.; Benattouche, Z.; Matallah-Boutiba, A.; Benchohra, M.; Moumen Chentouf, W.; Bouhadi, D.; Boutiba, Z. Antimicrobial activity of two marine algae *Ulva rigida* and *Ulva intestinalis* collected from Arzew gulf (Western Algeria). *J. Appl. Environ. Biol. Sci.* **2016**, *6*, 242–248.
109. Saviuc, C.; Ciubucă, B.; Dincă, G.; Bleotu, C.; Drumea, V.; Chifiriuc, M.C.; Lazăr, V. Development and sequential analysis of a new multi-agent, anti-acne formulation based on plant-derived antimicrobial and anti-inflammatory compounds. *Int. J. Mol. Sci.* **2017**, *18*, 175. [CrossRef]
110. Ruxton, C.H.; Jenkins, G. A novel topical ingredient derived from seaweed significantly reduces symptoms of acne vulgaris: A general literature review. *J. Cosmet. Sci.* **2012**, *64*, 219–226.
111. Treyvaud Amiguet, V.; Jewell, L.E.; Mao, H.; Sharma, M.; Hudson, J.B.; Durst, T.; Arnason, J.T. Antibacterial properties of a glycolipid-rich extract and active principle from Nunavik collections of the macroalgae *Fucus evanescens* C. Agardh (Fucaceae). *Can. J. Microbiol.* **2011**, *57*, 745–749. [CrossRef]
112. Choi, J.S.; Bae, H.J.; Kim, S.J.; Choi, I.S. In vitro antibacterial and anti-inflammatory properties of seaweed extracts against acne inducing bacteria, *Propionibacterium acnes*. *J. Environ. Biol.* **2011**, *32*, 313–318.
113. Lee, J.; Eom, S.; Lee, E.; Jung, Y.; Kim, H.; Jo, M.; Son, K.; Lee, H.; Kim, J.H.; Lee, M. In vitro antibacterial and synergistic effect of phlorotannins isolated from edible brown seaweed Eisenia bicyclis against acne-related bacteria. *Algae* **2014**, *29*, 47–55. [CrossRef]
114. Sebaaly, C.; Kassem, S.; Grishina, E.; Kanaan, H.; Sweidan, A.; Chmit, M.S.; Kanaan, H.M. Anticoagulant and antibacterial activities of polysaccharides of red algae Corallina collected from Lebanese coast. *J. Appl. Pharm. Sci.* **2014**, *4*, 30–37.

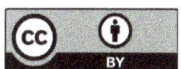

© 2019 by the authors. Licensee MDPI, Basel, Switzerland. This article is an open access article distributed under the terms and conditions of the Creative Commons Attribution (CC BY) license (http://creativecommons.org/licenses/by/4.0/).

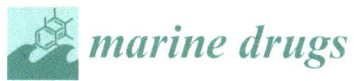

Review

Macroalgae as a Valuable Source of Naturally Occurring Bioactive Compounds for the Treatment of Alzheimer's Disease

Tosin A. Olasehinde [1,2,3,*], Ademola O. Olaniran [4] and Anthony I. Okoh [1,2]

1   Applied Environmental and Microbiology Research Group (AEMREG), Department of Biochemistry and Microbiology, University of Fort Hare, Eastern Cape, Alice 5700, South Africa; aokoh@ufh.ac.za
2   SAMRC Microbial Water Quality Monitoring Centre, University of Fort Hare, Eastern Cape, Alice 5700, South Africa
3   Nutrition and Toxicology Division, Food Technology Department, Federal Institute of Industrial Research, Oshodi, Lagos PMB 21023, Nigeria
4   Discipline of Microbiology, School of Life Sciences, College of Agricultural, Engineering and Science, University of Kwazulu-Natal, Durban 4001, South Africa; Olanirana@ukzn.ac.za
*   Correspondence: tosinolasehinde26@yahoo.com; Tel.: +27-810147782

Received: 20 September 2019; Accepted: 11 October 2019; Published: 25 October 2019

Abstract: Alzheimer's disease (AD) is a neurological condition that affects mostly aged individuals. Evidence suggests that pathological mechanisms involved in the development of AD are associated with cholinergic deficit, glutamate excitotoxicity, beta-amyloid aggregation, tau phosphorylation, neuro-inflammation, and oxidative damage to neurons. Currently there is no cure for AD; however, synthetic therapies have been developed to effectively manage some of the symptoms at the early stage of the disease. Natural products from plants and marine organisms have been identified as important sources of bioactive compounds with neuroprotective potentials and less adverse effects compared to synthetic agents. Seaweeds contain several kinds of secondary metabolites such as phlorotannins, carotenoids, sterols, fucoidans, and poly unsaturated fatty acids. However, their neuroprotective effects and mechanisms of action have not been fully explored. This review discusses recent investigations and/or updates on interactions of bioactive compounds from seaweeds with biomarkers involved in the pathogenesis of AD using reports in electronic databases such as Web of science, Scopus, PubMed, Science direct, Scifinder, Taylor and Francis, Wiley, Springer, and Google scholar between 2015 and 2019. Phlorotannins, fucoidans, sterols, and carotenoids showed strong neuroprotective potentials in different experimental models. However, there are no data from human studies and/or clinical trials.

Keywords: Alzheimer's disease; seaweeds; cholinesterases; beta-secretase; beta-amyloid aggregation; neuroprotection

1. Introduction

Macroalgae, also known as seaweeds, are marine organisms and reservoirs of natural biologically active compounds. Different classes of macroalgae include rhodophyta (red algae), chlorophyta (green algae), and phaeophyta (brown algae). There are over 4000 red, 900 green, and 1500 brown species of macroalgae all over the world [1]. Most of the brown macroalgae are able to thrive in temperate and cool waters while green and red algal species exist in tropical and subtropical waters [1]. Several species of macroalgae thrive in their habitat at extreme conditions due to their capacity to develop defense mechanism via the release of some secondary metabolites. Historically, seaweeds have been used traditionally, especially in Asian countries, as herbal medicine for the treatment of tumors, urinary disease, gastrointestinal problems, cough, boils, hemorrhoid, ulcers, asthma, and headaches [2]. The appreciable levels of iodine in some edible seaweeds also make them a good choice for the treatment of goiter [3,4]. Specifically, species such as *Ulva* spp., *Laminaria japonica*, *Porphyra* spp., and *Sargassum fusiforme* have been used for the treatment of scrofula (cervical tuberculosis), edema, and goiter [3]. Furthermore, a combination of *Ecklonia* spp. and *Sargassum* spp. are used as herbs in Chinese medicine for the treatment of tumors, liver cirrhosis, and spleen enlargement [5]. Seaweeds are commonly consumed locally as vegetables and in salad. Some species of macroalgae are consumed as part of a staple diet because they are rich in functionally active compounds such as phenolic compounds, alkaloids, sterols, omega-6 fatty acids, antioxidants, carotenoids, and phenolic compounds [6]. They are also used as ingredients for dietary supplements, nutraceuticals, and pharmaceuticals. Some of the applications of some macroalgal species can be seen in their use as ingredients for the production of flavor, meat, cereal, and dairy products [7]. Much attention has been on marine macroalgae for the development of new drugs, nutraceuticals, and dietary supplements due to their beneficial effects as antioxidant [8], anti-tumor [9], anti-inflammatory [10], antidiabetic [11], anti-hypertensive [12], and antibacterial [13] agents. Evidence has shown that macroalgal-derived compounds are capable of improving learning and memory function in neurodegenerative conditions [14]. The neuroprotective effects of biologically active compounds from some macroalgae against neurodegenerative diseases has been described by Alghazwi et al. [15].

Alzheimer's disease (AD) is the most common form of dementia and has become a major health problem among aged individuals [16]. AD is characterized by cholinergic dysfunction, cognitive impairment, memory loss, neuronal death, and behavioral disturbances. The pathogenesis of AD involves complex mechanisms and impairment of the neurological cascade involved in memory function. The early onset of this disease has been diagnosed in persons less than 65 years. However, more than 90% of cases diagnosed are associated with the late onset of AD and this occurs mostly in individuals above 65 years of age [17]. The development of early onset AD has been linked with genetic mutations, especially genes that are responsible for Aβ peptide production (amyloid precursor protein (APP gene)), preselinin 1 (PS1), and preselinin 2 (PS2) genes [18]. Evidence has shown that dysregulation in the expression of these genes may account for about 5–10% of diagnosed cases of early onset AD [17,18]. Furthermore, apolipoprotein E (APO-E) polymorphic alleles has been identified as a major genetic risk factor for the development of early onset and late onset AD [19]. APOε4 alleles have been shown to trigger cognitive decline and cerebral amyloid angiopathy in aged individuals [20]. APOE is produced in astrocytes in the central nervous system, and it is important in the regulation of lipid homeostasis and beta-amyloid (Aβ) metabolism. It also contributes to the formation of Aβ plaques and development of cerebral amyloid angiopathy [21]. Furthermore, APOε4 has also been linked to tau pathology [22]. The molecular mechanisms involved in the development of sporadic late onset of AD is not well known; however, previous reports have shown that it is linked to oxidative stress [23], loss of cholinergic signaling [24], accumulation of Aβ plaques [25], and formation of neurofibrillary tangles [26]. Moreover, a recent report has shown that hyperphosphorylation of tau proteins is a major causative factor involved in the development and progression of AD [27]. Hence, recent research investigations are considering tau pathology as a therapeutic strategy for the management of AD.

Previous experimental investigations have established that natural products could be effective in the management of Alzheimer's disease and have been suggested as an alternative therapeutic approach compared to synthetic agents [28–30]. The discovery of novel natural compounds from different species of marine macroalgae represents an important source of biologically active compounds with strong neuroprotective potentials. This present review report provides current knowledge on neuroprotective potentials of macroalgal-derived natural compounds and their effects on pathological mechanisms (oxidative stress-induced neurodegeneration, cholinergic dysfunction, and beta-secretase activities, as well as glutamate and metal-induced neurotoxicity and beta-amyloid aggregation) linked to Alzheimer's disease.

2. Methods

A literature search was done in different databases including Web of Science, Scopus, Scifinder, PubMed, Google scholar, Science direct, Springer, Taylor and Francis, and Wiley to identify reports published between 2015 and 2019 that are related to antioxidant activity and neuroprotective effects of macroalgal extracts and compounds as well as their modulatory effects on biomarkers linked with Alzheimer's disease. Articles revealing reports on the neuroprotective properties and modulatory effects of macroalgal extracts on biomolecules related to other neurodegenerative diseases such as Parkinson's disease, Huntington's disease, ischemia, and stroke were not considered in this study.

3. Etiology of AD

The occurrence of AD amongst aged individuals has been estimated to increase annually due to the complexity of its pathological mechanisms [31]. The etiology of AD is not well understood due to the multifactorial mechanisms underlying the disease process. Some of the factors that have been linked to the development and progression of AD include ageing, cholinergic deficit, Aβ aggregation, tau hyperphosphorylation, oxidative stress, neuro-inflammation, and diabetes. Figure 1 shows a complex cascade and set of mechanisms involving the development of AD. The cure for AD has not been discovered due to the complexity of the neuropathological mechanisms involved in the development and progression of the disease [32]. Fewer achievements have been attained in terms of effective treatment of the disease; however, much focus has been on early detection and prevention. Adequate diagnostic methods for AD is one of the challenging factors that has been encountered due to non-availability of reliable biomarkers. The current therapeutic approach used for the management of AD involves the use of cholinesterase inhibitors and the N-methyl-d-aspartate receptor antagonist. These drugs do not have the capacity to halt the progression of the disease. Effective therapeutic agents or disease modifying drugs that are capable of stopping or preventing the clinical symptoms of AD are currently under extensive investigation [33,34]. However, seaweed-derived compounds have shown great potential as an alternative strategy for the management of AD (Figure 1).

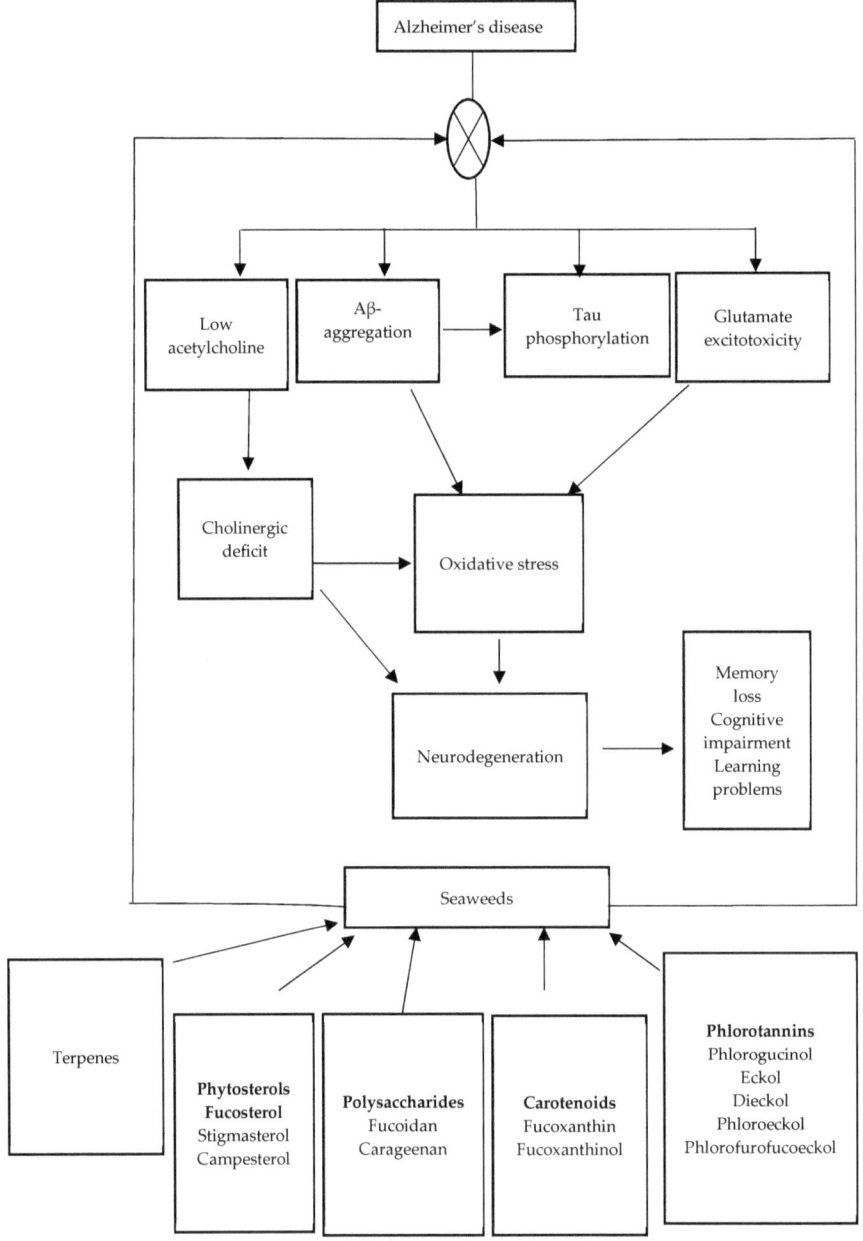

Figure 1. Mechanism of action of bioactive compounds from macroalgae against Alzheimer's disease.

4. Therapeutic Role of Some Macroalgae in the Management of AD

4.1. Evidence from In Vitro Studies

Some in vitro models have been used to determine the neuroprotective potentials of some macroalgal species against biomarkers of AD. Extracts derived from several species of macroalgae have been tested for their cholinesterase and beta-secretase (BACE-1) inhibitory activities. Neuronal cells have also been used as experimental models to determine the neuroprotective activities of macroalgal-derived compounds and extracts.

4.1.1. Cholinesterase Inhibitory Activity

Acetylcholinesterase (AChE) and butyrylcholinesterase (BChE) are important enzymes involved in the regulation of acetylcholine (ACh) in the synaptic cleft of neurons to promote cognitive function [35,36]. However, loss or rapid degradation of acetylcholine leads to cholinergic dysfunction and ultimately memory impairment [37,38]. Hence, cholinesterases have been developed to alleviate cholinergic deficit by restoring ACh levels and improving cognitive function [39,40]. Seaweed-derived biologically active compounds have been reported to exhibit inhibitory effects on enzymes associated with Alzheimer's disease (Table 1). Results from some in vitro studies from our laboratory revealed that aqueous-ethanol extracts rich in phlorotannins, phenolic acids, and flavonoids from *Ecklonia maxima*, *Gelidium pristoides*, *Gracilaria gracilis*, and *Ulva lactuca* exhibit acetylcholinesterase and butyrylcholinesterase inhibitory activities [41]. Furthermore, sulfated polysaccharides obtained from *Ulva rigida* as well as the aforementioned algal species also showed potent inhibitory effects on BChE and AChE in vitro [42,43]. Purified fractions of *Gelidiella acerosa* showed AChE and BChE inhibitory activity [44]. Phytol was identified in the fraction as the most effective constituent. In the same study, molecular docking analysis revealed that phytol tightly binds to the arginine residue at the active site of the enzyme, thereby changing its conformation and exerting its inhibitory effect. Rengasamy et al. [45] reported AChE inhibitory activity of *Codium duthieae*, *Amphiroa beauvoisii*, *Gelidium foliaceum*, *Laurencia complanata*, and *Rhodomelopsis africana*. *Hypnea musciformis* and *Ochtodes secundiramea* extracts showed weak inhibitory activity (less than 30% inhibition) on AChE. Jung et al. [46] also reported AChE and BChE inhibitory effects of methanol extracts of *Ecklonia cava*, *Ecklonia kurome*, and *Myelophycus simplex*. Glycoprotein isolated from *Undaria pinnatifida* showed dose responsive inhibitory effects on butyrylcholinesterase and acetylcholinesterase activities [47].

The IC_{50} values revealed that the glycoprotein exhibited higher inhibitory effect on AChE (63.56 µg/mL) than BChE (99.03 µg/mL). The enzyme inhibitory activities of the extracts were attributed to the presence of monoterpenes, which are reversible competitive inhibitors of the AChE. Shanmuganathan et al. [48] attributed the inhibitory effect of acetone extracts from *P. gymnospora* to alpha bisabolol.

In a recent study, fucosterol isolated from *Sargassum horridum* demonstrated potent inhibition against AChE activity [49]. Kinetic studies revealed that fucosterol showed competitive and non-competitive inhibition due to its high binding affinity to AChE compared to neostigmine. Choi et al. [50] reported that phlorofucofuroeckol isolated from *Ecklonia cava* exhibited potent inhibitory effects against BChE with an activity of over 100 fold higher than AChE inhibition.

4.1.2. BACE-1 Inhibitory Activity

BACE-1 has been identified as one of the prime therapeutic targets for the treatment of AD. It is a membrane-bound aspartyl protease that regulates Aβ production in the metabolism of amyloid precursor proteins. An increase in BACE-1 activity as well as elevated protein expression levels have been shown to trigger rapid production of Aβ protein and sporadic AD [51]. Cheng et al. [52] suggested that elevated levels of BACE-1 activity and increase in tumor necrosis factor (TNFa) expression may contribute to mild cognitive impairment and early events of AD. Furthermore, elevated BACE-1 activity also contributes to the increased number of plaques around the neurons and reduces cognitive ability of AD patients. High BACE-1 activity was also attributed to neurodegeneration and neurological decline in a transgenic mice model of AD [53]. The search for potent BACE-1 inhibitors has been a huge task as many inhibitors that have been developed have failed clinical tests. Some marine algal species have shown good potential as BACE-1 inhibitors (Table 1). Findings from our laboratory revealed that aqueous-ethanol extracts of *G. pristoides*, *E. maxima*, *U. lactuca*, and *G. gracilis* containing phlorotannins, flavonoids, and phenolic acids exhibited strong BACE-1 inhibitory activity with percentage inhibition of 97.2, 83.3, 86.9, and 91.2% at the highest concentration (120 µg/mL) [41]. In another study, fucoidan, ulvan, and carrageenan obtained from *E. maxima*, *U. lactuca*, and *G. pristoides* also inhibited BACE-1 activity with percentage inhibition of 87.1, 71.2, and 51.3%, respectively, at the highest concentration (5.0 mg/mL) [43]. Jung et al. [54] also reported the potency of fucosterol and fucoxanthin isolated from *Undaria pinnatifida* and *Ecklonia stolonifera*, respectively, against BACE-1 activity. Fucoxanthin and fucosterol showed mixed and non-competitive types of inhibition, respectively, and their inhibitory activities were attributed to strong binding to hydroxyl groups of specific amino acid residues at the active site of the enzyme. Seong et al. [55] elucidated that monoterpenoids obtained from *S. sagamianum* exhibited potent BACE-1 inhibitory activity in vitro. The isolated compounds, saraquinoic and sargahydroquinoic acids, as well as sargachromenol interacted with the catalytic aspartyl residues and allosteric sites, thereby initiating tight binding to the enzyme, hence reducing its activity. Phlorofucofuroeckol isolated from *E. cava* also reduced BACE-1 activity [50]. Rafiquzzaman et al. [47] isolated and purified glycoproteins from *Undaria pinnatifida* and investigated their inhibitory effects on BACE-1 activity. The glycoprotein exhibited a dose dependent inhibitory effect on BACE-1. An insilico investigation on BACE-1 inhibitory potentials of glycyrrhizin and its metabolites isolated from *Hizikia fusiformis* revealed that 18α-glycyrrhetinic acid and 18β-glycyrrhetinic acid showed inhibitory effects against BACE-1 activity [56]. Moreover, 18β-glycyrrhetinic acid showed two-fold potent inhibitory activity compared with quercetin. The inhibitory activity of these compounds were attributed to their strong capacity to bind to the amino acid residues at the active site of BACE-1 via hydrogen bonds.

Table 1. Cholinesterase and beta-secretase inhibitory activities of macroalgal-derived extracts and isolated compounds.

Class of Compounds	Components	Algal Source	Mechanism of Action	Reference
Crude extracts	Benzene:ethyl acetate fraction	*G. acerosa*	Inhibition of AChE	[44]
	Methanol extracts	*E. cava* *E. kurome*	Inhibition of AChE and BACE-1	
		M. simples	Inhibition of AChE	
Phlorotannins	Phlorofucofuroeckol	*E. cava*	Inhibition AChE, BChE, and BACE-1	[46]
Polysaccharides	Purified glycoprotein	*U. pinnatifida*	Inhibition of AChE, BChE and BACE-1"	[47]
Sterol	Fucosterol	*S. horridum*	Inhibition of AChE	[49]
Carotenoids	Fucoxanthin	*U. pinnatifida* *E. stolonifera*	Inhibition of BACE-1	[54]
	Sarahydroquinoic acid	*S. serratifolium*	Inhibition of BACE-1	[55]
Triterpenoid-saponin	Glycyrrhizin 18α-glycyrrhetinic acid 18β-glycyrrhetinic acid	*H. fusiformis*	Inhibition of AChE, BChE, and BACE-1	[56]

4.1.3. Action against Glutamate-Induced Neurotoxicity in Neuronal Cells

Glutamate is an important neurotransmitter responsible for memory, learning, and cognitive function. However, excess levels of glutamate activate NMDA receptors and trigger the production of Aβ peptide. Previous studies have highlighted two major pathways that trigger glutamate excitotoxicity; these include disruption of calcium homeostasis, which leads to the production of reactive oxygen species and neuronal death, as well as alterations in cysteine uptake due to high levels of glutamate [57]. This leads to imbalance of cystine homeostasis, limited levels of glutathione, and rapid production of reactive oxygen species. Hence, biologically active compounds capable of protecting the brain cells against glutamate excitotoxicity may be a good therapeutic intervention.

Macroalgae are good sources of compound with the capacity to attenuate glutamate excitotoxicity in neuronal cells. Acetone extracts from two edible seaweeds (*Saccahrina latissima* and *Fucus serratus*) improved cell viability in glutamate-induced neurotoxicity in SH-SY5Y cells [58]. Phlorofucofuroeckol isolated from *E. cava* protected neurons against cell death, improved mitochondrial dysfunction, and regulated intracellular production of reactive oxygen species (ROS) in PC12 cells [59].

4.1.4. Protection against Aβ-Induced Neurotoxicity

Accumulation of Aβ peptide is one of the hallmarks of AD pathology. Aβ is a pathogenic peptide released from amyloid precursor protein, which aggregates to form toxic plaques around the neurons [60]. Currently, no drug has been developed to combat Aβ aggregation and its pathological processes in AD. Some species of macroalgae have been identified as potential sources of compounds capable of attenuating Aβ-induced neurotoxicity in AD models (Table 2).

Crude extracts of some algal species have been reported to inhibit amyloid formation and cause dis-aggregation of matured beta-amyloid fibrils [48,61,62]. In a study carried out by Alghazwi et al. [63], some species of Australian brown, green, and red algae attenuated Aβ-induced toxicity in PC12 cells. Fucosterol from *Padina australis* was evaluated for its neuroprotective effects in SH-SY5Y cells treated with Aβ [64]. The result revealed that fucosterol ameliorated the neurotoxic effect of Aβ and triggered the downregulation of APP expression. Alghazwi et al. [65] also reported the neuroprotective effects of fucoidans isolated from *Undaria pinnatifida* and *Fucus vesiculosus* via their inhibitory effect on Aβ aggregation and Aβ$_{1-42}$-induced cytotoxicity in PC12 cells. In the same study, phlorotannins such as 7-phloroeckol, phlorofucofuroeckol, and dieckol also protected PC-12 cells against Aβ-induced neurotoxicity, reduced ROS production, and restored intracellular levels of Ca^{2+}. However, dieckol exhibited moderately weak neuroprotective effects compared to 7-phloroeckol and phlorofucofuroeckol. Furthermore, phloroglucinol isolated from *E. cava* reduced ROS generation caused by Aβ-induced neurotoxicity in HT-22 cells [66]. Another unique phlorotannin (eckmaxol) isolated from *E. maxima*, also exhibited anti-amyloidogenic activity [67] (Table 2). Furthermore, fucoxanthin and fucosterol also attenuated amyloid oligomer-induced neurotoxicity in neuronal cell line models [68–70]. Wei et al. [71] also showed that fucoidan inhibited apoptosis in PC12 cells via activation of caspases, prevention of cytochrome c release, and upregulation of X-linked inhibitor of apoptosis (XIAP) in Aβ-induced PC-12 cells.

Table 2. Macroalgae extracts and compounds and inhibition of beta-amyloid-induced neurotoxicity.

Class of Compounds	Components	Algal Source	Mechanism of Action	Reference
Crude extracts	Aqueous extracts	*A. esculenta*	Inhibition of amyloid formation	[61]
	Acetone extracts	*P. gymnospora*	Anti-aggregation and dis-aggregation of amyloid fibrils	[18]
	Ether/benzene extracts	*G. acerosa*	Prevention of Aβ$_{25-35}$ formation and dis-aggregation of pre-formed fibrils	[62]
Phlorotannins	Phloroglucinol	*E. cava*	Inhibition of Aβ-induced-cytotoxicity and protection against ROS accumulation in HT-22 cells	[64]
	Eckmaxol	*E. maxima*	Prevention of Aβ-induced neuronal apoptosis and decrease in intracellular ROS	[67]
Phytosterol	Fucosterol	*Padina australis*	Reduction of APP mRNA and inhibition of Aβ-induced neurotoxicity	[64]
		E. stolonifera	Attenuation of Aβ-induced cognitive dysfunction	[68]
Carotenoid	Fucoxanthin	*Sargassum horneri*	Attenuation of Aβ-oligomer-induced neurotoxicity in SYH-SY5Y cells	[69]
			Attenuation of Aβ-induced neurotoxicity in PC12-cells	[70]
Sulfated polysaccharides	Fucoidan	*U. pinnatifida*	Protection against Aβ$_{1-42}$-induced neuronal death in PC-12 cells	[65]
		F. vesiculosus	Inhibition of Aβ$_{25-35}$-induced neurotoxicity in PC-12 cells	[71]

4.1.5. Antioxidant Activity of Macroalgae and AD

Antioxidants have been identified as an effective therapeutic strategy for the delay of the progression of AD. This is due to the fact that elevated levels of ROS in the brain are associated with the progression of AD. Brain cells are highly susceptible to free radical attack due to high consumption of oxygen and lipid content as well as low antioxidant defense system. Hence, high levels of reactive oxygen species in brain cells may lead to lipid peroxidation, neurodegeneration, and ultimately cell death. Some species of macroalgae have been reported to exhibit neuroprotective effects via their antioxidant activities. Alghazwi et al. [15] reported the antioxidant activity of 49 compounds isolated from some brown, red, and green macroalgal species. Most of these compounds were identified as polysaccharides, phlorotannins, and terpenoids. Recent findings on the antioxidant activity of macroalgae revealed that some other algal species exhibit radical scavenging and metal chelating activities in vitro (Table 3 and Figure 2). Sathya et al. [72] reported the DPPH radical scavenging activity of methanol, ethylacetate, and dichloromethane extracts of *Cystoseira trinodis* with scavenging activity of 50%, 54%, and 69% respectively. The ethyl acetate and butanol fractions of *Sargassum fusiforme* were also reported to exhibit radical scavenging activity [73]. Methanol extracts of some *Gracilaria* spp., *Lesonia* spp., *Laminaria japonica*, and *Ascophyllum nodosum* also exhibited DPPH and ABTS radical scavenging activities and ferric reducing properties [74,75]. Furthermore, acetone extracts from *Ulva lactuca* and *Entermorpha intestinalis* [76], and ethanol and hexane extracts from *Pterocladiella capillacea* and *Osmindaria obtusiloba* [77] including aqueous extracts from *Ascophyllum nodosum*, *Bifurcaria bifurcate*, and *Fucus vesiculosus* [78] also exhibited potent antioxidant activity via their radical scavenging activities, ferric reducing properties, and inhibition of lipid oxidation. The antioxidant activities of these algal extracts were attributed to the presence of phlorotannins. Pinteus et al. [79] reported the antioxidant activity of the methanol and dichloromethane extracts of 27 red, green, and brown macroalgal species through their oxygen radical antioxidant capacity and DPPH radical scavenging activity. The study showed that the methanol extracts of the brown algal species exhibited the highest antioxidant activities. Similarly, out of the hexane, ethyl acetate, and methanol extracts of seven algal species reported by Chiboub et al. [80], only *Cytoseira sedoides* (hexane, ethyl acetate, and methanol), *Padina pavonica* (ethyl acetate extract), *Cladostephus spongiosum* (ethylacetate and methanol), and *Halopteris scoparia* (methanol extract) exhibited DPPH and ABTS radical scavenging activity above 50%.

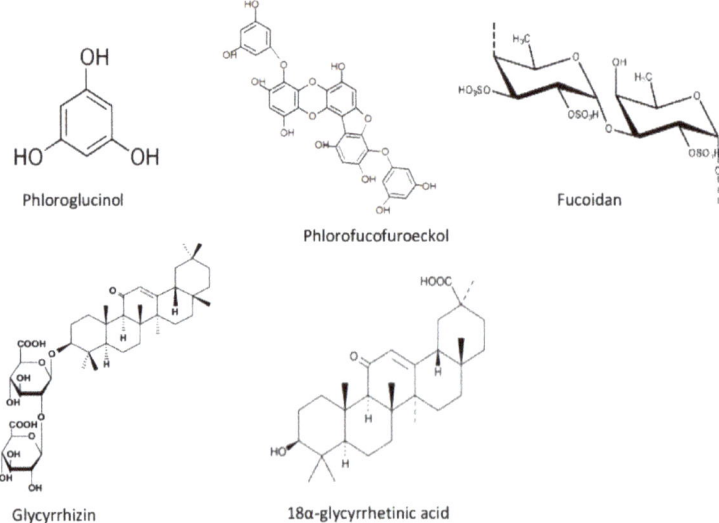

Figure 2. *Cont.*

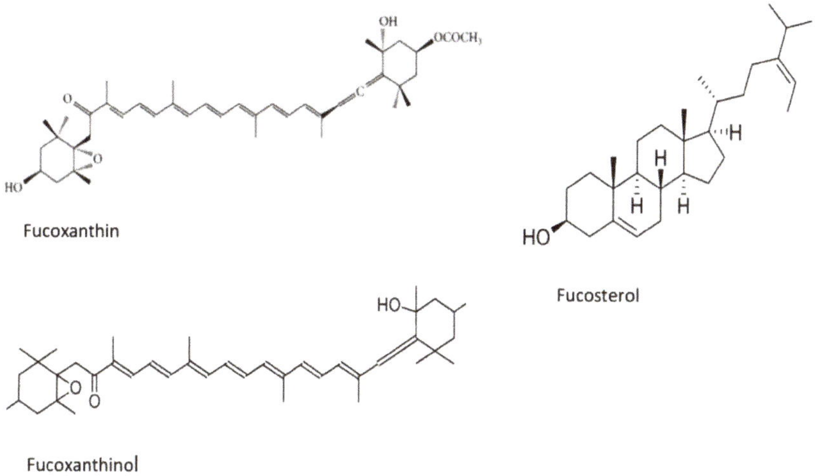

Figure 2. Chemical structures of some neuroprotective compounds in marine seaweeds.

Crude fucoidans extracted from *Sargassum* sp. also exhibited antioxidant activity via their ferric reducing antioxidant properties and hydroxyl radical scavenging activities [81]. Purified fractions of *H. elongata* and *Macrocytis pyrifera* extracts exhibited antioxidant activity and this effect was attributed to the presence of phenolic terpenes, flavonoid derivatives, and phlorotannins [82,83]. Phenolic rich extracts from *E. maxima, U. lactuca, U. rigida, G. gracilis,* and *G. pristoides* also attenuated Zn-induced neurotoxicity and protected hippocampal neuronal cells (HT-22) against neuronal damage via inhibition of apoptosis, reduction of nitric oxide and malondialdehyde production, and improvement of antioxidant status [84,85]. The neuroprotective effects of the phenolic extracts could be linked to the radical scavenging and metal chelating activities of some of the bioactive constituents, which include phloroglucinol, ferulic acid, dihydroxybenzoic acid, 3,7-dimethyl quercetin, 5,7-dimethoxyflavone, dihydronaringenin-O-sulfate, apigenin, 7,2,4-trihydroxyisoflavanol, and kaempferol 3-(6-acetyl galactoside)7-rhamnose [41,84,85]. Polysaccharides such as fucoidans, alginates isolated from *Sargassum* spp., *Laminaria japonica, Cystoseira trinodi,* and *Nizimuddinia zanardini* [86–91], as well as protein extracts obtained from *Ulva* spp. and *Gracilaria* spp. [92] also showed potent radical scavenging activities. Furthermore, the report of Mohibbullah et al. [93] revealed that *Porphyra yezoensis* (an edible red alga) extracts induced synaptogenesis, increased neuronal survivability, and prevented neuronal death due to its radical scavenging ability. The neuroprotective effect of the extracts was attributed to taurine, an active component that improved neuronal development and maturation. Some studies also showed that carotenoids such as fucoxanthin and fucoxanthinol isolated from brown alga *Himanthalia elongata* [94], *Sargassum horneri* [95], and *Undaria pinnatifida* [96] exhibit neuroprotection via their antioxidant activity, as revealed by their radical scavenging activities, inhibition of apoptosis, intracellular reactive oxygen species and malondialdehyde production, attenuation of mitochondria membrane dysfunction, and DNA fragmentation. Glycoprotein isolated from *U. pinnatifida* increased superoxide dismutase and xanthine oxidase activities in hippocampal neuronal cells, which suggest its ability to prevent neurodegeneration [47]. Table 3 shows recent findings on the antioxidant activities of different classes of algal extracts and compounds. Antioxidant activity has been linked with neuroprotective effects due to the ability of antioxidants to suppress neurodegeneration, prevent neuronal death, and halt the progression of AD. Hence macroalgae are good sources of antioxidants with neuroprotective effects.

Table 3. Antioxidant activity of macroalgal-derived extracts and compounds.

Class of Compounds	Components	Algal Source	Mechanism of Action	Reference
Crude extracts	Methanol extract	Ascophyllum nodosum	ABTS and DPPH scavenging activity	[74]
		Laminaria japonica Lessonia trabeculate Lessonia nigrescens	Ferric reducing antioxidant property	
		Gracilaria edulis Gracilaria corticata	DPPH, ABTS, and NO radical scavenging activities	[75]
		Myelophycus simplex	ABTS radical scavenging activity	[46]
		Ecklonia cava E. kurome	Attenuation of H2O2-induced oxidative damage in SH-SY5Y cells	
	Acetone extract	Ulva lactuca	DPPH and superoxide anion scavenging activity	[76]
		Entermorpha intestinalis	Ferric reducing antioxidant property	
	Ethanol/hexane extract	Pterocladiella capillacea	DPPH radical scavenging activity	[77]
		Osmindaria obtusiloba	Metal chelating activity	
	Aqueous extract	Ascophyllum nodosum Bifurcaria bifurcate Fucus vesiculosus	DPPH, ABTS, and hydroxyl radical scavenging activities Ferric reducing antioxidant capacity Inhibition of lipid oxidation	[78]
Phlorotannins	Phlorotannin extract	Macrocytis pyrifera	DPPH radical scavenging activity	[83]
Polysaccharides	Fucoidan	Sargassum glaucescens	ABTS and DPPH scavenging and metal chelating activities	[85]
		Sargassum polycystum	DPPH radical scavenging activity Ferric reducing antioxidant property	[87]
	Fucoidan and alginate	Cystoseira trinodis	Ferric reducing antioxidant property	[88]
	Fucoidan and alginate	Sargassum latifolium	Hydroxyl radical scavenging activity	[89]
	Sodium alginate	Nizimuddinia zanardini	DPPH radical scavenging activity	[90]
	Polysaccharides	Laminaria japonica	DPPH and oxygen radical scavenging activity	[91]
	Fucoidan	U. pinnatifida F. vesiculosus	Attenuation of hydrogen peroxide-induced oxidative stress and apoptosis in PC-12 cells	[65]
			Activation of superoxide dismutase and glutathione in Aβ-induced neurotoxicity in PC-12 cells	[71]
Proteins	Protein extracts	Ulva spp.	Ferric reducing antioxidant property	[92]
		Gracilaria spp.	Oxygen radical absorption capacity	
Carotenoids	Fucoxanthin	Himanthalia elongata	Ferric reducing antioxidant property DPPH radical scavenging activity	[94]
			Attenuation of H_2O_2-induced neuronal apoptosis and intracellular ROS	[95]
		Sargassum horneri	Reduced malondialdehyde levels and SOD activity in Aβ-induced cell death in PC12 cells	[70]
	Fucoxanthinol	Undaria pinnatifida	Attenuation of oxidative stress in rats' hippocampal neurons	[96]

4.2. Evidence from In Vivo Studies

Neuroprotective effects of macroalgal extracts and compounds have been determined using different targets, which include oxidative stress, cholinergic function, beta-amyloid aggregation, apoptosis, and behavioral studies in in vivo models.

4.2.1. Neuroprotective Activities of Some Macroalgal Extracts

Crude extracts of some macroalgal species have shown neuroprotective potentials against some markers of Alzheimer's disease in vivo. Syad and Devi [97] confirmed that benzene extracts of *G. acerosa* attenuated neurotoxicity induced by AB_{25-35} in Swedish mice brain. *G. acerosa* improved memory function by attenuating cholinergic dysfunction via inhibition of acetylcholinesterase and butyrylcholinesterase. The extracts also inhibited BACE-1 activity in vivo, hence suppressing Aβ neurotoxicity. In the same study, *G. acerosa* extract protected mouse brain against lipid peroxidation and reduced caspase 3-activity and Bax expression, which suggest its effect against neuronal death. Acute and sub-acute toxicity experiments carried out on the benzene extract did not show any toxic effects on different organs in Swedish mice. Furthermore, a phlorotannin-rich fraction of *Ishige foliacea*, an edible brown seaweed, was reported to improve memory function in scopolamine-induced rat brain via reduction of lipid peroxidation, increase in superoxide dismutase activity and glutathione levels, as well as upregulation of brain-derived neurotrophic factors (BNDF), cyclic-AMP response binding protein (CREB), and phosphorylated extracellular signal regulated kinase (ERK) [98]. Choi et al. [99] found that ethanol extracts of *U. pinnatifida* improved cognitive dysfunction in mouse brain. The results of the study indicate that treatment with ethanol extracts of *U. pinnatifida* caused repairing effects in memory and restored spine density and morphology via increase in latency time in the passive avoidance test and dendritic spine in hippocampal neurons of scopolamine-induced rats. Similarly, fucoidan enhanced spatial learning and memory, which was impaired by infusion of D-galactose in mice brain [71]. In the same study, D-galactose reduced acetylcholine levels and choline acetyltransferase activity while acetylcholinesterase activity was significantly high, which suggests cholinergic dysfunction. However, treatment with fucoidan (50 mg/kg) reversed the levels of acetylcholine as well as choline acetyltransferase and acetylcholinesterase activities, which indicates an improvement in cholinergic function. Similarly, the neuroprotective effect of a fucoidan (SFPS65) isolated from *Sargassum fusiforme* was found in scopolamine and sodium nitrate-induced rats investigated by Hu et al. [100]. The authors suggested that SFPS65A improved stepdown latency, which was disrupted by scopolamine, and mitigated shock number and total wrong frequency. SFPS65A also attenuated spatial learning and memory dysfunction caused by ethanol and sodium in mice brain.

4.2.2. Neuroprotective Effects of Macroalgal-Derived Compounds

Several compounds have been identified and isolated from macroalgae; however, only few have been tested against biomarkers of AD in vivo. Fucoidan present brown alga showed neuroprotective Aβ-induced neurotoxicity in a transgenic *Caenorhabditis elegans* AD model [101]. The result of the study revealed that fucoidan reduced Aβ accumulation by improving proteolysis and attenuation of Aβ-induced ROS production Oh et al. [68] investigated the effect of fucosterol isolated from *E. stolonifera* on Aβ-induced cognitive dysfunction, again in rats. The study showed that fucosterol may enhance cognitive function in aging-induced endoplasmic reticulum stress and memory impairment. Fucosterol attenuated Aβ-induced cognitive dysfunction via upregulation of BDNF–TRkB–ERK1/2 expression in rats' dentate gyrus. Lin et al. [102] evaluated the effect of fucoxanthin in scopolamine-induced memory impairment in rats' brains. Fucoxanthin reversed scopolamine-induced memory dysfunction via inhibition of acetylcholinesterase, and decrease in choline acetyltransferase activity and BDNF expression. Structure–activity analysis showed that fucoxanthin binds to the peripheral anionic site of AChE, hence decreasing the activity of the enzyme. Similarly, the study of Xiang et al. [103] revealed that fucoxanthin attenuated Aβ-induced cognitive impairment in mice brain. The inhibitory effects of fucoxanthin against Aβ oligomerization and aggregation was attributed to its hydrophobic interaction with the peptide, hence preventing conformational transition and self-aggregation of the Aβ peptide. Fucoxanthin also improved spatial learning and memory via the water maze tests and reversed the low levels of glutathione and superoxide dismutase and high levels of malondialdehyde in Aβ-induced mice. Furthermore, fucoxanthin activated the nuclear factor eythroid 2-related factor (NrF-2)-antioxidant response element (ARE) pathway and reversed upregulation of malondialdehyde and glutathione peroxidase activity in a rat model of traumatic brain injury, hence alleviating neurological deficits, neuronal apoptosis, brain lesion, and cerebral edema [104]. Yang et al. [66] reported that phloroglucinol isolated from *E. cava* attenuated cognitive deficit in mice brain. The study revealed that phloroglucinol may delay the onset or progression of AD due to its protective effects against the decrease in dendritic spine density, synaptophysin, and post synaptic density protein 95 (PSD-95). Yang et al. [105] also confirmed that oral administration of phloroglucinol improved impaired cognitive function in 5XFAD mice via reduction of 4-hydroxylnonenal, Aβ plaques, and pro-inflammatory cytokine production, as well as attenuation of glial reactivation.

5. Conclusions

This review provides evidence that macroalgae exhibit neuroprotective effects and could be important sources of biologically active compounds with therapeutic potential for the management of AD. Despite the identification of several macroalgal species and their various biological activities, only few have been explored for their neuroprotective effects against pathological mechanisms involved in Alzheimer's disease. The neuroprotective activities of some macroalgal-derived compounds and extracts via attenuation of cholinergic deficit, Aβ aggregation, oxidative damage to neurons, and glutamate excitation, which have been established in recent findings, could be a significant approach for the management and treatment of AD. However, further investigations are needed to explore other species. Macroalgal extracts with potential neuroprotective activities should be characterized and purified, and their active constituents should be isolated. Further studies are also required to determine the mechanisms of action of macroalgal compounds and investigate their structure–activity relationship. Future research works on the neuroprotective effects of macroalgae may also focus on other targets linked with AD such as serotonin, somatostatin, tau hyperphosphorylation, neuro-inflammation, and metal-induced neurotoxicity, which have not been reported. Furthermore, most studies have shown in vitro neuroprotective effects of some algal species while in vivo experimental models are few. Further works should be done to determine the mechanism of action of macroalgal compounds in in vivo AD models. Compounds which have been established to exhibit neuroprotective effects in vivo, should be tested further in clinical trials.

Author Contributions: T.A.O. searched databases, reviewed the cited literature, and wrote the manuscript. T.A.O., A.O.O., and A.I.O. read and approved the final manuscript.

Funding: We are grateful to the National Research Foundation of South Africa, the World Academy of Science, and the South African Medical Research Council for financial support.

Conflicts of Interest: The authors declare no conflict of interest.

References

1. Rengasamy, K.R.; Kulkarni, M.G.; Stirk, W.A.; van Staden, J. Advances in algal drug research with emphasis on enzyme inhibitors. *Biotechnol. Adv.* **2014**, *32*, 1364–1381. [CrossRef]
2. Hong, D.D.; Hien, H.T. Nutritional analysis of Vietnamese seaweeds for food and medicineNo Title. *Biofactors* **2008**, *22*, 323–325. [CrossRef]
3. Chengkui, Z.; Tseng, C.; Junfu, Z.; Chang, C.F. Chinese seaweeds in herbal medicineNo Title. *Hdrobiologia* **1984**, *116*, 152–154. [CrossRef]
4. Niazi, A.K.; Kalra, S.; Irfan, A.; Islam, A. Thyroidology over the ages. *Indian J. Endocrinol. Metab.* **2011**, *15*, S121–S126. [CrossRef] [PubMed]

5. Yang, Y. *Chinese Herbal Medicines: Comparisons and Characteristicstle*; Churchill Livingstone: London, UK, 2009; Volume 268.
6. Hamed, S.M.; El-Rhman, A.A.A.; Ibraheem, I.B.M. Role of marine macroalgae in plant protection & improvement for sustainable agriculture technology. *Beni-Suef Univ. J. Basic Appl. Sci.* **2018**, *7*, 104–110.
7. Wells, M.I.; Potin, P.; Craigie, J.S.; Raven, J.A.; Merchant, S.S.; Helliwell, K.E.; Smith, A.G.; Camire, M.E.; Brawley, S.H. Algae as nutritional and functional food sources: Revisiting our understanding. *J. Appl. Phycol.* **2017**, *29*, 949–982. [CrossRef]
8. Kelman, D.; Posner, E.K.; McDermid, K.J.; Tabandera, N.K.; Wright, P.R.; Wright, A.D. Antioxidant activity of Hawaiian marine algae. *Mar. Drugs* **2012**, *10*, 403–416. [CrossRef]
9. Moussavou, G.; Kwak, D.H.; Obiang-Obonou, B.F.; Maranguy, C.A.; Dinzouna-Boutamba, S.; Lee, D.H.; Pissibanganga, O.G.M.; Ko, K.; Seo, J.I.; Choo, Y.K. Anticancer effects of different seaweeds on human colon and breast cancers. *Mar. Drugs* **2014**, *12*, 4898–4911. [CrossRef]
10. Riahi, C.R.; Tarhouni, S.; Kharrat, R. Screening of anti-inflammatory and analgesic activities in marines macroalgae from Mediterranean Sea. *Arch. Inst. Pasteur Tunis* **2011**, *88*, 19–28.
11. Zhao, C.; Yang, C.F.; Liu, B.; Lin, L.; Sarker, S.D.; Nahar, L.; Yu, H.; Cao, H.; Xiao, J. Bioactive compounds from marine macroalgae and their hypoglycemic benefits. *Trends Foods Sci. Technol.* **2018**, *72*, 1–12. [CrossRef]
12. Tierney, M.S.; Croft, A.K.; Hayes, M. A review of antihypertensive and antioxidant activities in macroalgae. *Bot. Mar.* **2010**, *53*, 387–408. [CrossRef]
13. Pérez, M.J.; Falque, E.; Domingue, H. Antimicrobial action of compounds from marine seaweed. *Mar. Drugs* **2016**, *14*, 52. [CrossRef] [PubMed]
14. Pangestuti, R.; Kim, S.K. Neuroprotective effects of marine algae. *Mar. Drugs* **2011**, *9*, 803–818. [CrossRef] [PubMed]
15. Alghazwi, M.; Kan, Y.Q.; Zhang, W.; Gai, W.P.; Garson, M.J.; Smid, S. Neuroprotective activities of natural products from marine macroalgae during 1999–2015. *J. Appl. Phycol.* **2016**, *28*, 3599–3616. [CrossRef]
16. Paris, D.; Beaulieu-Abdelahad, D.; Bachmeier, C.; Reed, J.; Ait-Ghezala, G.; Bishop, A.; Chao, J.; Mathura, V.; Crawford, F.; Mullan, M. Anatabine lowers Alzheimer's Aβ production in vitro and in vivo. *Eur. J. Pharmacol.* **2011**, *670*, 384–391. [CrossRef] [PubMed]
17. Isik, A.T. Late onset Alzheimer's disease in older people. *Clin. Interv. Aging* **2010**, *5*, 307–311. [CrossRef]
18. Bekris, L.M.; Yu, C.; Bird, T.D.; Tsuang, T.W. Genetics of Alzheimer disease. *J. Geriatr. Psychiatry Neurol.* **2010**, *23*, 213–227. [CrossRef]
19. Yamazaki, Y.; Painter, M.M.; Bu, G.; Kanekiyo, T. Apolipoprotein E as a therapeutic target in Alzheimer's disease: A review of basic research and clinical evidence. *CNS Drugs* **2016**, *30*, 773–789. [CrossRef]
20. Liu, C.; Kanekiyo, T.; Xu, H.; Bu, G. Apolipoprotein E and Alzheimer disease: Risk, mechanisms, and Therapy. *Nat. Rev. Neurol.* **2013**, *9*, 106–118. [CrossRef]
21. Kim, J.; Basak, J.M.; Holtzman, D.M. The role of apolipoprotein E in Alzheimer's disease. *Neuron* **2009**, *63*, 287–303. [CrossRef]
22. Shi, Y.; Yamada, K.; Liddelow, S.A.; Smith, S.T.; Zhao, L.; Luo, W.; Tsai, R.M.; Spina, S.; Grinberg, L.T.; Rojas, J.C.; et al. ApoE4 markedly exacerbates tau-mediated neurodegeneration in a mouse model of tauopathy. *Nature* **2017**, *549*, 523–527. [CrossRef] [PubMed]
23. Zhao, Y.; Zhao, B. Oxidative stress and the pathogenesis of Alzheimer's disease. *Oxid. Med. Cell. Longev.* **2013**, *2013*, 316523. [CrossRef] [PubMed]
24. Haam, J.; Yakel, J.L. Cholinergic modulation of the hippocampal region and memory function. *J. Neurochem.* **2017**, *142*, 111–121. [CrossRef] [PubMed]
25. Sadigh-Eteghad, S.; Sabermarouf, B.; Majdi, A.; Talebi, M.; Farhoudi, M.; Mahmoudi, J. Amyloid-beta: A crucial factor in Alzheimer's disease. *Med. Princ. Pract.* **2015**, *24*, 1–10. [CrossRef] [PubMed]
26. Reas, X.E. Amyloid and tau pathology in normal cognitive aging. *J. Neurosci.* **2017**, *37*, 7561–7563. [CrossRef]
27. Kametani, F.; Hasegawa, M. Reconsideration of amyloid hypothesis and tau hypothesis in Alzheimer's disease. *Front. Neurosci.* **2018**, *12*, 25. [CrossRef]
28. Shal, B.; Ding, W.; Ali, H.; Kim, Y.S.; Khan, S. Anti-neuroinflammatory potential of natural products in attenuation of Alzheimer's disease. *Front. Pharmacol.* **2018**, *9*, 548. [CrossRef]
29. Olasehinde, T.A.; Olaniran, A.O.; Okoh, A. Therapeutic potentials of microalgae in the treatment of Alzheimer's disease. *Molecules* **2017**, *22*, 480. [CrossRef]

30. Oboh, G.; Nwanna, E.E.; Oyeleye, S.I.; Olasehinde, T.A.; Ogunsuyi, O.B.; Boligon, A.A. In vitro neuroprotective potentials of aqueous and methanol extracts from *Heinsia crinita* leaves. *Food Sci. Hum. Wellness* **2016**, *5*, 95–102. [CrossRef]
31. Qui, C.; Kivipelto, M.; Strauss, E. Epidemiology of Alzheimer's disease: Occurrence, determinants, and strategies toward intervention. *Dialogues Clin. Neurosci.* **2009**, *11*, 111–128.
32. Graham, W.V.; Bonito-Oliva, A.; Sakmar, T.P. Update on Alzheimer's disease therapy and prevention strategies. *Annu. Rev. Med.* **2017**, *68*, 413–430. [CrossRef] [PubMed]
33. Yiannopoulou, K.G.; Papageorgiou, S.G. Current and future treatments for Alzheimer's disease. *Ther. Adv. Neurol. Disord.* **2013**, *6*, 19–33. [CrossRef] [PubMed]
34. Frozza, R.L.; Lourenco, M.V.; de Felice, F.G. Challenges for Alzheimer's disease therapy: Insights from novel mechanisms beyond memory defects. *Front. Neurosci.* **2018**, *12*, 37. [CrossRef] [PubMed]
35. Oboh, G.; Olasehinde, T.A.; Ademosun, A.O. Essential oil from lemon peels inhibit key enzymes linked to neurodegenerative conditions and pro-oxidant induced lipid peroxidation. *J. Oleo Sci.* **2014**, *63*, 373–381. [CrossRef] [PubMed]
36. Olasehinde, T.A.; Odjadjare, E.C.; Mabinya, L.V.; Olaniran, A.O.; Okoh, A.I. *Chlorella sorokiniana* and *Chlorella minutissima* exhibit antioxidant potentials, inhibit cholinesterases and modulate disaggregation of β-amyloid fibrils. *Electron. J. Biotechnol.* **2019**, *40*, 1–9. [CrossRef]
37. Oboh, G.; Adewuni, T.M.; Ademosun, A.O.; Olasehinde, T.A. Sorghum stem extract modulates Na$^+$/K$^+$-ATPase, ecto-5′-nucleotidase, and acetylcholinesterase activities. *Comp. Clin. Pathol.* **2016**, *25*, 749–756. [CrossRef]
38. Oboh, G.; Oyeleye, S.I.; Akintemi, O.A.; Olasehinde, T.A. *Moringa oleifera* supplemented diet modulates nootropic-related biomolecules in the brain of STZ-induced diabetic rats treated with acarbose. *Metab. Brain Dis.* **2018**, *33*, 457–466. [CrossRef]
39. Oboh, G.; Adewuni, T.M.; Ademiluyi, A.O.; Olasehinde, T.A.; Ademosun, A.O. Phenolic constituents and inhibitory effects of *Hibiscus sabdariffa* L.(Sorrel) calyx on cholinergic, monoaminergic, and purinergic enzyme activities. *J. Diet. Suppl.* **2018**, *15*, 910–922. [CrossRef]
40. Oboh, G.; Ademosun, A.O.; Ogunsuyi, O.B.; Oyedola, E.T.; Olasehinde, T.A.; Oyeleye, S.I. In vitro anticholinesterase, antimonoamine oxidase and antioxidant properties of alkaloid extracts from kola nuts (*Cola acuminata* and *Cola nitida*). *J. Complement. Integr. Med.* **2018**. [CrossRef]
41. Olasehinde, T.A.; Olaniran, A.O.; Okoh, A.I. Aqueous–ethanol extracts of some South African seaweeds inhibit beta-amyloid aggregation, cholinesterases, and beta-secretase activities in vitro. *J. Food Biochem.* **2019**, *43*, e12870. [CrossRef]
42. Olasehinde, T.A.; Mabinya, L.V.; Olaniran, A.O.; Okoh, A.I. Chemical characterization of sulfated polysaccharides from *Gracilaria gracilis* and *Ulva lactuca* and their radical scavenging, metal chelating, and cholinesterase inhibitory activities. *Int. J. Food Prop.* **2019**, *22*, 100–110. [CrossRef]
43. Olasehinde, T.A.; Mabinya, L.V.; Olaniran, A.O.; Okoh, A.I. Chemical characterization, antioxidant properties, cholinesterase inhibitory and anti-amyloidogenic activities of sulfated polysaccharides from some seaweeds. *Bioact. Carbohydr. Diet. Fibre* **2019**, *18*, 100182. [CrossRef]
44. Syad, A.N.; Rajamohamed, B.S.; Shunmugaiah, K.P.; Devi, P.K. Neuroprotective effect of the marine macroalga *Gelidiella acerosa*: Identification of active compounds through bioactivity-guided fractionation. *Pharm. Biol.* **2016**, *54*, 2073–2081. [CrossRef] [PubMed]
45. Rengasamy, K.R.; Amoo, S.O.; Aremu, A.O.; Stirk, W.A.; Gruz, J.; Šubrtová, M.; Doležal, K.; Staden, J.V. Phenolic profiles, antioxidant capacity, and acetylcholinesterase inhibitory activity of eight South African seaweeds. *J. Appl. Phycol.* **2015**, *27*, 1599–1605. [CrossRef]
46. Jung, S.H.; Young, U.M.; Inho, K.; Suengmok, C.; Daeseok, H.; Changho, L. In vitro screening for anti-dementia activities of seaweed extracts. *J. Korean Soc. Food Sci. Nutr.* **2016**, *45*, 966–997.
47. Rafiquzzaman, S.M.; Ki, E.Y.; Lee, J.M.; Mohibbullah, M.; BadrulAlam, M.; Moon, S.; Kim, J.M.; Kong, S. Anti-Alzheimers and anti-inflammatory activities of a glycoprotein purified from the edible brown alga *Undaria pinnatifida*. *Food Res. Int.* **2015**, *77*, 118–124. [CrossRef]
48. Shanmuganathan, B.; Sheeja, M.D.; Sathya, S.; Devi, P.K. Antiaggregation potential of *Padina gymnospora* against the toxic Alzheimer's beta-amyloid peptide 25–35 and cholinesterase inhibitory property of its bioactive compounds. *PLoS ONE* **2015**, *10*, e0141708. [CrossRef]

49. Castro-Silva, E.S.; Bello, M.; Hernández-Rodríguez, M.; Correa-Basurto, J.; Murillo-Álvarez, J.I.; Rosales-Hernández, M.C.; Muñoz-Ochoa, M. Invitro and insilico evaluation of fucosterol from *Sargassum horridum* as potential human acetylcholinesterase inhibitor. *J. Biomol. Struc. Dyn.* **2018**. [CrossRef]
50. Choi, B.W.; Lee, H.S.; Shin, H.; Lee, B.H. Multifunctional activity of polyphenolic compounds associated with a potential for Alzheimer's disease therapy from *Ecklonia Cava*. *Phytother. Res.* **2015**, *29*, 549–553. [CrossRef]
51. Sathya, M.; Premkumar, P.; Karthick, C.; Moorthi, P.; Jayachandran, K.S.; Anusuyadevi, M. BACE1 in Alzheimer's disease. *Clin. Chim. Acta* **2012**, *24*, 171–178. [CrossRef]
52. Cheng, X.; He, P.; Lee, T.; Yao, H.; Li, R.; Shen, Y. High activities of BACE1 in brains with mild cognitive impairment. *Am. J. Pathol.* **2014**, *184*, 141–147. [CrossRef] [PubMed]
53. Rockenstein, E.; Mante, M.; Alford, M.; Adame, A.; Crews, L.; Hashimoto, M.; Esposito, L.; Mucke, L.; Masliah, E. High β-secretase activity elicits neurodegeneration in transgenic mice despite reductions in amyloid-β levels. *J. Biol. Chem.* **2005**, *280*, 32957–32967. [CrossRef] [PubMed]
54. Jung, H.A.; Ali, M.Y.; Choi, R.J.; Jeong, H.O.; Chung, H.Y.; Choi, J.S. Kinetics and molecular docking studies of fucosterol and fucoxanthin, BACE1 inhibitors from brown algae *Undaria pinnatifida* and *Ecklonia stolonifera*. *Food Chem. Toxicol.* **2016**, *89*, 104–111. [CrossRef] [PubMed]
55. Seong, S.H.; Ali, M.Y.; Kim, H.R.; Jung, H.A.; Choi, J.S. BACE1 inhibitory activity and molecular docking analysis of meroterpenoids from *Sargassum serratifolium*. *Bioorg. Med. Chem.* **2017**, *25*, 3964–3970. [CrossRef] [PubMed]
56. Wagle, A.; Seong, S.H.; Zhao, B.T.; Woo, M.H.; Jung, H.A.; Choi, J.S. Comparative study of selective in vitro and in silico BACE1 inhibitory potential of glycyrrhizin together with its metabolites, 18a-and 18b-glycyrrhetinic acid, isolated from *Hizikia fusiformis*. *Arch. Pharm. Res.* **2018**, *41*, 409–418. [CrossRef]
57. Dong, X.; Wang, Y.; Qin, Z. 2009. Molecular mechanisms of excitotoxicity and their relevance to pathogenesis of neurodegenerative diseases. *Acta Pharm. Sin.* **2009**, *30*, 379–387. [CrossRef]
58. Fernandes, F.; Barbosa, M.; Oliveira, A.P.; Azevedo, I.C.; Sousa-Pinto, I.; Valentão, P.; Andrade, P.B. The pigments of kelps (*Ochrophyta*) as part of the flexible response to highly variable marine environments. *J. Appl. Phycol.* **2016**, *28*, 3689–3696. [CrossRef]
59. Kim, J.J.; Kang, Y.J.; Shin, S.A.; Bak, D.H.; Lee, J.W.; Lee, K.B.; Yoo, Y.C.; Kim, D.K.; Lee, B.H.; Kim, D.W.; et al. Phlorofucofuroeckol improves glutamate-induced neurotoxicity through modulation of oxidative stress-mediated mitochondrial dysfunction in PC12 cells. *PLoS ONE* **2016**, *11*, 0163433. [CrossRef]
60. O'Brien, R.J.; Wong, B.C. Amyloid precursor protein processing and Alzheimer's disease. *Annu. Rev. Neurosci.* **2011**, *34*, 185–204. [CrossRef]
61. Giffin, J.C.; Richards, R.C.; Craft, C.; Jahan, N.; Leggiadro, C.; Chopin, T.; Szemerda, M.; MacKinnon, S.L.; Ewart, K.V. An extract of the marine alga *Alaria esculenta* modulates α-synuclein folding and amyloid formation. *Neurosci. Lett.* **2017**, *22*, 87–93. [CrossRef]
62. Syad, A.N.; Devi, K.P. Assessment of anti-amyloidogenic activity of marine red alga *G. acerosa* against Alzheimer's beta-amyloid peptide 25–35. *Neurol. Res.* **2015**, *37*, 14–22. [CrossRef] [PubMed]
63. Alghazwi, M.; Smid, S.; Zhang, W. In vitro protective activity of South Australian marine sponge and macroalgae extracts against amyloid beta ($A\beta_{1-42}$) induced neurotoxicity in PC-12 cells. *Neurotoxicol. Teratol.* **2018**, *68*, 72–83. [CrossRef] [PubMed]
64. Gan, S.Y.; Wong, L.Z.; Wong, J.W.; Tan, E.L. Fucosterol exerts protection against amyloid β-induced neurotoxicity, reduces intracellular levels of amyloid β and enhances the mRNA expression of neuroglobin in amyloid β-induced SH-SY5Y cells. *Int. J. Biol. Macromol.* **2019**, *121*, 207–213. [CrossRef] [PubMed]
65. Alghazwi, M.; Smid, S.; Karpiniec, S.; Zhang, W. Comparative study on neuroprotective activities of fucoidans from *Fucus vesiculosus* and *Undaria pinnatifida*. *Int. J. Biol. Macromol.* **2019**, *122*, 255–264. [CrossRef] [PubMed]
66. Yang, E.J.; Ahn, S.; Ryu, J.; Choi, M.; Choi, S.; Chong, Y.H.; Hyun, J.W.; Chang, M.; Kim, H.S. Phloroglucinol attenuates the cognitive deficits of the 5XFAD mouse model of Alzheimer's disease. *PLoS ONE* **2015**, *10*, e0135686. [CrossRef]
67. Wang, J.; Zheng, J.; Huang, C.; Zhao, J.; Lin, J.; Zhou, X.; Naman, C.B.; Wang, N.; Gerwick, W.H.; Wang, Q.; et al. Eckmaxol, a phlorotannin extracted from *Ecklonia maxima*, produces anti-β-amyloid oligomer neuroprotective effects possibly via directly acting on glycogen synthase kinase 3β. *ACS Chem. Neurosci.* **2018**, *9*, 1349–1356. [CrossRef]
68. Oh, J.H.; Choi, J.S.; Nam, T. Fucosterol from an edible brown alga *Ecklonia stolonifera* prevents soluble amyloid beta-induced cognitive dysfunction in aging rats. *Mar. Drugs* **2018**, *16*, 368. [CrossRef]

69. Lin, J.; Yu, J.; Zhao, J.; Zhang, K.; Zheng, J.; Wang, J.; Huang, C.; Zhang, J.; Yan, X.; Gerwick, W.H.; et al. Fucoxanthin, a marine carotenoid, attenuates β-amyloid oligomer-induced neurotoxicity possibly via regulating the PI3K/Akt and the ERK pathways in SH-SY5Y cells. *Oxid. Med. Cell. Longev.* **2017**, *2017*, 6792543. [CrossRef]
70. Zhao, X.; Zhang, S.; An, C.; Zhang, H.; Sun, Y.; Li, Y.; Pu, X. Neuroprotective effect of fucoxanthin on β-amyloid induced cell death. *J. Chin. Pharm. Sci.* **2015**, *24*, 467–470.
71. Wei, H.; Gao, Z.; Zheng, L.; Zhang, C.; Liu, Z.; Yang, Y.; Teng, H.; Hou, L.; Yin, Y.; Zou, X. Protective effects of fucoidan on Aβ25–35 and d-Gal-induced neurotoxicity in PC12 cells and d-Gal-induced cognitive dysfunction in mice. *Mar. Drugs* **2017**, *15*, 77. [CrossRef]
72. Sathya, R.; Kanaga, N.; Sankar, P.; Jeeva, S. Antioxidant properties of phlorotannins from brown seaweed *Cystoseira trinodis* (Forsskål) C. Agardh. *Arab. J. Chem.* **2017**, *10*, S2608–S2614. [CrossRef]
73. Li, Y.; Fu, X.; Duan, D.; Liu, X.; Xu, J.; Gao, X. Extraction and identification of phlorotannins from the brown alga, *Sargassum fusiforme* (Harvey) setchell. *Mar. Drugs* **2017**, *15*, 49. [CrossRef] [PubMed]
74. Yuan, Y.; Zhang, J.; Fan, J.; Clark, J.; Shen, P.; Li, Y.; Zhang, C. Microwave assisted extraction of phenolic compounds from four economic brown macroalgae species and evaluation of their antioxidant activities and inhibitory effects on α-amylase, α-glucosidase, pancreatic lipase and tyrosinase. *Food Res. Int.* **2018**, *113*, 288–297. [CrossRef] [PubMed]
75. Arulkumar, A.; Rosemary, T.; Paramasivam, S.; Rajendran, R.B. Phytochemical composition, in vitro antioxidant, antibacterial potential and GC-MS analysis of red seaweeds (*Gracilaria corticata* and *Gracilaria edulis*) from Palk Bay, India. *Biocatal. Agric. Biotechnol.* **2018**, *15*, 63–71. [CrossRef]
76. Kosanić, M.; Ranković, B.; Stanojković, T. Biological activities of two macroalgae from Adriatic coast of Montenegro. *Saudi J. Biol. Sci.* **2015**, *22*, 390–397. [CrossRef] [PubMed]
77. Alencar, D.B.; Carvalho, C.F.T.; Rebouças, R.H.; Santos, D.R.D.; Pires-Cavalcante, K.M.; Lima, R.L.; Baracho, B.M.; Bezerra, R.M.; Viana, F.A.; Vieira, R.H.; et al. Bioactive extracts of red seaweeds *Pterocladiella capillacea* and *Osmundaria obtusiloba* (Florideophyceae: Rhodophyta) with antioxidant and bacterial agglutination potential. *Asian Pac. J. Trop. Med.* **2016**, *9*, 372–379. [CrossRef] [PubMed]
78. Agregán, R.; Munekata, P.E.; Domínguez, R.; Carballo, J.; Franco, D.; Lorenzo, J.M. Proximate composition, phenolic content and in vitro antioxidant activity of aqueous extracts of the seaweeds *Ascophyllum nodosum*, *Bifurcaria bifurcata* and *Fucus vesiculosus*. Effect of addition of the extracts on the oxidative stability of canola oil under accelerated storage conditions. *Food Res. Int.* **2017**, *99*, 986–994.
79. Pinteus, S.; Silva, J.; Alves, C.; Horta, A.; Fino, N.; Inês, A. Rodrigues susana mendes rui pedrosa. cytoprotective effect of seaweeds with high antioxidant activity from the Peniche coast (Portugal). *Food Chem.* **2017**, *218*, 591–599. [CrossRef]
80. Chiboub, O.; Ktari, L.; Sifaoui, I.; López-Arencibia, A.; Batle, M.R.; Mejri, M.; Valladares, B.; Abderrabba, M.; Piñero, J.E.; Lorenzo-Morales, J. In vitro amoebicidal and antioxidant activities of some Tunisian seaweeds. *Exp. Parasit.* **2017**, *183*, 76–80. [CrossRef]
81. Hifney, A.F.; Fawzy, M.A.; Abdel-Gawad, K.M.; Gomaa, M. Industrial optimization of fucoidan extraction from *Sargassum* sp. and its potential antioxidant and emulsifying activities. *Food Hydrocoll.* **2016**, *54*, 77–88. [CrossRef]
82. Rajauria, G.; Foley, B.; Abu-Ghannam, N. Identification and characterization of phenolic antioxidant compounds from brown Irish seaweed *Himanthalia elongata* using LC-DAD–ESI-MS/MS. *Innov. Food Sci. Emerg. Technol.* **2016**, *37*, 261–268. [CrossRef]
83. Leyton, A.; Pezoa-Conte, R.; Barriga, A.; Buschmann, A.H.; Mäki-Arvela, P.; Mikkola, J.P.; Lienqueo, M.E. Identification and efficient extraction method of phlorotannins from the brown seaweed *Macrocystis pyrifera* using an orthogonal experimental design. *Algal Res.* **2016**, *16*, 201–208. [CrossRef]
84. Olasehinde, T.A.; Olaniran, A.O.; Okoh, A.I. Neuroprotective effects of some seaweeds against Zn–induced neuronal damage in HT-22 cells via modulation of redox imbalance, inhibition of apoptosis and acetylcholinesterase activity. *Metab. Brain Dis.* **2019**. [CrossRef] [PubMed]
85. Olasehinde, T.A.; Olaniran, A.O.; Okoh, A.I. Phenolic composition, antioxidant activity, anticholinesterase potential and modulatory effects of aqueous extracts of some seaweeds on β-amyloid aggregation and disaggregation. *Pharm. Biol.* **2019**, *57*, 460–469. [CrossRef] [PubMed]

86. Huang, C.; Wu, S.; Yang, W.; Kuan, A.; Chen, C. Antioxidant activities of crude extracts of fucoidan extracted from *Sargassum glaucescens* by a compressional-puffing hydrothermal extraction process. *Food Chem.* **2016**, *197*, 1121–1129. [CrossRef] [PubMed]
87. Palanisamy, S.; Vinosha, M.; Marudhupandi, T.; Rajasekar, P.; Prabhu, N.M. Isolation of fucoidan from *Sargassum polycystum* brown algae: Structural characterization, in vitro antioxidant and anticancer activity. *Int. J. Biol. Macromol.* **2017**, *102*, 405–412. [CrossRef] [PubMed]
88. Hifney, A.W.; Fawzy, M.A.; Abdel-Gawad, K.M.; Gomaa, M. Upgrading the antioxidant properties of fucoidan and alginate from *Cystoseira trinodis* by fungal fermentation or enzymatic pretreatment of the seaweed biomass. *Food Chem.* **2018**, *269*, 387–395. [CrossRef]
89. Gomaa, M.; Fawzy, M.A.; Hifney, A.F.; Abdel-Gawad, K.M. Use of the brown seaweed *Sargassum latifolium* in the design of alginate-fucoidan based films with natural antioxidant properties and kinetic modeling of moisture sorption and polyphenolic release. *Food Hydrocoll.* **2018**, *82*, 64–72. [CrossRef]
90. Khajouei, R.A.; Keramat, J.; Hamdami, N.; Delattre, C.; Laroche, C.; Gardarin, C.; Lecerf, D.; Desbrières, J.; Djelveh, G.; Michaud, P. Extraction and characterization of an alginate from the Iranian brown seaweed *Nizimuddinia zanardini*. *Int. J. Biol. Macromol.* **2018**, *118*, 1073–1081. [CrossRef]
91. Yao, Y.; Xiang, H.; You, L.; Cui, C.; Sun-Waterhouse, D.; Zhao, M. Hypolipidaemic and antioxidant capacities of polysaccharides obtained from *Laminaria japonica* by different extraction media in diet-induced mouse model. *Int. J. Food Sci. Tech.* **2017**, *52*, 2274–2281. [CrossRef]
92. Kazir, M.; Abuhassira, Y.; Robin, A.; Nahor, O.; Luo, J.; Israel, A.; Golberg, A.; Livney, Y.D. Extraction of proteins from two marine macroalgae, *Ulva* sp. and *Gracilaria* sp., for food application, and evaluating digestibility, amino acid composition and antioxidant properties of the protein concentrates. *Food Hydrocoll.* **2019**, *87*, 194–203. [CrossRef]
93. Mohibbullah, M.; Maqueshudul, M.; Bhuiyan, H.; Hannan, M.A.; Getachew, P.; Hong, Y.; Choi, J.; Choi, S.; Moon, S. The edible red alga *Porphyra yezoensis* promotes neuronal survival and cytoarchitecture in primary hippocampal neurons. *Cell. Mol. Neurobiol.* **2016**, *36*, 669–682. [CrossRef] [PubMed]
94. Rajauria, G.; Foley, B.; Abu-Ghannam, N. Characterization of dietary fucoxanthin from *Himanthalia elongata* brown seaweed. *Food Res. Int.* **2017**, *99*, 995–1001. [CrossRef] [PubMed]
95. Yu, J.; Lin, J.; Yu, R.; He, S.; Wang, Q.; Cui, W.; Zhang, J. Fucoxanthin prevents H_2O_2-induced neuronal apoptosis via concurrently activating the PI3-K/Akt cascade and inhibiting the ERK pathway. *Food Nutr. Res.* **2017**, *61*, 1304678. [CrossRef]
96. Mohibbullah, M.; Haque, M.N.; Khan, M.N.; Park, I.S.; Moon, I.S.; Hong, Y. Neuroprotective effects of fucoxanthin and its derivative fucoxanthinol from the phaeophyte *Undaria pinnatifida* attenuate oxidative stress in hippocampal neurons. *J. Appl. Phycol.* **2018**. [CrossRef]
97. Syad, A.N.; Devi, P.K. *Gelidiella acerosa* protects against Aβ 25–35-induced toxicity and memory impairment in Swiss Albino mice: An in vivo report. *Pharm. Biol.* **2017**, *55*, 1423–1435.
98. Um, Y.M.; Lim, D.W.; Son, H.J.; Cho, S.; Lee, C. Phlorotannin-rich fraction from *Ishige foliacea* brown seaweed prevents the scopolamine-induced memory impairment via regulation of ERK-CREB-BDNF pathway. *J. Funct. Foods* **2018**, *40*, 110–116. [CrossRef]
99. Choi, J.Y.; Mohibbullah, M.; Park, I.S.; Moon, I.S.; Hong, Y.K. An ethanol extract from the phaeophyte *Undaria pinnatifida* improves learning and memory impairment and dendritic spine morphology in hippocampal neurons. *J. Appl. Phycol.* **2018**, *30*, 129–136. [CrossRef]
100. Hu, P.; Li, Z.; Chen, M.; Sun, Z.; Ling, Y.; Jiang, J.; Huang, C. Structural elucidation and protective role of a polysaccharide from *Sargassum fusiforme* on ameliorating learning and memory deficiencies in mice. *Carbohydr. Polym.* **2016**, *139*, 150–158. [CrossRef]
101. Wang, X.; Yi, K.; Zhao, Y. Fucoidan inhibits amyloid-β-induced toxicity in transgenic *Caenorhabditis elegans* by reducing the accumulation of amyloid-β and decreasing the production of reactive oxygen species. *Food Funct.* **2018**, *9*, 552–560. [CrossRef]
102. Lin, J.; Huang, L.; Yu, J.; Xiang, S.; Wang, J.; Zhang, J.; Yan, X.; Cui, W.; He, S.; Wang, Q. Fucoxanthin, a marine carotenoid, reverses scopolamine-induced cognitive impairments in mice and inhibits acetylcholinesterase in vitro. *Mar. Drugs* **2016**, *14*, 67. [CrossRef] [PubMed]
103. Xiang, S.; Liu, F.; Lin, J.; Chen, H.; Huang, C.; Chen, L.; Zhou, Y.; Ye, L.; Zhang, K.; Jin, J.; et al. Fucoxanthin inhibits β-amyloid assembly and attenuates β-amyloid oligomer-induced cognitive impairments. *J. Agric. Food Chem.* **2017**, *65*, 4092–4102. [CrossRef] [PubMed]

104. Zhang, L.; Wang, H.; Fan, Y.; Gao, Y.; Li, X.; Hu, Z.; Ding, K.; Wang, Y.; Wang, X. Fucoxanthin provides neuroprotection in models of traumatic brain injury via the Nrf2-ARE and Nrf2-autophagy pathways. *Sci. Rep.* **2017**, *7*, 46763. [CrossRef] [PubMed]
105. Yang, E.J.; Mahmood, U.; Kim, H.; Choi, M.; Choi, Y.; Lee, J.; Cho, J.; Hyun, J.; Kim, Y.S.; Chang, M.; et al. Phloroglucinol ameliorates cognitive impairments by reducing the amyloid β peptide burden and pro-inflammatory cytokines in the hippocampus of 5XFAD mice. *Free Radic. Biol. Med.* **2018**, *126*, 221–234. [CrossRef]

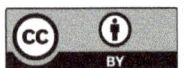

© 2019 by the authors. Licensee MDPI, Basel, Switzerland. This article is an open access article distributed under the terms and conditions of the Creative Commons Attribution (CC BY) license (http://creativecommons.org/licenses/by/4.0/).

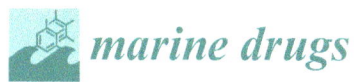

Review

Integral Utilization of Red Seaweed for Bioactive Production

Maria Dolores Torres, Noelia Flórez-Fernández and Herminia Domínguez *

Department of Chemical Engineering, Faculty of Sciences, University of Vigo, Campus Ourense, As Lagoas, 32004 Ourense, Spain; matorres@uvigo.es (M.D.T.); noelia.florez@uvigo.es (N.F.-F.)
* Correspondence: herminia@uvigo.es; Tel.: +34-988-387-082

Received: 8 May 2019; Accepted: 22 May 2019; Published: 28 May 2019

Abstract: The hydrocolloids carrageenan and agar are the major fraction industrially extracted and commercialized from red seaweeds. However, this type of macroalgae also contains a variety of components with nutritional, functional and biological properties. In the context of sustainability and bioeconomy, where the integral utilization of the natural resources is incentivized, the sequential separation and valorization of seaweed components with biological properties of interest for food, nutraceuticals, cosmeceuticals and pharmaceuticals is proposed. In this work, a review of the available conventional and alternative greener and efficient extraction for obtaining red seaweed bioactives is presented. The potential of emerging technologies for the production of valuable oligomers from carrageenan and agar is also commented, and finally, the sequential extraction of the constituent fractions is discussed.

Keywords: red seaweed; bioactives; extraction; biorefinery

1. Introduction

Seaweeds are widespread and traditionally used in Eastern countries for food and for medicinal purposes. In Western countries, despite being included recently in the diet, direct human consumption is still unusual, mainly being used for the production of hydrocolloids with thickening and gelling properties. Among seaweeds, red algae (Rhodophyta) contain high amounts of polysaccharides (floridean starch and sulfated galactans, such as carrageenans or agarans), proteins and derived peptides (phycobiliproteins, phycolectins and mycosporine-like amino acids), minerals and other valuable compounds, such as polyphenols and lipids [1,2]. The whole algae of red seaweeds have been traditionally used as food, while agars and carrageenans have been extracted for multiple purposes, namely for food, pharmaceutical applications and biotechnological applications.

The reader can find compilations on the chemical and nutritional characteristics of seaweeds as a feed livestock resource [3] and its health-promoting properties [4], including the anticancer [5] and antiviral [6] features. Additionally, there have been some interesting reviews on the use of red seaweeds for carrageenans [7], agar and carrageenan oligosaccharides [8]. The extraction technology, which influences the composition, structure and properties of the target solutes, is conventionally addressed using chemicals, in long term operation, and with high energy consumption [9]. The recent developments of blue biotechnology and novel extraction techniques meeting the requirements of low cost, sustainability, food-compatibility and industrial scale feasibility to obtain seaweed components [10], the systematical selection of operational variables of emerging extraction technologies [11] or the use of alternative solvents, such as ionic liquids [12], or supercritical CO_2 for macro and microalgae [13] have been reviewed. Scarcer studies are focused on the extraction of red seaweed components, such as carrageenan and agar fractions [9,14], photoprotective substances [15] and pigments [16]. Particular interest has been on the influence on the depolymerization of saccharidic and protein components, since both the type of extraction process and the operational conditions have to be controlled depending on the future uses [17]; however, further development and additional studies are still needed [18]. The mentioned studies are oriented to the selective extraction of some valuable fractions, but scarce information is found for the simultaneous utilization of the different components in a more rational scheme, following the philosophy of the biorefineries [19]. Biomass refineries, with a production scheme analogous to the petroleum refineries, are aimed at obtaining a wide range of products from renewable raw materials, including value added components for the food, cosmetic and pharmaceutical industries, as well as biofuels. These multistage multiproduct processes are based on the sequential fractionation of the biomass and on their subsequent physical, chemical or biotechnological transformation into the target final products. This sustainable approach adopts an integral utilization of resources, promoting the development of a marine bio-economy.

The present review presents an overview of the properties and potential applications of red seaweed bioactives, the specific technologies for extraction and also for the depolymerization of agar and carrageenan into oligosaccharides, as well as the potential of these techniques for the extraction of other red seaweed components. Both conventional and emerging extraction and depolymerization technologies are discussed with the aim of promoting the sustainability based on (i) the development of clean processes and (ii) the integral utilization and valorization of resources following the philosophy of biomass biorefineries.

2. Components: Properties and Extraction

2.1. Polysaccharides

Polysaccharides are the main components in marine algae according to their abundance and their current commercial value based on their technological features [4,20]. More recently, attention has been directed to their health benefits [21,22]. These polysaccharides, generally not digested by humans, are considered to be dietary fibers [23]. The composition, structure and rheological properties are influenced by the algal source, life-stage, growth, environment and by the extraction method [24]. Agars and carrageenans are major cell wall polysaccharides in red macroalgae, also known as galactans, accounting for up to 40–50% of the dry weight. They are highly anionic homopolysaccharides, composed of a backbone built from disaccharide blocks of D-galactose and 3,6-anhydrogalactose (L-AHG in agar and D-AHG in carrageenan) with different sulfation, methylation and pyruvation patterns that vary among species [21,25]. The high electronegative charge density from their sulfated esters favors the electrostatic interactions with specific proteins, determining their biological effects, which are also closely related to the structural features [20,26–28]. Proteins, minerals and lipids also confer red seaweed important structural value [29].

2.1.1. Agar

- Composition, structure, occurrence and properties

Agar is a linear polysaccharide composed of alternating (1,3) linked D-galactose and (1,4) linked 3,6-anhydro-L-galactose [25] and substituted in some degree by sulfate, methyl or pyruvate groups [30–32]. The molecular structure of agar polysaccharides, particularly the type and location of sulfate esters, appears to be species-specific [33]. Agar has two different constituents: agarose and agaropectin (Figure 1). Agarose is a neutral linear polysaccharide composed of three linked β-D-galactose and four linked 3,6-anhydro-α-L-galactose. Agaropectin is an acid polysaccharide containing sulfate groups, pyruvic acid, and D-glucuronic acid conjugated to agarobiose. Agarose accounts for up to 70% of the mixture and is responsible for gelling, whereas agaropectin is responsible for thickening characteristics. Different derived agarose molecules can be obtained from chemical or enzymatic degradation. Most of the corresponding hydrolysis products such as agarooligosaccharides (AOSs), neoagarooligosaccharides (NAOSs), neoagarobiose (NAB) and 3,6-anhydro-L-galactose (L-AHG) exhibit biological activities [34].

Agar is mainly found in the cell matrix of seaweeds of the order Gelidiales (*Gelidium* and *Pterocladia*) and Gracilariales (*Gracilaria* and *Hydropuntia*), which have become the major worldwide source. Its abundance and easier exploitation made *G. tenuistipitata* an economically important raw material for agar production [35]. In comparison with agars from *Gelidium* and *Pterocladia*, agars from *Gracilaria* can have higher degrees of sulfation, methoxylation and pyruvylation [31].

The agar properties are dependent on the species and environmental characteristics of the collection or cultivation area, such as season, life cycle and geographical features [36,37] and the storage, extraction processes and postharvest storage [24,32,38–41]. The quality of agar is determined by the type, pattern and degree of substitution as well as molecular weight, chemical composition (pyruvate, methyoxyl and sulfate) and physical properties (gel strength, gel syneresis, viscosity, gelling and melting temperatures) that determine its market value [30,32,42]. The agar gel strength, in terms of elastic modulus (G'), of systems formulated at 1.5% agar in milli-Q water is around 238 Pa at 25 °C, with gelling temperatures of 48 °C, and those agars with gel strengths greater than 6.9×10^4 Pa are referred to as high quality agars [24].

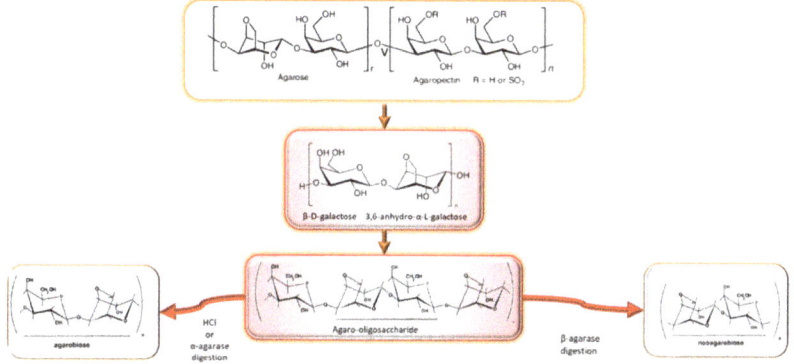

Figure 1. Scheme of the agar constituents (agarose and agaropectine) and different derived molecules with biological activities, adapted from [43,44].

Agar is a generally recognized as safe (GRAS) food additive in the United States and a food additive approved in Europe (E406). Agar cannot be digested in the gastrointestinal tract because humans lack α/β-agarases, but can be metabolized by intestinal bacteria to D-galactose [45]. Agar is demanded as gelling agent and stabilizing agent, and as cryoprotectants in the pharmaceutical, cosmetics and food industries [39,46–49]. The human food industry demands for 80% production, and biotechnological applications for the remaining 20% [50]. The importance of these products is based on high market demand for agar and the higher price compared to alginates and carrageenans [24,32,51]. It is used as a gelling, thickening and stabilizing agent in food formulations and it has also been used in microbiological media and in chromatographic techniques. Most native agars from *Gracilaria* are not bacteriological grade agar due to their high content of methoxyls, but they can be food and reactive grade [52].

- Extraction processes: conventional and emerging technologies

The storage conditions and duration before extraction affects the agar quality from *Gracilaria*, since seaweeds are susceptible to degradation by agarolytic enzymes and bacteria. Some species from temperate and cold water could be more resistant to hydrolysis during storage. Postharvest treatment with acid, alkali or formaldehyde is necessary to prevent enzymatic and microbial degradation [32,37,40,47,50,53]. Another factor requiring attention after harvesting algae is correct drying under 20% moisture and packing, and avoid wetting during the transporting and storage period, but dewatering pre-treatments have to be defined according to the species and to collection season [54].

Although *Gelidium* agar has better quality and is easily extracted with boiling water, the gelling ability of agars from *Gracilaria sp* can be enhanced by an alkali pretreatment to convert α-L-galactose 6 sulfate into 3,6-anhydro-α-L-galactose. This treatment reduces the sulfate content and improves the gelling properties as evidenced by higher gel strength, gelling, melting temperatures and viscosity [42]. Generally, the alkali-treatment was most effective for obtaining more galactose-rich hydrocolloids [24]. However, agar degradation and diffusion towards the aqueous medium could occur, reducing the extraction yield [29,55], although in some cases, no reduction was observed [24]. Alkaline pretreatment variables, such as alkaly type and concentration or heating time and temperature affected the yield and quality of the agar. Regardless the alkaline concentration, NaOH rendered agar with a higher quality than KOH [35,56]. Compilations of conditions are also found in [37], being the optimal in the range 5–7% NaOH, up to 80–100 °C for 0.5–3 h [29,35,46,48,50], but higher alkali concentrations (10%) [55], shorter times [57] and the application of several stages [53] have also been reported. An alternative pretreatment was proposed by Roleda [58], which consisted of soaking the *Gelidiella acerosa* air dried sample in 0.5% acetic acid for 1 h at 16–20 °C, then 1 h steam pressure at 15–20 psi and boiling at 100 °C. Freile-Pelegrín [59] proposed the cultivation of *Gracilaria cornes* under dark and salinity treatments (50 and 25% salinity) to replace the alkali treatment. Pigments, such as chlorophyll, carotenoids and phycoerythrobilin, can be leached out during the alkaline pretreatment and an alternative environmentally friendly scalable photobleaching process for *Gracilaria asiatica* and *Gracilaria lemaneiformis* with 3–5% NaOH and photobleaching for 5 h was proposed [60]. The pigments and the agar sulfate contents decreased during the photobleaching agar extraction process, and the gel strength increased during the photolysis.

The industrial agar extraction process is based on using hot water during several hours under conventional heating, a time-consuming process requiring high solvent consumption and generating large amounts of waste disposal. Therefore, water recycling has been suggested [36]. Compilations on agar yield (10–43.4%) can be found in [37]. Cold extraction with distilled water at room temperature was reported for *Gracilaria birdiae* [61], but agar extracts prepared at 20 °C showed a wider size distribution (1–30,000 kDa) [62]. For the chemical liquefaction of agarose, acid prehydrolysis has been commonly employed [63–65]. Mild conditions, such as low acid concentrations, low temperatures or short reaction times, result in even-numbered oligosaccharides due to the preferential cleavage of α-1,3-glycosidic linkages and the release of the acid-labile L-AHG at the reducing end converts even-numbered AOSs into odd-numbered ones. The released L-AHG is readily degraded into 5-hydroxymethylfurfural [65]. Table 1 summarizes some representative examples of the conventional and emerging technologies proposed for agar extraction. Another disadvantage of alkali treatment is the generation of effluents with environmental impact if not properly treated [66]. Enzymatic treatment could be a more ecofriendly alternative to improve the gel strength of agar. Shukla [67] proposed the use of sulfatase/sulfohydrolase to decrease the sulfate content and increase both the 3,6-anhydrogalactose content and gel strength of agar. However, the cost could not make the process commercially competitive with this sulfatase/sulfohydrolase compared to alkaline treatment [22].

Processes based on combined heat and ultrasound treatments would enable reducing the amount of time and energy needed. Martínez-Sanz et al., [29] observed a four-fold reduction in time without affecting the yields and properties of *Gelidium sesquipedale* agar-based extracts. The extracts also contained proteins, polyphenols and minerals, conferring antioxidant capacity to the browned softer gels. In contrast, an alkali pre-treatment could yield almost pure agars with higher molecular weights and crystallinities and resulted in stiffer gels, but lower extraction yields.

Microwave assisted extraction (MAE) allowed reducing the required 2–4 h for agar extraction in conventional processes to a very short period, consuming less energy and solvent volume and reducing waste disposal requirements [9,48]. Navarro and Stortz [68] used microwave assisted alkaline modification to improve the gelling properties of carrageenans from *Iridaea undulosa* and porphyran from *Porphyra columbina*. Substantial depolymerization of *Gracilaria vermiculophylla* agar was observed in microwave assisted extraction with lower values of viscosity and molecular weight (54 kDa against

111 kDa) and methylation degree than those obtained in conventional extraction [36]. Intermittent microwave treatment was proposed for the extraction of sulfated porphyran from *Porphyra dentata* with ethanol and the gelling capacity of extracted porphyran was not affected [69].

Other technologies have been proposed, such as ionic liquid-based extraction [12], radiation to increase the agar yield from *Gelidiella acerosa*, at 15 kGy yield increased, but the gel strength decreased and the sulfate level did not vary significantly [70].

Table 1. Some examples of technologies proposed for agar extraction.

Pretreatment/Extraction	Seaweed	Gel Properties	Reference
P: - E: Distilled water; pH 6.3–6.4; 100 °C, 1.5 h; ethanol precipitation	*Gracilaria cornes*	GS: (1.2–2.5) × 10^4; Tg: 39.2–41.8; Tm: 74.3–82.6; Mw: ND	[59]
P: 1–15% NaOH, 90 °C, 1 h, 0.025% HCl, 1 h E: Water, 100 °C, 2 h, ethanol precipitation	*Gracilaria verrucosa*	GS: (1.6–1.8, 2.6–2.7) × 10^4; Tg: 32–43; Tm: 49–80.5; Mw: ND	[55]
P: - E: Distilled water, 20–28 °C, 15 h, ethanol precipitation	*Gracilaria birdiae*	GS: ND; Tg: ND; Tm: ND; Mw: 1–30,000	[61]
P: - E: Water, 80–100 °C, 2–4 h; ethanol precipitation	*Hydropuntia cornea*	GS: (0.7–1.3) × 10^4; Tg: 25–32.1; Tm: 65–79; Mw: 342–371 kDa	[71]
^{1} P: 5–7% NaOH, 80–100 °C, 0.5–3 h E: Water, 80 °C, pH 6.2, 90 min, ethanol precipitation	*Gracilaria vermiculophylla*	GS: (0.9–1.2) × 10^5; Tg: 52–68; Tm: 92–95; Mw: ND	[37]
^{1} P: 1–5% NaOH, 30–85 °C, 1–2 h E: Water, 700–115 °C, 2–3 h, 1–2 stages, ethanol precipitation	*Gracilaria corticata*, *Gracilaria eucheumoides*, *Gracilaria cliftonii*, *Gracilaria lemaneiformis*	GS: (1.2–4.2) × 10^4; Tg: ~32; Tm: ~78; Mw: ND	[50,53,72,73]
P: 5% NaOH, 1–48 h, room temperature. Dil. H_2SO_4, 15 min E: Water, 100 °C, 1 h 30 min, ethanol precipitation	*Gracilaria manilaensis*	GS: (1–4.9) × 10^4; Tg: ND; Tm: ND; Mw: ND	[56]
P: - E: Pressurized water extraction, 120 °C, 15 min, ethanol precipitation	*Gracilaria vermiculophylla*	GS: 1.3 × 10^5; Tg: 40.7; Tm: 93.1; Mw: ND	[48]
P: Acetic acid, 16–20 °C, 1 h E: Steam pressure, 15–20 psi; ethanol precipitation	*Gelidiella acerosa*	GS: (4.9–6.9) × 10^4; Tg: 42–47; Tm: 90–98; Mw: ND	[58,74]
^{1} P: 2.5 M NaOH, 90 °C, 2 h E: Water, 90 °C, 2 h; ultrasound assisted, 30 min, 400 w, 24 kHz; ethanol precipitation	*Gelidium sesquipedale*	GS: (0.2–1.2) × 10^5; Tg: ND; Tm: ND; Mw: (2.5–11) × 10^5	[29]
^{1} P: 0.1 M NaOH, 22 °C E: Enzyme (60 °C, 12 h, pH 8) and ultrasound assisted extraction (60 °C, 30 min, 60 W); ethanol precipitation	*Gracilaria birdiae*	GS: ND; Tg: ND; Tm: ND; Mw: 20–45	[75]
P: - E: Protease digestion, 60 °C, 6 h, pH 5	*Gracilaria cornea*	GS: ND; Tg: ND; Tm: ND; Mw: ND	[76]
P: Radiation, at 5–15 kGy E: Water, 95–100 °C or pressure cooking 121 °C, 15 psi, 1 h; ethanol precipitation	*Gelidiella acerosa*	GS: (2.5–6.0) × 10^4; Tg: ND; Tm: ND; Mw: ND	[70]

^{1} Optional pretreatment; P: pretreatment conditions; E: extraction conditions; GS: gel strength (G′, elastic modulus at 25 °C, Pa); Tg: gelling temperature (°C); Tm: Melting temperature (°C); MW: Molecular weight (kDa); ND: not determined.

- Agarooligosaccharides: properties and production strategies

Two oligosaccharides can be formed depending on the moiety of end sugar, namely, agaro-oligosaccharides and neoagaro-oligosaccharides [77]. Neoagarobiose, α-L-3,6-anhydro-L-galactosyl-

(1→3)-β-D-galactopyranose, is the basic unit of neoagarooligosaccharides. Neoagarooligosaccha-rides were found to be safe up to 5000 mg/kg body weight in acute oral toxicity tests with rat and beagle dog models [45].

The biological activities of agar oligosaccharides include anti-microbial, antiviral [78], prebiotic [79], anti-tumoral, immunomodulatory, anti-inflammatory [76,80–87], glucosidase inhibitory [77], anticariogenic [34], hepatoprotective [83], antioxidant [77,83] and other properties of interest for skin care [45,77,84,85] (Figure 2). Liu et al. [86] summarized research progress on biological activities of agaro-oligosaccharide. Agaro-oligosaccharides display antioxidant effects which differ according to their degree of polymerization [77]; additionally, Kazłowski et al. [87] summarized the influence of the degree of polymerization (DP) of agar oligomers on their physiological activities. Agarose is biocompatible and has been used for neural and cartilage tissue repair [88] and for the preparation of biomaterials [89,90]. Due to its low cell adhesiveness and slow degradation rate, agarose was composited with fast degradable biomaterials for drug delivery, tissue engineering and wound healing [91].

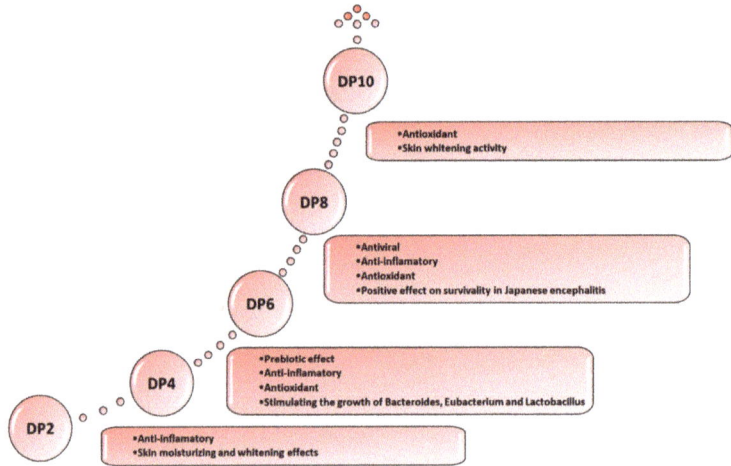

Figure 2. Influence of the depolymerization degree (DP) of agar oligomers on their biological properties [34,77,84,87,92,93].

Agaro-oligosaccharides (AOS) are conventionally prepared by acid hydrolysis of agars; however, this method produces substantial pollution and wastes. Alternative strategies have also been proposed using the same subsequent stages for purification, usually based on ultrafiltration, ethanolic precipitation, purification by chromatography and further in activated carbon [77,83,87].

Several acids have been used to hydrolyze agar. Chen [77] compared the use of hydrochloric acid, citric acid and cationic exchange resin; the latter avoided the neutralization step and offered higher yield of agaro-oligosaccharides with high DP (octaose and decaose) and low content of agarobiose. Hydrochloric acid hydrolysis produced DP lower than 6, whereas citric acid yielded small amount of oligosaccharides, mainly agarooctaose and agarodecaose.

Alternative methods have been used to hydrolyze agar, such as enzymatic, physical and chemical degradation. Enzymatic hydrolysis, which can be performed by agarases [77], show disadvantages such as the low activity, low stability and productivity, which limit their wide application in industry. However, chemical degradation, especially acid hydrolysis, is available for industrial preparation because of its simplicity, rapidity, low cost and high yield [77]. Different bacteria have been used as a source of agarolytic enzymes, i.e., *Flammeovirga pacifica* [83], *Streptomyces coelicolor* [45] or *Agarivorans* sp. JA-1 [84]. Agar oligosaccharides can be produced by hydrolysis using chemicals or agarolytic enzymes.

Since agarose comprises alternating L-AHG and D-galactose units linked by α-1,3- and β-1,4-glycosidic bonds, two types of agarases exist: α-agarases cleave the α-1,3 linkages of agarose endolytically and produce agaro-oligosaccharides AOSs as the reaction products. Neoagarooligosaccharides are prepared from agar by β-agarase hydrolysis, by cleaving the β-1,4-glycosidic linkages of agarose endolytically or exolytically, and also releases neoagarooligosaccharides with neoagarobiose or neogarobiose alone, respectively. Agaro-oligosaccharides obtained by enzymatic degradation exhibited high solubility percentages, water and oil absorption capacities, as well as considerable 2,2-diphenyl-1-picrylhydrazyl (DPPH) and 2,2′-azino-bis(3-ethylbenzothiazoline-6-sulphonic acid (ABTS$^+$) radical scavenging and ferric reducing antioxidant activities, depending on the degree hydrolysis [94]. Kazłowski et al. [44,87] prepared neoagaro-oligosaccharides by β-agarase digestion and agaro-oligosaccharides by HCl hydrolysis from agarose and observed that the enzymatically prepared oligosaccharides usually show a low DP and a broad range of bioactivities, whereas those from acid hydrolysis contain only oligosaccharides with odd numbers of sugar unit [83].

The agaro-oligosaccharides, obtained from commercial agarose through enzymatic hydrolysis, did not show improvement on its oil and water absorption capacities. Furthermore, a higher degree hydrolysis could lead to increase the reducing capacity and antiradical properties (Table 2).

Table 2. Examples of techniques for depolymerization of agar.

Depolymerization Technique	Seaweed or Polysaccharide	Activity	Reference
Acid (HCl, citric acid, and cationic exchange resin (solid acid))	Agar (C)	Antioxidant and -glucosidase inhibition	[77]
Enzymatic	Agarose (C) Gracilaria cornea Gracilaria lemaneiformis	Functional, antioxidant, skin whitening	[76,83,84,94]
Free-radical induced	Halymenia durvillei	ND	[95]
High-pressure homogenization	Halymenia durvillei	ND	[95]
Microwave assisted	Pyropia yezoensis	Antioxidant	[93]
Ultrasound assisted	Porphyra yezoensis Gracilaria birdiae	Anticoagulant, antioxidant	[75,96]

C: commercial; ND: not determined.

Zou et al. [93] prepared low molecular weight polysaccharides (3.2, 10.5, 29.0, and 48.8 kDa) from *Pyropia yezoensis* using microwave-assisted acid hydrolysis. The lower molecular weight (Mw) product (3.2 kDa) was the most efficient protecting wheat seedlings against salt stress. These authors also indicated that microwave irradiation accelerated the reaction rate. Stronger gels were also obtained using microwave assisted extraction when compared with gels produced applying the traditional method. The average sulfate content was similar to the obtained by the traditional method from *G. vermiculophylla* produced in the selected integrated multitrophic aquaculture (IMTA) system. However, radical depolymerization assisted by ultrasounds induced a loss of sulfate functions in addition to the shortening of the polysaccharides chain length [97]. It should be indicated that the microwave assisted extraction approach requires less energy and solvent than conventional processes, while generating fewer wastes.

Free-radical depolymerization of polysaccharides, based on the formation of free radicals ·OH by the Fenton reaction using a metallic catalyst, was proposed as a reproducible scalable technique for the degradation of polysaccharides without changes in structural features, producing an average molar mass of 1500 kDa [95].

High-pressure homogenization performed on the polysaccharide of *Halymenia durvillei* showed their feasibility and effectiveness and showed that an advantage of the degradation at high pressure was the ease and speed of the preparation [95].

It has been suggested that ultrasound promotes the extraction of other non-sulfated polysaccharides [75]. One of the fractions obtained by ultrasonic degradation of *Porphyra yezoensis* polysaccharides did not change the main structure of polysaccharides and enhanced the antioxidant properties of the agar fractions [96].

Combination of techniques was also useful, enzyme and ultrasound assisted extraction led to the same sulfated polysaccharides from *Gracilaria birdiae* [75], but the yield was higher when both techniques were jointly applied to alkaline treated seaweeds. Combined techniques were used in the extraction of pigments and sulfated polysaccharides from the red alga *G. verrucosa*. The method is easy to use, allows the extraction of pigments and agar highly quantitative in one step. Sulfated polysaccharides obtained were similar to agar extracted directly from dried material without any treatment. Compared to the common agar extraction method, enzyme mixtures tested for R-phycoerythrin can be proposed as pretreatment for agar extraction. However, Öğretmen and Duyar [98] observed that autoclave provided lower agar yields than water bath from Gelidium latifolium.

Agaro-oligosaccharide dried products show high thermal and pH stability; however, the drying step is highly relevant to other product properties, both functional (water solubility index, water absorption capacity and oil absorption capacity) and antioxidant (radical scavenger and reducing capacity). Kang et al. [94] observed the highest solubility index in spray dried products and the highest water and oil absorption capacities in freeze dried products, which showed minimal color deterioration and higher oxidative stability, whereas the oven drying could be more deleterious. Antiradical properties were high in freeze-dried and spray-dried oligosaccharide powders.

2.1.2. Carrageenan

- Composition, structure, occurrence and properties

Carrageenans are high-molecular-weight linear hydrophilic, sulfated galactans formed by alternate units of D-galactose and 3,6-anhydrogalactose alternately linked by α-1,3 and β-1,4 glycosidic linkages. They can be classified according to differences in their average molecular mass and to the number and the position of the sulfate ester groups and the occurrence of a 3,6 anhydro-ring in the α-linked galactose. The three types with higher commercial importance, namely κ-, ι- and λ-carrageenan, are presented in Figure 3.

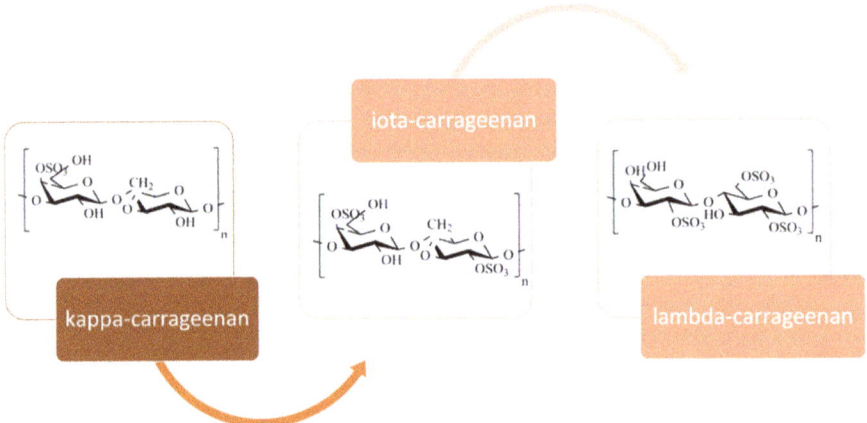

Figure 3. Repeating units in the main three types of carrageenan with commercial interest, adapted from Pereira [99].

Carrageenans are mainly obtained from the genus *Chondrus*, *Eucheuma*, *Gigartina*, *Iridae*, *Furcellaria* and *Hypnea*, and the expansion and increased demand led to the introduction of the cultivation of

Kappaphycus alvarezii and *Eucheuma denticulatum*, with a predominant content of k- and i-carrageenan, respectively, available all year [100]. *Chondrus crispus*, the original source, which contains a mixture of k- and λ- carrageenan, could be a model organism [101] and there is a renewed interest in the cultivation for cold water carrageenophytes, although the economics need to be carefully considered [102]. The differences in composition and molecular conformation determines the rheological profiles, gel properties and textures of carrageenans as well as the interactions with other gelling agents and food ingredients [103].

The three most commercially exploited carrageenans are kappa (κ-), iota (ι-) and lambda (λ-) carrageenans, which can be separately provided or as a well-defined mixture, since most of the seaweeds contain hybrid carrageenans [22]. Mu and nu carrageenans are the precursors in carrageenan, which are converted to kappa and iota, respectively, by means of alkaline modification. In the natural state, unmodified kappa and iota carrageenans account for around 30% mu and nu-carrageenans, remaining less than 5% after alkaline modification, randomly distributed within the repeating structures [103]. Origin, species or extraction processing conditions notably affect the type and quality of carrageenan isolated. The carrageenan types vary among species from the *Cystocloniaceae* family predominantly produce iota-carrageenans; the *Gigartinaceae* family lead to hybrid kappa-iota carrageenans and lambda-family carrageenans (sporophytic plants); the *Phyllophoraceae* family produces kappa-iota hybrid-carrageenans [104]. Commonly, κ-carrageenan is commercially isolated from *Kappaphycus alvarezii* red seaweed through a hot extraction process, whereas λ-carrageenan is more hygroscopic and it is usually extracted from red seaweeds of the genera *Gigartina* or *Chondrus* by drum dryer or alcohol precipitation process [105]. Concerning ι-carrageenan, it is commercially extracted from *Eucheuma denticulatum* by the freeze thaw or gel process [106]. The highest carrageenan yields can exceed 70% (dry basis) for some species such as *B. gelatinum*, *K. alvarezii* or *K. striatum*. Other species have values close to 30%, such as *E. denticulatum* or *C. crispus*. Sulfate content in carrageenans varies from 20% in κ-carrageenan, to 33% in ι-carrageenan and to 41% in λ-carrageenan [107]. It is well known that the carrageenans gelation process is affected by the biopolymer content, temperature, ionic strength of the solution and the cation type and content, being the most effective K^+ and Rb^+. In general, iota carrageenans form soft and elastic gels with higher gelling temperatures than κ-carrageenans [108]. In contrast, λ-carrageenan did not form gels, being used solely as thickening agent [109]. Gelling temperatures ranged from 32 to 36 °C for the κ-carrageenans, whereas ι-carrageenans exhibited values of 70–74 °C. Gel strengths, elastic modulus at 25 °C, varied between 4000–6500 Pa for alkali pre-treated samples [24].

Carrageenan is a natural ingredient, used for decades in food applications and generally recognized as safe (GRAS) by the Food and Drug Administration; furthermore, carrageenan and semi-refined carrageenan are food additives (E-407 and E407a, respectively) approved by European Food Safety Authority. The food viscosity specification is equivalent to an average molecular weight greater than 100 kDa, and commercial food carrageenan have Mw in the range 200–800 kDa [102,103]. Carrageenan is not degraded nor absorbed in the gastrointestinal tract [110–112] and should not contain low Mw fractions, poligeenan or degraded carrageenan, since it exhibits toxicological properties at high doses [110] and can induce gastrointestinal irritation and cancer in animal models [112] or can lead to cell death and inflammatory responses on human colonic epithelial cells [113,114], bacterial dysbiosis and shifted community composition [115] and decreased anti-inflammatory bacteria [116]. Further studies of its impact on digestive proteolysis, the colon microbiome and inflammation [117–119] and the effects on predisposed populations [119,120] are required. Carrageenans are also used for the pharmaceutical sector [106,107], based on anti-inflammatory [121], antiviral [6,122–126], anticoagulant [17,127], immunomodulatory [128], antitumoral [129], antioxidant [17,129,130], anti-angiogenic [97] and neuroprotective [129] activities. The biological properties of carrageenans have been reviewed in several publications [28,119,131–133].

Carrageenans are widely used as an inflammatory inducing agent in experimental animals [134], and have also been proposed for the immobilization and encapsulation of biocatalysts [135], for entrapping lactic bacteria and enzymes [136], for microencapsulation of probiotics in mixtures of k-carrageenan with carboxymethylcellulose [137]. Recent pharmaceutical applications are found in drug delivery and for tissue regeneration [138]. Carrageenans are highly biocompatible and are used as ingredients for films, beads, microparticles, nanoparticles, hydrogels, inhalable and injectable systems [107,108,139] used alone or in combination with other polymers, and its mucoadhesive properties have been exploited in the preparation of aerogel microparticles for mucosal drug delivery [140].

The role of carrageenans in agriculture has also been confirmed [141–148], since it stimulates growth [149] and increases defense responses against viruses [141,148] and abiotic stresses [93].

- Extraction processes: conventional and emerging technologies

Specific details of the commercial extraction processes are trade secrets for the manufacturers of carrageenan. The seaweed is usually dried quickly to prevent degradation during transportation to the processing facilities. The original method to produce the commercial carrageenans is based on washing to remove impurities, such as sand, epiphytes and salt and the carrageenan extraction in a hot aqueous solution, neutral or alkaline, filtration, recovery from the solution by alcohol precipitation, separation of the precipitate, drying and milling. However, this method is time and energy consuming, and has a low extraction efficiency. Alternatively, extraction of minerals, protein and lipids can be proposed, leaving in the raffinate the carrageenan and cellulose as a semi-refined low purity carrageenan. The main variables during extraction, namely temperature, pH, time and alkaline pre-treatment (alkaline agent, concentration and time), have to be optimized for each seaweed to maximize the structural and gelling properties [150,151]. The alkali pretreatment of red seaweed increases the ratio of ι- versus κ-hybrid [17], but usually, an excessive alkali content and prolonged treatment time can lower molecular mass and depressed gel properties [150]. Table 3 shows some representative examples of carrageenan extraction procedures.

Table 3. Carrageenan yields and extraction procedures.

Process [1]	Seaweed	Properties	Reference
[1] P: 6% KOH, 80 °C, 3 h E: Water, 90–105 °C, 1.5 h, ethanol precipitation	Hypnea musciformis, Kappaphycus alvarezii, Solieria chordalis	Y: 19–27; GS: (4–6.5) × 10^3; Tg: 32–36, 70–74	[24,152]
P: - E: Water, room temperature, 24 h, ethanol precipitation	Mastocarpus stellatus	Y: 15–30 BP: antioxidant, anti-coagulant activities	[17]
[1] P1,2: 3% KOH, 90 °C, 4 h E1: Water, room temp, 12 h, ethanol precipitation E2: Ultrasound assisted extraction, 15–30 min, 400–500 W, ethanol precipitation	Kappaphycus alvarezii, Euchema denticulatum, Hypnea musciformis	E1: Y: 30–40 E2: Y: 32–49, higher yield with shorter times BP: No differences in antioxidant features	[7,153]
P1: 3% KOH, 85 °C, 3.5 h E1: Water, 85 °C, 12 h, ethanol precipitation P2:- E2: Microwave assisted closed vessels, 85–105 °C, 10–20 min, ethanol precipitation	Hypnea musciformis, Solieria chordalis	E1: Y: 20–40 E2: Y: 15–25; higher desulfation degree; BP: antiviral	[152,154]
P, E: Alkali extraction, ethanol precipitation	Chondracanthus acicularis, Chondracanthus teedei, Gigartina pistillata, Chondrus crispus	Y: 15–45%	[104]

[1] Optionally, an alkaline pretreatment can be applied; P: pre-treatment conditions; E: extraction conditions; Y: yield (%); GS: gel strength (G′, elastic modulus at 25 °C, Pa); Tg: gelling temperature (° C); BP: biological properties.

Alternatively, low temperature has been proposed to extract low-molecular-weight carrageenans [155] and to maintain reducing, antiradical and anticoagulant activities, probably due to the higher sulfate content, which would be lost after hot-water, acid and alkali treatments [17].

Other options can lower time, energy demand and the consumption of water, chemicals and solvents. Among the novel extraction techniques to enhance the extraction efficiency are pressurized solvent extraction, microwave-, ultrasonic- and enzyme-assisted extractions [7,9,14].

Microwave-assisted extraction offers a reduction in time and energy consumption, thus enhancing the process efficiency [9]. Operating in closed vessel, more efficient desulfation was observed and the κ/ι hybrid carrageenan obtained was comparable to that extracted by the conventional technique [154]. Boulho et al. [152] did not observe significant differences in the carrageenan (predominantly iota-) yield from *Solieria chordalis*, were observed between MAE and conventional method under alkaline conditions, and the product showed antiviral activity against *Herpes simplex* virus type 1. Almutairi et al. [156] reported λ-carrageenan discoloration occurring during microwave irradiation for the aqueous solutions exposed to microwave heating.

The ultrasound assisted processes both alkaline and aqueous, shortened extraction times compared to the conventional method, avoiding degradation of labile compounds, showing a slight variation in sulfate, AG and Gal contents and viscosity [153]. Youssof et al. [7] reported that they doubled the yields attained in four–eight longer times with conventional extraction without affecting the chemical structure and molar mass distribution of carrageenans.

- Carraoligosaccharides: properties and production strategies

Oligocarrageenans are oligomers of sulfated galactose, usually DP 2–20 [148,157], prepared by depolymerization by acid hydrolysis. Despite the degraded carrageenan caused significant mucosal ulceration of the colon, associated to histopathological changes, epithelial thinning, slight erosion, cellular infiltration and other negative changes in animal organisms [143], carrageenan oligosaccharides exhibit several biological activities, influenced by their molecular weight and sulfation degree.

Carrageenan oligosaccharides show scavenging properties against reactive oxygen species [158], hydroxyl radicals, superoxide anion, nitric oxide and hydrogen peroxide [159]. They also present anti-inflammatory and immunomodulatory [6,131,160,161], anticoagulant [158], antimicrobial and antiviral [6,148,158,162–164] and healing [165] properties. They also showed anticarcinogenic action [158,166–169], with low cytotoxicity [167] and synergistic effects with conventional drugs, improving the immunocompetence damaged by these drugs. The oligocarrageenans promote plant growth by enhancing photosynthesis, nitrogen assimilation, embryogenesis, basal metabolism, cell division, regulation of phytohormone synthesis [170–173] and by increasing protection against viral, fungal and bacterial infections [147,148,174,175], partly due to the accumulation of compounds with antimicrobial activity [148].

Partial depolymerization by chemical or enzymatic hydrolysis to obtain a range of oligosaccharides is a common strategy for structural analysis and for characterization of activity [176,177]. The biological profile of the products may be influenced by the depolymerization method, since it affects their size and molecular weight. In addition, carrageenan or their derived oligosaccharides may also be chemically modified by oversulfation, desulfation, acetylation or phosphorylation to achieve better physicochemical and biological properties [28,160,164,176], i.e., the antioxidant [176] and antiviral [178] activities.

Acid hydrolysis has been considered as a common and rapid method. The presence of acid and oxidizing agents may induce carrageenan depolymerization through cleavage of glycosidic linkages, a process accelerated by dissolved oxygen, high temperature and low pH. In order to limit undesirable degradation, high temperature and short time mild acid hydrolysis is preferred [164]. Karlsson and Singh [179] reported that carrageenans were stable to desulfation during acid (pH 2) hydrolysis at 35 and 55 °C. Kalitnik et al. [161] used mild acid hydrolysis of *Chondrus armatus* κ-carrageenan under conditions avoiding excess destruction of 3,6-AGal and observed that mild and acid hydrolysis cause breakage of inside α-1,3 links, producing mainly odd-numbered oligosaccharides. Mild acid hydrolysis at 37 °C increased yields of even fractions in comparison with those obtained at 60 °C [180].

Enzymatic hydrolysis offers advantages due to its high efficiency under mild conditions, avoids the use of polluting chemicals, and the resulting oligosaccharides generated show higher homogeneity and lower polydispersity, thus providing compounds with improved and reproducible biological properties [107]. In addition, it avoids side reactions leading to undesired modifications of the native structure and the release of high amounts of monosaccharides and undesirable toxic products [8]. The enzymatic method, either using non-specific commercial enzymes or carragenases, is a relatively costly alternative. Carrageenases, produced only by marine gram negative bacterial species, are endohydrolases that hydrolyze the internal β-1,4 linkages in carrageenans [22,107,181]. Table 4 summarizes some representative examples of depolymerized carrageenans.

Microwave assisted degradation allowed a reduction in operation times and almost did not change the structure and constitutions of the λ-carrageenan [162], and κ-carrageenan [157] with antiviral properties. However, the special high-pressure equipment needed could be difficult to operate [162]. Operation in closed vessels and in open vessel was reported; additionally, operation in domestic devices could be proposed for acid hydrolysis [157].

During ozonation the depolymerization of polysaccharides causes chemical changes, as well as physicochemical and rheological modifications, since ozonation of κ-carrageenan leads to the formation of carbonyl, carboxyl or double bonds; however, the sulfate groups in k-carrageenans were maintained [177].

The ultrasound-assisted depolymerization of κ-carrageenan is simple, suitable for food applications and energy saving, since it is faster than thermal depolymerization at lower temperatures [158]. The susceptibility to ultrasound assisted degradation differs among the carrageenan types, being higher for κ- than for τ-carrageenans [182] and possibly occurs due to the ultrasonically induced breakage of non-covalent bonds in κ-carrageenan molecules [158].

Table 4. Examples of technologies used for extraction of carrageenan oligomers.

Depolymerization	Seaweed or Polyssaccharide	Properties	References
Acid hydrolysis	Carrageenan (C)	Mw: κ-, 510–4000; ι-, 110–3300; λ-, 660–5800	[179]
Acid hydrolysis	Eucheuma cottonii	DP: κ-, 6–20	[180]
Enzymatic	Chondrus armatus, Kappaphycus alvarezii, Tichocarpus crinitus	Mw: k-, 2.2–4.3	[176,178]
Enzymatic	Carrageenan (C)	Mw: k-, 681–798	[183]
High-Pressure	Halymenia durvillei	Mw: λ-, 260–1100	[95]
Irradiation	Carrageenan (C)	Mw: κ-, 8.5–32.1; ι-, 3.1–6.9; λ-, 2.7–6.5	[184]
Microwave assisted	Solieria chordalis, Chondrus ocellatus	Mw: λ-, 3–240 Mw: λ-, 650	[152,162]
Ozonization	Carrageenan (C)	Mw: k-, 10–200	[177]
Radical depolymerization	Halymenia durvillei	Mw: λ-, 3.3–890	[95]
Subcritical water extraction ionic liquids as catalyst	Kappaphycus alvarezii	Mw: k-, 10–60	[185]
Ultrasound assisted	Kappaphycus alvarezii, Eucheuma cottonii	Mw: k-, 545 Mw: k-, 160–240	[158,182]

C: commercial; Mw: Molecular weight (kDa); DP: degree of polymerization.

Carrageenan can be degraded by gamma irradiation, operating in different systems (solid, gel or solution) at ambient temperature and the molecular weights can be lowered to 8–100 kDa with a narrow distribution, but different yield and susceptibility to degradation occur for the different carrageenan types. Abad [184] reported the use of irradiation with gamma rays at room temperature to depolymerize polysaccharides with enhanced antioxidant properties [186]. Irradiated κ-carrageenan as incorporated as antioxidants in many food systems, but the toxicity of radiolytic products from irradiated κ-carrageenan have to be studied further [184].

Comparative studies have revealed that the method of depolymerization strongly influences the properties of carrageenan oligomers [178]. The chemical depolymerization (free radical or mild acid hydrolysis), produced oligomers with lower Mw (1.2–3.5 kDa) than the enzymatic depolymerization using a recombinant kappa-carrageenase from *Pseudoalteromonas carrageenovora*, yielding 2.2 kDa oligomers from *Chondrus armatus* and *Kappaphycus alvarezii* κ-carrageenans and 4.3 kDa oligomers from *Tichocarpus crinitus* κ/β-carrageenans. Low molecular weight derivatives obtained by mild acid hydrolysis showed higher antiviral activity than those obtained by free radical depolymerization, which were more active than those enzymatically prepared. Sun et al. [176] observed that mild acid hydrolysis caused higher saccharide degradation than H_2O_2 depolymerization and κ-carrageenase digestion; the original sulfate content was substantially retained and all the hydrolysates had stronger reducing power than the polysaccharide, with H_2O_2 hydrolysates being the most potent. After free radical treatment at 40 °C for 4 h, the low-molecular weight oligosaccharides from κ-carrageenan ranged from disaccharide to octasaccharide. The degradation with a κ-carrageenase hydrolyzing the β-1,4 linkages to a series of homologous, even-numbered oligosaccharides (An-G4S)n, yielding 2, 4, 6, 8 and 10 DP, being dominant the tetra- and hexasaccharides [176]. Whereas for H_2O_2 treatment, the scavenging ability increased with time as a result from the increment of –COOH groups, the scavenging ability of HCl hydrolysates and enzymatic hydrolysates decreased when the molecular weight decreased. Other combinations have been suggested, i.e., radical depolymerization, and high-pressure homogenization led to several samples of various and controlled molar masses of *Halymenia durvillei* [95].

2.2. Protein

The protein content in red algae, higher than in brown and green groups, accounts for 10–50% of the dry weight, being comparable or higher than in some foods [187,188] and the essential aminoacid content, accounting for 25–50% of the total amino acids, is similar as in other protein sources such as casein, ovalbumin and leguminous [3,189–191]. The protein contents differ according to the species and seasonal conditions [187,188], being the highest in *Porphyra*, followed by *Palmaria* sp. Nitrogen-to-protein conversion factors of 4.92, lower than for brown and green algae have been proposed [192,193] and algae may contain non-protein nitrogen, resulting in an overestimation of their protein content. Although the digestibility of proteins seems to be limited by the algae non-proteic fraction [187,189] they have been proposed for inclusion in diets of ruminants, hens, rabbit, poultry and pigs [3].

Red algae have a characteristic bright pink color caused by phycobiliproteins. Phycobiliproteins are covalently bound via cysteine amino acids to pigmented phycobilins [3,16]. They are classified into phycoerythrin (red) and phycocyanin (blue). The two types of phycoerythrin (PE) were named after the taxa of the organism form which they were first isolated: R-PE from Rhodophyta and B-PE from Bangiales. Phycocyanins are further subdivided into C-phycocyanin, R-phycocyanin, allophycocyanin or phycoerythrocyanin. Examples of phycobiliproteins found in red seaweeds are shown in Figure 4.

Phycobiliproteins are commercially used in foods, nutraceuticals, cosmetics as a colorant and for their therapeutic value, namely their antimicrobial, antioxidant, anti-inflammatory, neuroprotective, hepatoprotective, immunomodulating and anticarcinogenic properties [16,194–201]. They can improve the efficacy of standard anticancer drugs, lower their side effects [202] and act as photosensitizers for the treatment of tumoral cells [203]. They are also used as fluorescent markers in clinical diagnostics and immunological analysis.

The storage conditions influence the preservation of phycoerythrin (R-PE) and freezing was reported as the best preservation method [204]. Significant changes in phycoerythrin and phycocyanin were also observed after different culinary treatments [205]. Whereas drying and hydration did not affect the content of phycoerythrin, boiling and steaming caused lowered values.

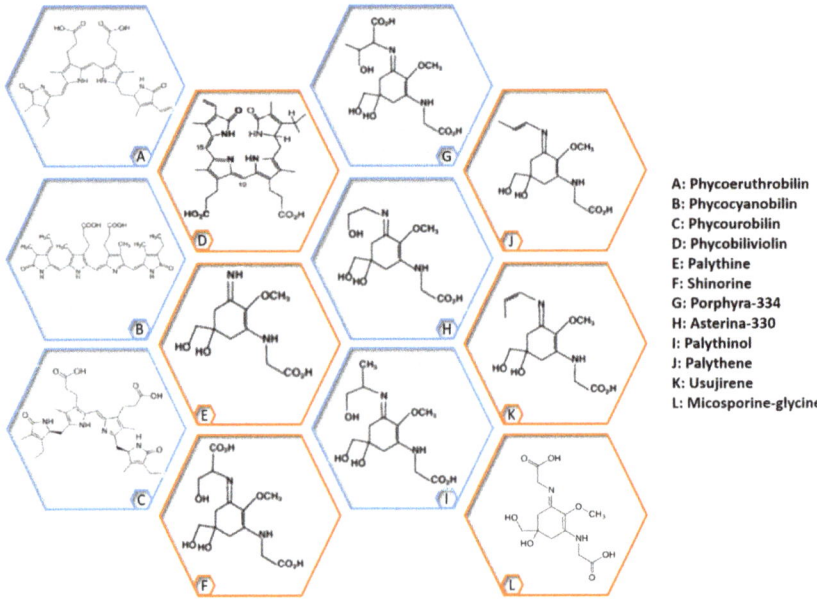

Figure 4. Structure of phycobiliproteins and micosporine-like-aminoacids, adapted from [16,188].

- Extraction processes: conventional and emerging technologies

Since the extraction of proteins from seaweeds is complicated by the presence of cell wall polysaccharides, the classical procedures are based on the use of buffer, osmotic shock, detergents or the application of alkali treatment, some examples are summarized in Table 5. Different physico-chemical and enzymatic pretreatments have been suggested to enhance the yields, such as repeated freeze-thaw cycles [201,206], or grinding in liquid nitrogen of the freeze-dried seaweeds [207] aided in the release of R-phycoerythrin. Their further purification from the crude extract has been usually addressed through ammonium sulfate precipitation [208] or also by sucrose step-gradient ultracentrifugation [209] followed by purification by gel filtration and by ion exchange chromatography [130,210–212].

The use of enzymes degrading the cell wall polysaccharides as an alternative method to improve the extraction and the solubilization of algal proteins [188], since firstly reported by Amano and Noda [213] suggested the use of a mixture of enzymes from the gut of abalone *Haliotis discus* and a commercial one to enhance the extraction of proteins from *Porphyra yezoensis*. Enzyme assisted extraction could improve the physicochemical characteristics, volatile compounds and organoleptic quality of plant proteins producing peptides and amino acids with less salt and carcinogenic compounds than acid hydrolysis [214]. Both the extraction efficiency and the composition of the extracts depended on the seaweed [215], but the influence of the type of enzyme is also determinant on yields, composition and properties. Whereas some cellulases enhanced the protein extraction yields when used alone [190,216], in other studies, polysaccharidases alone or in mixtures caused only a partial digestion of seaweed cell walls and did not improve the yields [217,218] and mixtures of cellulase with carrageenase or agarase were more favorable [201,217]. Proteolytic hydrolysis is usually proposed to obtain bioactive peptides; however, the protease treatments also enhanced the extraction of antioxidants from *Palmaria palmata* compared to carbohydrases and cold water extraction [190].

Table 5. Red seaweed protein extraction.

Technologies	Seaweed	Product	Properties	Reference
Accelerated solvent extraction (acetone or methanol)	Porphyra umbilicalis	Carbohydrate/ Phlorotannin extraction	Antioxidant	[219]
Carbohydrase hydrolysis under high hydrostatic pressure	Palmaria palmata, Solieria chordalis	Antioxidant peptides	Antioxidant	[220]
Enzyme hydrolysis with: protease, agarase, carrageenase, xylanase, cellulase	Gelidium pusillum Chondrus crispus, Gracilaria verrucosa, Palmaria palmata Osmundea pinnatifida, Codium tomentosum, Solieria chordalis	Antioxidant peptides, protein, phycobiliproteins, R-phycoerythrin	Antioxidant, α-glucosidase inhibition anti-inflammatory	[197,201, 215,216, 221–227]
Freezing and thawing	Porphyra haitanensis, Gelidium pusillum	Phycobiliproteins (R-PE and R-PC)	Antioxidant	[210,228]
Grinding freeze-dried seaweed in liquid nitrogen	Mastocarpus stellatus	R-phycoerythrin	Antioxidant	[207]
Homogenization in water or buffer	Chondrus crispus, Palmaria palmata, Heterosiphonia japonica, Gelidium pusillum	Phycobiliproteins (R-PE and R-PC)	Antioxidant, antidiabetic, antitumor	[130,189, 228,229]
Osmotic shock	Palmaria palmata, Polysiphonia urceolata	Bioactive peptides, R-phycoerythrin	Antioxidant, prevention of atherosclerosis	[210,223]
Subcritical water, optionally catalyst	Hypnea musciformis, Kappaphycus alvarezii	Protein, antioxidants, emulsifyiers	Antioxidant, emulsifyier	[230,231]
Ultrasound-assisted extraction	Palmaria palmata, Porphyra umbilicalis	Bioactive peptides R-PE and R-PC	Antioxidant	[215,219, 223,228]
Ultrasound-assisted extraction	Gelidium pusillum, Porphyra yezoensis	R-PE, R-PC, taurine	Antioxidant	[228,232]
Ultrasound and enzyme-assisted extraction	Osmundea pinnatifida, Codium tomentosum	Protein	Antioxidant, prebiotic effect	[215]

Additionally, it can be useful in combination with other intensification technologies. Le Guillard et al. [233] reported ultrasound-assisted extraction and ultrasound-assisted enzymatic hydrolysis with an enzymatic cocktail for the extraction of R-phycoerythrin from *Grateloupia turuturu*. They recommended the use of 22 °C to avoid R-PE destruction, and 40 °C when the objective was liquefaction. Enzymatic hydrolysis was combined with mechanical methods, namely, ultrasonication [201]. Suwal [220] reported on the use of a non-thermal high hydrostatic pressure (400 MPa, 20 min) processing combined with polysaccharidases to improve the extraction of proteins, polyphenols and polysaccharides from *Palmaria palmata* and *Solieria chordalis*; the effect of this technique being dependent on the seaweed species and the enzyme used. Mittal et al. [228] compared different pre-treatments for extraction of phycobiliproteins from *Gelidium pusillum* and observed a synergistic effect of ultrasonication when employed in combination with other conventional extraction methods, although ultrasonication alone was not efficient. However, Harrysson et al. [219] observed that the pH-shift protein extraction provided the highest protein yields and concentration in the extracts from *Porphyra umbilicalis*, compared to sonication. Fitzgerald et al. [223] used a papain digestion of crude *Palmaria palmate* protein obtained by osmotic shock and ultrasound assisted extraction, with the aim of obtaining bioactive peptides for the prevention of atherosclerosis and the hydrolysate was nontoxic.

Gereniu et al. [230] extracted protein from *Kappaphycus alvarezii* processed by pressurized hot water extraction. Whereas the hydrolysis efficiency increased from 150 °C to 270 °C, and decreased at 300 °C due to decomposition and protein denaturation, the highest foaming properties were attained at 150 °C, whereas the best emulsifying properties were found at 300 °C. Pangestuti et al. [231] proposed the hydrolysis of *Hypnea musciformis* using subcritical water extraction (120–270 °C) to obtain antioxidant and functional material. They found increased protein and sugar content at 120–150 °C, more marked at higher temperatures (180–210 °C), showing the highest antioxidant activity and thermostable emulsifying properties, which could be related to the increased solubility of protein, to the hydrolysis of oligosaccharides and the degradation of monosaccharides.

Wang et al. [232] reported on the use of ultrasound-assisted extraction during the purification of taurine from *Porphyra yezoensis*. This sulfur-containing amino acid can enhance seafood profile flavour. Homotaurine, an aminosulfonate compound present in different species, has shown in vitro and in vivo neuroprotective effect and could be a promising drug for both prevention of Alzheimer's disease [234]. Operating at 40 °C and 300 W, the ultrasonic process lowered the extraction time by nine compared to the conventional extraction.

2.3. Lipids and Fatty acids

In red seaweed, lipids and fatty acids are present in low amounts, generally 1–5% of the dry weight [235,236]; however, they contain significantly higher levels or polyunsaturated fatty acids than vegetables and have been proposed as a chemotaxonomic tool to differentiate macroalgae [237]. Macroalgae also contain various other lipids and lipid like compounds such as sterols, phospholipids and glycolipids, but red seaweeds have a high ω-3 fatty acids content, being a rich source of α-linolenic acid (ALA) [18:3(ω3)], AA, eicosapentaenoic acid (EPA) [20:5(n-3)], and docosahexaenoic acid (DHA) [22:6(ω3)]), and most species showed a nutritionally beneficial ω6/ω3 ratio [3,238,239] (Table 6). Some macroalgae present a low ω6/ω3 ratio, the ω3 polyunsaturated fatty acids (PUFAs) cannot be synthesized by humans and are thus obtained only through dietary sources. Their therapeutic, especially eicosapentaenoic acid (EPA), has been shown in the reduction of blood cholesterol, and in the protection against cardiovascular and coronary heart diseases [240], and they have anti-inflammatory, anti-thrombotic and anti-arrhythmic properties [241].

Total fatty acid concentrations vary among species, accounting for 1–8 in % of dry weight, showing significant differences in the fatty acid profiles [242], which can also be depending on the storage conditions (time and temperature) and the solvent also influences the yields and composition of the lipid extracts [242].

Kumari et al. [237] compiled the total lipid content and fatty acid distribution of different seaweeds and suggested that the variations observed between different species of the same genus was more likely to be due to the inter-specific/intra-generic variations rather than to geographical and environmental conditions as apparent from the minor variations found with the environmental parameters for the studied collection sites.

- Extraction processes: conventional and emerging technologies

The growing interest in PUFA-rich lipids from seaweeds for incorporation into foods has led to an increasing demand for novel extraction techniques with food grade solvents providing high extraction yields. Supercritical CO_2 extraction of bioactives (neutral lipids and antioxidants) from microalgae and seaweeds [243] is performed in a non-oxidizing atmosphere, which can prevent degradation. Drying and crushing are required stages despite the high energy consumption of the first stage. Chen and Chou [227] reported similar fatty acid profiles of different red seaweeds extracted by supercritical fluids extraction method; however, Cheung [244] observed increased proportions of *Hypnea charoides* PUFAs with operation pressure. The total fatty acid content and the EPA content in the extract produced by pH-shift was slightly reduced compared to that in the crude seaweed from *Porphyra umbilicalis* [219].

Patra et al. [245] reported the use of microwave assisted hydrodistillation to extract the volatile oil from *Porphyra tenera*, which showed radical scavenging properties comparable with BHT and α-tocopherol. Kumari et al. [246] reported on the application of sonication and buffer individually on the lipid extraction from *Gracilaria corticata* with analytical purposes. Table 6 shows the extraction yields and the PUFA ratio for different red seaweed genus obtained with conventional and alternative extraction technologies.

Table 6. Total lipid (TL) content, polyunsaturated fatty acids PUFA ratio and distribution in red seaweed extracts.

Seaweed Genus	Extraction	TL (mg/g fr. wt.)	PUFA/SFA	ω6/ω3	Reference
Acanthophora	CHF/M/PB	6.8–10.4	0.79–0.94	0.9–1.8	[237]
Asparagopsis	CSE (H)	3.0	0.06	0.62	[238]
Bangia	SFE	13.3 dw	2.8	2.22	[240]
Bornetia	CSE (H)	5.3	0.76	0.29	[238]
Botryocladia	CHF/M/PB	2.3–5.2	0.49–0.54	1.7–3.6	[237]
Coelarthrum	CHF/M/PB	7.7	0.67	5.7	[237]
Delisea	CSE (Et; DCM:M)	2.2	1.35	0.4	[242]
Galaxaura	SFE	19.8 dw	0.98	0.71	[240]
Gastroclonium	CHF/M/PB	4.3	0.59	5.1	[237]
Gelidiopsis	CHF/M/PB	5.5	0.84	0.8	[237]
Gelidiella	CHF/M/PB	6.7	0.98	0.6	[237]
Gracilaria	CHF/M/PB	2.9–9.7	0.15–2.13	0.6–1.9	[237]
Grateloupia	CHF/M/PB; SFE	5.0–6.4, 13.6 dw	0.74–1.4	0.5–1.9	[237,240]
Griffithsia	CHF/M/PB	4.2			[237]
Halymenia	CHF/M/PB; SFE	10–18.8 dw	1.37–1.8	1.7–5	[237,240]
Helmintocladia	SFE	19.7 dw	1.05	1	[240]
Hypnea	SCF: 50 °C, 37.9 MPa	5.8–7.8	0.31–0.43	0.8–16	[237,243]
Jania	CSE (H)	2	0.79	0.60	[238]
Jania	CHF/M/PB	12.2	0.32	2.9	[237]
Laurencia	CSE (Et; DCM:M)	5.4–16.0	0.41–1.08	0.4–1.7	[237,242]
Liagora	SFE	17.6–21.5 dw	0.94–1.43	0.42	[240]
Peyssonelia	CSE (H)	4.8	1.33	1.9	[238]
Porphyra	MAHD: 40 W, water	11.2–12.4 dw	2.4–2.5	1.2–9.1	[240,245]
Pterocladiella	CSE (H)	5.5	0.51	0.9	[238]
Pyropia	CHF/M/PB	7.0–7.7	1.23–1.76	0.7–1.4	[237]
Rhodymenia	CHF/M/PB	7.1	0.87	88.2	[237]
Sarconema	CHF/M/PB	4.3–9.8	0.27–1.04	2.4–2.5	[237]
Solieria	CHF/M/PB	9.0	0.35	0.8	[237]
Cryptonemia	CHF/M/PB	11.3	0.86–1.28	0.9–18.8	[237]
Odonthalia	CHF/M/PB	11.4	0.72	0.6	[237]
Polysiphonia	CHF/M/PB	9.6	0.53	1.1	[237]
Scinaia	CHF/M/PB	5.2–17 dw	0.23–1.86	1.1–5.3	[237,240]
Palmaria	CSE (Et; DCM:M)	14–46 dw	0.49–1.1	0.21–0.41	[241,247]
Vertebrata	CSE (Et; DCM:M)	13–18 dw	0.79	0.4	[247]

CSE: Conventional solvent extraction; CHF/M/PB: chloroform–methanol–phosphate buffer; Et: ether extraction; DCM:M: dichloromethane/methanol; H: hexane; MAHD: Microwave assisted hydrodistillation; SFE: Supercritical fluid extraction.

2.4. Extractives

The solvent influences the composition and activity as well as the mechanism of action of extracts [248]. Many studies aimed at the solvent extraction of polyphenols, flavonoids and carotenoids [249]. Organic solvents, such as ethanol, methanol, acetone or their mixtures such as chloroform:methanol, have been used for the extraction of antioxidant components, some illustrative examples are shown in Table 7. The choice of extracting solvents with different polarities can have a significant effect due to the different nature of compounds present in the seaweeds and also species–species differences. Intensification with ultrasound was suggested to enhance the solvent extraction process [250].

Supercritical fluid extraction with pure carbon dioxide can be favorable for the extraction of apolar compounds [13], the addition of a small amount of polar modifiers may increase the affinity of this solvent for relatively polar compounds. Zheng et al. [251] obtained extracts, mainly composed by sesquiterpenes, ketones, fatty acids, phenols and sterols from *Gloiopeltis tenax* by supercritical carbon dioxide extraction with ethanol as modifier, and reported remarkable antioxidant and antimicrobial activity. Ospina et al. [252] reported the extraction of *Gracilaria mammillaris* extracts compounds with antioxidant activity using supercritical CO_2 modified with ethanol.

When the simultaneous extraction of different components is addressed, the selection of the enzyme activities could be relevant, i.e., for the extraction of phenolics from *P. palmate*, protease provided higher contents than water extract, whereas some carbohydrases showed lower contents, an effect ascribed to their ability of proteases to liberate LMW peptides and amino acids by proteases, which could also enhance the scavenging activities of the extracts [190]. Combination of enzyme digestion with cellulase and hemicellulose, which disrupted or weakened the structural integrity of the seaweed cell wall and high hydrostatic pressure (HHP) increased the accessibility of enzymes, accelerating the release of intracellular polyphenols from *P. palmata*, and from *S. chordalis* [220]. In some cases, organic solvent extraction was more efficient than emerging techniques, i.e., for phenolics from *Osmundea pinnatifida*, and *Codium tomentosum* and was more efficient than hot water extraction or than enzyme or ultrasound assisted extraction [215]; however, the benefits of using greener solvents have to be considered.

Table 7. Examples of extraction of bioactives from red seaweeds.

Solvent	Seaweed	Activity	Reference
Ethanol (70–80%), methanol (80%), Acetone, ethyl acetate, chloroform:methanol (2:1) (80%), dimethyl sulfoxide (80%)	*Gracilaria changii*, *Gelidium amansii*, *Kappaphycus alvarezii*, *Osmundea pinnatifida*, *Codium tomentosum*, *Gracilaria lemaneiformis*	Antioxidant, glucose uptake regulation, anti-diabetic, neuroprotective, gastroprotective	[215,248,249, 253,254]
Enzyme (proteases, carbohydrases) assisted	*Parmaria palmate*	Antioxidant	[190]
Phosphate buffer	*G. amansii*	Antitumoral	[248]
Ultrasound-assisted	*Laurencia obtusa*	Antioxidant	[250]
Supercritical CO_2	*Gloiopeltis tenax*, *Gracilaria mammillaris*	Antioxidant, antimicrobial	[251,252]
Enzyme and high hydrostatic pressure	*Palmaria palmate*, *Solieria chordalis*	Antioxidant	[220]

Mycosporine-like amino acids are low-molecular-weight, water-soluble components with antioxidant and photoprotective properties found in red seaweeds. Since they have been reported as the strongest UVA-absorbing compounds in nature, they have been proposed as photoprotective materials for skin care products. The antioxidant and antiproliferative activities and mycosporine-like amino acid depended on locations varying in UV-exposure [255], with higher values summer and in shallow waters than in deeper waters [255,256]. Conventional extraction with organic solvents has been reported, i.e., methanol [255], but the ultrasound assistance was also proposed to obtain UV-absorbing compounds [257].

2.5. Minerals

Seaweeds are particularly rich in minerals and trace elements, showing ash contents, in the range 20–40% w/w, and could be a good source of K, Ca, Fe, Mg and other trace elements essential for human nutrition [246,258,259]. Seaweeds concentrate minerals due to their capacity to retain inorganic marine substances from seawater based on the characteristics of their cell surface polysaccharides [23], and contain 10–20 times the minerals of land plants. The Na/K ratios were below 1.5 and can be proposed for low sodium diets, since diets with a high Na/K ratio have been related to the incidence of hypertension.

Jaballi et al. [260] reported the ability of a mineral and antioxidant-rich extract from *Chondrus canaliculatus* to improve the toxicity caused by a fungicide in adult rat, being effective against hematotoxicity, genotoxicity and oxidative stress in the blood and bone and maintained osteomineral metabolism and bone histo-architecture.

3. Combined Extraction

Most of the proposed extraction processes are not selective and apart from the target compound, others can also be obtained. This could be illustrated with some examples. Extraction by enzymatic hydrolysis of R-phycoerythrin from *Gracilaria verrucosa* causes the release of a small amount of polysaccharides, which could be recovered in the coproduct [225]. Some intensification technologies also favor the simultaneous extraction of different components. During protein extraction, the mineral content in the extracts could be enhanced using accelerated solvent extraction produced extracts compared to that of conventional extracts, whereas the pH-shift-produced extracts had lower ash content than the whole biomass. Although the co-extraction of other compounds different from the target ones could difficult and make more expensive the purification stages, the presence of other high-value food components could confer additional value and synergistic functional and biological properties to the final product. This could occur, as fatty acids together with proteins could be of interest for producing multi-functional protein extracts [219].

Some authors proposed the use of more than one fraction, such as the sequential extraction of R-phycoerythrin and agar from *Gracilaria verrucosa* [226], Yuan et al. [254] proposed an initial extraction of the pigments for decolorization of *Gracilaria lemaneiformis* before agar production, allowing also to recover the removed fractions as natural antioxidants. Niu et al. [261] observed that after water extraction of proteins from *Gracilaria lemaneiformis* and further purification of R-phycoerythrin the remaining biomass was used for agar extraction. The yield of agar and its properties showed no significant difference from those obtained from the direct agar extraction from the dried algae. However, the R-phycoerythin recovery and purity were lower than when it was extracted from fresh algae. The most frequent approach consists on the valorization of the waste fractions after phycocolloid extraction as a source of protein. Cian et al. [262,263] reported the use of *Porphyra columbina* wastes to obtain proteins that after proteolystic digestion to produce fractions with immunosuppressive, antihypertensive and antioxidant actions.

Particularly interesting is the integral utilization of the raw material, following a biorefinery approach. In order to make use of all seaweed components requires a rational processing of the whole material, and the algal processing by-products according to the biorefinery concept to allow a complete utilization of biomass [19,264,265]. This alternative processing approach would provide different products and applications, favoring the economics of a process that would not rely exclusively on one product and could be adapted to the demand and needs of different sectors.

Figure 5 represents a general flow diagram for a multistage multipurpose biorefinery processing of red seaweeds. The suggested scheme is based on the initial production of food or feed products, with the final ones being destined to energetic and soil applications. It is desirable that biorefineries are designed in a flexible way allowing the possibility of processing different seaweeds, obtaining different products including those of high volume/low quality and those of high quality/low volume ones. If possible, it is also recommended to integrate food and non-food sectors. In the extraction stages, the utilization of more efficient greener technologies is recommended to enhance the yields and productivities, keeping the products quality and lowering energetic and operation costs.

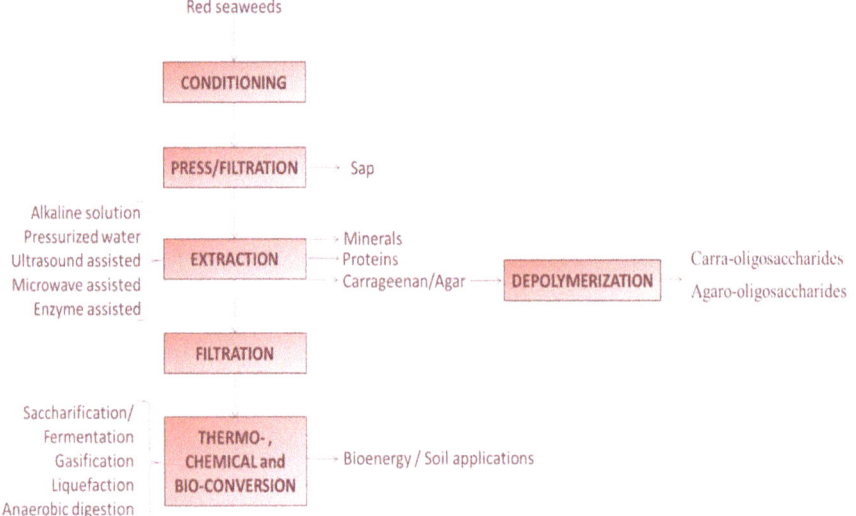

Figure 5. Simplified flow diagram of a red seaweed biorefinery.

Different authors proposed the utilization of agarophytic biomass for biorefinery including the energetic uses [266–270] and for the production of chemicals, such as 5-hydroxymethyl furfural, levulinic acid and formic acid from *K. alvarezii* [271]. However, in the present review, the valorization of bioactives is emphasized, and this type of seaweed is highly interesting, since they contain a high proportion of proteins, some being colorants (R-phycoerythrin, R-phycocyanin), fatty acids and minerals. Therefore, biotechnological, nutraceutical and pharmaceutical applications have been highlighted.

Even when the ethanol production was also considered in their approach, Baghel et al. [264], have designed a complete valorization of *Gracilaria corticata* bioactives, including phycobiliproteins, lipids and agar. The solid residue after phycocolloid extraction is still a good source of bioactives and has been explored in a number of studies. Based on the ingent amounts generated during industrial processing, their valorization would also report environmental benefits. Cian et al. [263] used this waste from *Porphyra columbina* to obtain low molecular weight peptides with angiotensin-converting-enzyme (ACE) inhibitory action, as well as antioxidant properties, which could also be due to some phenolic compounds. Laohakunjit [214] proposed the hydrolysis of *Gracilaria fisheri* residue after agar extraction and the protein hydrolysate was used to obtain free amino acids and odorant compounds valuable as an umami conferring tasting product.

Despite the fact that seaweed biorefineries have started to develop later than terrestrial ones, they offer environmental and economic advantages and show higher potential as a source of nutrients, hydrocolloids, pigments, bioactives and energy, and, based on their complex and exclusive composition, red seaweeds are particularly interesting for their cascading valorization in food, cosmetic and therapeutic applications.

4. Conclusions

The integral utilization of the valuable components from red seaweeds is a technologically feasible approach with environmental and economic advantages. Apart from gelling biopolymers, a number of bioactive compounds with nutritional, functional or biological features can be recovered from red macroalgae using conventional and greener technologies. The challenge is the sequential extraction of these components using emerging technologies for the integral valorization of this type of macroalgae. This opens new attractive alternatives to fulfill the growing market's demand for natural bioactive compounds of interest in the food, cosmetic, personal care, biomedical or pharmaceutical field.

Author Contributions: All the authors have read, approved, and made substantial contributions to the manuscript. H.D. conceived the study, built the database, made the drafting of the manuscript and the critical revision. M.D.T. made the drafting of the manuscript and the critical revision. N.F.-F. supported the drafting of the manuscript.

Funding: This research was funded by the Ministry of Science, Innovation and Universities of Spain (RTI2018-096376-B-I00). M.D.T. thanks the Spanish Ministry of Science, Innovation and Universities for her postdoctoral grant (IJCI-2016-27535), and N.F.-F. thanks Xunta de Galicia for her postdoctoral grant (ED481B 2018/071).

Conflicts of Interest: The authors declare no conflict of interest. The funders had no role in the design of the study; in the collection, analyses, or interpretation of data; in the writing of the manuscript, or in the decision to publish the results.

References

1. Cian, R.E.; Drago, S.R.; De Medina, F.S.; Martínez-Augustin, O. Proteins and carbohydrates from red seaweeds: Evidence for beneficial effects on gut function and microbiota. *Mar. Drugs* **2015**, *13*, 5358–5383. [CrossRef]
2. Dhanalakshmi, S.; Jayakumari, S.A. Perspective studies on marine red algae—*Hypnea valentiae*. *Drug Invent. Today* **2018**, *10*, 266–267.
3. Makkar, H.P.S.; Tran, G.; Heuzé, V.; Giger-Reverdin, S.; Lessire, M.; Lebas, F.; Ankers, P. Seaweeds for livestock diets: A review. *Anim. Feed Sci. Technol.* **2016**, *212*, 1–17. [CrossRef]
4. Sanjeewa, K.K.A.; Lee, W.W.; Jeon, Y.J. Nutrients and bioactive potentials of edible green and red seaweed in Korea. *Fish. Aquat. Sci.* **2018**, *21*, 19. [CrossRef]
5. Ruan, B.F.; Ge, W.W.; Lin, M.X.; Li, Q.S. A review of the components of seaweeds as potential candidates in cancer therapy. *Anti-Cancer Agents Med. Chem.* **2018**, *18*, 354–366. [CrossRef] [PubMed]
6. Shi, Q.; Wang, A.; Lu, Z.; Qin, C.; Hu, J.; Yin, J. Overview on the antiviral activities and mechanisms of marine polysaccharides from seaweeds. *Carbohydr. Res.* **2017**, *453*, 1–9. [CrossRef] [PubMed]
7. Youssouf, L.; Lallemand, L.; Giraud, P.; Soulé, F.; Bhaw-Luximon, A.; Meilhac, O.; D'Hellencourt, C.L.; Jhurry, D.; Couprie, J. Ultrasound-assisted extraction and structural characterization by NMR of alginates and carrageenans from seaweeds. *Carbohydr. Polym.* **2017**, *166*, 55–63. [CrossRef]
8. Cheong, K.L.; Qiu, H.M.; Du, H.; Liu, Y.; Khan, B.M. Oligosaccharides derived from red seaweed: Production, properties, and potential health and cosmetic applications. *Molecules* **2018**, *23*, 2451. [CrossRef]
9. Abdul Khalil, H.P.S.; Lai, T.K.; Tye, Y.Y.; Rizal, S.; Chong, E.W.N.; Yap, S.W.; Hamzah, A.A.; Nurul Fazita, M.R.; Paridah, M.T. A review of extractions of seaweed hydrocolloids: Properties and applications. *Express Polym. Lett.* **2018**, *12*, 296–317. [CrossRef]
10. Grosso, C.; Valentão, P.; Ferreres, F.; Andrade, P.B. Alternative and efficient extraction methods for marine-derived compounds. *Mar. Drugs* **2015**, *13*, 3182–3230. [CrossRef] [PubMed]
11. Ciko, A.M.; Jokić, S.; Šubarić, D.; Jerković, I. Overview on the application of modern methods for the extraction of bioactive compounds from marine macroalgae. *Mar. Drugs* **2018**, *16*, 348. [CrossRef] [PubMed]
12. Chew, K.W.; Juan, J.C.; Phang, S.M.; Ling, T.C.; Show, P.L. An overview on the development of conventional and alternative extractive methods for the purification of agarose from seaweed. *Sep. Sci. Technol.* **2018**, *53*, 467–480. [CrossRef]

13. Machmudah, S.; Wahyudiono Kanda, H.; Goto, M. Supercritical fluids extraction of valuable compounds from algae: Future perspectives and challenges. *Eng. J.* **2018**, *22*, 13–30. [CrossRef]
14. Xu, S.Y.; Huang, X.; Cheong, K.L. Recent advances in marine algae polysaccharides: Isolation, structure, and activities. *Mar. Drugs* **2017**, *15*, 388. [CrossRef] [PubMed]
15. Pangestuti, R.; Siahaan, E.A.; Kim, S.K. Photoprotective substances derived from marine algae. *Mar. Drugs* **2018**, *16*, 399. [CrossRef]
16. Aryee, A.N.; Agyei, D.; Akanbi, T.O. Recovery and utilization of seaweed pigments in food processing. *Curr. Opin. Food Sci.* **2018**, *19*, 113–119. [CrossRef]
17. Gómez-Ordóñez, E.; Jiménez-Escrig, A.; Rupérez, P. Bioactivity of sulfated polysaccharides from the edible red seaweed *Mastocarpus stellatus*. *Bioact. Carbohydr. Diet. Fibre* **2014**, *3*, 29–40. [CrossRef]
18. Abdul Khalil, H.P.S.; Suk, W.Y.; Owolabi, F.A.T.; Haafiz, M.K.M.; Fazita, M.; Deepu, G.; Hasan, M.; Samsul, R. Techno-functional properties of edible packaging films at different polysaccharide blends. *J. Phys. Sci.* **2019**, *30*, 23–41.
19. Torres, M.D.; Kraan, S.; Domínguez, H. Seaweed biorefinery. *Rev. Environ. Sci. Bio/Technol.* **2019**, *18*, 335–388. [CrossRef]
20. Meinita, M.D.N.; Kang, J.Y.; Jeong, G.T.; Koo, H.M.; Park, S.M.; Hong, Y.K. Bioethanol production from the acid hydrolysate of the carrageenophyte *Kappaphycus alvarezii* (cottonii). *J. Appl. Phycol.* **2012**, *24*, 857–862. [CrossRef]
21. Pomin, V.H. Structural and functional insights into sulfated galactans: A systematic review. *Glycoconj. J.* **2010**, *27*, 1–12. [CrossRef]
22. Schultz-Johansen, M.; Bech, P.K.; Hennessy, R.C.; Glaring, M.A.; Barbeyron, T.; Czjzek, M.; Stougaard, P.A. Novel enzyme portfolio for red algal polysaccharide degradation in the marine bacterium *Paraglaciecola hydrolytica* S66T encoded in a sizeable polysaccharide utilization locus. *Front. Microbiol.* **2018**, *9*, 839. [CrossRef]
23. Mabeau, S.; Fleurence, J. Seaweed in Food Products: Biochemical and Nutritional Aspects. *Trends Food Sci. Technol.* **1993**, *4*, 103–107. [CrossRef]
24. Rhein-Knudsen, N.; Ale, M.T.; Ajalloueian, F.; Yu, L.; Meyer, A.S. Rheological properties of agar and carrageenan from Ghanaian red seaweeds. *Food Hydrocoll.* **2017**, *63*, 50–58. [CrossRef]
25. Usov, A.I. Polysaccharides of the red algae. *Adv. Carbohydr. Chem. Biochem.* **2011**, *65*, 115–217.
26. Usov, A.I. Structural analysis of red seaweed galactans of agar and carrageenan groups. *Food Hydrocoll.* **1998**, *12*, 301–308. [CrossRef]
27. Lahaye, M. Developments on gelling algal galactans, their structure and physico-chemistry. *J. Appl. Phycol.* **2001**, *13*, 173–184. [CrossRef]
28. Campo, V.L.; Kawano, D.F.; Silva, D.B., Jr.; Carvalho, I. Carrageenans: Biological properties, chemical modifications and structural analysis—A review. *Carbohydr. Polym.* **2009**, *77*, 167–180. [CrossRef]
29. Martínez-Sanz, M.; Gómez-Mascaraque, L.G.; Ballester, A.R.; Martínez-Abad, A.; Brodkorb, A.; López-Rubio, A. Production of unpurified agar-based extracts from red seaweed *Gelidium sesquipedale* by means of simplified extraction protocols. *Algal Res.* **2019**, *38*, 101420. [CrossRef]
30. Lahaye, M.; Yaphe, W. The Chemical Structure of Agar from Gracilaria compressa (C. Agardh) Greville, G. cervicornis (Turner) J. Agardh, G. damaecornis J. Agardh and G. domingensis Sonder ex Kützing (Gigartinales, Rhodophyta). *Botanica Marina* **1989**, *32*, 369–378. [CrossRef]
31. Armisén, R. World-wide use and importance of *Gracilaria*. *J. Appl. Phycol.* **1995**, *7*, 231–243. [CrossRef]
32. Lee, W.K.; Lim, Y.Y.; Leow, A.T.C.; Namasivayam, P.; Abdullah, J.O.; Ho, C.L. Factors affecting yield and gelling properties of agar. *J. Appl. Phycol.* **2017**, *29*, 1527–1540. [CrossRef]
33. Craigie, J. Seaweed extract stimuli in plant science and agriculture. *J. Appl. Phycol.* **2011**, *23*, 371–393. [CrossRef]
34. Yun, E.J.; Yu, S.; Kim, K.H. Current knowledge on agarolytic enzymes and the industrial potential of agar-derived sugars. *Appl. Microbiol. Biotechnol.* **2017**, *101*, 5581–5589. [CrossRef]
35. Yarnpakdee, S.; Benjakul, S.; Kingwascharapong, P. Physico-chemical and gel properties of agar from *Gracilaria tenuistipitata* from the lake of Songkhla, Thailand. *Food Hydrocoll.* **2015**, *51*, 217–226. [CrossRef]
36. Sousa, A.M.M.; Morais, S.; Abreu, M.H.; Pereira, R.; Sousa-Pinto, I.; Cabrita, E.J.; Delerue-Matos, C.; Gonçalves, M.P. Structural, physical, and chemical modifications induced by microwave heating on native agar-like galactans. *J. Agric. Food Chem.* **2012**, *60*, 4977–4985. [CrossRef]

37. Vergara-Rodarte, M.A.; Hernández-Carmona, G.; Rodríguez-Montesinos, Y.E.; Arvizu-Higuera, D.L.; Riosmena-Rodríguez, R.; Murillo-Álvarez, J.I. Seasonal variation of agar from *Gracilaria vermiculophylla*, effect of alkali treatment time, and stability of its Colagar. *J. Appl. Phycol.* **2010**, *22*, 753–759. [CrossRef]
38. Marinho-Soriano, E.; Bourret, E. Effects of season on the yield and quality of agar from *Gracilaria* species (Gracilariaceae Rhodophyta). *Bioresour. Technol.* **2003**, *90*, 329–333. [CrossRef]
39. Marinho-Soriano, E.; Bourret, E. Polysaccharides from the red seaweed *Gracilaria dura* (Gracilariales, Rhodophyta). *Bioresour. Technol.* **2005**, *96*, 379–382. [CrossRef] [PubMed]
40. Romero, J.B.; Villanueva, R.D.; Montaño, M.N.E. Stability of agar in the seaweed *Gracilaria eucheumatoides* (Gracilariales, Rhodophyta) during postharvest storage. *Bioresour. Technol.* **2008**, *99*, 8151–8155. [CrossRef]
41. Chirapart, A.; Munkit, J.; Lewmanomont, K. Changes in yield and quality of agar from the agarophytes, *Gracilaria fisheri* and *G. tenuistipitata* var. liui cultivated in earthen ponds. *Kasetsart J. Nat. Sci.* **2006**, *40*, 529–540.
42. Arvizu-Higuera, D.L.; Rodríguez-Montesinos, Y.E.; Murillo-Alvarez, J.I.; Muñoz-Ochoa, M.; Hernández-Carmona, G. Effect of alkali treatment time and extraction time on agar from *Gracilaria vermiculophylla*. *J. Appl. Phycol.* **2008**, *20*, 515–519. [CrossRef]
43. Kohajdová, Z.; Karovičová, J.; Gajdošová, Ž. Importance of hydrocolloids in bakery industry. *Potravinarstvo* **2008**, *2*, 9–18.
44. Kazłowski, B.; Pan, C.L.; Ko, Y.T. Separation and quantification of neoagaro- and agaro-oligosaccharide products generated from agarose digestion by β-agarase and HCl in liquid chromatography systems. *Carbohydr. Res.* **2008**, *343*, 2443–2450. [CrossRef]
45. Hong, S.J.; Lee, J.H.; Kim, E.J.; Yang, H.J.; Park, J.S.; Hong, S.K. Toxicological evaluation of neoagarooligosaccharides prepared by enzymatic hydrolysis of agar. *Regul. Toxicol. Pharm.* **2017**, *90*, 9–21. [CrossRef]
46. Freile-Pelegrín, Y.; Robledo, D. Influence of alkali treatment on agar from *Gracilaria cornea* from Yucatán, México. *J. Appl. Phycol.* **1997**, *9*, 533–539.
47. Freile-Pelegrın, Y.; Murano, E. Agars from three species of *Gracilaria* (Rhodophyta) from Yucatan Peninsula. *Bioresour. Technol.* **2005**, *96*, 295–302. [CrossRef]
48. Sousa, A.M.M.; Alves, V.D.; Morais, S.; Delerue-Matos, C.; Gonçalves, M.P. Agar extraction from integrated multitrophic aquacultured *Gracilaria vermiculophylla*: Evaluation of a microwave-assisted process using response surface methodology. *Bioresour. Technol.* **2010**, *101*, 3258–3267. [CrossRef] [PubMed]
49. Villanueva, R.D.; Sousa, A.M.M.; Gonçalves, M.P.; Nilsson, M.; Hilliou, L. Production and properties of agar from the invasive marine alga, *Gracilaria vermiculophylla* (Gracilariales, Rhodophyta). *J. Appl. Phycol.* **2010**, *22*, 211–220. [CrossRef]
50. Kumar, V.; Fotedar, R. Agar extraction process for *Gracilaria cliftonii* (Withell, Millar, & Kraft, 1994). *Carbohydr. Polym.* **2009**, *78*, 813–819.
51. Saha, D.; Bhattacharya, S. Hydrocolloids as thickening and gelling agents in food: A critical review. *J. Food Sci. Technol.* **2010**, *47*, 587–590. [CrossRef]
52. Murano, E. Chemical structure and quality of agars from Gracilaria. *J. Appl. Phycol.* **1995**, *7*, 245–254. [CrossRef]
53. Yousefi, M.K.; Islami, H.R.; Filizadeh, Y. Effect of extraction process on agar properties of *Gracilaria corticata* (Rhodophyta) collected from the persian gulf. *Phycologia* **2013**, *52*, 481–487. [CrossRef]
54. Gallagher, J.A.; Turner, L.B.; Adams, J.M.M.; Barrento, S.; Dyer, P.W.; Theodorou, M.K. Species variation in the effects of dewatering treatment on macroalgae. *J. Appl. Phycol.* **2018**, *30*, 2305–2316. [CrossRef]
55. Rath, J.; Adhikary, S.P. Effect of alkali treatment on the yield and quality of agar from red alga *Gracilaria verrucosa* (Rhodophyta, Gracilariales) occurring at different salinity gradient of Chilika lake. *Indian J. Mar. Sci.* **2004**, *33*, 202–205.
56. Ahmad, R.; Surif, M.; Ramli, N.; Yahya, N.; Nor, A.R.M.; Bekbayeva, L.A. Preliminary study on the agar content and agar gel strength of *Gracilaria manilaensis* using different agar extraction processes. *World Appl. Sci. J.* **2011**, *15*, 184–188.
57. González-Leija, J.A.; Hernández-Garibay, E.; Pacheco-Ruíz, I.; Guardado-Puentes, J.; Espinoza-Avalos, J.; López-Vivas, J.M.; Bautista-Alcantar, J. Optimization of the yield and quality of agar from *Gracilariopsis lemaneiformis* (Gracilariales) from the Gulf of California using an alkaline treatment. *J. Appl. Phycol.* **2009**, *21*, 321–326. [CrossRef]

58. Roleda, M.Y.; Montaño, N.E.; Ganzon-Fortes, E.T.; Villanueva, R.D. Acetic acid pretreatment in agar extraction of Philippine *Gelidiella acerosa* (Forsskaal) Feldmann et Hamel (Rhodophyta, Gelidiales). *Bot. Mar.* **1997**, *40*, 63–69. [CrossRef]
59. Freile-Pelegrín, Y.; Robledo, D.; Pedersén, M.; Bruno, E.; Rönnqvist, J. Effect of dark and salinity treatment in the yield and quality of agar from *Gracilaria cornea* (Rhodophyceae). *Cienc. Mar.* **2002**, *28*, 289–296. [CrossRef]
60. Li, H.; Huang, J.; Xin, Y.; Zhang, B.; Jin, Y.; Zhang, W. Optimization and scale-up of a new photobleaching agar extraction process from *Gracilaria lemaneiformis*. *J. Appl. Phycol.* **2009**, *21*, 247–254. [CrossRef]
61. Maciel, J.S.; Chaves, L.S.; Souza, B.W.S.; Teixeira, D.I.A.; Freitas, A.L.P.; Feitosa, J.P.A.; de Paula, R.C.M. Structural characterization of cold extracted fraction of soluble sulfated polysaccharide from red seaweed *Gracilaria birdiae*. *Carbohydr. Polym.* **2008**, *71*, 559–565. [CrossRef]
62. Al-Alawi, A.; Chitra, P.; Al-Mamun, A.; Al-Marhubi, I.; Rahman, M.S. Characterization of red seaweed extracts treated by water, acid and alkaline solutions. *Int. J. Food Eng.* **2018**, *14*, 20170353. [CrossRef]
63. Kim, M.; Yim, J.H.; Kim, S.-Y.; Kim, H.S.; Lee, W.G.; Kim, S.J.; Kang, P.S.; Lee, C.-K. In vitro inhibition of influenza A virus infection by marine microalga-derived sulfated polysaccharide p-KG03. *Antivir. Res.* **2012**, *93*, 253–259. [CrossRef] [PubMed]
64. Lee, J.M.; Boo, S.M.; Mansilla, A.; Yoon, H.S. Unique repeat and plasmid sequences in the mitochondrial genome of *Gracilaria chilensis* (Gracilariales, Rhodophyta). *Phycologia* **2015**, *54*, 20–23. [CrossRef]
65. Park, S.Y.; Lee, E.S.; Han, S.H.; Lee, H.Y.; Lee, S. Antioxidative effects of two native berry species, *Empetrum nigrum* var. *japonicum* K. Koch and Rubus buergeri Miq., from the Jeju Island of Korea. *J. Food Biochem.* **2012**, *36*, 675–682.
66. Villanueva, R.; Montaño, M.N. Enhancement of carrageenan gel quality in the commercially important tropical seaweed *Eucheuma denticulatum* (Rhodophyta), with postharvest treatment in low-nutrient conditions. *Bot. Mar.* **2014**, *57*, 217–223. [CrossRef]
67. Shukla, M.K.; Kumar, M.; Prasad, K.; Reddy, C.R.K.; Jha, B. Partial characterization of sulfohydrolase from *Gracilaria dura* and evaluation of its potential application in improvement of the agar quality. *Carbohydr. Polym.* **2011**, *85*, 157–163. [CrossRef]
68. Navarro, D.A.; Stortz, C.A. Microwave-assisted alkaline modification of red seaweed galactans. *Carbohydr. Polym.* **2005**, *62*, 187–191. [CrossRef]
69. Wu, S.C.; Lin, Y.P.; King, V.A.E. Optimization of intermittent microwave-assisted extraction of sulfated porphyran from *Porphyra dentate*. *Trans. ASABE* **2014**, *57*, 103–110.
70. Villanueva, R.D.; Rumbaoa, R.O.; Gomez, A.V.; Loquias, M.M.; De La Rosa, A.M.; Montaño, N.E. γ-Irradiation in the extraction of agar from *Gelidiella acerosa* (Forsskaal) Feldmann et Hamel. *Bot. Mar.* **1998**, *41*, 199–202. [CrossRef]
71. Pereira-Pacheco, F.; Robledo, D.; Rodríguez-Carvajal, L.; Freile-Pelegrín, Y. Optimization of native agar extraction from *Hydropuntia cornea* from Yucatán, México. *Bioresour. Technol.* **2007**, *98*, 1278–1284. [CrossRef]
72. Villanueva, R.D.; Pagba, C.V.; Montaño, N.E. Optimized agar extraction from *Gracilaria eucheumoides* Harvey. *Bot. Mar.* **1997**, *40*, 369–372. [CrossRef]
73. Li, H.; Yu, X.; Jin, Y.; Zhang, W.; Liu, Y. Development of an eco-friendly agar extraction technique from the red seaweed *Gracilaria lemaneiformis*. *Bioresour. Technol.* **2008**, *99*, 3301–3305. [CrossRef] [PubMed]
74. Prasad, K.; Siddhanta, A.K.; Ganesan, M.; Ramavat, B.K.; Jha, B.; Ghosh, P.K. Agars of Gelidiella acerosa of west and southeast coasts of India. *Bioresour. Technol.* **2007**, *98*, 1907–1915. [CrossRef]
75. Fidelis, G.P.; Camara, R.B.G.; Queiroz, M.F.; Costa, M.S.S.P.; Santos, P.C.; Rocha, H.A.O.; Costa, L.S. Proteolysis, NaOH and ultrasound-enhanced extraction of anticoagulant and antioxidant sulfated polysaccharides from the edible seaweed, *Gracilaria birdiae*. *Molecules* **2014**, *19*, 18511–18526. [CrossRef] [PubMed]
76. Coura, C.O.; Souza, R.B.; Rodrigues, J.A.G.; Vanderlei, E.D.S.O.; De Araújo, I.W.F.; Ribeiro, N.A.; Frota, A.F.; Ribeiro, K.A.; Chaves, H.V.; Pereira, K.M.A.; et al. Mechanisms involved in the anti-inflammatory action of a polysulfated fraction from *Gracilaria cornea* in rats. *PLoS ONE* **2015**, *10*, e0119319. [CrossRef]
77. Chen, H.M.; Zheng, L.; Yan Agaro, X.J. Bioactivity research of oligosaccharides. *Food Technol. Biotechnol.* **2005**, *43*, 29–36.
78. Mazumder, S.; Ghosal, P.K.; Pujol, C.A.; Carlucci, M.J.; Damonte, E.B.; Ray, B. Isolation, chemical investigation and antiviral activity of polysaccharides from *Gracilaria corticata* (Gracilariaceae, Rhodophyta). *Int. J. Biol. Macromol.* **2002**, *31*, 87–95. [CrossRef]

79. Bhattarai, Y.; Kashyap, P.C. Agaro-oligosaccharides: A new frontier in the fight against coloncancer? *Am. J. Physiol.- Gastrointest. Liver Physiol.* **2016**, *310*, G335–G336. [CrossRef]
80. Enoki, T.; Okuda, S.; Kudo, Y.; Takashima, F.; Sagawa, H.; Kato, I. Oligosaccharides from agar inhibit pro-inflammatory mediator release by inducing heme oxygenase 1. *Biosci. Biotechnol. Biochem.* **2010**, *74*, 766–770. [CrossRef]
81. Enoki, T.; Tominaga, T.; Takashima, F.; Ohnogi, H.; Sagawa, H.; Kato, I. Anti-tumor-promoting activities of agaro-oligosaccharides on two-stage mouse skin carcinogenesis. *Biol. Pharm. Bull.* **2012**, *35*, 1145–1149. [CrossRef]
82. Higashimura, Y.; Naito, Y.; Takagi, T.; Mizushima, K.; Hirai, Y.; Harusato, A.; Ohnogi, H.; Yamaji, R.; Inui, H.; Nakano, Y.; et al. Oligosaccharides from agar inhibit murine intestinal inflammation through the induction of heme oxygenase-1 expression. *J. Gastroenterol.* **2013**, *48*, 897–909. [CrossRef]
83. Jin, M.; Liu, H.; Hou, Y.; Chan, Z.; Di, W.; Li, L.; Zeng, R. Preparation, characterization and alcoholic liver injury protective effects of algal oligosaccharides from *Gracilaria lemaneiformis*. *Food Res. Int.* **2017**, *100*, 186–195. [CrossRef]
84. Jang, M.K.; Lee, D.G.; Kim, N.Y.; Yu, K.H.; Jang, H.J.; Lee, S.W.; Jang, H.J.; Lee, Y.H. Purification and characterization of neoagarotetraose from hydrolyzed agar. *J. Microbiol. Biotechnol.* **2009**, *19*, 1197–1200.
85. Hehemann, J.H.; Correc, G.; Thomas, F.; Bernard, T.; Barbeyron, T.; Jam, M.; Helbert, W.; Michel, G.; Czjzek, M. Biochemical and structural characterization of the complex agarolytic enzyme system from the marine bacterium *Zobellia galactanivorans*. *J. Biol. Chem.* **2012**, *28*, 30571–30584. [CrossRef] [PubMed]
86. Liu, M.Y.; Mei, J.F.; Yi, Y.; Chen, J.S.; Ying, G.Q. Advances in study on biological activities of agaro-oligosaccharide. *Pharm. Biotechnol.* **2008**, *15*, 493–496.
87. Kazłowski, B.; Liang, C.; Yuan, P.; Ko, P. Monitoring and preparation of neoagaro- and agaro-oligosaccharide products by high performance anion exchange chromatography systems. *Carbohydr. Polym.* **2015**, *122*, 351–358. [CrossRef]
88. Tripathi, A.; Kathuria, N.; Kumar, A. Elastic and macroporous agarose–599 gelatin cryogels with isotropic and anisotropic porosity for tissue engineering. *J. Biomed. Mater. Res. Part A* **2009**, *90*, 680–694. [CrossRef]
89. Ramana Ramya, J.; Thanigai Arul, K.; Sathiamurthi, P.; Asokan, K.; Narayana Kalkura, S. Novel gamma irradiated agarose-gelatin-hydroxyapatite nanocomposite scaffolds for skin tissue regeneration. *Ceram. Int.* **2016**, *42*, 11045–11054. [CrossRef]
90. Gao, M.; Lu, P.; Bednark, B.; Lynam, D.; Conner, J.M.; Sakamoto, J.; Tuszynski, M.H. Templated agarose scaffolds for the support of motor axon regeneration into sites of complete spinal cord transection. *Biomaterials* **2013**, *34*, 1529–1536. [CrossRef]
91. Zhang, L.M.; Wu, C.X.; Huang, J.Y.; Peng, X.H.; Chen, P.; Tang, S.Q. Synthesis and characterization of a degradable composite agarose/HA hydrogel. *Carbohydr. Polym.* **2012**, *88*, 1445–1452. [CrossRef]
92. Hu, J.; Zhu, Y.; Tong, H.; Shen, X.; Chen, L.; Ran, J. A detailed study of homogeneous agarose/hydroxyapatite nanocomposites for load-bearing bone tissue. *Int. J. Biol. Macromol.* **2016**, *82*, 134–143. [CrossRef]
93. Zou, P.; Lu, X.; Jing, C.; Yuan, Y.; Lu, Y.; Zhang, C.; Meng, L.; Zhao, H.; Li, Y. Low-molecular-weightt polysaccharides from *Pyropia yezoensis* enhance tolerance of wheat seedlings (*Triticum aestivum* L.) to salt stress. *Front. Plant Sci.* **2018**, *9*, 427. [CrossRef] [PubMed]
94. Kang, O.L.; Ghani, M.; Hassan, O.; Rahmati, S.; Ramli, N. Novel agaro-oligosaccharide production through enzymatic hydrolysis: Physicochemical properties and antioxidant activities. *Food Hydrocoll.* **2014**, *42*, 304–308. [CrossRef]
95. Fenoradosoa, T.A.; Laroche, C.; Delattre, C.; Dulong, V.; Cerf, D.L.; Picton, L.; Michaud, P. Rheological behavior and non-enzymatic degradation of a sulfated galactan from *Halymenia durvillei* (Halymeniales, Rhodophyta). *Appl. Biochem. Biotechnol.* **2012**, *167*, 1303–1313. [CrossRef]
96. Zhou, C.; Yu, X.; Zhang, Y.; He, R.; Ma, H. Ultrasonic degradation, purification and analysis of structure and antioxidant activity of polysaccharide from *Porphyra yezoensis* Udea. *Carbohydr. Polym.* **2012**, *87*, 2046–2051. [CrossRef]
97. Poupard, N.; Badarou, P.; Fasani, F.; Groult, H.; Bridiau, N.; Sannier, F.; Bordenave-Juchereau, S.; Kieda, C.; Piot, J.M.; Grillon, C.; et al. Assessment of heparanase-mediated angiogenesis using microvascular endothelial cells: Identification of λ-Carrageenan derivative as a potent anti angiogenic agent. *Mar. Drugs* **2017**, *15*, 134. [CrossRef]

98. Öğretmen, Ö.Y.; Duyar, H.A. The effect of different extraction methods and pre-treatments on agar yield and physico-chemical properties of *Gelidium latifolium* (Gelidiaceae, Rhodophyta) from Sinop Peninsula Coast of Black Sea, Turkey. *J. Appl. Phycol.* **2018**, *30*, 1355–1360. [CrossRef]
99. Pereira, L.; Gheda, S.; Ribeiro-Claro, P. Analysis by vibrational spectroscopy of seaweed with potential use in food, pharmaceutical and cosmetic industries. *Int. J. Carbohydr. Chem.* **2013**, *2013*, 537202. [CrossRef]
100. Knudsen, N.R.; Ale, M.T.; Meyer, A.S. Seaweed hydrocolloid production: An update on enzyme assisted extraction and modification technologies. *Mar. Drugs* **2015**, *13*, 3340–3359. [CrossRef]
101. Collén, J.; Cornish, M.L.; Craigie, J.; Ficko-Blean, E.; Hervé, C.; Krueger-Hadfield, S.A.; Leblanc, C.; Michel, G.; Potin, P.; Tonon, T.; et al. *Chondrus crispus*—A present and historical model organism for red seaweeds. *Adv. Bot. Res.* **2014**, *71*, 53–89.
102. Pereira, L.; Critchley, A.T.; Amado, A.M.; Ribeiro-Claro, P.J.A. A comparative analysis of phycocolloids produced by underutilized versus industrially utilized carrageenophytes (Gigartinales, Rhodophyta). *J. Appl. Phycol.* **2009**, *21*, 599–605. [CrossRef]
103. Blakemore, W.R.; Harpell, A.R. Carrageenan. In *Food Stabilisers, Thickeners and Gelling Agents*; Imeson, A., Ed.; Blackwell Publishing Ltd.: Oxford, UK, 2009; pp. 73–94.
104. Pereira, L.; Meireles, F.; Gaspar, R. Population studies and carrageenan properties in eight gigartinales (Rhodophyta) from Iberian Peninsula. In *Seaweeds: Agricultural Uses, Biological and Antioxidant Agents*; Nova Science Publishers, Inc.: New York, NY, USA, 2014; pp. 115–134.
105. Vera, J.; Castro, J.; González, A.; Moenne, A. Seaweed polysaccharides and derived oligosaccharides stimulate defense responses and protection against pathogens in plants. *Mar. Drugs* **2011**, *9*, 2514–2525. [CrossRef]
106. Necas, J.; Bartosikova, L. Carrageenan: A review. *Vet. Med.* **2013**, *58*, 187–205. [CrossRef]
107. Ghanbarzadeh, M.; Golmoradizadeh, A.; Homaei, A. Carrageenans and carrageenases: Versatile polysaccharides and promising marine enzymes. *Phytochem. Rev.* **2018**, *17*, 535–571. [CrossRef]
108. Cunha, L.; Grenha, A. Sulfated seaweed polysaccharides as multifunctional materials in drug delivery applications. *Mar. Drugs* **2016**, *14*, 42. [CrossRef]
109. Van de Vijver, M.J.; He, Y.D.; van't Veer, L.J.; Dai, H.; Hart, A.A.; Voskuil, D.W.; Schreiber, G.J.; Peterse, J.L.; Roberts, C.; Marton, M.J.; et al. A gene-expression signature as a predictor of survival in breast cancer. *N. Engl. J. Med.* **2002**, *347*, 1999–2009. [CrossRef]
110. Cohen, S.M.; Ito, N. A critical review of the toxicological effects of carrageenan and processed *Eucheuma* seaweed on the gastrointestinal tract. *Crit. Rev. Toxicol.* **2002**, *32*, 413–444. [CrossRef]
111. Weiner, M.L. Food additive carrageenan: Part II: A critical review of carrageenan in vivo safety studies. *Crit. Rev. Toxicol.* **2014**, *44*, 244–269. [CrossRef]
112. Weiner, M.L. Parameters and pitfalls to consider in the conduct of food additive research, Carrageenan as a case study. *Crit. Rev. Toxicol.* **2016**, *87*, 31–44. [CrossRef]
113. Bhattacharyya, S.; Borthakur, A.; Dudeja, P.K.; Tobacman, J.K. Carrageenan induces cell cycle arrest in human intestinal epithelial cells in vitro. *J. Nutr.* **2008**, *138*, 469–475. [CrossRef]
114. Chen, M.; Schliep, M.; Willows, R.D.; Cai, Z.L.; Neilan, B.A.; Scheer, H. A red-shifted chlorophyll. *Science* **2010**, *329*, 1318–1319. [CrossRef]
115. Munyaka, P.M.; Sepehri, S.; Ghia, J.E.; Khafipour, E. Carrageenan gum and adherent invasive Escherichia coli in a piglet model of inflammatory bowel disease: Impact on intestinal mucosa-associated microbiota. *Front. Microbiol.* **2016**, *7*, 462. [CrossRef]
116. Shang, Q.; Sun, W.; Shan, X.; Jiang, H.; Cai, C.; Hao, J.; Li, G.; Yu, G. Carrageenan-induced colitis is associated with decreased population of anti-inflammatory bacterium, *Akkermansia muciniphila*, in the gut microbiota of C57BL/6J mice. *Toxicol. Lett.* **2017**, *279*, 87–95. [CrossRef]
117. Wei, W.; Feng, W.; Xin, G.; Tingting, N.; Zhanghe, Z.; Haimin, C.; Xiaojun, Y. Enhanced effect of κ-carrageenan on TNBS-induced inflammation in mice. *Int. Immunopharmacol.* **2016**, *39*, 218–228. [CrossRef]
118. Wu, W.; Wang, F.; Gao, X.; Niu, T.; Zhu, X.; Yan, X.; Chen, H. Synergistic effect of κ-carrageenan on oxazolone-induced inflammation in BALB/c mice. *BMC Gastroenterol.* **2016**, *16*, 41. [CrossRef]
119. David, S.; Shani Levi, C.; Fahoum, L.; Ungar, Y.; Meyron-Holtz, E.G.; Shpigelman, A.; Lesmes, U. Revisiting the carrageenan controversy: Do we really understand the digestive fate and safety of carrageenan in our foods? *Food Funct.* **2018**, *9*, 1344–1352. [CrossRef]

120. David, S.; Fahoum, L.; Rozen, G.; Shaoul, R.; Shpigelman, A.; Meyron-Holtz, E.G.; Lesmes, U. Reply to the Comment on "Revisiting the carrageenan controversy: Do we really understand the digestive fate and safety of carrageenan in our foods?". *Food Funct.* **2019**, *10*, 1763–1766. [CrossRef]
121. De Sousa Oliveira Vanderlei, E.; De Araújo, I.W.F.; Quinderé, A.L.G.; Fontes, B.P.; Eloy, Y.R.G.; Rodrigues, J.A.G.; Silva, A.A.R.E.; Chaves, H.V.; Jorge, R.J.B.; De Menezes, D.B.; et al. The involvement of the HO-1 pathway in the anti-inflammatory action of a sulfated polysaccharide isolated from the red seaweed *Gracilaria birdiae*. *Inflamm. Res.* **2011**, *60*, 1121–1130. [CrossRef]
122. Inic-Kanada, A.; Stein, E.; Stojanovic, M.; Schuerer, N.; Ghasemian, E.; Filipovic, A.; Marinkovic, E.; Kosanovic, D.; Barisani-Asenbauer, T. Effects of iota-carrageenan on ocular *Chlamydia trachomatis* infection in vitro and in vivo. *J. Appl. Phycol.* **2018**, *30*, 2601–2610. [CrossRef]
123. Talarico, L.B.; Zibetti, R.G.; Faria, P.C.; Scolaro, L.A.; Duarte, M.E.; Noseda, M.D.; Pujol, C.A.; Damonte, E.B. Anti-herpes simplex virus activity of sulfated galactans from the red seaweeds *Gymnogongrus griffithsiae* and *Cryptonemia crenulata*. *Int. J. Biol. Macromol.* **2004**, *34*, 63–71. [CrossRef]
124. Talarico, L.B.; Pujol, C.A.; Zibetti, R.G.; Faría, P.C.; Noseda, M.D.; Duarte, M.E.; Damonte, E.B. The antiviral activity of sulfated polysaccharides against dengue virus is dependent on virus serotype and host cell. *Antivir. Res.* **2005**, *66*, 103–110. [CrossRef]
125. Cáceres, P.J.; Carlucci, M.J.; Damonte, E.B.; Matsuhiro, B.; Zúñiga, E.A. Carrageenans from Chilean samples of *Stenogramme interrupta* (Phyllophoraceae): Structural analysis and biological activity. *Phytochemistry* **2000**, *53*, 81–86. [CrossRef]
126. Chattopadhyay, K.; Ghosh, T.; Pujol, C.A.; Carlucci, M.J.; Damonte, E.B.; Ray, B. Polysaccharides from *Gracilaria corticata*: Sulfation, chemical characterization and anti-HSV activities. *Int. J. Biol. Macromol.* **2008**, *43*, 346–351. [CrossRef]
127. Yuan, H.; Song, J.; Li, X.; Li, N.; Dai, J. Immunomodulation and antitumor activity of kappa-carrageenan oligosaccharides. *Cancer Lett.* **2006**, *243*, 228–234. [CrossRef]
128. Liu, J.; Hafting, J.; Critchley, A.T.; Banskota, A.H.; Prithiviraj, B. Components of the cultivated red seaweed *Chondrus crispus* enhance the immune response of *Caenorhabditis elegans* to *Pseudomonas aeruginosa* through the pmk-1, daf-2/daf-16, and skn-1 pathways. *Appl. Environ. Microbiol.* **2013**, *79*, 7343–7350. [CrossRef]
129. Souza, M.P.; Vaz, A.F.M.; Costa, T.B.; Cerqueira, M.A.; De Castro, C.M.M.B.; Vicente, A.A.; Carneiro-da-Cunha, M.G. Construction of a Biocompatible and Antioxidant Multilayer Coating by Layer-by-Layer Assembly of κ-Carrageenan and Quercetin Nanoparticles. *Food Bioprocess Technol.* **2018**, *11*, 1050–1060. [CrossRef]
130. Sun, L.; Wang, S.; Gong, X.; Zhao, M.; Fu, X.; Wang, L. Isolation, purification and characteristics of R-phycoerythrin from a marine macroalga *Heterosiphonia japonica*. *Protein Expr. Purif.* **2010**, *64*, 146–154. [CrossRef]
131. De Jesus Raposo, M.F.; De Morais, A.M.B.; De Morais, R.M.S.C. Marine polysaccharides from algae with potential biomedical applications *Mar. Drugs* **2015**, *13*, 2967–3028. [CrossRef] [PubMed]
132. Hayashi, L.; Reis, R.P. Cultivation of the red algae *Kappaphycus alvarezii* in Brazil and its pharmacological potential. *Braz. J. Pharmacogn.* **2012**, *22*, 748–752. [CrossRef]
133. Abdul Khalil, H.P.S.; Saurabh, C.K.; Tye, Y.Y.; Lai, T.K.; Easa, A.M.; Rosamah, E.; Fazita, M.R.N.; Syakir, M.I.; Adnan, A.S.; Fizree, H.M.; et al. Seaweed based sustainable films and composites for food and pharmaceutical applications: A review. *Renew. Sustain. Energy Rev.* **2017**, *77*, 353–362. [CrossRef]
134. Morris, C.E. How does fertility of the substrate affect intra-specific competition? Evidence and synthesis from self-thinning. *Ecol. Res.* **2003**, *18*, 287–305. [CrossRef]
135. Briones, A.V.; Sato, T. Encapsulation of glucose oxidase (GOD) in polyelectrolyte complexes of chitosan-carrageenan. *React. Funct. Polym.* **2010**, *70*, 19–27. [CrossRef]
136. Zhang, W.T.; Yue, C.; Huang, Q.W.; Yuan, K.; Yan, A.J.; Shi, S. Contents of eight saccharides in unprocessed and processed *Rehmannia glutinosa* and content changes at different processing time points. *Chin. Tradit. Herb. Drug.* **2016**, *47*, 1132–1136.
137. Dafe, A.; Etemadi, H.; Zarredar, H.; Mahdavinia, G.R. Development of novel carboxymethyl cellulose/k-carrageenan blends as an enteric delivery vehicle for probiotic bacteria. *Int. J. Biol. Macromol.* **2017**, *97*, 299–307. [CrossRef]
138. Li, L.; Ni, R.; Shao, Y.; Mao, S. Carrageenan and its applications in drug delivery. *Carbohydr. Polym.* **2014**, *103*, 1–11. [CrossRef] [PubMed]

139. Sahiner, N.; Sagbas, S.; Yllmaz, S. Microgels derived from different forms of carrageenans, kappa, iota, and lambda for biomedical applications. *MRS Adv.* **2017**, *2*, 2521–2527. [CrossRef]
140. Gonçalves, A.L.; Pires, J.C.M.; Simões, M. Biotechnological potential of *Synechocystis salina* co-cultures with selected microalgae and cyanobacteria: Nutrients removal, biomass and lipid production. *Bioresour. Technol.* **2016**, *200*, 279–286. [CrossRef]
141. Ghannam, A.; Abbas, A.; Alek, H.; Al-Waari, Z.; Al-Ktaifani, M. Enhancement of local plant immunity against tobacco mosaic virus infection after treatment with sulphated-carrageenan from redalga (*Hypnea musciformis*). *Physiol. Mol. Plant Pathol.* **2013**, *84*, 19–27. [CrossRef]
142. Mercier, L.; Lafitte, C.; Borderies, G.; Briand, X.; Esquerré-Tugayé, M.T.; Fournier, J. The algal polysaccharide carrageenans can act as an elicitor of plant defence. *New Phytol.* **2001**, *149*, 43–51. [CrossRef]
143. Nagorskaya, V.P.; Reunov, A.V.; Lapshina, L.A.; Ermak, I.M.; Barabanova, A.O. Inhibitory effect of κ/β-carrageenan from red alga *Tichocarpus crinitus* on the development of a potato virus X infection in leaves of *Datura stramonium* L. *Biol. Bull.* **2010**, *37*, 653–658. [CrossRef]
144. Sangha, J.S.; Ravichandran, S.; Prithiviraj, K.; Critchley, A.T.; Prithiviraj, B. Sulfated macroalgal polysaccharides λ-carrageenan and ι-carrageenan differentially alter *Arabidopsis thaliana* resistance to *Sclerotinia sclerotiorum*. *Physiol. Mol. Plant Pathol.* **2010**, *75*, 38–45. [CrossRef]
145. Sangha, J.S.; Khan, W.; Ji, X.; Zhang, J.; Mills, A.A.S.; Critchley, A.T.; Prithiviraj, B. Carrageenans, sulphated polysaccharides of red seaweeds, differentially affect *Arabidopsis thaliana* resistance to *Trichoplusia ni* (Cabbage looper). *PLoS ONE* **2011**, *6*, e26834. [CrossRef]
146. Sangha, J.S.; Kandasamy, S.; Khan, W.; Bahia, N.S.; Singh, R.P.; Critchley, A.T.; Prithiviraj, B. λ-Carrageenan suppresses tomato chlorotic dwarf viroid (TCDVd) replication and symptom expression in tomatoes. *Mar. Drugs* **2015**, *13*, 2875–2889. [CrossRef] [PubMed]
147. Shukla, P.S.; Borza, T.; Critchley, A.T.; Prithiviraj, B. Carrageenans from red seaweeds as promoters of growth and elicitors of defense response in plants. *Front. Mar. Sci.* **2016**, *3*, 81. [CrossRef]
148. Vera, J.; Castro, J.; Contreras, R.A.; González, A.; Moenne, A. Oligocarrageenans induce a long-term and broad-range protection against pathogens in tobacco plants (var. *Xanthi*). *Physiol. Mol. Plant Pathol.* **2012**, *79*, 31–39. [CrossRef]
149. Bi, Y.; Hu, Y.; Zhou, Z.G. Genetic variation of *Laminaria japonica* (Phaeophyta) populations in China as revealed by RAPD markers. *Acta Oceanol. Sin.* **2011**, *30*, 103–112. [CrossRef]
150. Azevedo, G.; Torres, M.D.; Sousa-Pinto, I.; Hilliou, L. Effect of pre-extraction alkali treatment on the chemical structure and gelling properties of extracted hybrid carrageenan from *Chondrus crispus* and *Ahnfeltiopsis devoniensis*. *Food Hydrocoll.* **2015**, *50*, 150–158. [CrossRef]
151. Hilliou, L.; Larotonda, F.D.S.; Abreu, P.; Ramos, A.M.; Sereno, A.M.; Goncalves, M.P. Effect of extraction parameters on the chemical structure and gel properties of κ/ι-hybrid carrageenans obtained from *Mastocarpus stellatus*. *Biomol. Eng.* **2006**, *23*, 201–208. [CrossRef] [PubMed]
152. Boulho, R.; Marty, C.; Freile-Pelegrín, Y.; Robledo, D.; Bourgougnon, N.; Bedoux, G. Antiherpetic (HSV-1) activity of carrageenans from the red seaweed *Solieria chordalis* (Rhodophyta, Gigartinales) extracted by microwave-assisted extraction (MAE). *J. Appl. Phycol.* **2017**, *29*, 2219–2228. [CrossRef]
153. Rafiquzzaman, S.M.; Ahmed, R.; Lee, J.M.; Noh, G.; Jo, G.A.; Kong, I.S. Improved methods for isolation of carrageenan from *Hypnea musciformis* and its antioxidant activity. *J. Appl. Phycol.* **2016**, *28*, 1265–1274. [CrossRef]
154. Vázquez-Delfín, E.; Robledo, D.; Freile-Pelegrín, Y. Microwave-assisted extraction of the Carrageenan from *Hypnea musciformis* (Cystocloniaceae, Rhodophyta). *J. Appl. Phycol.* **2014**, *26*, 901–907. [CrossRef]
155. Estevez, J.M.; Ciancia, M.; Cerezo, A.S. The system of low-molecular-weight carrageenans and agaroids from the room-temperature-extracted fraction of *Kappaphycus alvarezii*. *Carbohydr. Res.* **2000**, *325*, 287–299. [CrossRef]
156. Almutairi, F.M.; Adams, G.G.; Kök, M.S.; Lawson, C.J.; Gahler, R.; Wood, S.; Foster, T.J.; Rowe, A.J.; Harding, S.E. An analytical ultracentrifugation based study on the conformation of lambda carrageenan in aqueous solution. *Carbohydr. Polym.* **2013**, *97*, 203–209. [CrossRef]
157. Tang, F.; Chen, F.; Li, F. Preparation and potential in vivo anti-influenza virus activity of low molecular-weight k-carrageenans and their derivatives. *J. Appl. Polym. Sci.* **2013**, *127*, 2110–2115. [CrossRef]
158. Ratnawati, R.; Prasetyaningrum, A.; Wardhani, D.H. Kinetics and thermodynamics of ultrasound-assisted depolymerization of κ-carrageenan. *Bull. Chem. React. Eng. Catal.* **2016**, *11*, 48–58. [CrossRef]

159. Sokolova, R.V.; Ermakova, S.P.; Awada, S.M.; Zvyagintseva, T.N.; Kanaan, H.M. Composition, structural characteristics, and antitumor properties of polysaccharides from the brown algae *Dictyopteris polypodioides* and *Sargassum* sp. *Chem. Nat. Compd.* **2011**, *47*, 329–334. [CrossRef]
160. Hamias, R.; Wolak, T.; Huleihel, M.; Paran, E.; Levy-Ontman, O. Red alga polysaccharides attenuate angiotensin II-induced inflammation in coronary endothelial cells. *Biochem. Biophys. Res. Commun.* **2018**, *500*, 944–951. [CrossRef] [PubMed]
161. Kalitnik, A.A.; Marcov, P.A.; Anastyuk, S.D.; Barabanova, A.O.B.; Glazunov, V.P.; Popov, S.V.; Ovodov, Y.S.; Yermak, I.M. Gelling polysaccharide from *Chondrus armatus* and its oligosaccharides: The structural peculiarities and anti-inflammatory activity. *Carbohydr. Polym.* **2015**, *115*, 768–775. [CrossRef]
162. Wang, W.; Wang, S.-X.; Guan, H.-S. The antiviral activities and mechanisms of marine polysaccharides: An overview. *Marine Drugs* **2012**, *10*, 2795–2816. [CrossRef] [PubMed]
163. Yamada, T.; Ogamo, A.; Saito, T.; Watanabe, J.; Uchiyama, H.; Nakagawa, Y. Preparation and anti-HIV activity of low-molecular-weight carrageenans and their sulfated derivatives. *Carbohydr. Polym.* **1997**, *32*, 51–55. [CrossRef]
164. Yamada, S.; Kosugi, I.; Katano, H.; Fukui, Y.; Kawasaki, H.; Arai, Y.; Kurane, I.; Inoue, N. In vivo imaging assay for the convenient evaluation of antiviral compounds against cytomegalovirus in mice. *Antivir. Res.* **2010**, *88*, 45–52. [CrossRef]
165. Abad, L.V.; Kudo, H.; Saiki, S.; Nagasawa, N.; Tamada, M.; Katsumura, Y.; Aranilla, C.T.; Relleve, L.S.; De La Rosa, A.M. Radiation degradation studies of carrageenans. *Carbohydr. Polym.* **2009**, *78*, 100–106. [CrossRef]
166. Zhou, G.; Sun, Y.; Xin, H.; Zhang, Y.; Li, Z.; Xu, Z. In vivo antitumor and immunomodulation activities of different molecular weight lambda-carrageenans from *Chondrus ocellatus*. *Pharmacol. Res.* **2004**, *50*, 47–53. [CrossRef]
167. Raman, M.; Doble, M. κ-Carrageenan from marine red algae, *Kappaphycus alvarezii*—A functional food to prevent colon carcinogenesis. *J. Funct. Foods* **2015**, *15*, 354–364. [CrossRef]
168. Zhou, G.; Xin, H.; Sheng, W.; Sun, Y.; Li, Z.; Xu, Z. In vivo growth-inhibition of S180 tumor by mixture of 5-Fu and low molecular lambda-carrageenan from *Chondrus ocellatus*. *Pharmacol. Res.* **2005**, *51*, 153–157. [CrossRef]
169. Zhou, G.; Sheng, W.; Yao, W.; Wang, C. Effect of low molecular λ-carrageenan from Chondrus ocellatus on antitumor H-22 activity of 5-Fu. *Pharmacol. Res.* **2006**, *53*, 129–134. [CrossRef] [PubMed]
170. Lemonnier-Le Penhuizic, C.; Chatelet, C.; Kloareg, B.; Potin, P. Carrageenan oligosaccharides enhance stress-induced microspore embryogenesis in *Brassica oleracea* var. italica. *Plant Sci.* **2001**, *160*, 1211–1220. [CrossRef]
171. Muñoz, A.M.; Ponce, J.C.; Araya, J.V. Method to Stimulate Carbon Fixation in Plants with an Aqueous Solution of Oligo-Carrageenans Selected from Kappa1, Kappa2, Lambda or Iota. U.S. Patent 12/911,790, 5 May 2011.
172. Castro, J.; Vera, J.; González, A.; Moenne, A. Oligo-carrageenans stimulate growth by enhancing photosynthesis, basal metabolism, and cell cycle in tobacco plants (var. Burley). *J. Plant Growth Regul.* **2012**, *31*, 173–185. [CrossRef]
173. Saucedo, S.; Contreras, R.A.; Moenne, A. Oligo-carrageenan kappa increases C, N and S assimilation, auxin and gibberellin contents, and growth in *Pinus radiata* trees. *J. For. Res.* **2015**, *26*, 635–640. [CrossRef]
174. Abad, L.V.; Nasimova, I.R.; Relleve, L.S.; Aranilla, C.T.; De La Rosa, A.M.; Shibayama, M. Dynamic light scattering studies of irradiated kappa carrageenan. *Int. J. Biol. Macromol.* **2004**, *34*, 81–88. [CrossRef]
175. González, A.; Castro, J.; Vera, J.; Moenne, A. Seaweed oligosaccharides stimulate plant growth by enhancing carbon and nitrogen assimilation, basal metabolism, and cell division. *J. Plant Growth Regul.* **2013**, *32*, 443–448. [CrossRef]
176. Sun, Y.; Yang, B.; Wu, Y.; Liu, Y.; Gu, X.; Zhang, H.; Wang, C.; Cao, H.; Huang, L.; Wang, Z. Structural characterization and antioxidant activities of κ-carrageenan oligosaccharides degraded by different methods. *Food Chem.* **2015**, *178*, 311–318. [CrossRef]
177. Prasetyaningrum, A.; Jos, B.; Dharmawan, Y.; Octaviani, R.V.; Ratnawati, R. Chemical and spectral characterization of the ozonation products of κ-carrageenan. *MATEC Web Conf.* **2018**, *156*, 05006. [CrossRef]
178. Kalitnik, A.A.; Byankina Barabanova, A.O.; Nagorskaya, V.P.; Reunov, A.V.; Glazunov, V.P.; Solov'eva, T.F.; Yermak, I.M. Low molecular weight derivatives of different carrageenan types and their antiviral activity. *J. Appl. Phycol.* **2013**, *25*, 65–72. [CrossRef]

179. Karlsson, A.; Singh, S.K. Acid hydrolysis of sulphated polysaccharides. Desulphation and the effect on molecular mass. *Carbohydr. Polym.* **1999**, *38*, 7–15. [CrossRef]
180. Yang, B.; Yu, G.; Zhao, X.; Jiao, G.; Ren, S.; Chai, W. Mechanism of mild acid hydrolysis of galactan polysaccharides with highly ordered disaccharide repeats leading to a complete series of exclusively odd-numbered oligosaccharides. *FEBS J.* **2009**, *276*, 2125–2137. [CrossRef] [PubMed]
181. Chauhan, P.S.; Saxena, A. Bacterial carrageenases: An overview of production and biotechnological applications. *3 Biotech* **2016**, *6*, 146. [CrossRef]
182. Lii, C.Y.; Chen, C.H.; Yeh, A.I.; Lai, V.M.F. Preliminary study on the degradation kinetics of agarose and carrageenans by ultrasound. *Food Hydrocoll.* **1999**, *13*, 477–481. [CrossRef]
183. Hu, X.; Jiang, X.; Aubree, E.; Boulenguer, P.; Critchley, A.T. Preparation and in vivo antitumor activity of κ-carrageenan oligosaccharides. *Pharm. Biol.* **2006**, *44*, 646–650. [CrossRef]
184. Abad, L.V.; Relleve, L.S.; Racadio, C.D.T.; Aranilla, C.T.; De la Rosa, A.M. Antioxidant activity potential of gamma irradiated carrageenan. *Appl. Radiat. Isot.* **2013**, *79*, 73–79. [CrossRef]
185. Gereniu, C.R.N.; Saravana, P.S.; Chun, B.S. Recovery of carrageenan from Solomon Islands red seaweed using ionic liquid-assisted subcritical water extraction. *Sep. Purif. Technol.* **2018**, *196*, 309–317. [CrossRef]
186. Choi, E.M.; Kim, G.H.; Lee, Y.S. Atractylodes japonica root extract protects osteoblastic MC3T3-E1 cells against hydrogen peroxide-induced inhibition of osteoblastic differentiation. *Phytother. Res.* **2009**, *23*, 1537–1542. [CrossRef]
187. Fleurence, J. The enzymatic degradation of algal cell walls: A useful approach for improving protein accessibility? *J. Appl. Phycol.* **1999**, *11*, 313–314. [CrossRef]
188. Vieira, E.F.; Soares, C.; Machado, S.; Correia, M.; Ramalhosa, M.J.; Oliva-Teles, M.T.; Paula Carvalho, A.; Domingues, V.F.; Antunes, F.; Oliveira, T.A.C.; et al. Seaweeds from the Portuguese coast as a source of proteinaceous material: Total and free amino acid composition profile. *Food Chem.* **2018**, *269*, 264–275. [CrossRef] [PubMed]
189. Galland-Irmouli, A.V.; Fleurence, J.; Lamghari, R.; Luçon, M.; Rouxel, C.; Barbaroux, O.; Bronowicki, J.P.; Villaume, C.; Guéant, J.L. Nutritional value of proteins from edible seaweed *Palmaria palmata* (Dulse). *J. Nutr. Biochem.* **1999**, *10*, 353–359. [CrossRef]
190. Wang, T.; Jónsdóttir, R.; Kristinsson, H.G.; Hreggvidsson, G.O.; Jónsson, J.Ó.; Thorkelsson, G.; Ólafsdóttire, G. Enzyme-enhanced extraction of antioxidant ingredients from red algae *Palmaria palmata*. *LWT Food Sci. Technol.* **2010**, *43*, 1387–1393. [CrossRef]
191. Paiva, L.; Lima, E.; Patarra, R.F.; Neto, A.I.; Baptista, J. Edible Azorean macroalgae as source of rich nutrients with impact on human health. *Food Chem.* **2014**, *164*, 128–135. [CrossRef] [PubMed]
192. Guiry, M.D. The Seaweed Site: Information on Marine Algae. 2014. Available online: http://www.seaweed.ie/ (accessed on 26 April 2019).
193. Misurcová, L. Chemical Composition of Seaweeds. In *Handbook of Marine Macroalgae: Biotechnology and Applied Phycology*; Kim, S.K., Ed.; John Wiley & Sons: New York, NY, USA, 2012; p. 567.
194. Roman, B.L.; Pham, V.; Lawson, N.D.; Kulik, M.; Childs, S.; Lekven, A.C.; Garrity, D.M.; Moon, R.T.; Fishman, M.C.; Lechleider, R.J.; et al. Disruption of acvrl1 increases endothelial cell number in zebrafish cranial vessels. *Development* **2002**, *129*, 3009–3019.
195. Sekar, S.; Chandramohan, M. Phycobiliproteins as a commodity: Trends in applied research, patents and commercialization. *J. Appl. Phycol.* **2008**, *20*, 113–136. [CrossRef]
196. Fernández-Rojas, B.; Hernández-Juárez, J.; Pedraza-Chaverri, J. Nutraceutical properties of phycocyanin. *J. Funct. Foods* **2014**, *11*, 375–392. [CrossRef]
197. Chandra, R.; Parra-Saldivar, R.; Hafiz, M.N.I. Phycobiliproteins: A novel green tool from marine origin blue-green algae and red algae—A review. *Pept. Lett.* **2016**, *23*, 1–8. [CrossRef] [PubMed]
198. Manirafasha, E.; Ndikubwimana, T.; Zeng, X.; Lu, Y.; Jing, K. Phycobiliprotein: Potential microalgae derived pharmaceutical and biological reagent. *Biochem. Eng. J.* **2016**, *109*, 282–296. [CrossRef]
199. Jiang, L.; Wang, Y.; Yin, Q.; Liu, G.; Liu, H.; Huang, Y.; Li, B. Phycocyanin: A potential drug for cancer treatment. *J. Cancer* **2017**, *8*, 3416–3429. [CrossRef]
200. Hao, S.; Yan, Y.; Li, S.; Zhao, L.; Zhang, C.; Liu, L.; Wang, C. The in vitro anti-tumor activity of phycocyanin against non-small cell lung cancer cells. *Mar. Drugs* **2018**, *16*, 178. [CrossRef] [PubMed]
201. Mittal, R.; Raghavarao, K.S.M.S. Extraction of R-Phycoerythrin from marine macro-algae, *Gelidium pusillum*, employing consortia of enzymes. *Algal Res.* **2018**, *34*, 1–11. [CrossRef]

202. Gantar, M.; Dhandayuthapani, S.; Rathinavelu, A. Phycocyanin induces apoptosis and enhances the effect of topotecan on prostate cell line LNCaP. *J. Med. Food* **2012**, *15*, 1091–1095. [CrossRef]
203. Huang, B.; Wang, G.C.; Zeng, C.K.; Li, Z.G. The experimental research of R- phycoerythrin subunits on cancer treatment—A new photosensitizer in PDT. *Cancer Biother. Radiopharm.* **2002**, *17*, 35–42.
204. Munier, M.; Dumay, J.; Morançais, M.; Jaouen, P.; Fleurence, J. Variation in the biochemical composition of the edible seaweed *Grateloupia turuturu* Yamada harvested from two sampling sites on the brittany coast (France): The influence of storage method on the extraction of the seaweed pigment r-phycoerythrin. *J. Chem.* **2013**, *2013*, 568548. [CrossRef]
205. Pina, A.L.; Costa, A.R.; Lage-Yusty, M.A.; López-Hernández, J. An evaluation of edible red seaweed (*Chondrus crispus*) components and their modification during the cooking process. *LWT Food Sci. Technol.* **2014**, *56*, 175–180. [CrossRef]
206. Niu, J.F.; Wang, G.C.; Zhou, B.C.; Lin, X.Z.; Chen, C.S. Purification of R-phycoerythrin from *Porphyra haitanensis* (Bangiales, Rhodophyta) using expanded-bed absorption. *J. Phycol.* **2007**, *43*, 1339–1347. [CrossRef]
207. Nguyen, H.P.T.; Morançais, M.; Fleurence, J.; Dumay, J. *Mastocarpus stellatus* as a source of R-phycoerythrin: Optimization of enzyme assisted extraction using response surface methodology. *J. Appl. Phycol.* **2017**, *29*, 1563–1570. [CrossRef]
208. Wang, C.; Kim, J.H.; Kim, S.W. Synthetic biol-ogy and metabolic engineering for marine carotenoids: New opportunities and future prospects. *Mar. Drugs* **2014**, *12*, 4810–4832. [CrossRef] [PubMed]
209. Senthilkumar, N.; Suresh, V.; Thangam, R.; Kurinjimalar, C.; Kavitha, G.; Murugan, P.; Rengasamy, R. Isolation and characterization of macromolecular protein R-Phycoerythrin from *Portieria hornemannii*. *Int. J. Biol. Macromol.* **2013**, *55*, 150–160. [CrossRef]
210. Niu, J.F.; Wang, G.C.; Tseng, C.K. Method for large-scale isolation and purification of R-phycoerythrin from red alga *Polysiphonia urceolata* Grev. *Protein Expr. Purif.* **2006**, *49*, 23–31. [CrossRef] [PubMed]
211. Niu, J.-F.; Wang, G.-C.; Lin, X.-Z.; Cheng, Z. Large-scale recovery of C-phycocyanin from Spirulina platensis using expanded bed adsorption chromatography. *J. Chromatogr. B* **2007**, *850*, 267–276. [CrossRef]
212. Galland-Irmouli, A.V.; Pons, L.; Luçon, M.; Villaume, C.; Mrabet, N.T.; Guéant, J.L.; Fleurence, J. One-step purification of R-phycoerythrin from the red macroalga *Palmaria palmata* using preparative polyacrylamide gel electrophoresis. *J. Chromatogr. B Biomed. Sci. Appl.* **2000**, *739*, 117–123. [CrossRef]
213. Amano, H.; Noda, H. Proteins of protoplasts from red alga *Porphyra yezoensis*. *Nippon Suisan Gakkaishi* **1990**, *56*, 1859–1864. [CrossRef]
214. Laohakunjit, N.; Selamassakul, O.; Kerdchoechuen, O. Seafood-like flavour obtained from the enzymatic hydrolysis of the protein by-products of seaweed *Gracilaria* sp. *Food Chem.* **2014**, *158*, 162–170. [CrossRef]
215. Rodrigues, D.; Sousa, S.; Silva, A.; Amorim, M.; Pereira, L.; Rocha-Santos, T.A.P.; Gomes, A.M.P.; Duarte, A.C.; Freitas, A.C. Impact of enzyme- and ultrasound-assisted extraction methods on biological properties of red, brown, and green seaweeds from the Central West Coast of Portugal. *J. Agric. Food Chem.* **2015**, *63*, 3177–3188. [CrossRef]
216. Hardouin, K.; Burlot, A.S.; Umami, A.; Tanniou, A.; Stiger-Pouvreau, V.; Widowati, I.; Bedoux, G.; Bourgougnon, N. Biochemical and antiviral activities of enzymatic hydrolysates from different invasive French seaweeds. *J. Appl. Phycol.* **2014**, *26*, 1029–1042. [CrossRef]
217. Fleurence, J.; Massiani, L.; Guyader, O.; Mabeau, S. Use of enzymatic cell wall degradation for improvement of protein extraction from *Chondrus crispus*, *Gracilaria verrucosa* and *Palmaria palmata*. *J. Appl. Phycol.* **1995**, *7*, 393–397. [CrossRef]
218. Denis, C.; Le Jeune, H.; Gaudin, P.; Fleurence, J. An evaluation of methods for quantifying the enzymatic degradation of red seaweed Grateloupia turuturu. *J. Appl. Phycol.* **2009**, *21*, 153–159. [CrossRef]
219. Harrysson, H.; Hayes, M.; Eimer, F.; Carlsson, N.G.; Toth, G.B.; Undeland, I. Production of protein extracts from Swedish red, green, and brown seaweeds, *Porphyra umbilicalis* Kützing, *Ulva lactuca* Linnaeus, and *Saccharina latissima* (Linnaeus) J. V. Lamouroux using three different methods. *J. Appl. Phycol.* **2018**, *30*, 3565–3580. [CrossRef]
220. Suwal, S.; Perreault, V.; Marciniak, A.; Tamigneaux, É.; Deslandes, É.; Bazinet, L.; Jacques, H.; Beaulieu, L.; Doyen, A. Effects of high hydrostatic pressure and polysaccharidases on the extraction of antioxidant compounds from red macroalgae, *Palmaria palmata* and *Solieria chordalis*. *J. Food Eng.* **2019**, *252*, 53–59. [CrossRef]

221. Fleurence, R.L.; Iglesias, C.P.; Torgerson, D.J. Economic evaluations of interventions for the prevention and treatment of osteoporosis: A structured review of the literature. *Osteoporos Int.* **2005**, *17*, 29–40. [CrossRef] [PubMed]
222. Dumay, J.; Clément, N.; Morançais, M.; Fleurence, J. Optimization of hydrolysis conditions of *Palmaria palmata* to enhance R-phycoerythrin extraction. *Bioresour. Technol.* **2013**, *131*, 21–27. [CrossRef]
223. Fitzgerald, C.; Gallagher, E.; O'Connor, P.; Prieto, J.; Mora-Soler, L.; Grealy, M.; Hayes, M. Development of a seaweed derived platelet activating factor acetylhydrolase (PAF-AH) inhibitory hydrolysate, synthesis of inhibitory peptides and assessment of their toxicity using the Zebrafish larvae assay. *Peptides* **2013**, *50*, 119–124. [CrossRef]
224. Harnedy, P.A.; O'Keeffe, M.B.; FitzGerald, R.J. Fractionation and identification of antioxidant peptides from an enzymatically hydrolysed *Palmaria palmata* protein isolate. *Food Res. Int.* **2017**, *100*, 416–422. [CrossRef]
225. Mensi, F.; Ksouri, J.; Seale, E. A statistical approach for optimization of R-phycoerythrin extraction from the red algae Gracilaria verrucosa by enzymatic hydrolysis using central composite design and desirability function. *J. Appl. Phycol.* **2012**, *24*, 915–926. [CrossRef]
226. Mensi, F. Agar yield from R-phycoerythrin extraction by-product of the red alga *Gracilaria verrucosa*. *J. Appl. Phycol.* **2019**, *31*, 741–751. [CrossRef]
227. Lee, D.; Nishizawa, M.; Shimizu, Y.; Saeki, H. Anti-inflammatory effects of dulse *Palmaria palmata* resulting from the simultaneous water-extraction of phycobiliproteins and chlorophyll a. *Food Res. Int.* **2017**, *100*, 514–521. [CrossRef] [PubMed]
228. Mittal, R.; Tavanandi, H.A.; Mantri, V.A.; Raghavarao, K.S.M.S. Ultrasound assisted methods for enhanced extraction of phycobiliproteins from marine macro-algae, *Gelidium pusillum*. *Ultrason. Sonochem.* **2017**, *38*, 92–103. [CrossRef] [PubMed]
229. Corey, P.; Kim, J.K.; Garbary, D.J.; Prithiviraj, B.; Duston, J. Bioremediation potential of *Chondrus crispus* (Basin Head) and *Palmaria palmata*: Effect of temperature and high nitrate on nutrient removal. *J. Appl. Phycol.* **2012**, *24*, 441–448. [CrossRef]
230. Gereniu, C.R.N.; Saravana, P.S.; Getachew, A.T.; Chun, B.S. Characteristics of functional materials recovered from Solomon Islands red seaweed (*Kappaphycus alvarezii*) using pressurized hot water extraction. *J. Appl. Phycol.* **2017**, *29*, 1609–1621. [CrossRef]
231. Pangestuti, R.; Getachew, A.T.; Siahaan, E.A.; Chun, B.-S. Characterization of functional materials derived from tropical red seaweed Hypnea musciformis produced by subcritical water extraction systems. *J. Appl. Phycol.* **2019**. [CrossRef]
232. Wang, F.; Guo, X.Y.; Zhang, D.N.; Wu, Y.; Wu, T.; Chen, Z.G. Ultrasound-assisted extraction and purification of taurine from the red algae *Porphyra yezoensis*. *Ultrason. Sonochem.* **2015**, *24*, 36–42. [CrossRef]
233. Le Guillard, C.; Dumay, J.; Donnay-Moreno, C.; Bruzac, S.; Ragon, J.-Y.; Fleurence, J.; Bergé, J.-P. Ultrasound-assisted extraction of R-phycoerythrin from Grateloupia turuturu with and without enzyme addition. *Algal Res.* **2015**, *12*, 522–528. [CrossRef]
234. Caltagirone, C.; Ferrannini, L.; Marchionni, N.; Nappi, G.; Scapagnini, G.; Trabucchi, M. The potential protective effect of tramiprosate (homotaurine) against Alzheimer's disease: A review. *Aging Clin. Exp. Res.* **2012**, *24*, 580–587.
235. Khotimchenko, S.V. Fatty acids of species in the genus *Codium*. *Botanica Marina* **2003**, *46*, 456–460. [CrossRef]
236. Holdt, S.L.; Kraan, S. Bioactive compounds in seaweed; functional food applications and legislation. *J. Appl. Phycol.* **2011**, *23*, 543–597. [CrossRef]
237. Kumari, S.; Vardhana, S.; Cammer, M.; Curado, S.; Santos, L.; Sheetz, M.P.; Dustin, M.L. T lymphocyte myosin IIA is required for Maturation of the immunological synapse. *Front. Immunol.* **2012**, *3*, 230. [CrossRef]
238. Pereira, L.C.C.; da Silva, N.I.S.; da Costa, R.M.; Asp, N.E.; da Costa, K.G.; Vila Concejo, A. Seasonal changes in oceanographic processes at an equatorial macrotidal beach in northen Brazil. *Cont. Shelf Res.* **2012**, *43*, 95–106. [CrossRef]
239. Kumari, P.; Bijo, A.J.; Mantri, V.A.; Reddy, C.R.K.; Jha, B. Fatty acid profiling of tropical marine macroalgae: An analysis from chemotaxonomic and nutritional perspectives. *Phytochemistry* **2013**, *86*, 44–56. [CrossRef]
240. Chen, C.Y.; Chou, H.N. Screening of red algae filaments as a potential alternative source of eicosapentaenoic acid. *Mar. Biotechnol.* **2002**, *4*, 189–192. [CrossRef]
241. Kumari, P.; Kumar, M.; Gupta, V.; Reddy, C.R.K.; Jha, B. Tropical marine macroalgae as potential sources of nutritionally important PUFAs. *Food Chem.* **2010**, *120*, 749–757. [CrossRef]

242. Schmid, M.; Kraft, L.G.K.; van der Loos, L.M.; Kraft, G.T.; Virtue, P.; Nichols, P.D.; Hurd, C.L. Southern Australian seaweeds: A promising resource for omega-3 fatty acids. *Food Chem.* **2018**, *265*, 70–77. [CrossRef] [PubMed]
243. Crampon, C.; Boutin, O.; Badens, E. Supercritical carbon dioxide extraction of molecules of interest from microalgae and seaweeds. *Ind. Eng. Chem. Res.* **2011**, *50*, 8941–8953. [CrossRef]
244. Cheung, P.C.K. Temperature and pressure effects on supercritical carbon dioxide extraction of n-3 fatty acids from red seaweed. *Food Chem.* **1999**, *65*, 399–403. [CrossRef]
245. Patra, J.K.; Lee, S.W.; Kwon, Y.S.; Park, J.G.; Baek, K.H. Chemical characterization and antioxidant potential of volatile oil from an edible seaweed *Porphyra tenera* (Kjellman, 1897). *Chem. Cent. J.* **2017**, *11*, 34. [CrossRef]
246. Kumari, P.; Reddy, C.R.K.; Jha, B. Comparative evaluation and selection of a method for lipid and fatty acid extraction from macroalgae. *Anal. Biochem.* **2011**, *415*, 134–144. [CrossRef]
247. Mæhre, H.K.; Malde, M.K.; Eilertsen, K.E.; Elvevoll, E.O. Characterization of protein, lipid and mineral contents in common Norwegian seaweeds and evaluation of their potential as food and feed. *J. Sci. Food Agric.* **2014**, *94*, 3281–3290. [CrossRef]
248. Chen, Y.H.; Tu, C.J.; Wu, H.T. Growth-inhibitory effects of the red alga *Gelidium amansii* on cultured cells. *Biol. Pharm. Bull.* **2004**, *27*, 180–184. [CrossRef]
249. Chan, P.T.; Matanjun, P.; Yasir, S.M.; Tan, T.S. Antioxidant activities and polyphenolics of various solvent extracts of red seaweed, *Gracilaria changii*. *J. Appl. Phycol.* **2015**, *27*, 2377–2386. [CrossRef]
250. Topuz, O.K.; Gokoglu, N.; Yerlikaya, P.; Ucak, I.; Gumus, B. Optimization of antioxidant activity and phenolic compound extraction conditions from red seaweed (*Laurencia obtusa*). *J. Aquat. Food Prod. Technol.* **2016**, *25*, 414–422. [CrossRef]
251. Zheng, J.; Chen, Y.; Yao, F.; Chen, W.; Shi, G. Chemical composition and antioxidant/antimicrobial activities in supercritical carbon dioxide fluid extract of *Gloiopeltis tenax*. *Mar. Drugs* **2012**, *10*, 2634–2647.
252. Ospina, M.; Castro-Vargas, H.I.; Parada-Alfonso, F. Antioxidant capacity of Colombian seaweeds: 1. Extracts obtained from *Gracilaria mammillaris* by means of supercritical fluid extraction. *J. Supercrit. Fluids* **2017**, *128*, 314–322. [CrossRef]
253. Kang, J.Y.; Chun, B.S.; Lee, M.C.; Choi, J.S.; Choi, I.S.; Hong, Y.K. Anti-inflammatory Activity and Chemical Composition of Essential Oil Extracted with Supercritical CO2 from the Brown Seaweed *Undaria pinnatifida*. *J. Essent. Oil Bear. Pl.* **2016**, *19*, 46–51. [CrossRef]
254. Yuan, S.; Duan, Z.; Lu, Y.; Ma, X.; Wang, S. Optimization of decolorization process in agar production from *Gracilaria lemaneiformis* and evaluation of antioxidant activities of the extract rich in natural pigments. *3 Biotech* **2018**, *8*, 8. [CrossRef]
255. Yuan, Y.V.; Westcott, N.D.; Hu, C.; Kitts, D.D. Mycosporine-like amino acid composition of the edible red alga, Palmaria palmata (Dulse) harvested from the west and east coasts of Grand Manan Island, New Brunswick. *Food Chem.* **2009**, *112*, 321–328. [CrossRef]
256. Aguilera, J.; Bischof, K.; Karsten, U.; Hanelt, D.; Wiencke, C. Seasonal variation in ecophysiological patterns in macroalgae from an Arctic fjord. II. Pigment accumulation and biochemical defense systems against high light stress. *Mar. Biol.* **2002**, *140*, 1087–1095.
257. Bedoux, G.; Hardouin, K.; Marty, C.; Taupin, L.; Vandanjon, L.; Bourgougnon, N. Chemical characterization and photoprotective activity measurement of extracts from the red macroalga *Solieria chordalis*. *Bot. Mar.* **2014**, *57*, 291–301. [CrossRef]
258. Rupérez, P. Mineral content of edible marine seaweeds. *Food Chem.* **2002**, *79*, 23–26. [CrossRef]
259. Kraan, S. Mass-cultivation of carbohydrate rich macroalgae, a possible solution for sustainable biofuel production. *Mitig. Adapt. Strateg. Glob. Chang.* **2013**, *18*, 27–46. [CrossRef]
260. Jaballi, I.; Saad, H.B.; Bkhairia, I.; Cherif, B.; Kallel, C.; Boudawara, O.; Droguet, M.; Magné, C.; Hakim, A.; Amara, I.B. Cytoprotective effects of the red marine alga *Chondrus canaliculatus* against Maneb-Induced hematotoxicity and bone oxidative damages in adult rats. *Biol. Trace Elem. Res.* **2018**, *184*, 99–113. [CrossRef] [PubMed]
261. Niu, Y.F.; Zhang, M.H.; Li, D.W.; Yang, W.D.; Liu, J.S.; Bai, W.B. Improvement of neutral lipid and polyunsaturated fatty acid biosynthesis by overexpressing a type 2 diacylglycerol acyltransferase in marine diatom *Phaeodactylum tricornutum*. *Mar. Drugs* **2013**, *11*, 4558–4569. [CrossRef] [PubMed]
262. Cian, R.; Martínez, O.; Drago, S. Bioactive properties of peptides obtained by enzymatic hydrolysis from protein byproducts of *Porphyra columbina*. *Food Res. Int.* **2012**, *49*, 364–372. [CrossRef]

263. Cian, R.E.; Vioque, J.; Drago, S.R. Enzyme proteolysis enhanced extraction of ACE inhibitory and antioxidant compounds (peptides and polyphenols) from *Porphyra columbiana* residual cake. *J. Appl. Phycol.* **2013**, *25*, 1197–1206. [CrossRef]
264. Baghel, R.S.; Trivedi, N.; Reddy, C.R. A simple process for recovery of a stream of products from marine macroalgal biomass. *Bioresour. Technol.* **2016**, *203*, 160–165. [CrossRef]
265. Gajaria, T.K.; Suthar, P.; Baghel, R.S.; Balar, N.B.; Sharnagat, P.; Mantri, V.A.; Reddy, C.R.K. Integration of protein extraction with a stream of byproducts from marine macroalgae: A model forms the basis for marine bioeconomy. *Bioresour. Technol.* **2017**, *243*, 867–873. [CrossRef]
266. Kumar, S.; Gupta, R.; Kumar, G.; Sahoo, D.; Kuhad, R.C. Bioethanol production from Gracilaria verricosa, a red alga, in a biorefinery approach. *Bioresour. Technol.* **2013**, *135*, 150–156. [CrossRef] [PubMed]
267. Baghel, R.R.S.; Trivedi, N.; Gupta, V.; Neori, A.; Reddy, C.R.K.; Lali, A.; Jha, B. Biorefining of marine macroalgal biomass for production of biofuel and commodity chemicals. *Green Chem.* **2015**, *17*, 2436–2443. [CrossRef]
268. Tan, I.S.; Lee, K.T. Enzymatic hydrolysis and fermentation of seaweed solid wastes for bioethanol production: An optimization study. *Energy* **2014**, *78*, 53–62. [CrossRef]
269. Francavilla, M.P.; Manara, P.; Kamaterou, M.; Monteleone, M.; Zabanioutou, A. Cascade approach of red macroalgae *Gracilaria gracilis* sustainable valorization by extraction of phycobiliproteins and pyrolysis of residue. *Bioresour. Technol.* **2015**, *184*, 305–313. [CrossRef] [PubMed]
270. Ingle, K.; Vitkin, E.; Robin, A.; Yakhini, Z.; Mishori, D.; Golberg, A. Macroalgae biorefinery from *Kappaphycus alvarezii*: Conversion, modeling and performance prediction for India and Philippines as examples. *BioEnergy Res.* **2018**, *11*, 22–32. [CrossRef]
271. Mondal, D.; Sharma, M.; Prasad, K.; Meena, R.; Siddhanta, A.; Ghosh, P. Fuel intermediates, agricultural nutrients and pure water from *Kappaphycus alvarezii* seaweed. *RSC Adv.* **2013**, *3*, 17989–17997. [CrossRef]

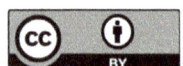

© 2019 by the authors. Licensee MDPI, Basel, Switzerland. This article is an open access article distributed under the terms and conditions of the Creative Commons Attribution (CC BY) license (http://creativecommons.org/licenses/by/4.0/).

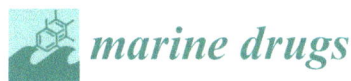

Review

Prebiotics from Seaweeds: An Ocean of Opportunity?

Paul Cherry [1,2,3], Supriya Yadav [2], Conall R. Strain [2,3], Philip J. Allsopp [1], Emeir M. McSorley [1], R. Paul Ross [3,4] and Catherine Stanton [2,3,*]

1. Nutrition Innovation Centre for Food and Health, Ulster University, Cromore Road, Coleraine, Co. Londonderry BT52 1SA, UK; paul.cherry@ucc.ie (P.C.); pj.allsopp@ulster.ac.uk (P.J.A.); em.mcsorley@ulster.ac.uk (E.M.M.)
2. Teagasc Food Research Centre, Moorepark, Fermoy, P61 C996 Co. Cork, Ireland; 18supriya@gmail.com (S.Y.); conall.strain@teagasc.ie (C.R.S.)
3. APC Microbiome Ireland, University College Cork, T12 YT20 Cork, Ireland; p.ross@ucc.ie
4. College of Science, Engineering and Food Science, University College Cork, T12 K8AF Cork, Ireland
* Correspondence: catherine.stanton@teagasc.ie; Tel.: +353-(0)-254-2606

Received: 1 May 2019; Accepted: 29 May 2019; Published: 1 June 2019

Abstract: Seaweeds are an underexploited and potentially sustainable crop which offer a rich source of bioactive compounds, including novel complex polysaccharides, polyphenols, fatty acids, and carotenoids. The purported efficacies of these phytochemicals have led to potential functional food and nutraceutical applications which aim to protect against cardiometabolic and inflammatory risk factors associated with non-communicable diseases, such as obesity, type 2 diabetes, metabolic syndrome, cardiovascular disease, inflammatory bowel disease, and some cancers. Concurrent understanding that perturbations of gut microbial composition and metabolic function manifest throughout health and disease has led to dietary strategies, such as prebiotics, which exploit the diet-host-microbe paradigm to modulate the gut microbiota, such that host health is maintained or improved. The prebiotic definition was recently updated to "a substrate that is selectively utilised by host microorganisms conferring a health benefit", which, given that previous discussion regarding seaweed prebiotics has focused upon saccharolytic fermentation, an opportunity is presented to explore how non-complex polysaccharide components from seaweeds may be metabolised by host microbial populations to benefit host health. Thus, this review provides an innovative approach to consider how the gut microbiota may utilise seaweed phytochemicals, such as polyphenols, polyunsaturated fatty acids, and carotenoids, and provides an updated discussion regarding the catabolism of seaweed-derived complex polysaccharides with potential prebiotic activity. Additional in vitro screening studies and in vivo animal studies are needed to identify potential prebiotics from seaweeds, alongside untargeted metabolomics to decipher microbial-derived metabolites from seaweeds. Furthermore, controlled human intervention studies with health-related end points to elucidate prebiotic efficacy are required.

Keywords: seaweed; gut microbiota; prebiotics; dietary fibre; complex polysaccharides; polyphenols; polyunsaturated fatty acids; carotenoids; phytochemicals

---

1. Introduction

Seaweeds are an underexploited and sustainable crop which offer a rich source of bioactive compounds, including novel dietary fibres, polyphenols, fatty acids, and carotenoids [1,2]. Epidemiological evidence comparing Japanese and Western diets have correlated seaweed consumption (5.3 g/day in Japan) with decreased incidence of chronic disease [3], while the purported efficacies of seaweed phytochemicals have led to potential functional food and nutraceutical applications which aim to protect against cardiometabolic and inflammatory risk factors associated with non-communicable diseases, such as obesity, type two diabetes, metabolic syndrome, cardiovascular disease, inflammatory bowel disease, and some cancers [1].

Current understanding of mutualistic diet-host-microbe interactions has generated efforts to exploit diet to maintain health status, and to prevent or overcome non-communicable diseases, where an imbalance of gut microbiota composition and metabolic function manifests during the onset and pathophysiology of gastrointestinal, neurological, and cardio-metabolic diseases, often congruent with intestinal inflammation and compromised gut barrier function [4,5]. As such, it has become pertinent to explore dietary strategies which modulate gut microbial composition and function to improve host health. This includes the use of prebiotics as fermentable substrates to enable selective gut commensal metabolism.

The prebiotic definition was recently updated to "a substrate that is selectively utilised by host microorganisms conferring a health benefit" [6], which includes the inhibition of pathogens, immune system activation, and vitamin synthesis and provides opportunity to explore the prebiotic efficacy of non-complex polysaccharide components such polyphenols, phytochemicals, and polyunsaturated fatty acids (PUFAs) [6]. It is also recognised that other microbial species have the potential to catabolise prebiotics, besides the classical examples of *Bifidobacterium* and *Lactobacillus* [6], courtesy of culture-independent techniques, such as 16S rRNA next generation sequencing and whole genome shotgun metagenomic sequencing which have provided taxonomic classification to identify microbial abundance/diversity and inferred or identified metabolic function [7].

Given that previous discussion regarding the prebiotic potential of seaweed components has focused solely upon the saccharolytic fermentation of complex polysaccharides and the physiological effects of short chain fatty acid metabolites (SCFAs) [3,8,9], scope exists to explore the prebiotic potential of other phytochemical components derived from seaweeds, namely polyphenols, carotenoids, and PUFAs, applicable to both human and animal health.

This review aims to provide an updated discussion regarding the fermentation and potential prebiotic effect of seaweed polysaccharides and oligosaccharides, based on recent evidence from in vitro fermentation studies and in vivo animal models, and to postulate how other seaweed phytochemicals, such as polyphenols, PUFAs, and carotenoids, may interact with the gut microbiota to manipulate microbial composition and/or function to elicit bioactivities pertained to a prebiotic. The latter provides new opportunities to complete prebiotic screening studies using in vitro techniques and pre-clinical animal models to understand how parent compound biotransformation into endogenously-derived or gut microbiota-derived metabolites impact bioaccessibility and bioavailability to influence gut microbial community structure and function, conducive to a prebiotic effect. Evidence from clinical trials with health-related end-points and mechanistic insight is imperative to substantiate health claims associated with a prebiotic effect.

2. Complex Polysaccharides

Seaweeds contain 2.97–71.4% complex polysaccharides [2,3], which include alginate, fucoidan, and laminarin in brown seaweeds; xylan and sulphated galactans, such as agar, carrageenan, and porphyran in red seaweeds; whilst ulvan and xylan are found in green seaweeds. The monosaccharide composition of the major brown, red, and green seaweed glycans are presented in Table 1, Table 2, Table 3, respectively. Whilst no human study to date has explored prebiotic sources from seaweeds, several in vitro studies [10–13], and in vivo animal studies [14,15], have explored the prebiotic potential seaweeds and their polysaccharide components.

Seaweed polysaccharides are atypical in structure to terrestrial glycans, and are understood to resist gastric acidity, host digestive enzymes, and gastrointestinal absorption [8]. Seaweed glycans may, therefore, serve as fermentation substrates for specific gut microbial populations or facilitate substrate cross-feeding of partially broken-down intermediates, such as oligosaccharides and metabolic cross-feeding of SCFAs to cause indirect proliferation of specific bacteria [16–20]. The physiological effects of SCFAs, primarily acetate, propionate, and butyrate, include the reduction of luminal pH to inhibit pathogens, the provision of energy sources to colonocytes, and the activation of free fatty acid receptors; where acetate and propionate are ligands for anorexigenic pathways in appetite regulation and can inhibit the rate limiting step of hepatic cholesterol synthesis via 3-hydroxy-3-methylglutaryl CoA reductase inhibition [21–23].

To facilitate saccharolytic fermentation in the colon, the gut microbiota must express functional carbohydrate active enzymes (CAZymes) to catabolise seaweed glycans as carbon sources within the colonic digesta. The repertoire of CAZymes expressed by the human gut microbiota includes glycoside hydrolase and polysaccharide lyase families to facilitate degradation via hydrolysis and elimination reactions, respectively [24–26]. Whole genome sequencing has previously identified gene clusters which encode the catabolic machinery responsible for the breakdown of prebiotics, which includes the CAZyme families responsible for the catabolism of inulin, lactulose, fructo-oligosaccharides, xylo-oligosaccharides, and galacto-oligosaccharides by human gut commensal strains, including *Bifidobacterium longum* NCC2705, *Bifidobacterium adolescentis* ATCC 15703, *Streptococcus thermophilus* LMD9, *Eubacterium rectale* ATCC 33656, *Bacteroides vulgatus* ATCC 8482, and *Fecalibacterium prausnitzii* KLE1255 [27].

Based on open source data from the Carbohydrate-Active enZYmes Database [28], Tables 1–3 detail the CAZyme families which may exert specificity for seaweed glycans and highlights the gut bacterial populations which have demonstrable evidence for seaweed glycan utilisation. This is dominated by *Bacteroides*, which have extensive glycolytic versatility [26,29]. This may explain why in vitro batch culture fermentation data of seaweeds and seaweed glycans indicate the proliferation of *Bacteroides*; whilst the degradation of complex seaweed glycans by *Bacteroides* could also facilitate the cross-feeding of oligosaccharides, monosaccharides, and SCFAs for gut commensals deemed beneficial to health, including *Bifidobacterium*.

In vitro fermentation studies are frequently used as screening tools to model colonic fermentation and determine substrate utilisation by an ex vivo faecal inoculum, with seaweed as a sole carbon source. An overview of recent in vitro fermentation studies which have evaluated the fermentation of whole seaweeds or extracted complex polysaccharide components by the human gut microbiota is presented in Table 4 (brown seaweeds), Table 5 (red seaweeds), and Table 6 (green seaweeds). These tables include differences in study methodologies, for example, test substrate dosage; the use of an in vitro digestion before the fermentation experiment (declared within the methods section of the cited research paper); how the inoculum was prepared; duration of the faecal fermentation experiment; microbial enumeration method; and the analytical technique used to ascertain metabolite changes during the fermentation. The use of an in vitro digestion before in vitro fermentation is often used to determine whether a substrate is resistant to endogenous digestive enzymes and small intestinal absorption, and to provide the fraction of a dietary component which is bioaccessible in the colon [30]. The lack of an in vitro digestion before fermentation experiments may cause false positive results, given that low molecular weight components present in seaweed extracts, normally absorbed in the small intestine, are used as fermentation substrates for the ex vivo microbiota. Table 7 highlights data from in vivo rodent studies which have evaluated the potential prebiotic effect of seaweeds and seaweed glycans.

Table 1. Potential degradation of brown seaweed glycans by the human gut microbiota.

	Carbohydrate		Carbohydrate-Active Enzyme (CAZyme)	Evidenced Glycolytic Bacteria	Reference
Alginate	1,4-β-D-mannuronic acid α-L-guluronic acid		PL6 Alginate lyase PL6 MG-specific alginate lyase	*Bacteroides clarus* *Bacteroides eggerthii*	[31–36]
			PL15 Alginate lyase PL15 Oligoalginate lyase	*Bacteroides ovatus* *Bacteroides thetaiotaomicron* *Bacteroides xylanisolvens*	
			PL17 Alginate lyase PL17 Oligoalginate lyase	*Bacteroides clarus* *Bacteroides eggerthii*	
Fucoidan	Sulphated 1,2-1,3-1,4-α-L-fucose		GH29 α-L-fucosidase GH29 α-1,3/1,4-L-fucosidase	Not determined	[37]
			GH95 α-L-fucosidase GH95 α-1,2-L-fucosidase		
Laminarin	1,3-1,6-β-glucose		GH16 β-glucanase GH16 β-1,3-1,4-glucanase GH16 endo-1,3-β-glucanase	*Bacteroides distasonis* *Bacteroides fragilis* *Bacteroides thetaiotaomicron*	[10,38]

PL, Polysaccharide Lyase family; GH, Glycoside Hydrolase family. Potential glycolytic bacteria were identified using the Carbohydrate-Active enZYmes Database [28].

Table 2. Potential degradation of red seaweed glycans by the human gut microbiota.

Carbohydrate		Carbohydrate-Active Enzyme (CAZyme)	Evidenced Glycolytic Bacteria	Reference
Agar (Galactan)	1,3-β-D-galactose 1,4-3,6-anhydro-α-L-galactose	GH2 β-galactosidase	*Bacteroidetes plebeius*	[39–42]
		GH16 β-agarase		
		GH86 β-agarase		
		GH117 1,3-α-3,6-anhydro-L-galactosidase		
Carrageenan (Galactan)	1,4-β-D-galactose 1,3-α-D-galactose 3,6-anhydro-D-galactose	GH2 β-galactosidase	*Bacteroides plebeius*	[41,43]
		GH117 1,3-α-3,6-anhydro-L-galactosidase		
Porphyran (Galactan)	Sulphated 1,3-β-D-galactose 1,4-α-L-galactose-6-sulfate 3,6-anhydro-α-L-galactose	GH16 β-porphyranase GH86 β-porphyranase	*Bacteroides plebeius*	[41,44,45]
Xylan	1,3-1,4-β-D-xylose	GH3 xylan 1,4-β-xylosidase	Not determined	[46–49]
		GH5 endo-1,4-β-xylanase		
		GH10 endo-1,4-β-xylanase		
		GH10 endo-1,3-β-xylanase		
		GH11 endo-β-1,4-xylanase		
		GH11 endo-β-1,3-xylanase		
		GH43 β-xylosidase		
		GH43 xylanase		
		GH43 β-1,3-xylosidase		
		GH67 xylan α-1,2-glucuronidase		
		GH115 xylan α-1,2-glucuronidase		
		CE1–CE7 and CE12 acetyl xylanesterases		

PL, Polysaccharide Lyase family; GH, Glycoside Hydrolase family. Potential glycolytic bacteria were identified using the Carbohydrate-Active enZYmes Database [28].

Table 3. Potential degradation of green seaweed glycans by the human gut microbiota.

	Carbohydrate	Carbohydrate-Active Enzyme (CAZyme)	Evidenced Glycolytic Bacteria	Reference
Ulvan	Sulphated 1,4-β-D-Glucuronic acid α-L-Rhamnose 1,4-β-D-xyloglucan	GH78 α-L-rhamnosidase	Not determined	[50,51]
		GH145 α-L-rhamnosidase		
Xylan	1,3-β-D-xylose	GH10 endo-1,3-β-xylanase,	Not determined	[52]
		GH11 endo-β-1,3-xylanase		
		GH43 β-1,3-xylosidase		

PL, Polysaccharide Lyase family; GH, Glycoside Hydrolase family. Potential glycolytic bacteria were identified using the Carbohydrate-Active enZYmes Database [28].

2.1. Brown Seaweed Polysaccharides

Brown seaweeds are commonly used as food ingredients owing to their commercial abundance [53]. The anti-obesogenic effects of brown seaweeds are reported in mice, where supplementation of 5% (w/w) *Saccorhiza polyschides* extract, containing 12% dietary fibre, reduced body weight gain and fat mass of mice with diet-induced obesity [54]. The anti-obesogenic effect was attributed to the fermentation of alginate and fucoidan complex polysaccharide components, owing to reduced microbial bile salt hydrolase activity; however, no gut microbial compositional data were provided. Elsewhere, the in vitro evidence (Table 4) indicates that whole brown seaweeds and their extracted complex polysaccharide components are fermented by the ex vivo faecal microbiota, with increased production of acetate, propionate, butyrate, and total SCFAs reported during fermentation experiments. A corresponding increase in populations, such as *Bifidobacterium*, *Bacteroides*, *Lactobacillus*, *Roseburia*, *Parasutterella*, *Fusicatenibacter*, *Coprococcus*, *Fecalibacterium* is also reported [55–57].

2.1.1. Alginate

Alginates are composed of 1,4-linked α-L-guluronic (G) and β-D-mannuronic acid (M) residues to form GM, GG and MM blocks, and represent 17–45% dry weight of brown seaweeds [58]. The colloidal properties of alginates have wide application in food processing, biotechnology, medicine and pharmaceutical industries [59], while degraded sodium alginate is an approved item of "foods with specified uses", under the categories of "Foods that act on cholesterol plus gastrointestinal conditions" and "Foods that act on blood cholesterol levels" in Japan [60]. The presence of water soluble alginate oligosaccharides in the faeces of pigs fed alginate is indicative of alginate lyase activity by the luminal or mucus adherent gut microbiota [61], although an adaptation period of > 39 days is reported for the degradation of G blocks by the porcine microbiota whilst M blocks are readily degraded [62].

The capacity for alginate to modulate the gut microbiota of Japanese individuals was highlighted over 20 years ago [63], where alginate supplementation (30 kDa, 10 g/day, n = 8) significantly increased faecal *Bifidobacterium* populations in healthy male volunteers after both one and two weeks, alongside significantly increased acetic and propionic acids after two weeks. Deleterious metabolites, including faecal sulphide, phenol, p-cresol, indole, ammonia and skatole were significantly reduced compared to the control (free living) diet. Notably, faecal *Bifidobacterium* counts and SCFA concentrations returned to baseline in the week after alginate diet cessation, which highlights the transient nature of the gut microbiota and the need for greater powered long-term human intervention studies.

Subsequent in vitro fermentation studies have indicated that alginate is fermented by the human gut microbiota, for example, a 24 h in vitro fermentation of a 212 kDa alginate increased total bacterial populations, although no statistical increase in individual *Bifidobacterium*, *Bacteroides/Prevotella*, *Lactobacillus/Enterococcus*, *Eubacterium rectale/Clostridium coccoides*, or *Clostridium histolyticum* populations were observed [11]. Acetic acid, propionic acid and total SCFAs were significantly increased after 24 h fermentation with the 212 kDa alginate, while alginate of 97 kDa increased total SCFA and acetate production after 10 h of fermentation. Alginates of 38 kDa, and 97 kDa did not change microbial abundance, although the authors could not correlate molecular weight with fermentation patterns.

Alginate oligosaccharides (AOS) (~3.5 kDa) can be obtained via acidic or enzymatic hydrolysis of alginate polysaccharides [58], and enzymatically derived AOS has promoted the growth of *Bifidobacterium bifidum* ATCC 29521, *Bifidobacterium longum* SMU 27001 and *Lactobacilli*, in vitro [64,65]. Supplementation of 2.5% AOS for two weeks significantly increased faecal *Bifidobacterium*. in rats compared to control and 5% FOS supplemented diets (13-fold and 4.7-fold increase, respectively), while faecal *Lactobacillus* were 5-fold greater in rats who consumed AOS compared to FOS. *Enterobacteriaceae* and *Enterococcus* populations were significantly decreased following AOS supplementation. Elsewhere, the hydrolysis of alginate, mannuronic acid oligosaccharides (MO) and guluronic oligosaccharides (GO) during a 48 h batch culture fermentation with the faecal microbiota of Chinese individuals demonstrated increased production of acetate, propionate, butyrate, and total SCFAs compared to the substrate-free control, where GO generated the greatest increase [36]. Subsequent strain isolation from the stools of individuals who demonstrated alginate degradation during fermentation identified *Bacteroides xylanisovlens* G25, *Bacteroides thetaiotomicron* A12, *Bacteroides ovatus* A9, and *Bacteroides ovatus* G19 as strains capable of hydrolysing alginate and AOS, where *Bacteroides ovatus* G19 expressed α-1,4-guluronanlyase and β-1,4-mannuronanlyase CAZymes [34].

A *Bacteroides xylanisolvens* strain with 99% similarity to *Bacteroides xylanisolvens* XB1A was recently isolated from the stool of a Chinese individual and the alginate lyase gene expressed was 100% homologous to the alginate lyase of *Bacteroides ovatus* strain ATCC 8483 [33]. The preceding in vitro fermentation study demonstrated increased production of acetate, propionate, butyrate, and total SCFAs compared to the soluble starch control vessel following a 72 h fermentation of alginate.

Alginate lyase depolymerises alginate polysaccharides to lower molecular weight oligosaccharides via β-elimination, and is most commonly expressed by marine bacteria, including *Flammeovirga*, *Vibrio*, *Pseudoalteromonas*, *Glaciecola chathamensis* S18K6, and *Zobellia galactanivorans* [65–69], while the terrestrial bacteria *Paenibacillus* sp. Strain MY03 was recently reported to possess genes encoding alginate lyase and agarase enzymes [70]. The acquisition of genes encoding alginate lyase enzymes by human gut *Bacteroides* is a suggested consequence of horizontal gene transfer from the marine environment [31,71], where seaweed consumption may have provided a vector to exert a selective pressure to induce diet-driven adaptations of the gut microbiota [35,72–76]. Recent work by Matthieu et al. [35] suggests that an alginate degradation system within the genome of human gut *Bacteroides* was a result of ancient acquisition, where the polysaccharide utilisation loci encodes PL6 and PL17 alginate lyase enzymes and hypothetical proteins responsible for alginate recognition, internalisation, and catabolism, including bacterial ABC transporter proteins to facilitate alginate uptake across the bacterial membrane [77]. Nevertheless, in vivo rodent studies have demonstrated that seaweed glycans are fermented even though animals have never been exposed to dietary seaweeds before the intervention, which suggests that the gut microbiome contains genes for CAZymes which can degrade seaweed glycans when expressed.

2.1.2. Laminarin

Laminarin is a water-soluble storage polysaccharide consisting of 1,3- or 1,6-β-glucose with an average molecular weight of 5 kDa [78] and accounts for 10–35% of the dry weight of brown seaweeds [58]. One in vitro batch culture fermentation of laminarin demonstrated increased *Bifidobacteria* and *Bacteroides* after 24 h [79], while another demonstrated increased propionate and butyrate production after 24 h [14]. A subsequent in vivo rat study (143 mg laminarin per kg body weight per day for 14 days) indicated that laminarin was not selectively fermented by *Lactobacillus* and

Bifidobacterium, but could modify jejunal, ileal, caecal and colonic mucus composition, secretion, and metabolism to protect against bacterial translocation. The authors suggest that increased luminal acidity and/or catabolism of laminarin by mucolytic commensals could elicit such effects, which corroborates the evidence that a complex polysaccharide-rich diet maintains mucus layer integrity to promote gut barrier function [80,81]. Future studies regarding intestinal mucus modulation by laminarin may wish to characterise gut microbiota compositional and functional changes following laminarin ingestion, to detect the abundance and metabolic activity of glycan degraders, such as *Bacteroides* [82,83] or mucolytic species associated with health, such as *Akkermansia muciniphila* or *Ruminococcus* [84,85]. Elsewhere, laminarin increased L-cell GLP-1 secretion to attenuate diet-induced obesity in mice, and improved glucose homeostasis and insulin sensitivity [86]. The authors suggested that the observed cytosolic Ca^{2+} cascade caused GLP-1 secretion, which is in agreement with GPR41/43 receptor activation by SCFAs produced by gut microbial fermentation [87,88], however, data obtained to assess laminarin-induced changes to gut microbiota composition and metabolic output is needed to ascribe a prebiotic effect in this study.

The abundance of glycoside hydrolase and β-glucosidase enzymes expressed by the human gut microbiota may have the capacity to catabolise laminarin [24,89–91], for example, a *Bacteroides cellulosyliticus* WH2 human gut isolate was able to grow on laminarin-supplemented minimal media in vitro, (incidentally it did not grow on alginate, carrageenan, or porphyran) [92]; however, the molecular mechanisms by which human gut *Bacteroides* breakdown laminarin are likely distinct from those responsible for the degradation of mix linked β 1,3- 1,4- glucans, such as those found in cereals (e.g., by $BoGH16_{MLG}$) [93].

2.1.3. Fucoidan

Fucoidans are water soluble polysaccharides composed of sulphated 1,2- or 1,3- or 1,4-α-L-fucose which exist as structural polysaccharides in brown seaweeds and occupy 5–20% of algal dry weight [58,94]. The structural heterogeneity of fucoidan encompasses varying degrees of branching, sulphate content, polydispersity, and irregular monomer patterns, which can include fucose, uronic acid, galactose, xylose, arabinose, mannose, and glucose residues [9,59,95].

A recent in vitro fermentation study of fucoidan (<30 kDa) extracted from *Laminaria japonica* demonstrated a greater increase in *Bifidobacterium* and *Lactobacillus* following 24 h and 48 h fermentation relative to >30 kDa fucoidan [12], while fucoidan from *Ascophyllum nodosum* (1330 kDa) and *Laminaria japonica* (310 kDa) were shown to increase *Lactobacillus* and *Ruminococcaceae*, respectively, in the caecal microbiota of mice gavaged with 100 mg/kg/day [96]. Fucoidan also reduced serum LPS-binding protein levels in this study—indicative of a reduced antigen load and reduced inflammatory response. In contrast, fucoidan with a fucose-rich and highly sulphated fucoidan extracted from *Cladosiphon okamuranus* was not fermented by the rat gut microbiota [97].

While the purported bioactivities of fucoidan include anti-obesogenic, anti-diabetic, anti-microbial, and anti-cancer properties [98], there is limited evidence to implicate a role for the gut microbiota with such bioactivities, and studies are needed to evaluate the structure-dependent fermentation of fucoidan to ascribe a prebiotic effect. For the latter, this is surprising given the myriad of α-fucosidase enzymes present in the human gut bacterial glycobiome.

Table 4. In vitro fermentation of brown seaweeds with human faecal inoculum.

Seaweed	Substrate	Dose	Use of a Simulated In Vitro Digestion Before Fermentation?	Experimental Parameters	Microbial Enumeration	Microbial Changes	Metabolomics Analysis Technique	Metabolite Changes	Reference
Ecklonia radiata	Crude fraction (CF) Phlorotannin-enriched fraction (PF) Low-molecular weight polysaccharide fraction (LPF) High-molecular weight polysaccharide fraction (HPF)	1.5% (w/v)	Yes CF = 71.5% digestible PF = 87.3% digestible LPF = 86.1% digestible HPF = non-digestible	10% (w/v) pooled inoculum (n = 3) 24 h	qPCR	↑*Bifidobacterium* ↑*Lactobacillus* (LPF) ↑ *F. prausnitzii* ↑ *C. coccoides* ↑*Firmicutes* (CF, LPF) ↑ *Bacteroidetes* ↑*E. coli* (CF, PF, LPF, HPF) ↓ *Enterococcus* (CF, PF)	GC-FID	↑Acetate (CF) ↑Propionate (CF, LPF, HPF) ↑Butyrate (CF, LPF, HPF) ↑Total SCFA (CF, LPF, HPF)	[56]
Ecklonia radiata	Water extract (WE) Acid extract (AE) Celluclast enzyme extract (CEE) Alcalase enzyme extract (AEE) Free sugar fraction (FF) Polysaccharide fraction (PF) Seaweed residue (SR) Seaweed powder (SP)	1.5% (w/v)	No-digestibility unknown	10% (w/v) pooled inoculum (n = 3) 24 h	qPCR	= *F. prausnitzii* = *C. leptum* = *R. bromii* ↑ Total bacteria (CEE, AEE, WE, FF) ↑*Bifidobacterium* ↑*Bacteroidetes* ↑*Lactobacillus* ↑ *C. coccoides* (CEE) ↑ *E. coli* ↑ *Enterococcus* (WE, AE, CEE, AEE, FF, PF, SP)	GC-FID	↑ Acetate ↑ Propionate (WE, AE, CEE, AEE, FF, PF, SP) ↑Total SCFA	[57]
Sargassum muticum	*Sargassum muticum* Alcalase enzyme extract (SAE)	1% (w/v)	Yes-non-digestible (% digestible undisclosed)	10% (w/v) single inoculum 24 h	FISH	= *Bifidobacterium* = *Lactobacillus* = *Clostridium histolyticum* ↑ *Bacteroides*/*Prevotella* ↑ *C.coccoides*/*E.rectale*	HPLC	↑Total SCFA	[99]
Sargassum thunbergii	Polysaccharide extract	0.3% (w/v)	No-digestibility unknown	20% (w/v) pooled inoculum (n = 3) 24 h	16S rRNA NGS	↑ Bacteroidetes ↑Bacteroidetes:Firmicutes ratio ↑ *Bifidobacterium* ↑ *Roseburia* ↑ *Parasutterella* ↑ *Fusicatenibacter* ↑ *Coprococcus* ↑ *Faecalibacterium*	GC-MS	↑Acetate ↑Propionate ↑Butyrate ↑Valerate ↑Total SCFA	[55]
-	Alginate	5% (w/v)	No-digestibility unknown	10% (w/v) single inoculum 72 h	16S rRNA DGGE 16S rRNA NGS	↑*Bacteroides*	GC-FID	↑Propionate ↑Butyrate ↑Total SCFA	[33]

Table 4. Cont.

Seaweed	Substrate	Concentration	Digestibility	Inoculum/Time	Method	Microbial Changes	SCFA Method	SCFA Changes	Ref
-	Alginate (A), Mannuronic acid oligosaccharides (MO), Guluronic acid oligosaccharides (GO), Propylene glycol alginate sodium sulphate (PSS)	5 g/L (A), 8 g/L (MO, GO, PSS)	No—digestibility unknown	10% (w/v) single inoculum 48 h	16S rRNA DGGE	Detection of *Bacteroides xylanisolvens*, *Clostridium clostridioforme*/*Clostridium symbiosum*, *Bacteroides fragoldii*, *Shigella flexneri*/*E.coli*, *E.fergusonii*, and *Bacteroides ovatus*	HPLC	A, MO, GO: ↑Acetate ↑Propionate ↑Butyrate ↑Total SCFA	[96]
Ascophyllum nodosum	Sulphated polysaccharide extract	9 mg/mL	Yes—non-digestible (% digestible undisclosed)	10% (w/v) pooled inoculum (n = 4) 24 h	16S rRNA NGS	↑*Bacteroides* ↑*Phascolarctobacterium* ↑*Oscillospira* ↑*Faecalibacterium*	GC-FID	↑Acetate ↑Propionate ↑Butyrate ↑Total SCFA	[100]
Laminaria digitata	Crude polysaccharide extract (CE), Depolymerised crude polysaccharide extract (DE)	1% (w/v)	Yes—non-digestible (% digestible undisclosed)	20% (w/v) pooled inoculum (n = 3) 48 h	16S rRNA NGS	↑*Parabacteroides* (CE, DE) ↑*Fibrobacter* (CE) ↓*Streptococcus* ↓*Ruminococcus* ↑*Lachnospiraceae* UC (DE) ↓*Peptostreptococcaceae* IS (DE) ↓*Dialister* (CE, DE) ↑γ B38UC (CE)	GC-FID	↑Acetate (CE, DE) ↑Propionate (CE, DE) ↑Butyrate (CE, DE) ↑Total SCFA (CE, DE)	[101]
-	Laminarin	1% (w/v)	No—digestibility unknown	10% (w/v) pooled inoculum (n = 5) 24 h	qPCR	↑*Bifidobacterium* ↑*Bacteroides*	HPLC	↑Acetate ↑Propionate ↑Total SCFA	[79]

qPCR, Quantitative PCR; GC-FID, Gas Chromatography with Flame Ionisation Detector; FISH, Flourescence in situ Hybridisation; 16S rRNA NGS, 16S rRNA Next Generation Sequencing; HPLC, High Performance Liquid Chromatography; GC-MS, Gas Chromatography-Mass Spectrometry; 16S rRNA DGGE, 16S rRNA Denaturing Gradient Gel Electrophoresis; 16S rRNA NGS, 16S rRNA Next Generation Sequencing; GC-FID, Gas Chromatography with Flame Ionisation Detector; HPLC, High Performance Liquid Chromaography; 16S rRNA Next Generation Sequencing; qPCR, Quantitative PCR; GC-FID, Gas Chromatography with Flame Ionisation Detector; HPLC, High Performance Liquid Chromatography; SCFA, Short Chain Fatty Acid; =, no statistical difference compared to the control; ↑, significant increase compared to the control; ↓ significant decrease compared to the control. Microbial and metabolite changes with abbreviations in parentheses indicate the substrate(s) which exerted the effect. If no abbreviations in parenthesis are presented, then all of the seaweed substrates tested exerted the effect.

2.2. Red Seaweed Polysaccharides

2.2.1. Galactans (Carrageenan, Agar, and Porphyran)

Red seaweeds, such as *Gelidium* spp. and *Gracilaria* spp., are used in the commercial production of agar and carrageenan food additives, including thickening, stabilizing and encapsulation agents [53]. A summary of evidence from recent in vitro fermentation experiments using red seaweed-derived substrates are presented in Table 5.

Carrageenans are composed of sulphated 1,4-β-D-galactose, 1,3-α-D-galactose, and 3,6-anhydro-D-galactose [43], and constitutes 30–75% dry weight of red seaweeds [58]. In rats fed 2.5% *Chondrus crispus*, of which carrageenan is a major polysaccharide component, faecal *Bifidobacterium breve*, and acetate, propionate, and butyrate SCFAs were significantly increased alongside a significant decrease in the pathogens *Clostridium septicum* and *Streptococcus pneumonia*, as compared to the basal diet [15]. Furthermore, a 1:1 mixture of polysaccharide extracts from *Kappaphycus alvarezii* (containing carrageenan) and *Sargassum polycystum* (brown seaweed) has lowered serum lipids in rats [39]. In a study by Li et al. [34], β-carrageenase activity in a *Bacteroides uniforms* 38F6 isolate complex of *Bacteroides xylanisolvens* and *Escherichia coli* hydrolysed κ-carrageenan oligosaccharides into 4-O-sulfate-D-galactose, κ-carratriose, κ-carrapentaose, and κ-carraheptaose, which could facilitate cross-feeding to promote the growth of *Bifidobacterium* populations.

Agar is composed of sulphated 1,3-β-D-galactose and 1,4- 3,6-anhydro-α-L-galactose [40] and can be fractionated into agarose and agaropectin [8]. Low molecular weight agar of 64.64 kDa has demonstrated a bifidogenic effect alongside increased acetate and propionate SCFA concentrations after 24 h in vitro fermentation with human stool inoculum [11], while mice fed with 2.5% (w/v) neoagarose oligosaccharides for 7 days demonstrated increased caecal and faecal *Lactobacillus* and *Bifidobacterium* [102]. The utilisation of agaro-oligosaccharides was noted in vitro by *Bacteroides uniforms* L8, isolated from Chinese individuals, which secreted a β-agarase CAZyme to breakdown agarooligosaccharides into agarotriose and subsequently facilitated the growth of *Bifidobacterium infantis* and *Bifidobacterium adolescentis* via the cross feeding of agarotriose [103].

Porphyran is made up of sulphated 1,3-β-D-galactose, 1,4-α-L-galactose-6-sulfate and 3,6-anhydro-α-L-galactose [41,104,105]. An in vitro faecal fermentation study indicated that porphyran did not significantly increase SCFAs, but stimulated *Lactobacillus* and *Bacteroides* populations [79]. While pure cultures of *Bifidobacterium breve*, *Bifidobacterium longum*, *Bifidobacterium infantis*, *Bifidobacterium adolescentis*, but not *Bifidobacterium bifidum*, were able to ferment dried *Porphyra yezoensis* (Nori), containing a low protein content (25%), whereas Nori with a high protein content (41%) was not fermented [105]. It is likely that carbohydrate content was highest in the low protein Nori, thus seasonal- and species-variation and in seaweed macronutrient content should be considered a determinant factor for the fermentability of whole seaweeds [106–109].

Evidence for the horizontal transfer of genes for porphyranase and agarase CAZymes from the marine bacteria, *Zobellia galactanivorans*, to *Bacteroides plebeius* of Japanese individuals is indicative of diet-driven adaptations of the human gut microbiome [41,44]; however, the North American counterparts in this study did not consume seaweeds and the gut microbiota of these individuals did not express such CAZymes. This may mean that the fermentation of seaweed polysaccharides, such as porphyran and agar, requires exposure to, and acquisition of, specific CAZymes usually present in the marine environment [73]. Red seaweed galactans are emerging prebiotic candidates given the commercial availability of red seaweed hydrocolloids and the potential gut modulatory effects of oligosaccharides obtained from red seaweeds. Nevertheless, further in vivo evidence is needed, given the purported pro-inflammatory effects of low molecular weight carrageenan [110–112].

2.2.2. Xylan

Xylan, composed of 1,3-1,4-β-D-xylose, is a major constituent of red seaweeds, such as *Palmaria palmata* [46]. A previous in vitro faecal fermentation study of xylan derived from *P. palmata*, reported that xylose was fermented after six h alongside a 58:28:14 ratio of acetate, propionate, and butyrate SCFAs (total SCFAs were 107 mM/L) [113]. This study did not ascertain bacterial compositional data, and thus a knowledge gap is presented given that xylans and xylooligosaccharides (XOS) extracted from terrestrial plants, such as wheat husks and maize, are mooted as potential prebiotics owing to evidence of bifidogenesis, improved plasma lipid profile, and positive modulation of immune function markers in healthy adults [114,115]. Given that human gut *Bacteroides* express a repertoire of xylanase and xylosidase CAZymes [116], investigations regarding the capacity of the human gut microbiota to catabolise red seaweed xylans and XOS are suggested.

Table 5. In vitro fermentation of red seaweeds with human faecal inoculum.

Seaweed	Substrate	Dose	Use of a Simulated in vitro Digestion Before Fermentation?	Experimental Parameters	Microbial Enumeration	Microbial Changes	Metabolomics Analysis Technique	Metabolite Changes	Reference
Kappaphycus alvarezii	Whole Seaweed (WS)	1% (w/v)	Yes–non-digestible (% digestible undisclosed)	10% (w/v) single inoculum 24 h	FISH	↑*Bifidobacterium* ↓*Clostridium coccoides*/ *Eubacterium rectale*	HPLC	↑Total SCFA	[13]
Osmundea pinnatifida	*Osmundea pinnatifida* Viscozyme extract (OVE)	1% (w/v)	Yes–non-digestible (% digestible undisclosed)	10% (w/v) single inoculum 24 h	FISH	=*Bifidobacterium* =*Lactobacillus* =*Clostridium histolticum*	HPLC	↑Total SCFA	[99]
Gracilaria rubra	Polysaccharide extract (PE)	1% (w/v)	Yes–non-digestible (% digestible undisclosed)	10% (w/v) pooled inoculum (n = 4) 24 h	16S rRNA NGS	↑*Bacteroides* ↑*Prevotella* ↑*Phascolarctobacterium* ↓Firmicutes:Bacteroidetes	GC-FID	↑Acetate ↑Propionate ↑Isobutyrate ↑Total SCFA	[117]
-	Porphyran	1% (w/v)	No–digestibility unknown	10% (w/v) pooled inoculum (n = 5) 24 h	qPCR	↑*Bifidobacterium* ↑*Bacteroides*	HPLC	=Acetate =Propionate =Butyrate =Total SCFA	[79]

FISH, Flourescence in situ Hybridisation; 16S rRNA NGS, 16S rRNA Next Generation Sequencing; qPCR, Quantitative PCR; GC-FID, Gas Chromatography with Flame Ionisation Detector; HPLC, High Performance Liquid Chromatography; SCFA, Short Chain Fatty Acid; =, no statistical difference compared to the control; ↑, significant increase compared to the control; ↓ significant decrease compared to the control. Microbial and metabolite changes with abbreviations in parenthesis indicate the substrate(s) which exerted the effect. If no abbreviations in parenthesis are presented, then all of the seaweed substrates tested exerted the effect.

2.3. Green Seaweed Polysaccharides

Ulvan

Ulvans are water-soluble cell wall polysaccharides that account for 8–29% dry weight of green seaweeds, and are composed of sulphated 1,3-α-L-rhamnose, 1,4-β-D-glucuronic acid, and 1,4-β-D-xyloglucan [51]. Previous reports indicate that *Ulva lactuca* and ulvan polysaccharides are poorly fermented by the human gut microbiota [8,95,118], while an in vitro fermentation study of *Enteromorpha* spp. With a human faecal inoculum reported no difference in *Enterococcus*, *Lactobacillus*, and *Bifidobacterium* populations compared to the control; only an increase in *Enterobacter* after 24 h and 48 h of fermentation (Table 6) [12]. In contrast, a recent in vitro faecal fermentation study indicated that Ulvan stimulated the growth of *Bifidobacterium* and *Lactobacillus* populations and promoted the production of lactate and acetate [79]. Further, a murine study showed that *Enteromorpha* (EP) and *Enteromorpha* polysaccharides (PEP) ameliorated inflammation associated with Loperamide-induced constipation in mice [119], where alpha diversity, Firmicutes, and Actinobacteria were increased in the faecal microbiota of seaweed-supplemented mice compared to the constipated control. Bacteroidetes and Proteobacteria were decreased, while Bacteroidales family S24-7 and *Prevotellaceae* were increased in EP and PEP, respectively. Current evidence for the fermentation of green seaweeds and their polysaccharides is limited and fermentation may require specific α-L-rhamnosidase activity by gut commensals [50]. More experimental evidence is needed to understand the impact of ulvans and ulvan-oligosaccharides in the human and animal diet.

2.4. Future Prospective–Obtaining Oligosaccharides

Enzyme technologies are reported to increase the extraction yield and reduce the molecular weight of bioactive components obtained from seaweeds, with examples of enhanced prebiotic activity when commercially available cellulases or seaweed-specific enzymes were used to hydrolyse polysaccharides [99,120]. Despite limited commercial availability of seaweed-specific enzymes, an avenue for functional oligosaccharide production is presented if efforts to develop commercially viable saccharolytic enzymes from microorganisms (primarily marine). Examples of such glycoside hydrolases include fucoidanase from *Sphingomonas paucimobilis* PF-1 [121]; ulvan lyase from *Alteromonas* spp. [122] and the family *Flavobacteriaceae* [123]; β-agarase from *Cellulophaga omnivescoria* W5C [124] and *Cellvibrio PR1* [125]; alginate lyase from *Flammeovirga* [126], and *Paenibacillus* [70]; and laminarinase from *Clostridiium thermocellum* [127]. Factors which influence the stability and efficacy of such hydrolytic enzymes may include metal ion interaction, or thermostability at the high temperatures needed to prevent gelling of polysaccharides. Recent insight into the production of agarose oligosaccharides and neoagarose oligosaccharides from agar exemplify this [128].

Table 6. In vitro fermentation of green seaweeds with human faecal inoculum.

Seaweed	Substrate	Dose	Use of a Simulated in vitro Digestion Before Fermentation?	Experimental Parameters	Microbial Enumeration	Microbial Changes	Metabolomics Analysis Technique	Metabolite Changes	Reference
Enteromorpha prolifera	Polysaccharide extract (PE)	0.2 g in 9.5 mL 0.8 g in 9.5mL	Yes-non-digestible (% digestible undisclosed)	10.5% (w/v) pooled inoculum (n = 3) 12, 24, and 48 h	Microbial culture	↑Enterobacter (0.2 PE and 0.8 PE at 24 h and 48 h) = Enterococcus = Lactobacillus = Bifidobacterium	GC-FID	= Acetate = Butyrate = Lactate	[12]
-	Ulvan	1% (w/v)	No-digestibility unknown	10% (w/v) pooled inoculum (n = 5) 24 h	qPCR	↑Bifidobacterium ↑Lactobacillus	HPLC	↑ Acetate ↑ Lactate	[79]

qPCR, Quantitative PCR; GC-FID, Gas Chromatography with Flame Ionisation Detector; HPLC, High Performance Liquid Chromatography; =, no statistical difference compared to the control; ↑, significant increase compared to the control; ↓ significant decrease compared to the control. Microbial and metabolite changes with abbreviations in parenthesis indicate the substrate(s) which exerted the effect. If no abbreviations in parenthesis are presented, then all of the seaweed substrates tested exerted the effect.

Table 7. Impact of seaweeds on the rodent gut microbiota.

Animal	Substrate	Dose	Duration	Biological Sample	Microbial Changes	Metabolite Changes	Reference
30 Male Sprague-Dawley Rats	Chondrus crispus Whole Seaweed (WS)	0.5% (w/w) 2.5% (w/w)	21 days	Faeces	↑Bifidobacterium ↑Legionella ↑Sutterella ↑Blautia ↑Holdemania ↑Shewanella ↑Agaritomans ↓Streptococcus ↑Bifidobacterium breve (2.5% WS)	↑ Acetate ↑ Propionate (2.5% WS) ↑ Butyrate ↑ Total SCFA	[15]
24 Male Sprague-Dawley Rats	Ecklonia radiata Whole Seaweed (WS) Ecklonia radiata Polysaccharide Fraction (PF)	5% (w/w) WS 5% (w/w) PF	7 days	Caecum	↑F. prausnitzii ↑ E. coli (PF) ↓ Enterococcus (WS) ↓Lactobacillus ↓Bifidobacterium ↑ Firmicutes:Bacteroidetes	↑ Acetate ↑ Propionate ↑ Butyrate (PF) ↓ Valerate ↓ Hexanoate ↑ Total SCFA ↓ i-Butyrate ↓ i-Valerate ↓ phenol ↓ p-cresol	[129]
18 Male Wistar Rats	Alginate (A) Laminarin (L) Fucoidan (F)	2% (w/w)	14 days	Caecum	↑Bacteroides (Bacteroides capillosus) Presence of Enterrhabdus (A) ↑ Proteobacteria. Presence of Lachnospiracea, Parabacteroides (Parabacteroides distasonis) and Parasutterella (L) Not fermented (F)	↑ Propionate (L) ↑ Total SCFA (A, L)	[97]

Table 7. Cont.

	Substrate	Dose	Duration	Sample	Microbiota changes	Metabolite changes	Ref
16 Male C57 BL/6 Mice	*Saccorhiza polyschides* extract (BAE)	High fat diet + 5% (w/w) BAE	8 months	Faeces		↓ Secondary bile acids	[54]
18 Male Wistar Rats	Alginate (A) Laminarin (L)	2% (w/w)	14 days	Caecum	↑*Lactobacillus* ↑*Porphyromonas* ↑*Coprobacillus* ↑*Oscillibacter valencigenes* ↓ *Parabacteroides* (L) ↑ *Catabacter honkongensis* ↑ *Stomatobaculum longum* ↓ *Adlercreuzia* (A) ↓ *Helicobacter* (A, L)	↓ Faecal bile salt hydrolase activity ↑ Lactic acid (L) = Acetate = Propionate = Butyrate = Total SCFA ↓ Indole	[30]
18 Male C57BL/6 mice	*Ascophyllum nodosum* Fucoidan (FuA) *Laminaria japonica* Fucoidan (FuL)	100 mg/kg/day	6 weeks	Caecum	↑*Lactobacillus* ↑*Anaeroplasma* ↑*Ruminococcaceae* ↓ *Alsitipes* ↑*Thalassospira* (FuA) ↓ *Clostridiales* ↓ *Akkermansia* (FuL) ↓ *Candidatus* ↓ *Arthromitus* ↓ *Peptococcus* ↓ *Lachnospiraceae Incertae Sedis* (FuA, FuL)	-	[96]
15 Male Wistar rats	*Ascophyllum nodosum* seaweed crude polysaccharide (SCP) SCP *Lactobacillus plantarum* hydrolysate (SCPH Lp) SCP *Enterococcus faecis* hydrolysate (SCPH Ef) Alginate (A) Hydrolysed Alginate (HA)	0.2 g per 180–200 g rat weight	4 days	Faeces	-	↑ Acetate (HA > A > SCPH Lp > SCPH Ef) ↑ Propionate (HA = A = SCPH Lp = SCPH Ef) ↑ Butyrate (HA = A = SCPH Lp = SCPH Ef) (relative to day zero)	[131]
32 Female Kunming mice	*Enteromorpha prolifera* (EP) *Enteromorpha* polysaccharide extract (PEP)	1:5 (w/w)	7 days	Faeces	↑Alpha diversity (EP) ↑*Bacteroidales* S24-7 (EP) ↑ *Prevotellaceae* (PEP) ↑ Firmicutes ↑Actinobacteria (EP, PEP) ↓ Bacteroidetes ↓ Proteobacteria (EP, PEP)	-	[119]

SCFA, Short Chain Fatty Acid; =, no statistical difference compared to the control; ↑, significant increase compared to the control; ↓ significant decrease compared to the control. Microbial and metabolite changes with abbreviations in parenthesis indicate the substrate(s) which exerted the effect. If no abbreviations in parenthesis are presented, then all of the seaweed substrates tested exerted the effect.

3. Polyphenols

Seaweeds are rich in polyphenols, such as catechins, flavonols, and phlorotannins. Red and green seaweeds are a source of bromophenols, phenolic acids, and flavonoids [132], while phlorotannins are the most abundant polyphenol in brown seaweeds. Most research to date concerns the bioactivity of phlorotannins, a class of polyphenol unique to brown algae comprised of phloroglucinol monomers and categorised as eckols, fucols, fuhalols, ishofuhalols, phloroethols, or fucophloroethols [132]. The purported bioactivities of seaweed polyphenols are associated with the mitigation of risk factors pertained to type 2 diabetes and cardiovascular disease, including hyperglycemia, hyperlipidemia, inflammation and oxidative stress [133–137], and also anti-microbial activity [138]. Owing to heterogeneity in both molecular weight and the level of isomerisation, characterisation of polyphenols is difficult [139–141], and a paucity of information exists regarding the endogenous digestion and microbial catabolism of seaweed polyphenols, with a scarce mechanistic understanding of how they may exert health benefits via the gut microbiota.

Most polyphenols of plant origin must undergo intestinal biotransformation by endogenous enzymes and the gut microbiota prior to absorption across enterocytes. These enzymatic transformations include the elimination of glycosidic bonds, for example, flavonoids are converted to glycones (sugars) and aglycones (non-sugars–polyphenols) by endogenous β-glucosidases in the small intestine [142]. The transport of aglycones to the liver via the portal vein results in phase II biotransformation (coupling reactions, chiefly hepatic conjugation to O-glucuronides and O-sulfates) to facilitate urinary and biliary elimination. Phase II metabolites are absorbed into the systemic circulation, or excreted in bile and re-enter the duodenum (hepatic recycling), where subsequent glucuronidase, glycosidase, or sulphatase-mediated deconjugation by the colonic microbiota may favour aglycone reabsorption [143].

Approximately 90–95% of dietary polyphenols reach the colon intact [144], where biotransformation and metabolism by the gut microbiota occurs via hydrolysis, reduction, decarboxylation, demethylation, dehydroxylation, isomerisation, and fission [145], to produce low-molecular weight compounds with less chemical heterogeneity than the polyphenol parent compound [142]. It is suggested that a complex network of gut microbial species is necessary for full biotransformation of polyphenols, whereas simple reactions, such as deglycosylation, can be achieved by individual gut strains. Furthermore, the bioactivities associated with dietary polyphenol intake may be dependent on the catabolic capacity and composition of the gut microbiota, owing to the biological activity of metabolites rather than the parent polyphenol compound present in food [146,147], while a synergistic effect between prebiotic polyphenols and probiotic bacteria may occur [6].

The identification of bacteria which possess the metabolic capabilities to utilise polyphenols was previously identified in *Eubacterium oxidoreducens*, which could catabolise gallate, pyrogallol, phloroglucinol and quercetin [148]. Quercetin biotransformation by *Eubacterium ramulus* has also been identified [149], and multiple human gut microbes which possess phenolic enzymes capable of breaking down glycosides, glucuronides, sulphates, esters, and lactones was summarised by Selma et al. [145]. Such microorganisms included *E. coli* with β-glucuronidase activity; *Eubacterium*, *Bacteroides*, and *Clostridium* with β-glucosidase activity; *Lactobacillus*, *Eubacterium*, *Clostridium* , *Butyrbacterium*, *Streptococcus*, and *Methylotrophicum* with demethylase activity; and *E. coli*, *Bifidobacterium*, *Lactobacillus*, *Bacteroides*, *Streptococcus* , *Ruminococcus*, and *Enterococcus* with esterase activity. There is also evidence for α-L-Rhamnosidase mediated hydrolysis of rutinose, present on glycosylated polyphenols (rhamnoglycosides), to produce aglycones, by species, such as *Bacteroides thetaiotaomicron* [50], *Bifidobacterium dentium* [150], *Bifidobacterium catenulatum* [151], *Bifidobacterium pseudocatenulatum* [151], and *Lactobacillus plantarum* [152].

Current knowledge regarding the fate of seaweed polyphenols in the human gastrointestinal tract is scarce; however, it is understood that the limited absorption of *Ascophyllum nodosum* polyphenols from small intestinal enterocytes to the portal vein may facilitate the conjugation of polyphenols to methylated, glucuronidated, or sulphated forms rather than hydrolysis to aglycones [153,154].

Subsequently, unabsorbed conjugated polyphenols are available for biotransformation by the colonic microbiota, then potentially absorbed across the colonocytes. Indeed, Corona et al. [154], observed a reduction of total polyphenol contents of an *Ascophyllum nodosum* polyphenol extract, high molecular weight fraction (>10 kDa), and low molecular weight fraction (1–10 kDa) following in vitro digestion and batch culture fermentation; although anti-genotoxic activity against H_2O_2 induced DNA damage of HT-29 cells was increased (to a greater extent by the high molecular weight fraction). This study did not assess the microbiota composition, however, elsewhere, an in vitro fermentation of an *Ecklonia radiata* phlorotannin extract significantly increased *Bacteroidetes*, *Clostridium coccoides*, *E. coli*, and *Fecalibacterium prausnitzii*, but decreased *Bifidobacterium* and *Lactobacillus* populations after 24 h fermentation [56]. More in vitro digestion studies would be useful to understand the stability of seaweed polyphenols as extracts or within the seaweed matrix [155,156]. These studies may be complemented by studies which use ileostomy patient cohorts to determine structural changes to seaweed polyphenols following upper GI digestion in vivo to indicate polyphenol bioaccessibility in the colon [157].

A recent review highlighted the potential for dietary polyphenols to modulate the gut microbiota by increasing *Bifidobacterium*, *Lactobacillus*, *Bacteroides*, *Enterococcus*, *Akkermansia muciniphila*, and *Fecalibacterium prausnitzii* populations [158]. This review did not include any studies which assessed modulation of the gut microbiota by seaweed polyphenols and, therefore, a research opportunity is presented. Inter-individual variation of gut microbiota composition and function is the key determinant for gut microbiota-mediated biotransformation of phenolic compounds to bioactive metabolites [159,160]. Therefore, identification of bacterial species or strains with the ability to catabolise seaweed polyphenols and their respective catabolic machinery is needed to understand if seaweed polyphenols could be prebiotic [161,162]. Moreover, considering that gut microbiota-derived secondary metabolites reach a peak plasma concentration much later than the original aglycone or hepatic conjugates, controlled nutrikinetic studies could elude how dietary polyphenols from seaweeds interact with host-microbiota metabolism [163,164]. Identification of faecal, urinary, serum, or tissue biomarkers via untargeted and targeted metabolomics approaches, and the use of stable isotope studies, may also indicate variation in synthesis, bioavailability, metabolism, and excretion of polyphenols and associated metabolites. While integration of dose response studies alongside metagenomics and metabolomics analyses, akin to those conducted for berry and wine polyphenols, could elude how much seaweed polyphenol is required to have an impact, if any, on gut microbial composition, metabolic function, and host health [165,166].

4. Other Seaweed Phytochemicals

4.1. Carotenoids

Carotenoids are lipid soluble compounds which function within the photosynthetic machinery of seaweeds to produce pigments. Fucoxanthin is the predominant carotenoid in brown seaweeds [167], while lutein, β-carotene, astaxanthin, echinenone, violaxanthin, neoxanthin, and zeaxanthin are found in red and green seaweeds. Carotenoids are used as food colouring additives, while the application of fucoxanthin as functional food ingredients is suggested, owing to putative anti-oxidant, anti-inflammatory, anti-cancer, anti-obesity, and anti-diabetic bioactivities [168–173].

While some carotenoids are absorbed by enterocytes and converted into vitamin A and retinoid derivatives by endogenous beta-carotene oxygenase 1 (BCO1) and beta-carotene dioxygenase 2 (BCO2) enzymes [174,175], the bioavailability of carotenoids in the blood is reported as 10–40% [176], which has led to suggestions that carotenoids could be fermented by the gut microbiota [174,177]. The only evidence to date has demonstrated that male C57BL/6J mice supplemented with 0.04% (w/w) astaxanthin during an eight-week pilot study had increased abundance of caecal *Bifidobacterium* [178], whereas *Proteobacteria* and *Bacteroides* were significantly increased in the caecum of BCO2 knockout mice; however, analysis of health biomarkers was not reported. Given the differences in microbiota composition between wild type and BCO2 knockout mice in this study, there is scope to investigate how carotenoids and their endogenous derivatives interact with the gut microbiota. Looking ahead, the use of in vitro models of gastrointestinal digestion and colonic fermentation would be useful to assess whether there is a direct substrate to microbiota effect or a host–microbe effect [179].

4.2. Polyunsaturated Fatty Acids (PUFAs)

The lipid content of seaweed ranges from 1–5% dry weight, which includes n-3 PUFAs, such as eicosapentanoic acid (EPA) and docosahexaenoic acid (DHA) [180,181]. The n-3 PUFA are associated with the anti-inflammatory activity to reduce cardiovascular disease risk and may also exert beneficial effects on brain function and behaviour, as mediated by the microbiota-gut-brain axis [182]. Dietary EPA and DHA intake are reported to improve microbial diversity, reduce the Firmicutes/Bacteroidetes ratio, reduce LPS-producing bacteria, and increase populations of *Bifidobacterium*, *Lachnospiraceae*, and lipopolysaccharide (LPS)-suppressing bacteria in both humans and animal models [182–184]. Although the evidence to date has focused on fish-derived n-3 PUFA, great scope exists to evaluate the prebiotic effect of n-3 PUFA obtained from seaweeds.

5. Fermented Foods

Fermented foods are understood to have improved nutritional and functional properties owing to bioactive or bioavailable components [185]. Seaweeds (mainly kelp) are a common vegetable ingredient in the fermented food, Kimchi. The microbial content of kimchi provides a source of probiotics, nutrients, and bioactive metabolites, which are reported to have anti-microbial, anti-oxidant, and anti-obesogenic activities [186–188]. One randomised controlled trial (RCT) observed that consumption of a seaweed Kimchi made from *L. japonica* for four weeks promoted the growth and survival of gut microbial lactic acid bacteria in humans [189], whilst another RCT concluded that consumption of 1.5 g/day fermented *L. japonica* containing 5.56% γ-aminobutyric acid (GABA) (*Lactobacillus brevis* BJ2 culture) was associated with a reduction in oxidative stress in healthy adults over four weeks, indicated by decreased serum γ-glutamyltransferse (GGT) and malondialdehyde, and increased antioxidant activity of superoxide dismutase and catalase compared to the placebo [190]. The latter study indicates that foods containing fermented brown seaweeds, such as *L. japonica*, may offer a novel source of GABA enriched ingredients, which are associated with hypotensive and anti-inflammatory effects [188]. Anti-oxidant, anti-diabetic, and anti-hypertensive efficacies are also reported for Korean rice wine fermented with *L. japonica* [191], while *Sargassum* fermented with a starter culture of *Enterococcus faecium* was reported to contain higher soluble polyphenol and mannuronic acid-rich alginate contents [192], which may increase the provision of microbiota accessible components for colonic fermentation.

Reports of the functional properties of fermented foods containing red seaweeds are scarce; however, examples of red seaweed fermented foods include a fermented *Porphyra yezoensis* seaweed sauce, which used the marine halophilic lactic acid bacteria, *Tetragenococcus halophilus*, as a starter culture [193]; a *Gracilaria domingensis* aqueous extract applied as a texture modifier in fermented milks as a non-animal alternative to gelatin [194]; and carrageenan as a salt replacer in the production of fat-free cheese [195].

Given the availability of red, brown, and green seaweeds both commercially and locally [196], the production of seaweed-containing fermented foods could be a cost-effective alternative to bioactive component extraction. Nevertheless, an understanding of how live bacteria and bacterial metabolites present in fermented foods contribute towards health is required [185].

6. Seaweeds and Animal Health

Seaweeds also have a historical use as animal feed ingredients [197]. The capacity for seaweeds to modulate the gut microbiota of monogastrics, such as pigs and hens, is presented in Tables 8 and 9, respectively, which complements the recent evidence for the application of seaweed bioactives in monogastric animal feed [198]. Table 8 shows limited evidence that the β-glucan, laminarin, may increase *Lactobacillus* populations but not *Bifidobacterium* populations. While there is scarce evidence for the selective stimulation of health-associated bacteria in pigs by the sulphated fucose, fucoidan. Only one recent study has evaluated the effect of dietary alginate on the porcine microbiota, where the genera *Ruminococcus*, *Roseburia* and *Lachnospira*, and an unclassified bacterium of the *F16* family were increased, alongside a significant decrease in the genus *Blautia*, the family *Clostridiaceae*, and an unclassified bacterium of *RF39* family [199]. In Table 9, recent evidence indicates that hens fed *Chondrus crispus* and *Sarcodiotheca gaudichaudii* red seaweeds may increase ceacal SCFA concentrations and modulate populations of *Bifidobacterium longum*, *Lactobacillus acidophilus*, *Streptococcus salivarius*, and *Clostridium perfringens* [200,201]; however, a bidirectional change in microbial composition was dose dependent and has only been assessed in two studies to date. Given the use of pigs as an animal model of humans [202], data from in vivo monogastric studies which are designed to evaluate the prebiotic potential of dietary seaweeds and seaweed-derived components could provide insight into the potential for human applications.

Tables 10 and 11 summarise recent studies which have examined the impact of seaweed diets on the ruminant microbiota of cows and sheep, respectively, with the potential application of reducing methane production. Despite demonstrating decreased methane production, the cow rumen in vitro fermentation studies presented in Table 10 did not assess microbiota compositional changes, thus a knowledge gap is presented to understand which bacteria (if any), are increased or decreased, and are associated with a reduction in methane production. Table 11 shows that methanogenic bacteria and methane production were significantly decreased compared to the basal grass substrate control following the in vitro fermentation of sheep rumen with the red seaweed *Asparagopsis taxiformis* [203]. While sheep given an ad libitum diet of *Ascophyllum nodosum* brown seaweed (1%, 3%, or 5% w/w) for 21 days demonstrated a dose-dependent decrease in propionate and butyrate SCFAs and a dose-dependent increase in acetate [204], while several bacteria were significantly decreased, including *Prevotella copri*, *Roseburia*, and *Coprococcus*, while *Blautia producta* and the family *Veillonellaceae* were significantly increased compared to the basal diet. Moreover, the specific case of seaweed-fed North Ronaldsay sheep highlights how isolated organisms of the ruminant microbiome, such as *Prevotella*, *Clostridium butyricum*, *Butyrivibrio fibrisolvens*, and Spirochaetes have adapted to hydrolyse alginate laminarin, and fucoidan [205,206]. However, there is a paucity of evidence to implicate any health benefits attributed to a seaweed diet in these animals.

Table 8. Impact of seaweeds on the porcine gut microbiota.

Animal	Seaweed Component	Dose	Duration	Biological Sample	Microbial Changes	Metabolite Changes	Reference
20 pregnant gilts and 48 piglets	Laminarin/Fucoidan Extract	10 g/day	Gestation (day 83) to weaning (day 28)	Faeces (Sow) Colonic digesta (Piglet)	Sows (parturition): ↓ Enterobacteriaceae = Lactobacilli Piglets (birth, 48h after birth, weaning): = Enterobacteriaceae = Lactobacilli	-	[207]
200 pigs	*Ecklonia cava* Whole Seaweed	0.05% (w/w) 0.1% (w/w) 0.15% (w/w)	28 days	Caecum	↑*Lactobacillus* ↓ *E. coli* = Total Anaerobes	-	[208]
24 pigs	Laminarin/Fucoidan Extract (SD) Laminarin/Fucoidan Wet Seaweed (WS)	5.37 Kg/tonne SD 26.3 Kg/tonne WS	21 days	Ileum Caecum Colon	= *Bifidobacteria* = *Lactobacillus* = *Enterobacterium* (SD, WS) ↑*Lactobacillus agilis* (colon)	-	[209]
48 pigs	Laminarin Extract	300 ppm	32 days	Faeces	↑*Lactobacillus* = *Bifidobacteria*	= Acetate ↓ Propionate = Butyrate = Valerate = i-Butyrate = i-Valerate	[210]
48 pigs	β-glucan	250 g/tonne 150 g/tonne	29 days	Ileum Caecum Proximal Colon Distal Colon	= *Lactobacilli* = *Bifidobacteria* ↑ *Lactobacillus* diversity	-	[211]
168 pigs	Laminarin (L) Fucoidan (F)	240 mg/kg F 150 mg/kg L 300 mg/kg L 150 mg/kg L and 240 mg/kg F 300 mg/kg L and 240 mg/kg F	35 days	Faeces	= *E. coli* = *Bifidobacteria* ↑ *Lactobacilli*	= Acetate = Propionate = Butyrate = Valerate = i-Butyrate = i-Valerate = Total SCFA	[212]

Table 8. Cont.

Animal	Seaweed Component	Dose	Duration	Biological Sample	Microbial Changes	Metabolite Changes	Reference
9 pigs	Alginate	5.14% (w/w)	84 days	Faeces	= Diversity ↑ Unclassified F16 family ↓ Clostridiaceae ↓ Unclassified RF39 (Mollicutes) ↑ Ruminococcus ↑ Roseburia ↑ unclassified F16 genus (TM7) ↓ Lachnospira ↓ Blautia	-	[199]

=, no statistical difference compared to the control; ↑, significant increase compared to the control; ↓ significant decrease compared to the control. Microbial and metabolite changes with abbreviations in parenthesis indicate the substrate(s) which exerted the effect. If no abbreviations in parenthesis are presented, then all of the seaweed substrates tested exerted the effect.

Table 9. Impact of seaweeds on the hen gut microbiota.

Animal	Seaweed Component	Dose	Duration	Biological Sample	Microbial Changes	Metabolite Changes	Reference
160 laying hens	Chondrus crispus Whole Seaweed (CC) Sarcodiotheca gaudichaudii Whole Seaweed (SG)	0.5% (w/w) 1% (w/w) 2% (w/w)	30 days	Ileum Caecal digesta	↑Bifidobacterium longum (CC2, SG1, SG2) ↑Streptococcus salivarius (CC1, CC2, SG2) ↓Clostridium perfringens (CC1, CC2, SG1, SG2) ↓Lactobacillus acidophilus (CC1, CC2)	↑ Acetate (CC1, SG1) ↑ Propionate (CC2) ↑ Butyrate (SC2)	[200]
96 laying hens	Chondrus crispus Whole Seaweed (CC) Sarcodiotheca gaudichaudii Whole Seaweed (SG)	Control diet + 2% (w/w) seaweed Control diet + 4% (w/w) seaweed	28 days	Caecum	↑Lactobacillus acidophilus (CC4) ↓Bifidobacterium longum (SG2, SG4, CC4) ↓ Streptococcus salivarius (SG2, SG4, CC2, CC4) ↑ Bacteroidetes (SG4, CC2, CC4)	↑ Propionate (CC4)	[201]

=, no statistical difference compared to the control; ↑, significant increase compared to the control; ↓ significant decrease compared to the control. Microbial and metabolite changes with abbreviations in parenthesis indicate the substrate(s) which exerted the effect. If no abbreviations in parenthesis are presented, then all of the seaweed substrates tested exerted the effect.

Table 10. In vitro fermentation of seaweeds with cow rumen inoculum.

Seaweed	Substrate	Experimental Parameters	Dose (w/v)	Microbial Enumeration	Microbial Changes	Metabolomics Analysis Technique	Metabolite Changes	Reference
Ascophyllum nodosum (AN) Laminaria digitata (LD)	Whole Seaweed	50% pooled inoculum (n = 4) 24 h	0.5 g/L 1 g/L 2 g/L	-	-	GC-FID	↑Propionate ↑Butyrate (LD) ↓ BCFA ↓Methane	[213]
Asparagopsis taxiformis	Whole Seaweed	20% pooled inoculum (n = 4) 72 h	0.5% 1% 2% 5% 10%	-	-	GC-FID	↓ Total gas production ↓ Methane ↓ Acetate ↑ Propionate ↑ Butyrate (2%, 10%) ↓ Total SCFA (5%, 10%)	[214]
Ulva sp. Laminaria ochroleuca Saccharina latissima Gigartina sp. Gracilaria vermiculophylla	Whole Seaweed	20% pooled inoculum (n = 2) 24 h	25%	-	-	GC-FID	↓ Methane	[215]
Brown seaweed by-products (BSB)	-	50% (v/v) single inoculum 0, 3, 6, 9, 12, and 24 h	2% 4%	-	-	GC-FID	↓ Ammonia (3, 9, 12 and 24 h) ↓ Total SCFA (24 h)	[216]

GC-FID, Gas Chromatography; =, no statistical difference compared to the control; ↑, significant increase compared to the control; ↓ significant decrease compared to the control. Microbial and metabolite changes with abbreviations in parenthesis indicate the substrate(s) which exerted the effect. If no abbreviations in parenthesis are presented, then all of the seaweed substrates tested exerted the effect.

Table 11. Impact of seaweeds on the sheep rumen microbiota.

Seaweed	Dose	Experimental Parameters	Microbial Enumeration	Microbial Changes	Metabolomics Analysis Technique	Metabolite Changes	Reference
Asparagopsis taxiformis Whole Seaweed	2%	in vitro batch culture fermentation 20% (v/v) pooled sheep rumen fluid inoculum (n = 4) 48 and 72 h	16S rRNA NGS qPCR	↓Methanogens ↓Bacteroidetes/Firmicutes ratio ↓ mcrA gene expression	GC-MS	↓Total Gas ↓Methane ↑Hydrogen	[203]
Ascophyllum nodosum Whole Seaweed	1% 3% 5%	Rams (n = 8) 21 days *ad libitum*	16S rRNA NGS	↓ undefined TM7-1 ↓undefined *Coriobacteriaceae* ↓*Roseburia* ↓*Coprococcus* ↓*Prevotella copri* ↓*Blautia producta* ↑ *Entodinium species 1* ↑*Veillonellaceae*	GC-FID	Dose dependent: ↑Acetate ↓Propionate ↓Butyrate PICRUSt: ↑Butanoate metabolism ↑Fatty acid metabolism ↓Glycerophospholipid metabolism	[204]

16S rRNA NGS, 16S rRNA Next Generation Sequencing; qPCR, Quantitative PCR; GC-FID, Gas Chromatography; =, no statistical difference compared to the control; ↑, significant increase compared to the control; ↓ significant decrease compared to the control. Microbial and metabolite changes with abbreviations in parenthesis indicate the substrate(s) which exerted the effect. If no abbreviations in parenthesis are presented, then all of the seaweed substrates tested exerted the effect.

7. Conclusions

Current evidence regarding the prebiotic effects of seaweeds is dominated by complex polysaccharide components. This is because prebiotic research was previously focused on saccharolytic fermentation by the gut microbiota. Accumulating evidence from in vitro and in vivo animal studies provides encouraging data regarding the utilisation of red seaweed galactans and brown seaweed glycans, such as alginates and laminarins, with minor evidence for fucoidan and the green seaweed polysaccharide, ulvan.

Given that the most recent definition of prebiotic places non-complex polysaccharide components in vogue, an opportunity is presented to explore how other seaweed phytochemicals, including polyphenols, carotenoids, and PUFAs, are metabolised by host microbial populations to benefit host health. Future investigations should consider the use of in vitro screening studies and in vivo animal studies to identify putative prebiotic compounds from seaweeds via the identification of host organisms which utilise seaweed components and the bioactive metabolites produced (via untargeted metabolomics). Furthermore, controlled human intervention studies with health-related end points to elucidate prebiotic efficacy are required.

Author Contributions: Conceptualization, P.C., S.Y., C.R.S., C.S, P.J.A., E.M.M., R.P.R.; writing—original draft preparation, P.C., S.Y., and C.R.S X.X.; writing—review and editing, P.C., S.Y., C.R.S., C.S, P.J.A., E.M.M., and R.P.R.; funding acquisition, C.S, P.J.A., E.M.M., and R.P.R.

Funding: This research was funded by The Department of Agriculture Food and the Marine (FIRM) under the National Development Plan 2007–2013, Project number 13F511 (PREMARA); and Science Foundation of Ireland—funded Centre for Science, Engineering and Technology, and APC Microbiome Ireland. Paul Cherry is in receipt of a Department for Employment and Learning Northern Ireland Postgraduate studentship.

Acknowledgments: Please see the above funding section.

Conflicts of Interest: The authors declare no conflict of interest.

References

1. Brown, E.S.; Allsopp, P.J.; Magee, P.J.; Gill, C.I.; Nitecki, S.; Strain, C.R.; McSorley, E.M. Seaweed and human health. *Nutr. Rev.* **2014**, *72*, 205–216. [CrossRef] [PubMed]
2. Cherry, P.; O'Hara, C.; Magee, P.J.; McSorley, E.M.; Allsopp, P.J. Risks and benefits of consuming edible seaweeds. *Nutr. Rev.* **2019**. [CrossRef] [PubMed]
3. De Jesus Raposo, M.F.; de Morais, A.M.; de Morais, R.M. Emergent sources of prebiotics: Seaweeds and microalgae. *Mar. Drugs* **2016**, *14*, 27. [CrossRef] [PubMed]
4. Thursby, E.; Juge, N. Introduction to the human gut microbiota. *Biochem. J.* **2017**, *474*, 1823–1836. [CrossRef] [PubMed]
5. Schippa, S.; Conte, M.P. Dysbiotic events in gut microbiota: Impact on human health. *Nutrients* **2014**, *6*, 5786–5805. [CrossRef] [PubMed]
6. Gibson, G.R.; Hutkins, R.; Sanders, M.E.; Prescott, S.L.; Reimer, R.A.; Salminen, S.J.; Scott, K.; Stanton, C.; Swanson, K.S.; Cani, P.D.; et al. Expert consensus document: The International Scientific Association for Probiotics and Prebiotics (ISAPP) consensus statement on the definition and scope of prebiotics. *Nat. Rev. Gastroenterol. Hepatol.* **2017**, *14*, 491–502. [CrossRef] [PubMed]
7. Arnold, J.W.; Roach, J.; Azcarate-Peril, M.A. Emerging technologies for gut microbiome research. *Trends Microbiol.* **2016**, *24*, 887–901. [CrossRef]
8. O'Sullivan, L.; Murphy, B.; McLoughlin, P.; Duggan, P.; Lawlor, P.G.; Hughes, H.; Gardiner, G.E. Prebiotics from marine macroalgae for human and animal health applications. *Mar. Drugs* **2010**, *8*, 2038–2064. [CrossRef]
9. Zaporozhets, T.S.; Besednova, N.N.; Kuznetsova, T.A.; Zvyagintseva, T.N.; Makarenkova, I.D.; Kryzhanovsky, S.P.; Melnikov, V.G. The prebiotic potential of polysaccharides and extracts of seaweeds. *Russ. J. Mar. Biol.* **2014**, *40*, 1–9. [CrossRef]
10. Devillé, C.; Damas, J.; Forget, P.; Dandrifosse, G.; Peulen, O. Laminarin in the dietary fibre concept. *J. Sci. Food Agric.* **2004**, *84*, 1030–1038. [CrossRef]

11. Ramnani, P.; Chitarrari, R.; Tuohy, K.; Grant, J.; Hotchkiss, S.; Philp, K.; Campbell, R.; Gill, C.; Rowland, I. In vitro fermentation and prebiotic potential of novel low molecular weight polysaccharides derived from agar and alginate seaweeds. *Anaerobe* **2012**, *18*, 1–6. [CrossRef] [PubMed]
12. Kong, Q.; Dong, S.; Gao, J.; Jiang, C. In vitro fermentation of sulfated polysaccharides from *E. prolifera* and *L. japonica* by human fecal microbiota. *Int. J. Biol. Macromol.* **2016**, *91*, 867–871. [CrossRef] [PubMed]
13. Bajury, D.M.; Rawi, M.H.; Sazali, I.H.; Abdullah, A.; Sarbini, S.R. Prebiotic evaluation of red seaweed (*Kappaphycus alvarezii*) using in vitro colon model. *Int. J. Food Sci. Nutr.* **2017**, *68*, 821–828. [CrossRef] [PubMed]
14. Devillé, C.; Gharbi, M.; Dandrifosse, G.; Peulen, O. Study on the effects of laminarin, a polysaccharide from seaweed, on gut characteristics. *J. Sci. Food Agric.* **2007**, *87*, 1717–1725. [CrossRef]
15. Liu, J.; Kandasamy, S.; Zhang, J.; Kirby, C.W.; Karakach, T.; Hafting, J.; Critchley, A.T.; Evans, F.; Prithiviraj, B.J.B.C.; Medicine, A. Prebiotic effects of diet supplemented with the cultivated red seaweed Chondrus crispus or with fructo-oligo-saccharide on host immunity, colonic microbiota and gut microbial metabolites. *BMC Complement. Altern. Med.* **2015**, *15*, 279. [CrossRef] [PubMed]
16. Rose, D.J.; Keshavarzian, A.; Patterson, J.A.; Venkatachalam, M.; Gillevet, P.; Hamaker, B.R. Starch-entrapped microspheres extend in vitro fecal fermentation, increase butyrate production, and influence microbiota pattern. *Mol. Nutr. Food Res.* **2009**, *53*, S121–S130. [CrossRef] [PubMed]
17. Timm, D.A.; Stewart, M.L.; Hospattankar, A.; Slavin, J.L. Wheat dextrin, psyllium, and inulin produce distinct fermentation patterns, gas volumes, and short-chain fatty acid profiles in vitro. *J. Med. Food* **2010**, *13*, 961–966. [CrossRef]
18. Belenguer, A.; Duncan, S.H.; Calder, A.G.; Holtrop, G.; Louis, P.; Lobley, G.E.; Flint, H.J. Two routes of metabolic cross-feeding between Bifidobacterium adolescentis and butyrate-producing anaerobes from the human gut. *Appl. Environ. Microbiol.* **2006**, *72*, 3593–3599. [CrossRef]
19. Macfarlane, G.T.; Macfarlane, S. Bacteria, colonic fermentation, and gastrointestinal health. *J. AOAC Int.* **2012**, *95*, 50–60. [CrossRef]
20. Ríos-Covián, D.; Ruas-Madiedo, P.; Margolles, A.; Gueimonde, M.; de los Reyes-Gavilán, C.G.; Salazar, N. Intestinal short chain fatty acids and their link with diet and human health. *Front. Microbiol.* **2016**, *7*, 185. [CrossRef]
21. Byrne, C.S.; Chambers, E.S.; Morrison, D.J.; Frost, G. The role of short chain fatty acids in appetite regulation and energy homeostasis. *Int. J. Obes. (2005)* **2015**, *39*, 1331–1338. [CrossRef] [PubMed]
22. Gunness, P.; Gidley, M.J. Mechanisms underlying the cholesterol-lowering properties of soluble dietary fibre polysaccharides. *Food Funct.* **2010**, *1*, 149–155. [CrossRef] [PubMed]
23. Den Besten, G.; van Eunen, K.; Groen, A.K.; Venema, K.; Reijngoud, D.-J.; Bakker, B.M. The role of short-chain fatty acids in the interplay between diet, gut microbiota, and host energy metabolism. *J. Lipid Res.* **2013**, *54*, 2325–2340. [CrossRef] [PubMed]
24. Tasse, L.; Bercovici, J.; Pizzut-Serin, S.; Robe, P.; Tap, J.; Klopp, C.; Cantarel, B.I.; Coutinho, P.M.; Henrissat, B.; Leclerc, M.; et al. Functional metagenomics to mine the human gut microbiome for dietary fiber catabolic enzymes. *Genome Res.* **2010**, *20*, 1605–1612. [CrossRef] [PubMed]
25. El Kaoutari, A.; Armougom, F.; Leroy, Q.; Vialettes, B.; Million, M.; Raoult, D.; Henrissat, B. Development and validation of a microarray for the investigation of the CAZymes encoded by the human gut microbiome. *PLoS ONE* **2013**, *8*, e84033. [CrossRef] [PubMed]
26. Ndeh, D.; Gilbert, H.J. Biochemistry of complex glycan depolymerisation by the human gut microbiota. *FEMS Microbiol. Rev.* **2018**, *42*, 146–164. [CrossRef] [PubMed]
27. Cecchini, D.A.; Laville, E.; Laguerre, S.; Robe, P.; Leclerc, M.; Doré, J.; Henrissat, B.; Remaud-Siméon, M.; Monsan, P.; Potocki-Véronèse, G. Functional metagenomics reveals novel pathways of prebiotic breakdown by human gut bacteria. *PLoS ONE* **2013**, *8*, e72766. [CrossRef] [PubMed]
28. Cantarel, B.L.; Coutinho, P.M.; Rancurel, C.; Bernard, T.; Lombard, V.; Henrissat, B. The Carbohydrate-Active EnZymes database (CAZy): An expert resource for Glycogenomics. *Nucleic Acids Res.* **2009**, *37*, D233–D238. [CrossRef]
29. Benitez-Paez, A.; Gomez Del Pulgar, E.M.; Sanz, Y. the glycolytic versatility of bacteroides uniformis CECT 7771 and its genome response to oligo and polysaccharides. *Front. Cell. Infect. Microbiol.* **2017**, *7*, 383. [CrossRef]

30. Brodkorb, A.; Egger, L.; Alminger, M.; Alvito, P.; Assunção, R.; Ballance, S.; Bohn, T.; Bourlieu-Lacanal, C.; Boutrou, R.; Carrière, F.; et al. INFOGEST static in vitro simulation of gastrointestinal food digestion. *Nat. Protoc.* **2019**, *14*, 991–1014. [CrossRef]
31. Thomas, F.; Barbeyron, T.; Tonon, T.; Genicot, S.; Czjzek, M.; Michel, G. Characterization of the first alginolytic operons in a marine bacterium: From their emergence in marine Flavobacteriia to their independent transfers to marine Proteobacteria and human gut Bacteroides. *Environ. Microbiol.* **2012**, *14*, 2379–2394. [CrossRef] [PubMed]
32. Brownlee, I.A.; Allen, A.; Pearson, J.P.; Dettmar, P.W.; Havler, M.E.; Atherton, M.R.; Onsoyen, E. Alginate as a source of dietary fiber. *Crit. Rev. Food Sci. Nutr.* **2005**, *45*, 497–510. [CrossRef] [PubMed]
33. Bai, S.; Chen, H.; Zhu, L.; Liu, W.; Yu, H.D.; Wang, X.; Yin, Y. Comparative study on the in vitro effects of Pseudomonas aeruginosa and seaweed alginates on human gut microbiota. *PLoS ONE* **2017**, *12*, e0171576. [CrossRef] [PubMed]
34. Li, M.; Shang, Q.; Li, G.; Wang, X.; Yu, G. Degradation of marine algae-derived carbohydrates by bacteroidetes isolated from human gut microbiota. *Mar. Drugs* **2017**, *15*, 92. [CrossRef] [PubMed]
35. Mathieu, S.; Touvrey-Loiodice, M.; Poulet, L.; Drouillard, S.; Vincentelli, R.; Henrissat, B.; Skjåk-Bræk, G.; Helbert, W. Ancient acquisition of "alginate utilization loci" by human gut microbiota. *Sci. Rep.* **2018**, *8*, 8075. [CrossRef] [PubMed]
36. Li, M.; Li, G.; Shang, Q.; Chen, X.; Liu, W.; Pi, X.; Zhu, L.; Yin, Y.; Yu, G.; Wang, X. In vitro fermentation of alginate and its derivatives by human gut microbiota. *Anaerobe* **2016**, *39*, 19–25. [CrossRef] [PubMed]
37. Zhang, J.J.; Zhang, Q.B.; Wang, J.; Shi, X.L.; Zhang, Z.S. Analysis of the monosaccharide composition of fucoidan by precolumn derivation HPLC. *Chin. J. Oceanol. Limnol.* **2009**, *27*, 578–582. [CrossRef]
38. Salyers, A.A.; Palmer, J.K.; Wilkins, T.D. Laminarinase (beta-glucanase) activity in Bacteroides from the human colon. *Appl. Environ. Microbiol.* **1977**, *33*, 1118–1124.
39. Dousip, A.; Matanjun, P.; Sulaiman, M.R.; Tan, T.S.; Ooi, Y.B.H.; Lim, T.P.J.o.A.P. Effect of seaweed mixture intake on plasma lipid and antioxidant profile of hypercholesterolaemic rats. *J. Appl. Phycol.* **2014**, *26*, 999–1008. [CrossRef]
40. Lahaye, M.; Rochas, C. Chemical-structure and physicochemical properties of agar. *Hydrobiologia* **1991**, *221*, 137–148. [CrossRef]
41. Hehemann, J.H.; Correc, G.; Barbeyron, T.; Helbert, W.; Czjzek, M.; Michel, G. Transfer of carbohydrate-active enzymes from marine bacteria to Japanese gut microbiota. *Nature* **2010**, *464*, 908–912. [CrossRef] [PubMed]
42. Rebuffet, E.; Groisillier, A.; Thompson, A.; Jeudy, A.; Barbeyron, T.; Czjzek, M.; Michel, G. Discovery and structural characterization of a novel glycosidase family of marine origin. *Environ. Microbiol.* **2011**, *13*, 1253–1270. [CrossRef] [PubMed]
43. Weiner, M.L. Food additive carrageenan: Part II: A critical review of carrageenan in vivo safety studies. *Crit. Rev. Toxicol.* **2014**, *44*, 244–269. [CrossRef] [PubMed]
44. Hehemann, J.H.; Kelly, A.G.; Pudlo, N.A.; Martens, E.C.; Boraston, A.B. Bacteria of the human gut microbiome catabolize red seaweed glycans with carbohydrate-active enzyme updates from extrinsic microbes. *Proc. Natl. Acad. Sci. USA* **2012**, *109*, 19786–19791. [CrossRef] [PubMed]
45. Zhang, Q.B.; Qi, H.M.; Zhao, T.T.; Deslandes, E.; Ismaeli, N.M.; Molloy, F.; Critchley, A.T. Chemical characteristics of a polysaccharide from Porphyra capensis (Rhodophyta). *Carbohydr. Res.* **2005**, *340*, 2447–2450. [CrossRef] [PubMed]
46. Usov, A.I. Polysaccharides of the Red Algae. *Adv. Carbohydr. Chem. Biochem.* **2011**, *65*, 115–217. [CrossRef] [PubMed]
47. Mirande, C.; Kadlecikova, E.; Matulova, M.; Capek, P.; Bernalier-Donadille, A.; Forano, E.; Bera-Maillet, C. Dietary fibre degradation and fermentation by two xylanolytic bacteria Bacteroides xylanisolvens XB1AT and Roseburia intestinalis XB6B4 from the human intestine. *J. Appl. Microbiol.* **2010**, *109*, 451–460. [CrossRef]
48. Hong, P.Y.; Iakiviak, M.; Dodd, D.; Zhang, M.L.; Mackie, R.I.; Cann, I. Two new xylanases with different substrate specificities from the human gut bacterium bacteroides intestinalis DSM 17393. *Appl. Environ. Microbiol.* **2014**, *80*, 2084–2093. [CrossRef]
49. Despres, J.; Forano, E.; Lepercq, P.; Comtet-Marre, S.; Jubelin, G.; Chambon, C.; Yeoman, C.J.; Miller, M.E.B.; Fields, C.J.; Martens, E.; et al. Xylan degradation by the human gut Bacteroides xylanisolvens XB1A(T) involves two distinct gene clusters that are linked at the transcriptional level. *BMC Genom.* **2016**, *17*. [CrossRef]

50. Munoz-Munoz, J.; Cartmell, A.; Terrapon, N.; Henrissat, B.; Gilbert, H.J. Unusual active site location and catalytic apparatus in a glycoside hydrolase family. *Proc. Natl. Acad. Sci. USA* **2017**, *114*, 4936–4941. [CrossRef]
51. Lahaye, M.; Robic, A. Structure and functional properties of ulvan, a polysaccharide from green seaweeds. *Biomacromolecules* **2007**, *8*, 1765–1774. [CrossRef] [PubMed]
52. Liang, W.-S.; Liu, T.C.; Chang, C.-J.; Pan, C.-L. Bioactivity of β-1,3-xylan Extracted from Caulerpa lentillifera by Using Escherichia coli ClearColi BL21(DE3)-β-1,3-xylanase XYLII. *J. Food Nutr. Res.* **2015**, *3*, 437–444. [CrossRef]
53. Usman, A.; Khalid, S.; Usman, A.; Hussain, Z.; Wang, Y. Chapter 5—algal polysaccharides, novel application, and outlook. In *Algae Based Polymers, Blends, and Composites*, 1st ed.; Zia, K.M., Zuber, M., Ali, M., Eds.; Elsevier: Amsterdam, The Netherlands, 2017; Volume 1, pp. 115–153. [CrossRef]
54. Huebbe, P.; Nikolai, S.; Schloesser, A.; Herebian, D.; Campbell, G.; Glüer, C.-C.; Zeyner, A.; Demetrowitsch, T.; Schwarz, K.; Metges, C.C.; et al. An extract from the Atlantic brown algae Saccorhiza polyschides counteracts diet-induced obesity in mice via a gut related multi-factorial mechanisms. *Oncotarget* **2017**, *8*, 73501–73515. [CrossRef] [PubMed]
55. Fu, X.; Cao, C.; Ren, B.; Zhang, B.; Huang, Q.; Li, C. Structural characterization and in vitro fermentation of a novel polysaccharide from Sargassum thunbergii and its impact on gut microbiota. *Carbohydr. Polym.* **2018**, *183*, 230–239. [CrossRef] [PubMed]
56. Charoensiddhi, S.; Conlon, M.A.; Vuaran, M.S.; Franco, C.M.M.; Zhang, W. Polysaccharide and phlorotannin-enriched extracts of the brown seaweed Ecklonia radiata influence human gut microbiota and fermentation in vitro. *J. Appl. Phycol.* **2017**, *29*, 2407–2416. [CrossRef]
57. Charoensiddhi, S.; Conlon, M.A.; Vuaran, M.S.; Franco, C.M.M.; Zhang, W. Impact of extraction processes on prebiotic potential of the brown seaweed Ecklonia radiata by in vitro human gut bacteria fermentation. *J. Funct. Foods* **2016**, *24*, 221–230. [CrossRef]
58. Vera, J.; Castro, J.; Gonzalez, A.; Moenne, A. Seaweed polysaccharides and derived oligosaccharides stimulate defense responses and protection against pathogens in plants. *Mar. Drugs* **2011**, *9*, 2514–2525. [CrossRef] [PubMed]
59. García-Ríos, V.; Ríos-Leal, E.; Robledo, D.; Freile-Pelegrin, Y. Polysaccharides composition from tropical brown seaweeds. *Phycol. Res.* **2012**, *60*, 305–315. [CrossRef]
60. Maeda-Yamamoto, M. Development of functional agricultural products and use of a new health claim system in Japan. *Trends Food Sci. Technol.* **2017**, *69*, 324–332. [CrossRef]
61. Jonathan, M.C.; Bosch, G.; Schols, H.A.; Gruppen, H. Separation and identification of individual alginate oligosaccharides in the feces of alginate-fed pigs. *J. Agric. Food Chem.* **2013**, *61*, 553–560. [CrossRef]
62. Jonathan, M.; Souza da Silva, C.; Bosch, G.; Schols, H.; Gruppen, H. In vivo degradation of alginate in the presence and in the absence of resistant starch. *Food Chem.* **2015**, *172*, 117–120. [CrossRef] [PubMed]
63. Terada, A.; Hara, H.; Mitsuoka, T. Effect of dietary alginate on the fecal microbiota and fecal metabolic activity in humans. *Microb. Ecol. Health Dis.* **1995**, *8*, 259–266. [CrossRef]
64. Wang, Y.; Han, F.; Hu, B.; Li, J.; Yu, W. In vivo prebiotic properties of alginate oligosaccharides prepared through enzymatic hydrolysis of alginate. *Nutr. Res.* **2006**, *26*, 597–603. [CrossRef]
65. Han, W.; Gu, J.; Cheng, Y.; Liu, H.; Li, Y.; Li, F. Novel Alginate Lyase (Aly5) from a Polysaccharide-degrading marine bacterium, Flammeovirga sp. Strain MY04: Effects of module truncation on biochemical characteristics, alginate degradation patterns, and oligosaccharide-yielding properties. *Appl. Environ. Microbiol.* **2016**, *82*, 364–374. [CrossRef] [PubMed]
66. Chen, X.-L.; Dong, S.; Xu, F.; Dong, F.; Li, P.-Y.; Zhang, X.-Y.; Zhou, B.-C.; Zhang, Y.-Z.; Xie, B.-B. Characterization of a New Cold-Adapted and Salt-Activated Polysaccharide Lyase Family 7 Alginate Lyase from Pseudoalteromonas sp. SM0524. *Front. Microbiol.* **2016**, *7*, 1120. [CrossRef]
67. Dong, Q.; Ruan, L.; Shi, H. Genome sequence of a high agarase-producing strain Flammeovirga sp. SJP92. *Stand. Genom. Sci.* **2017**, *12*, 13. [CrossRef]
68. Xu, F.; Dong, F.; Wang, P.; Cao, H.Y.; Li, C.Y.; Li, P.Y.; Pang, X.H.; Zhang, Y.Z.; Chen, X.L. Novel molecular insights into the catalytic mechanism of marine bacterial alginate lyase AlyGC from polysaccharide lyase family 6. *J. Biol. Chem.* **2017**, *292*, 4457–4468. [CrossRef]
69. Zhu, B.; Sun, Y.; Ni, F.; Ning, L.; Yao, Z. Characterization of a new endo-type alginate lyase from Vibrio sp. NJU-03. *Int. J. Biol. Macromol.* **2018**, *108*, 1140–1147. [CrossRef]

70. Liu, H.; Cheng, Y.; Gu, J.; Wang, Y.; Li, J.; Li, F.; Han, W. Draft genome sequence of Paenibacillus sp. Strain MY03, a terrestrial bacterium capable of degrading multiple marine-derived polysaccharides. *Genome Announc.* **2017**, *5*. [CrossRef]
71. Mathieu, S.; Henrissat, B.; Labre, F.; Skjåk-Bræk, G.; Helbert, W. Functional exploration of the polysaccharide lyase family PL6. *PLoS ONE* **2016**, *11*, e0159415. [CrossRef]
72. Cantarel, B.L.; Lombard, V.; Henrissat, B. Complex carbohydrate utilization by the healthy human microbiome. *PLoS ONE* **2012**, *7*, e28742. [CrossRef] [PubMed]
73. Hehemann, J.-H.; Boraston, A.B.; Czjzek, M. A sweet new wave: Structures and mechanisms of enzymes that digest polysaccharides from marine algae. *Curr. Opin. Struct. Biol.* **2014**, *28*, 77–86. [CrossRef] [PubMed]
74. Martin, M.; Barbeyron, T.; Martin, R.; Portetelle, D.; Michel, G.; Vandenbol, M. The cultivable surface microbiota of the brown alga Ascophyllum nodosum is enriched in macroalgal-polysaccharide-degrading bacteria. *Front Microbiol* **2015**, *6*, 1487. [CrossRef] [PubMed]
75. Singh, R.P.; Reddy, C.R.K. Unraveling the functions of the macroalgal microbiome. *Front. Microbiol.* **2015**, *6*, 1488. [CrossRef] [PubMed]
76. Bhattacharya, T.; Ghosh, T.S.; Mande, S.S. global profiling of carbohydrate active enzymes in human gut microbiome. *PLoS ONE* **2015**, *10*, e0142038. [CrossRef] [PubMed]
77. Maruyama, Y.; Itoh, T.; Kaneko, A.; Nishitani, Y.; Mikami, B.; Hashimoto, W.; Murata, K. Structure of a Bacterial ABC Transporter Involved in the Import of an Acidic Polysaccharide Alginate. *Structure* **2015**, *23*, 1643–1654. [CrossRef]
78. Kadam, S.U.; O'Donnell, C.P.; Rai, D.K.; Hossain, M.B.; Burgess, C.M.; Walsh, D.; Tiwari, B.K. Laminarin from Irish Brown Seaweeds Ascophyllum nodosum and Laminaria hyperborea: Ultrasound Assisted Extraction, Characterization and Bioactivity. *Mar. Drugs* **2015**, *13*, 4270–4280. [CrossRef]
79. Seong, H.; Bae, J.-H.; Seo, J.S.; Kim, S.-A.; Kim, T.-J.; Han, N.S. Comparative analysis of prebiotic effects of seaweed polysaccharides laminaran, porphyran, and ulvan using in vitro human fecal fermentation. *J. Funct. Foods* **2019**, *57*, 408–416. [CrossRef]
80. Brownlee, I.A.; Havler, M.E.; Dettmar, P.W.; Allen, A.; Pearson, J.P. Colonic mucus: Secretion and turnover in relation to dietary fibre intake. *Proc. Nutr. Soc.* **2003**, *62*, 245–249. [CrossRef]
81. Desai, M.S.; Seekatz, A.M.; Koropatkin, N.M.; Kamada, N.; Hickey, C.A.; Wolter, M.; Pudlo, N.A.; Kitamoto, S.; Terrapon, N.; Muller, A.; et al. A dietary fiber-deprived gut microbiota degrades the colonic mucus barrier and enhances pathogen susceptibility. *Cell* **2016**, *167*, 1339–1353. [CrossRef]
82. Salyers, A.A.; Vercellotti, J.R.; West, S.E.; Wilkins, T.D. Fermentation of mucin and plant polysaccharides by strains of Bacteroides from the human colon. *Appl. Environ. Microbiol.* **1977**, *33*, 319–322.
83. Salyers, A.A.; West, S.E.; Vercellotti, J.R.; Wilkins, T.D. Fermentation of mucins and plant polysaccharides by anaerobic bacteria from the human colon. *Appl. Environ. Microbiol.* **1977**, *34*, 529–533. [PubMed]
84. Tailford, L.E.; Crost, E.H.; Kavanaugh, D.; Juge, N. Mucin glycan foraging in the human gut microbiome. *Front. Genet.* **2015**, *6*, 81. [CrossRef] [PubMed]
85. Dao, M.C.; Everard, A.; Aron-Wisnewsky, J.; Sokolovska, N.; Prifti, E.; Verger, E.O.; Kayser, B.D.; Levenez, F.; Chilloux, J.; Hoyles, L.; et al. Akkermansia muciniphila and improved metabolic health during a dietary intervention in obesity: Relationship with gut microbiome richness and ecology. *Gut* **2016**, *65*, 426. [CrossRef] [PubMed]
86. Yang, L.; Wang, L.; Zhu, C.; Wu, J.; Yuan, Y.; Yu, L.; Xu, Y.; Xu, J.; Wang, T.; Liao, Z.; et al. Laminarin counteracts diet-induced obesity associated with glucagon-like peptide-1 secretion. *Oncotarget* **2017**, *8*, 99470–99481. [CrossRef]
87. Tolhurst, G.; Heffron, H.; Lam, Y.S.; Parker, H.E.; Habib, A.M.; Diakogiannaki, E.; Cameron, J.; Grosse, J.; Reimann, F.; Gribble, F.M. Short-chain fatty acids stimulate glucagon-like peptide-1 secretion via the G-protein-coupled receptor FFAR2. *Diabetes* **2012**, *61*, 364–371. [CrossRef]
88. Everard, A.; Cani, P.D. Gut microbiota and GLP-1. *Rev. Endocr. Metab. Disord.* **2014**, *15*, 189–196. [CrossRef]
89. Dabek, M.; McCrae, S.I.; Stevens, V.J.; Duncan, S.H.; Louis, P. Distribution of beta-glucosidase and beta-glucuronidase activity and of beta-glucuronidase gene gus in human colonic bacteria. *FEMS Microbiol. Ecol.* **2008**, *66*, 487–495. [CrossRef]
90. Gloux, K.; Berteau, O.; El oumami, H.; Béguet, F.; Leclerc, M.; Doré, J. A metagenomic β-glucuronidase uncovers a core adaptive function of the human intestinal microbiome. *Proc. Natl. Acad. Sci. USA* **2011**, *108*, 4539–4546. [CrossRef]

91. Michalska, K.; Tan, K.; Li, H.; Hatzos-Skintges, C.; Bearden, J.; Babnigg, G.; Joachimiak, A. GH1-family 6-P-β-glucosidases from human microbiome lactic acid bacteria. *Acta Crystallogr. Sect. D Biol. Crystallogr.* **2013**, *69*, 451–463. [CrossRef]
92. McNulty, N.P.; Wu, M.; Erickson, A.R.; Pan, C.; Erickson, B.K.; Martens, E.C.; Pudlo, N.A.; Muegge, B.D.; Henrissat, B.; Hettich, R.L.; et al. Effects of diet on resource utilization by a model human gut microbiota containing Bacteroides cellulosilyticus WH2, a symbiont with an extensive glycobiome. *PLoS Biol.* **2013**, *11*, e1001637. [CrossRef] [PubMed]
93. Tamura, K.; Hemsworth, G.R.; Déjean, G.; Rogers, T.E.; Pudlo, N.A.; Urs, K.; Jain, N.; Davies, G.J.; Martens, E.C.; Brumer, H. Molecular mechanism by which prominent human gut bacteroidetes utilize mixed-linkage beta-glucans, major health-promoting cereal polysaccharides. *Cell Rep.* **2017**, *21*, 417–430. [CrossRef] [PubMed]
94. Li, B.; Lu, F.; Wei, X.; Zhao, R. Fucoidan: Structure and Bioactivity. *Molecules* **2008**, *13*, 1671–1695. [CrossRef] [PubMed]
95. Jiao, G.; Yu, G.; Zhang, J.; Ewart, H.S. Chemical structures and bioactivities of sulfated polysaccharides from marine algae. *Mar. Drugs* **2011**, *9*, 196–223. [CrossRef] [PubMed]
96. Shang, Q.; Shan, X.; Cai, C.; Hao, J.; Li, G.; Yu, G. Dietary fucoidan modulates the gut microbiota in mice by increasing the abundance of Lactobacillus and Ruminococcaceae. *Food Funct.* **2016**, *7*, 3224–3232. [CrossRef]
97. An, C.; Yazaki, T.; Takahashi, H.; Kuda, T.; Kimura, B. Diet-induced changes in alginate- and laminaran-fermenting bacterial levels in the caecal contents of rats. *J. Funct. Foods* **2013**, *5*, 389–394. [CrossRef]
98. Collins, K.G.; Fitzgerald, G.F.; Stanton, C.; Ross, R.P. Looking beyond the terrestrial: The potential of seaweed derived bioactives to treat non-communicable diseases. *Mar. Drugs* **2016**, *14*. [CrossRef]
99. Rodrigues, D.; Walton, G.; Sousa, S.; Rocha-Santos, T.A.P.; Duarte, A.C.; Freitas, A.C.; Gomes, A.M.P. In vitro fermentation and prebiotic potential of selected extracts from seaweeds and mushrooms. *LWT Food Sci. Technol.* **2016**, *73*, 131–139. [CrossRef]
100. Chen, L.; Xu, W.; Chen, D.; Chen, G.; Liu, J.; Zeng, X.; Shao, R.; Zhu, H. Digestibility of sulfated polysaccharide from the brown seaweed Ascophyllum nodosum and its effect on the human gut microbiota in vitro. *Int. J. Biol. Macromol.* **2018**, *112*, 1055–1061. [CrossRef]
101. Strain, C.R.; Collins, K.C.; Naughton, V.; McSorley, E.M.; Stanton, C.; Smyth, T.J.; Soler-Vila, A.; Rea, M.C.; Ross, P.R.; Cherry, P.; et al. Effects of a polysaccharide-rich extract derived from Irish-sourced Laminaria digitata on the composition and metabolic activity of the human gut microbiota using an in vitro colonic model. *Eur. J. Nutr.* **2019**. [CrossRef]
102. Hu, B.; Gong, Q.; Wang, Y.; Ma, Y.; Li, J.; Yu, W. Prebiotic effects of neoagaro-oligosaccharides prepared by enzymatic hydrolysis of agarose. *Anaerobe* **2006**, *12*, 260–266. [CrossRef] [PubMed]
103. Li, M.; Li, G.; Zhu, L.; Yin, Y.; Zhao, X.; Xiang, C.; Yu, G.; Wang, X. Isolation and characterization of an agaro-oligosaccharide (AO)-hydrolyzing bacterium from the gut microflora of Chinese individuals. *PLoS ONE* **2014**, *9*, e91106. [CrossRef] [PubMed]
104. Zhang, Q.; Li, N.; Liu, X.; Zhao, Z.; Li, Z.; Xu, Z. The structure of a sulfated galactan from Porphyra haitanensis and its in vivo antioxidant activity. *Carbohydr. Res.* **2004**, *339*, 105–111. [CrossRef] [PubMed]
105. Muraoka, T.; Ishihara, K.; Oyamada, C.; Kunitake, H.; Hirayama, I.; Kimura, T. Fermentation Properties of Low-Quality Red Alga Susabinori Porphyra yezoensis by Intestinal Bacteria. *Biosci. Biotechnol. Biochem.* **2008**, *72*, 1731–1739. [CrossRef] [PubMed]
106. Rioux, L.-E.; Turgeon, S.L.; Beaulieu, M. Effect of season on the composition of bioactive polysaccharides from the brown seaweed Saccharina longicruris. *Phytochemistry* **2009**, *70*, 1069–1075. [CrossRef] [PubMed]
107. Kravchenko, A.O.; Byankina Barabanova, A.O.; Glazunov, V.P.; Yakovleva, I.M.; Yermak, I.M. Seasonal variations in a polysaccharide composition of Far Eastern red seaweed Ahnfeltiopsis flabelliformis (Phyllophoraceae). *J. Appl. Phycol.* **2018**, *30*, 535–545. [CrossRef]
108. Skriptsova, A.V. Seasonal variations in the fucoidan content of brown algae from Peter the Great Bay, Sea of Japan. *Russ. J. Mar. Biol.* **2016**, *42*, 351–356. [CrossRef]
109. Medcalf, D.G.; Lionel, T.; Brannon, J.H.; Scott, J.R. Seasonal variation in the mucilaginous polysaccharides from Ulva lactuca. *Bot. Mar.* **1975**, *18*, 67–70. [CrossRef]

110. Shang, Q.; Sun, W.; Shan, X.; Jiang, H.; Cai, C.; Hao, J.; Li, G.; Yu, G. Carrageenan-induced colitis is associated with decreased population of anti-inflammatory bacterium, Akkermansia muciniphila, in the gut microbiota of C57BL/6J mice. *Toxicol. Lett.* **2017**, *279*, 87–95. [CrossRef]
111. Bhattacharyya, S.; Liu, H.; Zhang, Z.; Jam, M.; Dudeja, P.K.; Michel, G.; Linhardt, R.J.; Tobacman, J.K. Carrageenan-induced innate immune response is modified by enzymes that hydrolyze distinct galactosidic bonds. *J. Nutr. Biochem.* **2010**, *21*, 906–913. [CrossRef]
112. Younes, M.; Aggett, P.; Aguilar, F.; Crebelli, R.; Filipič, M.; Frutos, M.J.; Galtier, P.; Gott, D.; Gundert-Remy, U.; Kuhnle, K.K.; et al. Re-evaluation of carrageenan (E 407) and processed Eucheuma seaweed (E 407a) as food additives. *EFSA J.* **2018**, *16*, e05238. [CrossRef]
113. Lahaye, M.; Michel, C.; Barry, J.L. Chemical, physicochemical and in-vitro fermentation characteristics of dietary fibres from Palmaria palmata (L.) Kuntze. *Food Chem.* **1993**, *47*, 29–36. [CrossRef]
114. Childs, C.E.; Roytio, H.; Alhoniemi, E.; Fekete, A.A.; Forssten, S.D.; Hudjec, N.; Lim, Y.N.; Steger, C.J.; Yaqoob, P.; Tuohy, K.M.; et al. Xylo-oligosaccharides alone or in synbiotic combination with Bifidobacterium animalis subsp. lactis induce bifidogenesis and modulate markers of immune function in healthy adults: A double-blind, placebo-controlled, randomised, factorial cross-over study. *Br. J. Nutr.* **2014**, *111*, 1945–1956. [CrossRef] [PubMed]
115. Lecerf, J.M.; Depeint, F.; Clerc, E.; Dugenet, Y.; Niamba, C.N.; Rhazi, L.; Cayzeele, A.; Abdelnour, G.; Jaruga, A.; Younes, H.; et al. Xylo-oligosaccharide (XOS) in combination with inulin modulates both the intestinal environment and immune status in healthy subjects, while XOS alone only shows prebiotic properties. *Br. J. Nutr.* **2012**, *108*, 1847–1858. [CrossRef] [PubMed]
116. Mirande, C.; Mosoni, P.; Bera-Maillet, C.; Bernalier-Donadille, A.; Forano, E. Characterization of Xyn10A, a highly active xylanase from the human gut bacterium Bacteroides xylanisolvens XB1A. *Appl. Microbiol. Biotechnol.* **2010**, *87*, 2097–2105. [CrossRef] [PubMed]
117. Di, T.; Chen, G.; Sun, Y.; Ou, S.; Zeng, X.; Ye, H. In vitro digestion by saliva, simulated gastric and small intestinal juices and fermentation by human fecal microbiota of sulfated polysaccharides from Gracilaria rubra. *J. Funct. Foods* **2018**, *40*, 18–27. [CrossRef]
118. Andrieux, C.; Hibert, A.; Houari, A.-M.; Bensaada, M.; Popot, F.; Szylit, O. Ulva lactuca is poorly fermented but alters bacterial metabolism in rats inoculated with human fecal flora from methane and non-methane producers. *J. Sci. Food Agric.* **1998**, *77*, 25–30. [CrossRef]
119. Ren, X.; Liu, L.; Gamallat, Y.; Zhang, B.; Xin, Y. Enteromorpha and polysaccharides from enteromorpha ameliorate loperamide-induced constipation in mice. *Biomed. Pharmacother.* **2017**, *96*, 1075–1081. [CrossRef]
120. Charoensiddhi, S.; Conlon, M.A.; Franco, C.M.M.; Zhang, W. The development of seaweed-derived bioactive compounds for use as using enzyme technologies. *Trends Food Sci. Technol.* **2017**, *70*, 20–33. [CrossRef]
121. Kim, W.J.; Park, J.W.; Park, J.K.; Choi, D.J.; Park, Y.I. Purification and Characterization of a Fucoidanase (FNase S) from a Marine Bacterium Sphingomonas paucimobilis PF-1. *Mar. Drugs* **2015**, *13*, 4398–4417. [CrossRef]
122. Coste, O.; Malta, E.-j.; López, J.C.; Fernández-Díaz, C. Production of sulfated oligosaccharides from the seaweed Ulva sp. using a new ulvan-degrading enzymatic bacterial crude extract. *Algal Res.* **2015**, *10*, 224–231. [CrossRef]
123. Barbeyron, T.; Lerat, Y.; Sassi, J.F.; Le Panse, S.; Helbert, W.; Collen, P.N. Persicivirga ulvanivorans sp. nov., a marine member of the family Flavobacteriaceae that degrades ulvan from green algae. *Int. J. Syst. Evol. Microbiol.* **2011**, *61*, 1899–1905. [CrossRef] [PubMed]
124. Ramos, K.R.M.; Valdehuesa, K.N.G.; Nisola, G.M.; Lee, W.K.; Chung, W.J. Identification and characterization of a thermostable endolytic beta-agarase Aga2 from a newly isolated marine agarolytic bacteria Cellulophaga omnivescoria W5C. *New Biotechnol.* **2018**, *40*, 261–267. [CrossRef] [PubMed]
125. Xie, Z.; Lin, W.; Luo, J. Comparative Phenotype and Genome Analysis of Cellvibrio sp. PR1, a Xylanolytic and Agarolytic Bacterium from the Pearl River. *BioMed Res. Int.* **2017**, *2017*, 6304248. [CrossRef] [PubMed]
126. Cheng, Y.; Wang, D.; Gu, J.; Li, J.; Liu, H.; Li, F.; Han, W. Biochemical characteristics and variable alginate-degrading modes of a novel bifunctional endolytic alginate lyase. *Appl. Environ. Microbiol.* **2017**, *83*. [CrossRef] [PubMed]
127. Kislitsyn, Y.A.; Samygina, V.R.; Dvortsov, I.A.; Lunina, N.A.; Kuranova, I.P.; Velikodvorskaya, G.A. Crystallization and preliminary X-ray diffraction studies of the family 54 carbohydrate-binding module from

laminarinase (beta-1,3-glucanase) Lic16A of Clostridium thermocellum. *Acta Crystallogr. Sect. F Struct. Biol. Commun.* **2015**, *71*, 217–220. [CrossRef]
128. Xu, X.Q.; Su, B.M.; Xie, J.S.; Li, R.K.; Yang, J.; Lin, J.; Ye, X.Y. Preparation of bioactive neoagaroligosaccharides through hydrolysis of Gracilaria lemaneiformis agar: A comparative study. *Food Chem.* **2018**, *240*, 330–337. [CrossRef]
129. Charoensiddhi, S.; Conlon, M.A.; Methacanon, P.; Franco, C.M.M.; Su, P.; Zhang, W. Gut health benefits of brown seaweed Ecklonia radiata and its polysaccharides demonstrated in vivo in a rat model. *J. Funct. Foods* **2017**, *37*, 676–684. [CrossRef]
130. Nakata, T.; Kyoui, D.; Takahashi, H.; Kimura, B.; Kuda, T. Inhibitory effects of laminaran and alginate on production of putrefactive compounds from soy protein by intestinal microbiota in vitro and in rats. *Carbohydr. Polym.* **2016**, *143*, 61–69. [CrossRef]
131. Kaewmanee, W.; Suwannaporn, P.; Huang, T.C.; Al-Ghazzewi, F.; Tester, R.F. In vivo prebiotic properties of Ascophyllum nodosum polysaccharide hydrolysates from lactic acid fermentation. *J. Appl. Phycol.* **2019**. [CrossRef]
132. Gomez-Guzman, M.; Rodriguez-Nogales, A.; Algieri, F.; Galvez, J. potential role of seaweed polyphenols in cardiovascular-associated disorders. *Mar. Drugs* **2018**, *16*, 250. [CrossRef] [PubMed]
133. Lee, D.H.; Park, M.Y.; Shim, B.J.; Youn, H.J.; Hwang, H.J.; Shin, H.C.; Jeon, H.K. Effects of Ecklonia cava polyphenol in individuals with hypercholesterolemia: A pilot study. *J. Med. Food* **2012**, *15*, 1038–1044. [CrossRef] [PubMed]
134. Lopes, G.; Andrade, P.B.; Valentao, P. Phlorotannins: Towards new pharmacological interventions for diabetes mellitus type 2. *Molecules* **2016**, *22*, 56. [CrossRef] [PubMed]
135. Murray, M.; Dordevic, A.L.; Ryan, L.; Bonham, M.P. An emerging trend in functional foods for the prevention of cardiovascular disease and diabetes: Marine algal polyphenols. *Crit. Rev. Food Sci. Nutr.* **2018**, *58*, 1342–1358. [CrossRef] [PubMed]
136. Murugan, A.C.; Karim, M.R.; Yusoff, M.B.; Tan, S.H.; Asras, M.F.; Rashid, S.S. New insights into seaweed polyphenols on glucose homeostasis. *Pharm. Biol.* **2015**, *53*, 1087–1097. [CrossRef] [PubMed]
137. Fernando, I.P.; Kim, M.; Son, K.T.; Jeong, Y.; Jeon, Y.J. Antioxidant activity of marine algal polyphenolic compounds: A mechanistic approach. *J. Med. Food* **2016**, *19*, 615–628. [CrossRef] [PubMed]
138. Eom, S.H.; Kim, Y.M.; Kim, S.K. Antimicrobial effect of phlorotannins from marine brown algae. *Food Chem. Toxicol. Int. J. Publ. Br. Ind. Biol. Res. Assoc.* **2012**, *50*, 3251–3255. [CrossRef] [PubMed]
139. Heffernan, N.; Brunton, N.P.; FitzGerald, R.J.; Smyth, T.J. Profiling of the molecular weight and structural isomer abundance of macroalgae-derived phlorotannins. *Mar. Drugs* **2015**, *13*, 509–528. [CrossRef]
140. Melanson, J.E.; MacKinnon, S.L. Characterization of Phlorotannins from Brown Algae by LC-HRMS. *Methods Mol. Biol.* **2015**, *1308*, 253–266. [CrossRef]
141. Montero, L.; Sanchez-Camargo, A.P.; Garcia Canas, V.; Tanniou, A.; Stiger-Pouvreau, V.; Russo, M.; Rastrelli, L.; Cifuentes, A.; Herrero, M.; Ibanez, E. Anti-proliferative activity and chemical characterization by comprehensive two-dimensional liquid chromatography coupled to mass spectrometry of phlorotannins from the brown macroalga Sargassum muticum collected on North-Atlantic coasts. *J. Chromatogr. A* **2016**, *1428*, 115–125. [CrossRef]
142. Lewandowska, U.; Szewczyk, K.; Hrabec, E.; Janecka, A.; Gorlach, S. Overview of metabolism and bioavailability enhancement of polyphenols. *J. Agric. Food Chem.* **2013**, *61*, 12183–12199. [CrossRef] [PubMed]
143. Opara, E.I.; Chohan, M. culinary herbs and spices: Their bioactive properties, the contribution of polyphenols and the challenges in deducing their true health benefits. *Int. J. Mol. Sci.* **2014**, *15*, 19183–19202. [CrossRef] [PubMed]
144. Clifford, M.N. Diet-derived phenols in plasma and tissues and their implications for health. *Planta Med.* **2004**, *70*, 1103–1114. [CrossRef] [PubMed]
145. Selma, M.V.; Espín, J.C.; Tomás-Barberán, F.A. Interaction between phenolics and gut microbiota: Role in human health. *J. Agric. Food Chem.* **2009**, *57*, 6485–6501. [CrossRef] [PubMed]
146. Williamson, G.; Clifford, M.N. Role of the small intestine, colon and microbiota in determining the metabolic fate of polyphenols. *Biochem. Pharmacol.* **2017**, *139*, 24–39. [CrossRef] [PubMed]
147. Espin, J.C.; Gonzalez-Sarrias, A.; Tomas-Barberan, F.A. The gut microbiota: A key factor in the therapeutic effects of (poly)phenols. *Biochem. Pharmacol.* **2017**, *139*, 82–93. [CrossRef] [PubMed]

148. Krumholz, L.R.; Bryant, M.P. Eubacterium oxidoreducens sp. nov. requiring H2 or formate to degrade gallate, pyrogallol, phloroglucinol and quercetin. *Arch. Microbiol.* **1986**, *144*, 8–14. [CrossRef]
149. Schneider, H.; Blaut, M. Anaerobic degradation of flavonoids by Eubacterium ramulus. *Arch. Microbiol.* **2000**, *173*, 71–75. [CrossRef]
150. Bang, S.H.; Hyun, Y.J.; Shim, J.; Hong, S.W.; Kim, D.H. Metabolism of rutin and poncirin by human intestinal microbiota and cloning of their metabolizing alpha-L-rhamnosidase from Bifidobacterium dentium. *J. Microbiol. Biotechnol.* **2015**, *25*, 18–25. [CrossRef]
151. Amaretti, A.; Raimondi, S.; Leonardi, A.; Quartieri, A.; Rossi, M. Hydrolysis of the rutinose-conjugates flavonoids rutin and hesperidin by the gut microbiota and bifidobacteria. *Nutrients* **2015**, *7*, 2788–2800. [CrossRef]
152. Delgado, S.; Florez, A.B.; Guadamuro, L.; Mayo, B. Genetic and biochemical characterization of an oligo-alpha-1,6-glucosidase from Lactobacillus plantarum. *Int. J. Food Microbiol.* **2017**, *246*, 32–39. [CrossRef] [PubMed]
153. Corona, G.; Ji, Y.; Anegboonlap, P.; Hotchkiss, S.; Gill, C.; Yaqoob, P.; Spencer, J.P.E.; Rowland, I. Gastrointestinal modifications and bioavailability of brown seaweed phlorotannins and effects on inflammatory markers. *Br. J. Nutr.* **2016**, *115*, 1240–1253. [CrossRef] [PubMed]
154. Corona, G.; Coman, M.M.; Guo, Y.; Hotchkiss, S.; Gill, C.; Yaqoob, P.; Spencer, J.P.E.; Rowland, I. Effect of simulated gastrointestinal digestion and fermentation on polyphenolic content and bioactivity of brown seaweed phlorotannin-rich extracts. *Mol. Nutr. Food Res.* **2017**, *61*. [CrossRef] [PubMed]
155. Sadeghi Ekbatan, S.; Sleno, L.; Sabally, K.; Khairallah, J.; Azadi, B.; Rodes, L.; Prakash, S.; Donnelly, D.J.; Kubow, S. Biotransformation of polyphenols in a dynamic multistage gastrointestinal model. *Food Chem.* **2016**, *204*, 453–462. [CrossRef] [PubMed]
156. Oliveira, A.; Pintado, M. Stability of polyphenols and carotenoids in strawberry and peach yoghurt throughout in vitro gastrointestinal digestion. *Food Funct.* **2015**, *6*, 1611–1619. [CrossRef] [PubMed]
157. Brown, E.M.; Nitecki, S.; Pereira-Caro, G.; McDougall, G.J.; Stewart, D.; Rowland, I.; Crozier, A.; Gill, C.I. Comparison of in vivo and in vitro digestion on polyphenol composition in lingonberries: Potential impact on colonic health. *BioFactors* **2014**, *40*, 611–623. [CrossRef]
158. Dueñas, M.; Muñoz-González, I.; Cueva, C.; Jiménez-Girón, A.; Sánchez-Patán, F.; Santos-Buelga, C.; Moreno-Arribas, M.V.; Bartolomé, B. A survey of modulation of gut microbiota by dietary polyphenols. *BioMed Res. Int.* **2015**, *2015*, 850902. [CrossRef]
159. Tomas-Barberan, F.A.; Selma, M.V.; Espin, J.C. Interactions of gut microbiota with dietary polyphenols and consequences to human health. *Curr. Opin. Clin. Nutr. Metab. Care* **2016**. [CrossRef]
160. Duda-Chodak, A.; Tarko, T.; Satora, P.; Sroka, P. Interaction of dietary compounds, especially polyphenols, with the intestinal microbiota: A review. *Eur. J. Nutr.* **2015**, *54*, 325–341. [CrossRef]
161. Nunez-Sanchez, M.A.; Gonzalez-Sarrias, A.; Romo-Vaquero, M.; Garcia-Villalba, R.; Selma, M.V.; Tomas-Barberan, F.A.; Garcia-Conesa, M.T.; Espin, J.C. Dietary phenolics against colorectal cancer—From promising preclinical results to poor translation into clinical trials: Pitfalls and future needs. *Mol. Nutr. Food Res.* **2015**, *59*, 1274–1291. [CrossRef]
162. Ozdal, T.; Sela, D.A.; Xiao, J.; Boyacioglu, D.; Chen, F.; Capanoglu, E. The Reciprocal Interactions between Polyphenols and Gut Microbiota and Effects on Bioaccessibility. *Nutrients* **2016**, *8*, 78. [CrossRef] [PubMed]
163. Van Duynhoven, J.; Vaughan, E.E.; Jacobs, D.M.; Kemperman, R.A.; van Velzen, E.J.; Gross, G.; Roger, L.C.; Possemiers, S.; Smilde, A.K.; Dore, J.; et al. Metabolic fate of polyphenols in the human superorganism. *Proc. Natl. Acad. Sci. USA* **2011**, *108*, 4531–4538. [CrossRef] [PubMed]
164. Rubio, L.; Macia, A.; Motilva, M.J. Impact of various factors on pharmacokinetics of bioactive polyphenols: An overview. *Curr. Drug Metab.* **2014**, *15*, 62–76. [CrossRef] [PubMed]
165. Feliciano, R.P.; Mills, C.E.; Istas, G.; Heiss, C.; Rodriguez-Mateos, A. Absorption, metabolism and excretion of cranberry (Poly)phenols in humans: A dose response study and assessment of inter-individual variability. *Nutrients* **2017**, *9*, 268. [CrossRef] [PubMed]
166. Dueñas, M.; Cueva, C.; Muñoz-González, I.; Jiménez-Girón, A.; Sánchez-Patán, F.; Santos-Buelga, C.; Moreno-Arribas, M.V.; Bartolomé, B. Studies on modulation of gut microbiota by wine polyphenols: From isolated cultures to omic approaches. *Antioxidants* **2015**, *4*, 1–21. [CrossRef]
167. Rajauria, G.; Foley, B.; Abu-Ghannam, N. Characterization of dietary fucoxanthin from Himanthalia elongata brown seaweed. *Food Res. Int.* **2017**, *99*, 995–1001. [CrossRef]

168. Christaki, E.; Bonos, E.; Giannenas, I.; Florou-Paneri, P. Functional properties of carotenoids originating from algae. *J. Sci. Food Agric.* **2013**, *93*, 5–11. [CrossRef]
169. Mikami, K.; Hosokawa, M. Biosynthetic pathway and health benefits of fucoxanthin, an algae-specific xanthophyll in brown seaweeds. *Int. J. Mol. Sci.* **2013**, *14*, 13763–13781. [CrossRef]
170. Lopes-Costa, E.; Abreu, M.; Gargiulo, D.; Rocha, E.; Ramos, A.A. Anticancer effects of seaweed compounds fucoxanthin and phloroglucinol, alone and in combination with 5-fluorouracil in colon cells. *J. Toxicol. Environ. Health* **2017**, *80*, 776–787. [CrossRef]
171. Maeda, H.; Tsukui, T.; Sashima, T.; Hosokawa, M.; Miyashita, K. Seaweed carotenoid, fucoxanthin, as a multi-functional nutrient. *Asia Pac. J. Clin. Nutr.* **2008**, *17*, 196–199. [CrossRef]
172. Woo, M.N.; Jeon, S.M.; Kim, H.J.; Lee, M.K.; Shin, S.K.; Shin, Y.C.; Park, Y.B.; Choi, M.S. Fucoxanthin supplementation improves plasma and hepatic lipid metabolism and blood glucose concentration in high-fat fed C57BL/6N mice. *Chem. Biol. Interact.* **2010**, *186*, 316–322. [CrossRef] [PubMed]
173. Kulczyński, B.; Gramza-Michałowska, A.; Kobus-Cisowska, J.; Kmiecik, D. The role of carotenoids in the prevention and treatment of cardiovascular disease—Current state of knowledge. *J. Funct. Foods* **2017**, *38*, 45–65. [CrossRef]
174. Bohn, T.; McDougall, G.J.; Alegria, A.; Alminger, M.; Arrigoni, E.; Aura, A.M.; Brito, C.; Cilla, A.; El, S.N.; Karakaya, S.; et al. Mind the gap-deficits in our knowledge of aspects impacting the bioavailability of phytochemicals and their metabolites—A position paper focusing on carotenoids and polyphenols. *Mol. Nutr. Food Res.* **2015**, *59*, 1307–1323. [CrossRef]
175. Widjaja-Adhi, M.A.K.; Lobo, G.P.; Golczak, M.; Von Lintig, J. A genetic dissection of intestinal fat-soluble vitamin and carotenoid absorption. *Hum. Mol. Genet.* **2015**, *24*, 3206–3219. [CrossRef] [PubMed]
176. Rein, M.J.; Renouf, M.; Cruz-Hernandez, C.; Actis-Goretta, L.; Thakkar, S.K.; da Silva Pinto, M. Bioavailability of bioactive food compounds: A challenging journey to bioefficacy. *Br. J. Clin. Pharmacol.* **2013**, *75*, 588–602. [CrossRef] [PubMed]
177. Bohn, T. Chapter 9 Metabolic Fate of Bioaccessible and Non-bioaccessible Carotenoids. In *Non-Extractable Polyphenols and Carotenoids: Importance in Human Nutrition and Health*, 1st ed.; Saura-Calixto, F., Pérez-Jiménez, J., Eds.; The Royal Society of Chemistry: London, UK, 2018; pp. 165–200. [CrossRef]
178. Lyu, Y.; Wu, L.; Wang, F.; Shen, X.; Lin, D. Carotenoid supplementation and retinoic acid in immunoglobulin A regulation of the gut microbiota dysbiosis. *Exp. Biol. Med.* **2018**, *243*, 613–620. [CrossRef] [PubMed]
179. Kamiloglu, S.; Capanoglu, E. Chapter 10 models for studying polyphenols and carotenoids digestion, bioaccessibility and colonic fermentation. In *Non-Extractable Polyphenols and Carotenoids: Importance in Human Nutrition and Health*, 1st ed.; Saura-Calixto, F., Pérez-Jiménez, J., Eds.; The Royal Society of Chemistry: London, UK, 2018; pp. 201–219. [CrossRef]
180. Van Ginneken, V.J.T.; Helsper, J.P.F.G.; de Visser, W.; van Keulen, H.; Brandenburg, W.A. Polyunsaturated fatty acids in various macroalgal species from north Atlantic and tropical seas. *Lipids Health Dis.* **2011**, *10*, 104. [CrossRef] [PubMed]
181. Robertson, R.C.; Guihéneuf, F.; Bahar, B.; Schmid, M.; Stengel, D.B.; Fitzgerald, G.F.; Ross, R.P.; Stanton, C. The Anti-Inflammatory Effect of Algae-Derived Lipid Extracts on Lipopolysaccharide (LPS)-Stimulated Human THP-1 Macrophages. *Mar. Drugs* **2015**, *13*, 5402–5424. [CrossRef]
182. Costantini, L.; Molinari, R.; Farinon, B.; Merendino, N. Impact of Omega-3 fatty acids on the gut microbiota. *Int. J. Mol. Sci.* **2017**, *18*, 2645. [CrossRef]
183. Menni, C.; Zierer, J.; Pallister, T.; Jackson, M.A.; Long, T.; Mohney, R.P.; Steves, C.J.; Spector, T.D.; Valdes, A.M. Omega-3 fatty acids correlate with gut microbiome diversity and production of N-carbamylglutamate in middle aged and elderly women. *Sci. Rep.* **2017**, *7*, 11079. [CrossRef]
184. Robertson, R.C.; Kaliannan, K.; Strain, C.R.; Ross, R.P.; Stanton, C.; Kang, J.X. Maternal omega-3 fatty acids regulate offspring obesity through persistent modulation of gut microbiota. *Microbiome* **2018**, *6*, 95. [CrossRef] [PubMed]
185. Marco, M.L.; Heeney, D.; Binda, S.; Cifelli, C.J.; Cotter, P.D.; Foligne, B.; Ganzle, M.; Kort, R.; Pasin, G.; Pihlanto, A.; et al. Health benefits of fermented foods: Microbiota and beyond. *Curr. Opin. Biotechnol.* **2017**, *44*, 94–102. [CrossRef] [PubMed]
186. Chilton, S.N.; Burton, J.P.; Reid, G. Inclusion of fermented foods in food guides around the world. *Nutrients* **2015**, *7*, 390–404. [CrossRef] [PubMed]

187. Tamang, J.P.; Shin, D.H.; Jung, S.J.; Chae, S.W. Functional properties of microorganisms in fermented foods. *Front. Microbiol.* **2016**, *7*, 578. [CrossRef] [PubMed]
188. Wilburn, J.R.; Ryan, E.P. Chapter 1—Fermented foods in health promotion and disease prevention: An overview. In *Fermented Foods in Health and Disease Prevention*; Frias, J., Martinez-Villaluenga, C., Peñas, E., Eds.; Academic Press: Boston, MA, USA, 2017; pp. 3–19. [CrossRef]
189. Ko, S.J.; Kim, J.; Han, G.; Kim, S.K.; Kim, H.G.; Yeo, I.; Ryu, B.; Park, J.W. Laminaria japonica combined with probiotics improves intestinal microbiota: A randomized clinical trial. *J. Med. Food* **2014**, *17*, 76–82. [CrossRef] [PubMed]
190. Kang, Y.M.; Lee, B.J.; Kim, J.I.; Nam, B.H.; Cha, J.Y.; Kim, Y.M.; Ahn, C.B.; Choi, J.S.; Choi, I.S.; Je, J.Y. Antioxidant effects of fermented sea tangle (Laminaria japonica) by Lactobacillus brevis BJ20 in individuals with high level of gamma-GT: A randomized, double-blind, and placebo-controlled clinical study. *Food Chem. Toxicol. Int. J. Publ. Br. Ind. Biol. Res. Assoc.* **2012**, *50*, 1166–1169. [CrossRef] [PubMed]
191. Choi, J.S.; Seo, H.J.; Lee, Y.R.; Kwon, S.J.; Moon, S.H.; Park, S.M.; Sohn, J.H. Characteristics and in vitro Anti-diabetic Properties of the Korean Rice Wine, Makgeolli Fermented with Laminaria japonica. *Prev. Nutr. Food Sci.* **2014**, *19*, 98–107. [CrossRef] [PubMed]
192. Shobharani, P.; Nanishankar, V.H.; Halami, P.M.; Sachindra, N.M. Antioxidant and anticoagulant activity of polyphenol and polysaccharides from fermented Sargassum sp. *Int. J. Biol. Macromol.* **2014**, *65*, 542–548. [CrossRef] [PubMed]
193. Uchida, M.; Miyoshi, T.; Yoshida, G.; Niwa, K.; Mori, M.; Wakabayashi, H. Isolation and characterization of halophilic lactic acid bacteria acting as a starter culture for sauce fermentation of the red alga Nori (Porphyra yezoensis). *J. Appl. Microbiol.* **2014**, *116*, 1506–1520. [CrossRef]
194. Tavares Estevam, A.C.; Alonso Buriti, F.C.; de Oliveira, T.A.; Pereira, E.V.; Florentino, E.R.; Porto, A.L. Effect of Aqueous Extract of the Seaweed Gracilaria domingensis on the Physicochemical, Microbiological, and Textural Features of Fermented Milks. *J. Food Sci.* **2016**, *81*, C874–C880. [CrossRef]
195. Blaszak, B.B.; Gozdecka, G.; Shyichuk, A. Carrageenan as a functional additive in the production of cheese and cheese-like products. *Acta Sci. Polonorum. Technol. Aliment.* **2018**, *17*, 107–116. [CrossRef]
196. Bixler, H.J.; Porse, H.J. A decade of change in the seaweed hydrocolloids industry. *J. Appl. Phycol.* **2011**, *23*, 321–335. [CrossRef]
197. Makkar, H.P.S.; Tran, G.; Heuzé, V.; Giger-Reverdin, S.; Lessire, M.; Lebas, F.; Ankers, P. Seaweeds for livestock diets: A review. *Anim. Feed Sci. Technol.* **2016**, *212*, 1–17. [CrossRef]
198. Overland, M.; Mydland, L.T.; Skrede, A. Marine macroalgae as sources of protein and bioactive compounds in feed for monogastric animals. *J. Sci. Food Agric.* **2018**, *99*, 13–24. [CrossRef] [PubMed]
199. Umu, O.C.; Frank, J.A.; Fangel, J.U.; Oostindjer, M.; da Silva, C.S.; Bolhuis, E.J.; Bosch, G.; Willats, W.G.; Pope, P.B.; Diep, D.B. Resistant starch diet induces change in the swine microbiome and a predominance of beneficial bacterial populations. *Microbiome* **2015**, *3*, 16. [CrossRef] [PubMed]
200. Kulshreshtha, G.; Rathgeber, B.; Stratton, G.; Thomas, N.; Evans, F.; Critchley, A.; Hafting, J.; Prithiviraj, B. Feed supplementation with red seaweeds, Chondrus crispus and Sarcodiotheca gaudichaudii, affects performance, egg quality, and gut microbiota of layer hens. *Poult. Sci.* **2014**, *93*, 2991–3001. [CrossRef] [PubMed]
201. Kulshreshtha, G.; Rathgeber, B.; MacIsaac, J.; Boulianne, M.; Brigitte, L.; Stratton, G.; Thomas, N.A.; Critchley, A.T.; Hafting, J.; Prithiviraj, B. Feed Supplementation with Red Seaweeds, Chondrus crispus and Sarcodiotheca gaudichaudii, Reduce Salmonella Enteritidis in Laying Hens. *Front. Microbiol.* **2017**, *8*, 567. [CrossRef]
202. Litten-Brown, J.C.; Corson, A.M.; Clarke, L. Porcine models for the metabolic syndrome, digestive and bone disorders: A general overview. *Animal* **2010**, *4*, 899–920. [CrossRef]
203. Machado, L.; Tomkins, N.; Magnusson, M.; Midgley, D.J.; de Nys, R.; Rosewarne, C.P. In Vitro Response of Rumen Microbiota to the Antimethanogenic Red Macroalga Asparagopsis taxiformis. *Microb. Ecol.* **2018**, *75*, 811–818. [CrossRef]
204. Zhou, M.; Hünerberg, M.; Chen, Y.; Reuter, T.; McAllister, T.A.; Evans, F.; Critchley, A.T.; Guan, L.L. Air-Dried Brown Seaweed, Ascophyllum nodosum, Alters the Rumen Microbiome in a Manner That Changes Rumen Fermentation Profiles and Lowers the Prevalence of Foodborne Pathogens. *mSphere* **2018**, *3*, e00017-18. [CrossRef]

205. Orpin, C.G.; Greenwood, Y.; Hall, F.J.; Paterson, I.W. The rumen microbiology of seaweed digestion in Orkney sheep. *J. Appl. Bacteriol.* **1985**, *58*, 585–596. [CrossRef] [PubMed]
206. Williams, A.G.; Withers, S.; Sutherland, A.D. The potential of bacteria isolated from ruminal contents of seaweed-eating North Ronaldsay sheep to hydrolyse seaweed components and produce methane by anaerobic digestion in vitro. *Microb. Biotechnol.* **2013**, *6*, 45–52. [CrossRef] [PubMed]
207. Heim, G.; O'Doherty, J.V.; O'Shea, C.J.; Doyle, D.N.; Egan, A.M.; Thornton, K.; Sweeney, T. Maternal supplementation of seaweed-derived polysaccharides improves intestinal health and immune status of suckling piglets. *J. Nutr. Sci.* **2015**, *4*, e27. [CrossRef] [PubMed]
208. Choi, Y.; Hosseindoust, A.; Goel, A.; Lee, S.; Jha, P.K.; Kwon, I.K.; Chae, B.-J. Effects of Ecklonia cava as fucoidan-rich algae on growth performance, nutrient digestibility, intestinal morphology and caecal microflora in weanling pigs. *Asian Australas. J. Anim. Sci.* **2017**, *30*, 64–70. [CrossRef] [PubMed]
209. Murphy, P.; Dal Bello, F.; O'Doherty, J.; Arendt, E.K.; Sweeney, T.; Coffey, A. The effects of liquid versus spray-dried Laminaria digitata extract on selected bacterial groups in the piglet gastrointestinal tract (GIT) microbiota. *Anaerobe* **2013**, *21*, 1–8. [CrossRef]
210. Heim, G.; Walsh, A.M.; Sweeney, T.; Doyle, D.N.; O'Shea, C.J.; Ryan, M.T.; O'Doherty, J.V. Effect of seaweed-derived laminarin and fucoidan and zinc oxide on gut morphology, nutrient transporters, nutrient digestibility, growth performance and selected microbial populations in weaned pigs. *Br. J. Nutr.* **2014**, *111*, 1577–1585. [CrossRef] [PubMed]
211. Murphy, P.; Dal Bello, F.; O'Doherty, J.; Arendt, E.K.; Sweeney, T.; Coffey, A. Analysis of bacterial community shifts in the gastrointestinal tract of pigs fed diets supplemented with β-glucan from Laminaria digitata, Laminaria hyperborea and Saccharomyces cerevisiae. *Animal* **2013**, *7*, 1079–1087. [CrossRef]
212. Walsh, A.M.; Sweeney, T.; O'Shea, C.J.; Doyle, D.N.; 'Doherty, J.V.O. Effect of supplementing varying inclusion levels of laminarin and fucoidan on growth performance, digestibility of diet components, selected fecal microbial populations and volatile fatty acid concentrations in weaned pigs. *Anim. Feed Sci. Technol.* **2013**, *183*, 151–159. [CrossRef]
213. Belanche, A.; Ramos-Morales, E.; Newbold, C.J. In vitro screening of natural feed additives from crustaceans, diatoms, seaweeds and plant extracts to manipulate rumen fermentation. *J. Sci. Food Agric.* **2016**, *96*, 3069–3078. [CrossRef]
214. Kinley, R.D.; de Nys, R.; Vucko, M.J.; Machado, L.; Tomkins, N.W. The red macroalgae Asparagopsis taxiformis is a potent natural antimethanogenic that reduces methane production during in vitro fermentation with rumen fluid. *J. Anim. Prod. Sci.* **2016**, *56*, 282–289. [CrossRef]
215. Maia, M.R.; Fonseca, A.J.; Oliveira, H.M.; Mendonca, C.; Cabrita, A.R. The potential role of seaweeds in the natural manipulation of rumen fermentation and methane production. *Sci. Rep.* **2016**, *6*, 32321. [CrossRef] [PubMed]
216. Hong, Z.S.; Kim, E.J.; Jin, Y.C.; Lee, J.S.; Choi, Y.J.; Lee, H.G. Effects of supplementing brown seaweed by-products in the diet of Holstein cows during transition on ruminal fermentation, growth performance and endocrine responses. *Asian Australas. J. Anim. Sci.* **2015**, *28*, 1296–1302. [CrossRef] [PubMed]

© 2019 by the authors. Licensee MDPI, Basel, Switzerland. This article is an open access article distributed under the terms and conditions of the Creative Commons Attribution (CC BY) license (http://creativecommons.org/licenses/by/4.0/).

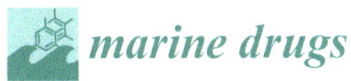

Review

Current Research on the Bioprospection of Linear Diterpenes from *Bifurcaria bifurcata*: From Extraction Methodologies to Possible Applications

Adriana C.S. Pais [1], Jorge A. Saraiva [2], Sílvia M. Rocha [2], Armando J.D. Silvestre [1] and Sónia A.O. Santos [1,*]

1. CICECO-Aveiro Institute of Materials, Chemistry Department, University of Aveiro, 3810-193 Aveiro, Portugal; a.c.p.s@ua.pt (A.C.S.P.); armsil@ua.pt (A.J.D.S.)
2. QOPNA/LAQV & REQUIMTE, Chemistry Department, University of Aveiro, 3810-193 Aveiro, Portugal; jorgesaraiva@ua.pt (J.A.S.); smrocha@ua.pt (S.M.R.)
* Correspondence: santos.sonia@ua.pt; Tel.: +351-234-370-711

Received: 23 August 2019; Accepted: 26 September 2019; Published: 28 September 2019

Abstract: Marine resources are considered as a very promising source of bioactive molecules, and macroalgae in particular have gained special attention, due to their structurally diverse composition. Particular interest has been devoted to the brown macroalga *Bifurcaria bifurcata*, due to their abundance in bioactive linear diterpenes. In this appraisal, a thorough review concerning the methodologies used in the extraction, fractionation, and identification of diterpenes from *B. bifurcata* is provided and discussed in detail. An exhaustive compilation of the mass spectra and nuclear magnetic resonance (NMR) data are also provided. The in vitro and *in chemico* assays already performed to assess different biological activities attributed to *B. bifurcata* diterpenes are also reviewed, emphasizing the use of isolated components, enriched fractions, or crude extracts. The associated major strengths and challenges for the exploitation of *B. bifurcata* diterpenes for high-value applications are critically discussed.

Keywords: *Bifurcaria bifurcata*; linear diterpenes; extraction; identification; biological activities; macroalgae; high value applications

---

1. Introduction

Marine resources have been seen as a promising source of added value molecules, an alternative of finite fossil resources, allowing for the boost of concepts such as biorefinery, circular economy, and blue economy [1–3]. In recent years, an increase in marine biotechnology investments has been observed around the world, with macroalgae being an object of particular interest, mainly due to their high productivity, wide diversity, and heterogeneous composition, notably with a high abundance of bioactive compounds [4]. In fact, besides the high content of polysaccharides, macroalgae have shown to be particularly rich in secondary metabolites with a wide range of biological activities, which can be exploited as functional ingredients, or in cosmetic and pharmaceutical formulations [4,5]. However, macroalgae metabolism, and consequently composition, is modulated by, among other factors, salinity, temperature, pressure, sunlight, geographic origin, and season of collection [6,7].

Macroalgae are ecologically and commercially important, being significant primary producers in oceanic aquatic foods chains [6]. These marine resources have been recognized to be a valuable source of polysaccharides, minerals, polyunsaturated fatty acids and vitamins, and, in some species, of phenolic compounds and terpenes [6,8,9].

Special attention has been devoted to brown macroalgae in particular, due to the presence of specific components, such as fucoidan, phlorotannins, or even fucoxanthin, for which promising bioactivities have been described, namely antitumor, antioxidant, and antihypertensive activities, among others [10–12].

Notwithstanding, brown macroalgae have attracted an increasing attention due to the presence of other compounds, such as some linear diterpenes commonly found in the Sargassaceae family, and particularly in *Bifurcaria bifurcata* species [13]. Compared to their cyclic congeners, these are quite rare in nature. In addition, a wide variety of promising biological activities have been attributed to these components. Although a detailed revision of the different linear diterpenes already identified in *B. bifurcata* has been previously reported [14], an overview of the *B. bifurcata* diterpenes' properties together with information about how these components can be extracted and identified is needed in order to boost their exploitation. In this vein, the purpose of this paper is to review the different extraction and characterization methodologies used to extract and identify linear diterpenes from *B. bifurcata* as well as the current findings on their biological properties. The major challenges and strengths for the exploitation of this fraction of *B. bifurcata* are also discussed.

2. *Bifurcaria bifurcata* General Characteristics and Linear Diterpenes Chemical Families

B. bifurcata is a brown macroalga, and due to its morphology it is classified as a cylindrical species [15] and can be scientifically classified as follows [16]:

- Empire: Eukaryota
- Kingdom: Chromista
- Phylum: Ochrophyta
- Class: Phaeophyceae
- Subclass: Fucophycidae
- Order: Fucales
- Family: Sargassaceae
- Genus: *Bifurcaria*

This brown macroalga lives in rock pools on the lower and middle tidal, needing shores for its settlement, and is distributed along the coast of the Northern Atlantic, between Morocco and Northwestern Ireland [17]. About 56% of the published (and here reviewed) studies concerning the linear diterpenes fraction of *B. bifurcata* use samples from the coast of France (Figure 1), which may be associated with the high abundance of this macroalga on that area [8,17–37].

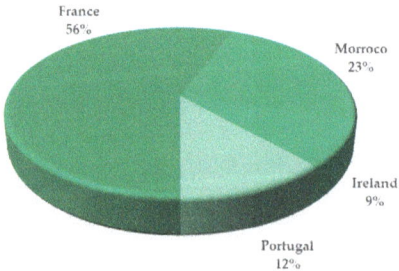

Figure 1. Distribution, in percentage, of the studies on *B. bifurcata* linear diterpenes and/or on related biological activities, according to the sampling location. The percentages presented in this graphic were determined considering the number of samples of each geographical location in all published studies here reviewed. (Analyzing Institute for Scientific Information (ISI) Web of Knowledge, keywords: *Bifurcaria bifurcata*, diterpenes; timespan: 1980–2019).

Additionally, all studies reviewed here have used wild samples of *B. bifurcata*, with the exception of the work of Santos et al. [38], in which *B. bifurcata* was collected from the Portuguese coast and cultivated in a land-based aquaculture system for three weeks at constant controlled conditions.

Concerning the different sampling locals as well as the exposure to different environmental factors, it is expected that this variety of B. bifurcata presents diverse compositions.

Linear Diterpenes Families of B. bifurcata

Phaeophyceae's class members are, in general, widely known for their ability to produce a large variety of terpenoids [4]. Terpene's chemical structures can be considered as being formed by multiple isoprene (C_5H_8) units (although being biosynthesized from isoprene derived activated precursors, as described below), and are relatively complex and extremely diverse, since they can have a linear, monocyclic, or bicyclic structure, among others, with different unsaturation degrees and patterns, as well as different levels of oxygenation [39,40]. This diversity can result in different chemical and biological properties [41]. Terpenes may be classified by the number of isoprene units that integrate the molecule, being grouped into hemi- (C_5), mono- (C_{10}), sesqui- (C_{15}), di- (C_{20}), sester- (C_{25}), tri- (C_{30}), tetra- (C_{40}), and polyterpenes, depending on the number of isoprene units [39,40].

Meroditerpenes (which correspond to a complex of terpenic and aromatic parts, and can be subdivided into linear, cyclic, and rearranged terpenoids) and linear diterpenes are the major terpenoids described in Sargassaceae family [40]. Linear (or acyclic) diterpenes, like all isoprenoids, are biosynthesized from isopentenyl diphosphate (IPP) and dimethylallyl diphosphate (DMAPP), which are formed via classical mevalonate (MVA) pathway from the condensation of acetyl-CoA or via 1-deoxy-D-xylulose 5-phosphate/2-C-methyl-D-erythritol 4-phosphate (DOXP/MEP) pathway, from the intermediates pyruvate and D-glyceraldehyde-3-phosphate (GAP) [42]. These linear terpenes are made up of a C_{16} backbone with four double bonds and generally with five non-substituted methylene groups. According to the main chemical characteristics, linear diterpenes are arranged in three families: A (C-12 oxidized compounds) (Figure 2); B (two subfamilies: on the one hand, B1 corresponds to C-13 oxidized molecules bearing an OH group, while on the other hand B2 are compounds with a ketone functionality at C-13 position) (Figures 3 and 4, respectively); and C (which are the non C-12/C-13 oxidized compounds) (Figure 5). These four groups of compounds (A, B1, B2, and C) have metabolic precursors, which are 12-(S)-hydroxygeranylgeraniol (bifurcadiol) (**1**), eleganediol ((S)-13-hydroxygeranylgeraniol) (**9**), eleganonole (13-oxogeranylgeraniol or (S)-13-ketogeranylgeraniol) (**15**), and geranylgeraniol (**39**), respectively [14].

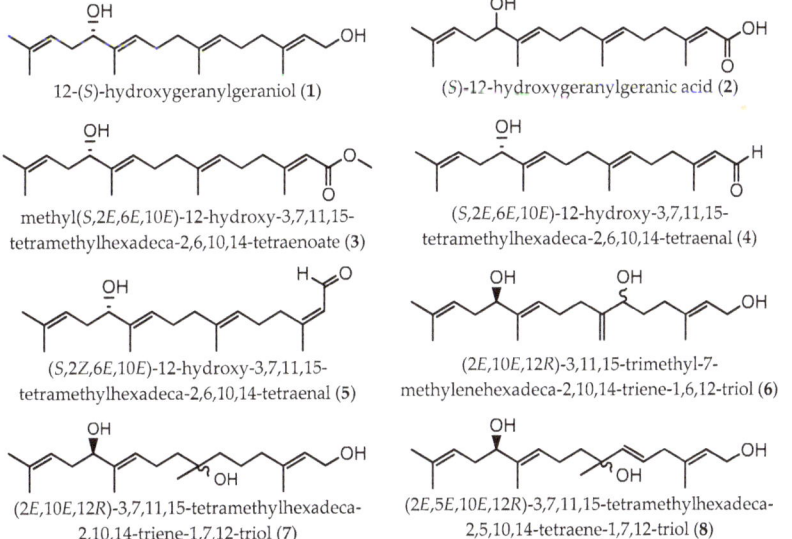

Figure 2. Chemical structures of acyclic diterpenes identified in *B. bifurcata*, belonging to family A.

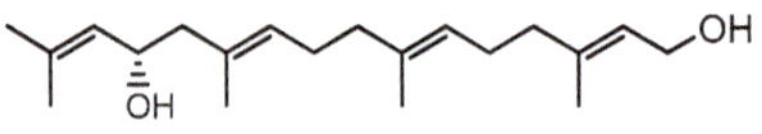

Eleganediol (**9**)

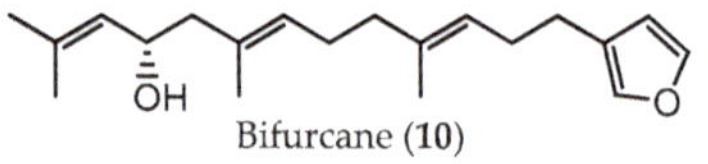

Bifurcane (**10**)
(*S*)-13-hydroxyfuranoditerpene

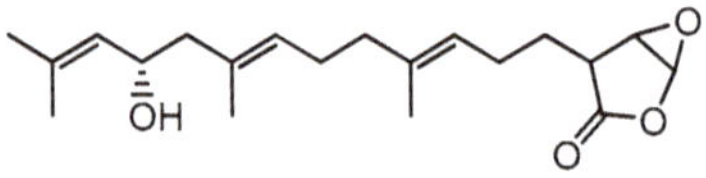

Epoxyeleganolactone (**11**)

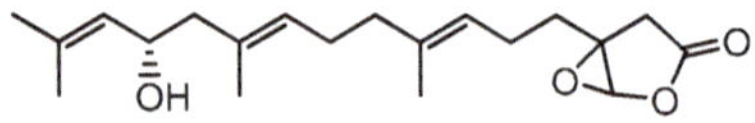

5-((*S*,3*E*,7*E*)-10-hydroxy-4,8,12-trimethyltrideca-3,7,11-trien-1-yl)-2,6-dioxabicyclo[3.1.0]hexan-3-one (**12**)

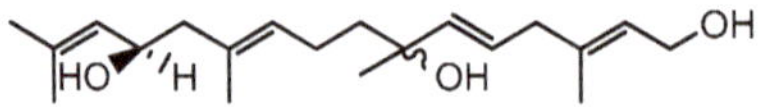

(2*E*,5*E*,10*E*,13*R*)-3,7,11,15-tetramethylhexadeca-2,5,10,14-tetraene-1,7,13-triol (**13**)

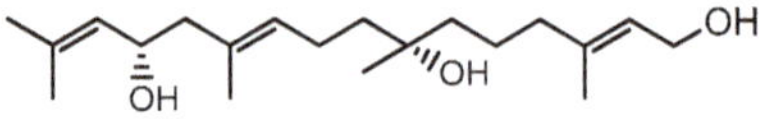

Bifurcatriol (**14**)

Figure 3. Chemical structures of acyclic diterpenes identified in *B. bifurcata*, belonging to family B1.

Linear diterpenes belonging to these 4 groups, have already been found in samples of *B. bifurcata* from different geographical origins and exposed to different external factors, which, as mentioned above, have a high influence on the macroalgae's chemical composition [6,7]. The detailed list of the linear diterpenes (and their content when available) already identified in *B. bifurcata* is depicted in Table 1. It must be highlighted that, due to the variation of sampling origin, season of collection, and thus different abiotic factors, together with the different extraction and characterization methodologies used by the different authors, it is not possible to establish correlations between these factors, conditions, or methodologies and the linear diterpenes profile detected.

Biard et al. reported for the first time the presence of linear diterpenes in *B. bifurcata* extracts, namely eleganolone (**15**), the major component (2% of dry weight (dw)), and two derivatives (**16** (0.06% of dw) and **9** (0.28% of dw)) [19,20]. The eleganolone (**15**) content in two samples from Brittany, France was also determined by Maréchal et al. and Hellio et al., which accounted 0.06% and 0.47% of dw, respectively. This difference could be related with the effect of several external factors, including season and sampling local, among others [23,36].

Le Lann et al. identified four distinct chemical profiles in extracts of *B. bifurcata*, collected during summer 2009 and winter 2010, from six regions along the Western coast of Britany, France, evidencing the high dependence of diterpenes composition on the sampling site and environmental factors. Eleganolone (**15**) was also identified as the major compound in both winter and summer seasons from these macroalgae samples, whereas bifurcanone (**18**) was only found during winter. The eleganediol (**9**), bifurcane (**10**), eleganolone (**15**), and bifurcanone (**18**) contents were shown to be also influenced by season and environmental factors [17].

In fact, eleganediol (**9**) [19,23,24,26,28,29,31,33,36,37], bifurcane (**10**) [29–31,36], and eleganolone (**15**) [20–24,26–28,30,31,36,37] have been described in several studies concerning *B. bifurcata* from France, together with other linear diterpenes, namely formyleleganolone (**35**) and bibifuran (**36**) [34]. The highest eleganediol (**9**) and bifurcane (**10**) contents (1.12% and 0.37% of dw, respectively) were described by Maréchal et al. [36]. Furthermore, 12-(*S*)-hydroxygeranylgeraniol (**1**) was only found in samples of *B. bifurcata* collected from Morocco, corresponding to 0.71% of dw studied by Hellio et al. [23,43–46].

In addition to bifurcane (**10**) and bibifuran (**36**), other *B. bifurcata* constituents are characterized by the presence of a furan ring in their structure, such as bifurcanone (**18**) and eleganolonebutenolide (**32**), which belong to B2 subfamily (C-13 oxidized molecule bearing an alcohol). Epoxyeleganolactone (**11**), which is a diterpene from B1 subfamily (with a ketone functionality at C-13 position), presents a C-2 epoxylactone [28–30].

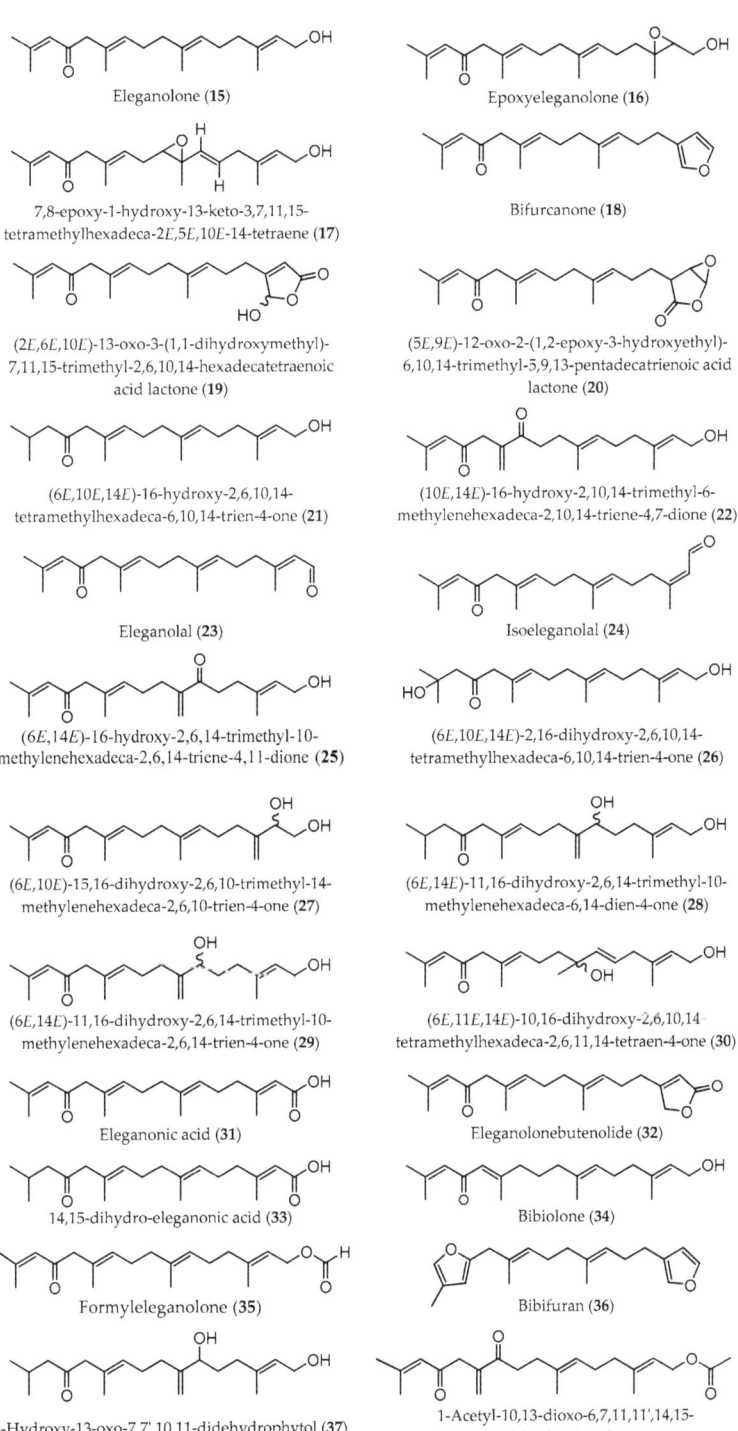

Figure 4. Chemical structures of acyclic diterpenes identified in *B. bifurcata*, belonging to subfamily B2.

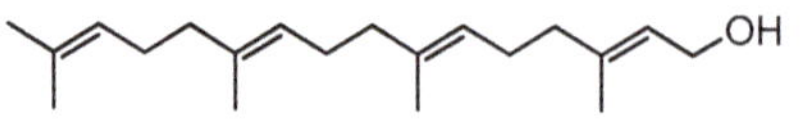

Geranylgeraniol (**39**)

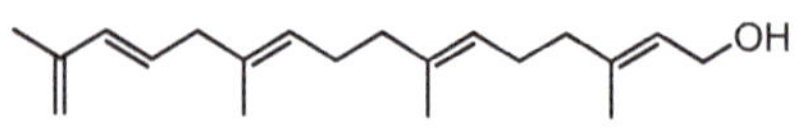

(2*E*,6*E*,10*E*,13*E*)-3,7,11,15-tetramethylhexadeca-2,6,10,13,15-pentaen-1-ol (**40**)

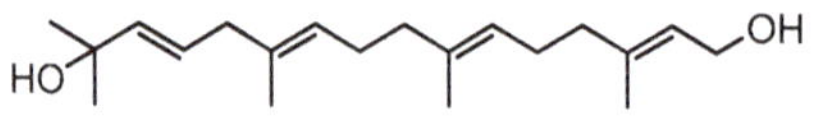

Bifurcanol (**41**)

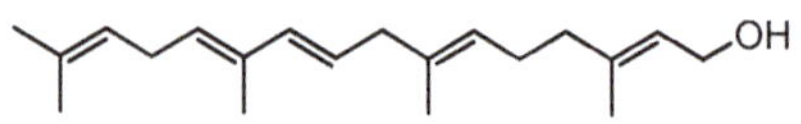

6,7,9,10,11,12,14,15-Tetrahydrophytol (**42**)

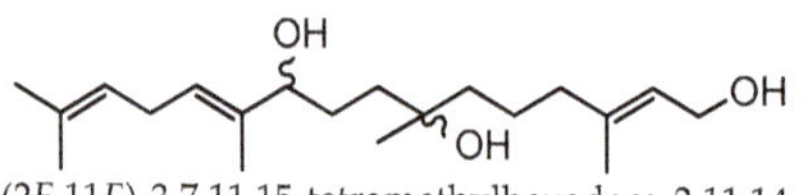

(2*E*,11*E*)-3,7,11,15-tetramethylhexadeca-2,11,14-triene-1,7,10-triol (**43**)

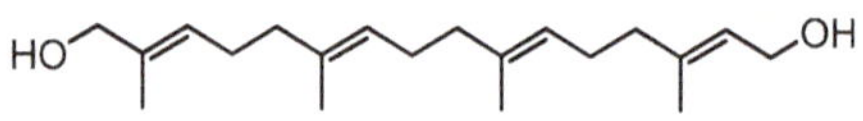

16-Hydroxygeranylgeraniol (**44**)

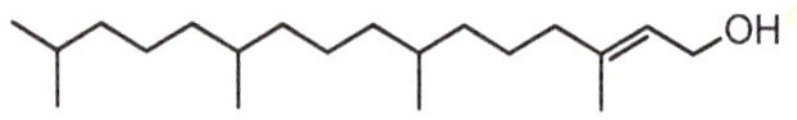

Phytol (**45**)

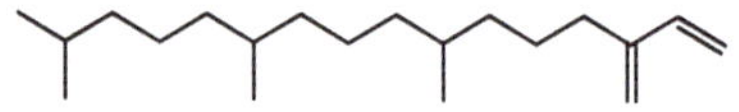

Neophytadiene (**46**)

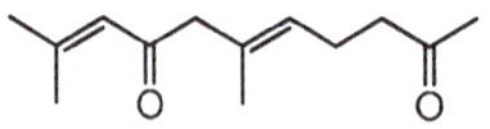

(*E*)-6,10-dimethylundeca-5,9-diene-2,8-dione (**47**)

Figure 5. Chemical structures of acyclic diterpenes identified in *B. bifurcata*, belonging to family C.

Some of the identified compounds have an acidic character due to the presence of a carboxylic group at C-1, such as the case of (*S*)-12-hydroxygeranylgeranic (**2**), eleganonic (**31**), and 14,15-dihydro-eleganonic acids (**33**) [30,34,43,47]. Semmak et al. reported the highest (*S*)-12-hydroxygeranylgeranic acid (**2**) content on *B. bifurcaria* from Morocco, which accounted 0.17% of dw [47].

Culioli et al. reported for the first time the presence of (*E*)-6,10-dimethylundeca-5,9-diene-2,8-dione (**47**) (0.01% of dw) in *B. bifurcata*, which resulted from the oxidative cleavage of the C-6 double bond of eleganolone (**15**) [33]. In addition, two pairs of isomers were also isolated from *B. bifurcata*, namely (*S*,2*E*,6*E*,10*E*)-12-hydroxy-3,7,11,15-tetramethylhexadeca-2,6,10,14-tetraenal (**4**) and (*S*,2*Z*,6*E*,10*E*)-12-hydroxy-3,7,11,15-tetramethylhexadeca-2,6,10,14-tetraenal (**5**), and eleganolal (**23**) (0.12% of dw) and isoeleganolal (**24**) (0.08% of dw) [32,46].

Several diterpenes were identified and quantified in a detailed study of the lipophilic fraction of a short-term cultivated *B. bifurcata*, collected in May, from Ria de Aveiro, Portugal, namely 6-hydroxy-13-oxo-7,7′,10,11-didehydrophytol (**37**) (0.06% of dw), 1-acetyl-10,13-dioxo-6,7,11,11′,14,15-tridehydrophytol (**38**) (0.10% of dw), geranylgeraniol (**39**) (0.01% of dw), 6,7,9,10,11,12,14,15-tetrahydrophytol (**42**) (0.01% of dw), phytol (**45**) (0.003% of dw), and neophytadiene (**46**) (0.01% of dw) [38]. Compounds **37**, **38**, **45**, and **46** were identified for the first time as constituents of this macroalga species, whereas compounds **39** [23,31,36,37] and **42** [46] had already been identified in samples from different geographical origins, namely from Morocco and France. A higher geranylgeraniol (**39**) content was verified by Hellio et al. in *B. bifurcata* from Morocco (0.12% of dw) than those determined by Culioli et al. and Maréchal et al. (0.01% and 0.02% of dw, respectively) in samples from Brittany, France and from Portugal [23,32,36,38].

Table 1. Linear diterpenes extracted from *B. bifurcata*, and the respective pretreatment, extraction, purification/fractionation and identification/analysis methodologies used, and time of collection/geographical origin.

Extraction Methodology	EY [a]	Sample Pretreatment	Fractionation/Purification	Identification/Analysis	Compound (Content [b])	Time of Collection/Geographical Origin	Ref
EtOAc S–L extraction	1.70	Freeze-dried	Chromatography (on Silica gel) eluted with EtOAc-*n*-heptane (4:1) and monitored at 270 nm; Bio-guided fractionation: chromatography (on a Lobar RP-8 co umn) with EtOH-H_2O; Fr. purification with MeCN-H_2O or EtOAc-$CHCl_3$.	(^1H and ^{13}C) NMR, MS	9 (0.06) 15 (0.07) 18 (0.11) 19 (0.03) 20 (0.02)	July to August/Roscoff, Brittany, France	[28]
EtOAc S–L extraction	N.D.	Freeze-dried	LC using Silica gel with a solvent gradient from DCM to DCM-MeOH (80:20); CC (on Silica gel) with solvent gradient DCM-MeOH (100:0 to 97:3) HPLC (RP18 column) with a gradient elution (from H_2O-MeCN (60:40), H_2O-MeCN (80:20) to MeOH)	HRESIMS, 1D and 2D NMR	10 15 18 21 27 31 32 33 34 41	September/Roscoff, Brittany, France	[30]
EtOAc S–L extraction, at RT	4.80	Freeze-dried and ground	Successive flash and CC (on Silica gel), eluting with cyclohexane—EtOAc mixture; Bio-guided fractionation: CC (on Silica gel), with cyclohexane-EtOAc	HREIMS, (^1H and ^{13}C) NMR	15 (0.004)	November to September/Basse-Normandie, France	[21]
EtOAc S–L extraction, at RT	N.D.	Freeze-dried and ground	Flash chromatography eluting with a H_2O-MeOH mixture of increasing polarity (95:5–0:100 in 30 minutes)	2D NMR, HPLC-DAD-MS-SPE-NMR	15	June/Cap Lévi, English Channel, France	[22]
EtOAc S–L extraction, at RT	4.8	Freeze-dried and ground	CC (on Silica gel) eluted with a solvent gradient from DCM to DCM-MeOH (80:20) UV-ESI-DAD–HPLC (using a Kromasil RP18 column) eluted with a solvent gradient H_2O-MeCN-MeOH	(^1H and ^{13}C) NMR, HRESI(+)MS	35 (0.002) 36 (0.001) 44 (0.0004)	September/Roscoff, Brittany, France	[34]
$CHCl_3$ S–L extraction	N.D.	Freeze-dried	Normal and reverse phase flash CC and RP18 HPLC	1D and 2D NMR, HRMS	9 10	May/Kilkee, County Clare of Ireland	[48]
$CHCl_3$–EtOH S–L extraction	1.52	Freeze-dried and ground	Partitioning between H_2O and Et_2O; Et_2O-soluble material: CC (on Silica gel) eluted with hexane-EtOAc (2:3); HPLC (EtOA.–isooctane, 2:3), with RI monitoring	IR, (^1H and ^{13}C) NMR, EIMS	1 (0.86)	–/Atlantic coast Morocco	[45]

Table 1. Cont.

Extraction Methodology	EY [a]	Sample Pretreatment	Fractionation/Purification	Identification/Analysis	Compound (Content [b])	Time of Collection/Geographical. Origin	Ref
EtOAc S-L extraction	1.70	Freeze-dried	Chromatography (on Silica gel) eluted with EtOAc-n-heptane (4:1) and monitored at 270 nm; Bio-guided fractionation: chromatography (on a Lobar RP-8 column) with EtOH-H$_2$O; Fr. purification with MeCN-H$_2$O or EtOAc-CHCl$_3$.	(^{1}H and ^{13}C) NMR, MS	9 (0.06) 15 (0.07) 18 (0.11) 19 (0.03) 20 (0.02)	July to August/Roscoff, Brittany, France	[28]
EtOAc S-L extraction	N.D.	Freeze-dried	LC using Silica gel with a solvent gradient from DCM to DCM-MeOH (80:20); CC (on Silica gel) with solvent gradient DCM-MeOH (100:0 to 97:3) HPLC (RP18 column) with a gradient elution (from H$_2$O-MeCN (60:40), H$_2$O-MeCN (80:20) to MeOH)	HRESIMS, 1D and 2D NMR	10 15 18 21 27 31 32 33 34 41	September/Roscoff, Brittany, France	[30]
EtOAc S-L extraction, at RT	4.80	Freeze-dried and ground	Successive flash and CC (on Silica gel), eluting with cyclohexane—EtOAc mixture; Bio-guided fractionation: CC (on Silica gel), with cyclohexane-EtOAc	HREIMS, (^{1}H and ^{13}C) NMR	15 (0.004)	November to September/Basse-Normandie, France	[21]
EtOAc S-L extraction, at RT	N.D.	Freeze-dried and ground	Flash chromatography eluting with a H$_2$O-MeOH mixture of increasing polarity (95:5–0:100 in 30 minutes)	2D NMR, HPLC-DAD-MS-SPE-NMR	15	June/Cap Lévi, English Channel, France	[22]
EtOAc S-L extraction, at RT	4.8	Freeze-dried and ground	CC (on Silica gel) eluted with a solvent gradient from DCM to DCM-MeOH (80:20) UV-ESI-DAD-HPLC (using a Kromasil RP18 column) eluted with a solvent gradient H$_2$O-MeCN-MeOH	(^{1}H and ^{13}C) NMR, HRESI(+)MS	35 (0.002) 36 (0.001) 44 (0.0004)	September/Roscoff, Brittany, France	[34]
CHCl$_3$ S-L extraction	N.D.		Normal and reverse phase flash CC and RP18 HPLC	1D and 2D NMR, HRMS	9 10	May/Kilkee, County Clare of Ireland	[48]
CHCl$_3$-EtOH S-L extraction	1.52	Freeze-dried and ground	Partitioning between H$_2$O and Et$_2$O; Et$_2$O-soluble material: CC (on Silica gel) eluted with hexane-EtOAc (2:3); HPLC (EtOAc–isooctane, 2:3), with RI monitoring	IR, (^{1}H and ^{13}C) NMR, EIMS	1 (0.86)	-/Atlantic coast Morocco	[45]
CHCl$_3$-MeOH S-L extraction, at RT	5.53	Shade-dried and ground	Partitioning in the mixture MeOH-isooctane (1:1); MeOH phase: dissolved in the mixture MeOH-CHCl$_3$-H$_2$O (4:3:1); Organic phase: CC (on Silica gel) eluted with a solvent gradient from isooctane to EtOAc and then from EtOAc to MeOH.	HREIMS, (^{1}H and ^{13}C) NMR	1 (0.37) 6 (0.01) 7 (0.004)	December/Oualidia, Morocco	[44]

Table 1. Cont.

Extraction Methodology	EY [a]	Sample Pretreatment	Fractionation/Purification	Identification/Analysis	Compound (Content [b])	Time of Collection/Geographical Origin	Ref
$CHCl_3$- MeOH S-L extraction; Et_2O S-L extraction of aqueous phase	1.95 g ext	Freshly collected	Open CC (on Silica gel) eluted with hexane to EtOAc (2:3); HPLC (eluent EtOAc-isooctane, 2:3).	IR, UV, (^1H and ^{13}C) NMR, EIMS, HRMS	2 (0.17) 40 (0.02)	-/Morocco	[47]
$CHCl_3$-MeOH S-L extraction	2.63	Shade-dried	Partitioning in the mixture MeOH-isooctane (1:1); MeOH extract: dissolution in the mixture MeOH–$CHCl_3$–H_2O (4:3:1); Organic extract: fractionation on silica gel column eluted with EtOAc and EtOAc-MeOH (98:2 and 95:5); HPLC on C-18 reversed-phase column, eluting with MeCN-H_2O (1:1 and/or 2:3).	HRMS, IR, (^1H and ^{13}C) NMR	8 43	-/Oualidia, Morocco	[49]
$CHCl_3$-MeOH S-L extraction, at RT $CHCl_3$–H_2O L-L extraction	6.92	Air-dried and ground	MeOH extract: defatting with n-hexane; CC (on Silica gel) using mixtures of $CHCl_3$-MeOH (from $CHCl_3$ to $CHCl_3$-MeOH, 1:1).	HPLC	9 13 15 21 25 26 27 28 29 30 39	July/Quiberon, Brittany, France	[37]
$CHCl_3$- MeOH S-L extraction, at RT	3.11	Shade-dried and ground	CC (on Silica gel) eluted with a solvent gradient from cyclohexane to E:OAc and then from EtOAc to MeOH; HPLC on an analytical C-18 reverse-phase column (eluent, MeCN-H_2O), with RI monitoring	HREIMS, IR, (^1H and ^{13}C) NMR	9 (0.15) 13 (0.0001) 15 (0.40) 21 (0.01) 25 (0.0001) 26 (0.0003) 27 (0.0002) 28 (0.0001) 29 (0.0005) 30 (0.0005) 39 (0.008) 47 (0.01)	July/Quiberon, Brittany, France	[24]

Table 1. *Cont.*

Extraction Methodology	EY [a]	Sample Pretreatment	Fractionation/Purification	Identification/Analysis	Compound (Content [b])	Time of Collection/Geographical Origin	Ref
Et$_2$O S–L extraction, at RT	1.65	Freeze-dried and powder	Partitioning between H$_2$O and Et$_2$O; Et$_2$O-soluble material: CC (on Silica gel) eluted with a solvent gradient from hexane to EtOAc; HPLC (eluent, EtOAc–isooctane), with RI monitoring	HRMS, EIMS, IR, (^{1}H and ^{13}C) NMR	1 (0.33–0.34) 2 (0.07–0.10) 9 (0.10–0.12; 0.36–0.38) 15 (0.29–0.32) 40 (0.03) 41 (0.01,0.04–0.05)	January to December/Atlantic coast of Morocco	[43]
Et$_2$O S–L extraction	2.94 3.15	Air-dried and ground	CC (on Silica gel) eluted with a gradient from isooctane to EtOAc; HPLC (eluent, isooctane-EtOAc); Semi-preparative and then analytical normal-phase HPLC with RI-monitoring.	1D and 2D NMR	1 (0.71) 39 (0.12) 9 (0.14) 15 (0.47) 21 (0.01) 22 (0.01) 25 (0.02)	November/Oualidia, Morocco December/Quiberon, Brittany, France	[25]
Et$_2$O S–L extraction, at RT	2.94	Shade-dried and ground	CC (on Silica gel) eluted with a solvent gradient from isooctane to EtOAc Semi-preparative normal phase HPLC (eluent, EtOAc-isooctane), with RI monitoring	HRMS, (^{1}H and ^{13}C) NMR	1 (0.71) 2 (0.03) 3 (0.08) 4 (0.01) 5 (0.004) 39 (0.12) 42 (0.01)	December/Oualidia, Morocco	[46]
Et$_2$O S–L extraction	N.D.	Freeze-dried	Preparative HPLC (DCM-EtOAc, 90:10)	UV, IR, (^{1}H and ^{13}C) NMR, MS	9 (0.28) 16 (0.06)	–/Loire-Atlantique, France	[19]
Et$_2$O S–L extraction	N.D.	Shade-dried	Separation in different fractions		9 15	–/Brittany, France	[26]
Et$_2$O S–L extraction, at RT, for 48h	2.2–2.9	Air-dried and ground	CC (on Silica gel) eluted with a solvent gradient from isooctane to EtOAc; Normal-phase HPLC (eluent, isooctane-EtOAc, 2:3), with RI-monitoring	IR, UV, HRMS, 1D and 2D NMR	9 (1.12) 10 (0.37) 15 (0.06) 39 (0.02)	July to June/Roscoff, Brittany, France	[36]
Et$_2$O S–L extraction, at RT	2.40	Freeze-dried and ground	Partitioning between H$_2$O and Et$_2$O; Et$_2$O-soluble material: CC (on Silica gel) eluted with hexane-EtAc (1:1); HPLC (EtOAc–isooctane), with RI monitoring.	HRMS, EIMS, IR, (^{1}H and ^{13}C) NMR	9 (0.15) 10 (0.23) 11 (0.03)	July to August/Roscoff, Brittany, France	[29]

Table 1. Cont.

Extraction Methodology	EY [a]	Sample Pretreatment	Fractionation/Purification	Identification/Analysis	Compound (Content [b])	Time of Collection/Geographical Origin	Ref
Et$_2$O S-L extraction, at RT	3.15	Shade-dried and ground	CC (on Silica gel) eluted with a solvent gradient from isooctane to EtOAc; Semi-preparative normal-phase HPLC (eluent, EtOAc-isooctane), with RI monitoring	HRMS, EIMS, IR, (^{1}H and ^{13}C) NMR.	9 (0.06) 15 (0.01) 21 (0.01) 22 (0.02) 25 (0.03)	December/Quiberon and Roscoff, Brittany, France	[31]
	2.40		CC (on Silica gel) eluted with a solvent gradient from hexane to Et$_2$O; HPLC (EtOAc- isooctane, 2:3), with RI monitoring.		9 (0.04) 10 (0.06) 11 (0.01) 12 (0.007) 15 (0.003)		
Et$_2$O S-L extraction	N.D.	Dried	LC using Silica gel; HPLC of the most polar fraction;	IR, MS, NMR	9 25 47	-/Quiberon, Brittany, France	[33]
Et$_2$O S-L extraction, at RT	N.D.	Crushed and freeze-dried	Insoluble impurities and pigments elimination with isooctane and EtOH-H$_2$O, respectively; TLC (eluted with Et$_2$O-petroleum ether, 50:50 or DCM-EtOAc 70:30); CC (on Silica gel, eluted with Et$_2$O-petroleum ether, 75:25) Semi-preparative HPLC	UV, IR, (^{1}H and ^{13}C) NMR, MS	15 (2)	-/Loire-Atlantique, France	[29]
Et$_2$O S-L extraction (3x) (3h at 20°C)	3.67	Freeze-dried and powder	CC (on Silica gel) eluted with a solvent gradient from hexane to Et$_2$O More polar fr.. HPLC with DCM-EtOAc (90:10)	IR, UV, MS, (^{1}H and ^{13}C) NMR	15 17 (0.01)	January to December/Piriac, France	[27]
Et$_2$O S-L extraction	N.D.	Dried	LC using Silica gel; HPLC of the less polar fr.; Semi-preparative normal-phase HPLC (EtOAc-isooctane, 1:1).	IR, MS, NMR	23 (0.12) 24 (0.08) 39 (0.01)	-/El Jadida, Morocco	[32]
DCM S-L extraction, at RT; MeOH S-L extraction	9.06	Freeze-dried	Modified Kupchan method: partitioning between (90:10) MeOH-H$_2$O and n-hexane; MeOH-H$_2$O phase: partitioning between (65:35) MeOH-H$_2$O and CHCl$_3$; Fractionation by flash chromatography (on Silica gel), with EtOAc-n-hexane (80:20) DAD and ELSD-HPLC (using a reverse-phase column), eluent gradient (55:45) MeCN-H$_2$O for 13 min, increasing to 100% MeCN in 5 min, maintaining for 20 min (rt = 16.3 min)	IR, 1D and 2D NMR, HRMS, VCD	14 (0.007)	May/Kilkee, County Clare of Ireland	[50]

Table 1. Cont.

Extraction Methodology	EY [a]	Sample Pretreatment	Fractionation/Purification	Identification/Analysis	Compound (Content [b])	Time of Collection/Geographical Origin	Ref
MeOH S-L extraction		Freeze-dried	VLC (on Silica gel) eluted with cyclohexane-EtOAc (1:2);	(^{1}H, ^{13}C, APT, COSY, HMBC and HSQC) NMR	15 (0.002)	May to June/Peniche, Portugal	[51]
DCM S-L extraction	0.95		Semi-preparative reverse phase HPLC (gradient of H_2O-MeCN)		23 (9.5 × 10^{-5})		
			PTLC over Silica gel (n-hexane-EtOAc, 7:3)				
DCM Soxhlet extraction (9 h)	3.92	Freeze-dried and ground		GC-MS	37 (0.06) 38 (0.10) 39 (0.01) 42 (0.01) 45 (0.003) 46 (0.01)	May/Ria de Aveiro, Portugal	[38]

[a]—% (w/w); [b]—when available, % of dw; ^{1}H—proton; ^{13}C—carbon; 1D and 2D—one and two dimensional; APT—attached proton test; CC—column chromatography; COSY—correlated spectroscopy; DAD—diode array detector; DCM—dichloromethane; EIMS—electron ionization mass spectrometry; ELSD—evaporative light scattering detector; ESI—electrospray ionization; Et_2O—diethyl ether; EtOAc—ethyl acetate; EtOH—ethanol; EY—extraction yield; ext.—extract; fr.—fraction; HMBC—heteronuclear multiple bond correlation; HPLC—high performance liquid chromatography; HRMS—high resolution mass spectrometry; HSQC—heteronuclear single quantum coherence; IR—infrared spectroscopy; LC—liquid chromatography; L–L—liquid-liquid; MeCN—acetonitrile; MeOH—methanol; MS—mass spectrometry; N.D.—nondeterminate; NMR—nuclear magnetic resonance; PTLC—plate thin layer chromatography; Ref—reference; RI—refractive index detector; rt—retention time; RP—reverse phase; RT—room temperature; S–L—solid–liquid; SPE—solid phase extraction; TLC—thin-layer chromatography; UV—ultraviolet spectroscopy; VCD—vibrational circular dichroism; VLC—Vacuum liquid chromatography.

3. Characterization of Linear Diterpenes from B. bifurcata

The bioprospection of linear diterpenes from B. bifurcata involves a sequential approach, including extraction, fractionation, identification, and quantification steps. Hence, in the following subchapters the methodologies already used to extract, fractionate, and characterize these bioactive compounds will be described.

3.1. Extraction and Fractionation Methodologies

Sample drying and milling are the first steps in the analysis of active compounds from plant raw materials. Macroalgae sample drying is a preliminary step that is often carried out prior to milling and extraction steps, and could be done by air drying (in the shade or not) [23,24,26,31,36,37,44,46,49,52] or by freeze-drying [8,19–22,27–30,34,35,38,43,50,51,53–55]. Notwithstanding, Semmak et al. have obtained linear diterpenes from freshly collected B. bifurcata [47]. The sample drying step is very important, especially when nonpolar extraction solvents are used, in order to avoid moisture contents that can diminish the extraction efficiency. Contrarily, when polar solvents [methanol (MeOH), ethanol (EtOH), ethyl acetate (EtOAc), among others] or solvent mixtures [hexane/acetone, hexane/acetonitrile (MeCN), etc.] are used, the use of wet samples can be considered [56]. Notwithstanding, it must be highlighted that when freshly collected macroalga is used, the moisture content is uncontrolled, which, consequently, compromises the extraction reproducibility.

The milling step could also have an important influence in the extraction, specifically in the compounds diffusion from the matrix to the solvent, since by decreasing the particles size, the surface area increases, improving the compounds diffusion [56,57]. Thus, the biomass is often ground prior to extraction [8,21–24,27,29,31,34–38,43–46,51,54,55,58,59]. Extraction is considered one of the most relevant steps, being a mass transport phenomenon, where components are transferred from the plant matrix to a solvent up to their equilibrium concentration [56]. The extraction efficacy is affected by several factors, such as the technique used to the sample drying, the particle size, the extraction solvent (or mixtures), temperature, and extraction time [60]. The different extraction conditions that have been applied to extract linear diterpenes from B. bifurcata are summarized in Table 1.

It should be highlighted that the effect of different solvents, extraction time, or even temperature used is difficult to critically compare, on one hand due to the different geographical origin or season of macroalgae sampling in each study, and, on the other hand, by the lack of accurate diterpenes quantification in many studies. Notwithstanding, an overview of the most commonly applied conditions will be reported and discussed.

Conventional solid–liquid extraction with continuous stirring (maceration) has been amongst the most used extraction methodology to obtain linear diterpenes from B. bifurcata [19–24,26–34,36,37,43–51]. The extraction yields (EY) obtained by maceration ranged from 0.95% to 9.06% (w/w) [21,23,24,27–29, 31,34,36,37,43–47,49–51]. This wide range could be a consequence of the different solvents used and/or the different geographical origins. The conventional Soxhlet extraction has also been shown to be efficient in extracting these compounds from B. bifurcata (EY of 3.92% ± 0.09% (w/w)) [38]. Diethyl ether (Et$_2$O) and EtOAc were the most used solvents, resulting in variable EYs, 1.65%–3.67% and 1.70%–4.80% (w/w), respectively [19–23,26–34,36,43,46,52]. Moreau et al., Ortalo-Magné et al., Semmak et al., among others, selected a mixture of chloroform–methanol (CHCl$_3$:MeOH) to extract different linear diterpenes from B. bifurcata, resulting in EYs from 2.63% to 6.92% (w/w) [24,37,44,47,49], while other authors have selected different mixtures of solvents (such as EtOH:CHCl$_3$, leading to EY of 1.52% (w/w)) [45].

Despite being a very important variable, most of studies did not specify the extraction time applied. Concerning the Soxhlet extraction with dichloromethane (DCM), an extraction time of 9 h was reported to be effective in the extraction of linear diterpenes from B. bifurcata [38]. Similarly, Combaut et al. carried out three consecutive solid–liquid extractions, also using Et$_2$O with an extraction time of 3 h, resulting in a EY of 3.67% (w/w) [27]. However, considerably higher extraction times were also used, such as in the study published by Maréchal et al., where an Et$_2$O solid–liquid extraction during

48 h also proved to be efficient in obtaining B. bifurcata linear diterpenes, with extraction yields ranging from 2.2% to 2.9% (w/w) [36].

Most of the diterpenes described in Table 1 were extracted from B. bifurcata at room temperature [21–24,27,29,31,32,34–37,43,44,46,50,59,61]. It is not clear from the reported data to what extent B. bifurcata diterpenes are thermosensitive, however their extraction by Soxhlet have been shown to be successful. Soxhlet extraction with DCM, at temperatures close to 40 °C, allowed researchers to extract about 1.9 g of diterpenes kg^{-1} of macroalga dw [38].

It should be highlighted that most of the studies concerning the extraction of diterpenes from B. bifurcata were carried out with analytical and bioprospection purposes, justifying the use of conventional methodologies with organic and often hazardous solvents. However, the exploitation of these bioactive components to high-value applications deserves the development and optimization of environmentally friendly and sustainable extraction approaches. Actually, the extraction of diterpenes from this macroalga species has been characterized by long operating times, and therefore high energetic consumption and the use of organic solvents, for which toxicity might compromise the exploitation of these fraction/extracts in food, nutraceutical, or pharmaceutical fields. New and promising environmental friendly extraction techniques have been developed to extract bioactive components from biomass, for example, ultrasound assisted extraction, microwave-assisted extraction, high pressure extraction, among others [57,60]. Due to the small amount of organic solvents used or even the possibility of their replacement by water, they are recognized as green (or eco-friendly) technologies [60,62]. In addition, these emerging technologies aim to shorten the extraction time, intensifying the mass transfer process, as well as to increase the extraction yields, resulting also in higher extracts quality and reducing the energy consumption [63]. Therefore the exploitation of these emerging technologies should allow researchers to widen the field of applications of B. bifurcata linear diterpenes fractions/extracts.

Fractionation and, in some cases, purification steps have been performed after extraction. Some authors have obtained enriched fractions by applying successive extraction methodologies [37,54,55,61] or even isolated compounds by fractionation with column chromatography (CC), followed, in most cases, by HPLC fractionation [20,23,24,27,29–31,34,36,43–47,49,51].

Usually, "bio-guided fractionation" has been applied as a strategy to isolate the main constituent of the most active fraction [21,28,35]. Although, Nardella et al. applied a new strategy to accelerate the discovery of new bioactive compounds, combining two-dimensional (2D) NMR analysis with high performance liquid chromatography with diode array detection coupled to mass spectrometry and solid phase extraction (HPLC-DAD-MS-SPE-NMR) to identify eleganolone (15). The authors called this new strategy "pharmacophoric deconvolution", which proved to be three times faster and to require less starting raw material than "bio-guided fractionation" [22].

3.2. Instrumental Analysis: Identification and Quantification

The identification of linear diterpenes from B. bifurcata has frequently been performed using spectroscopic techniques, such as infrared spectroscopy (IR), ultraviolet spectroscopy (UV), one (1D) and 2D (^{1}H and ^{13}C) NMR and high resolution mass spectrometry (HRMS) [19,20,24,27–34,36,43–47,49,51]. In fact, both NMR and mass spectrometry (MS) analysis can be expeditious ways to identify these components, since unique spectroscopic profiles can be recorded for each compound.

For example, Maréchal et al. obtained an Et_2O extract, with 2.2% to 2.9% of algal dw, and identified and quantified eleganediol (9) through IR, UV, HRMS, and 1D and 2D NMR [36]. Taking into account the MS data obtained by Biard et al., the mass spectrum of compound 9 presents a molecular ion $[M]^+$ at m/z 306 representing the chemical formula $C_{20}H_{34}O_2$ and also other characteristic product ions, namely $[M - H_2O]^+$ at m/z 288 [19]. Additionally, they carried out ^{13}C NMR analysis for its identification [19]. Valls et al. have also identified 9 by ^{1}H (360 MHz, deuterated chloroform ($CDCl_3$); 200 MHz, deuterated benzene (C_6D_6)), ^{13}C (90 MHz, $CDCl_3$; 50 MHz, C_6D_6), and distortionless enhancement by polarization transfer (DEPT) NMR [29].

Culioli et al. identified the chemical formula of methyl(S,2E,6E,10E)-12-hydroxy-3,7,11, 15-tetramethylhexadeca-2,6,10,14-tetraenoate (3) ($C_{21}H_{34}O_3$), (S,2E,6E,10E)-12-hydroxy-3,7,11, 15-tetramethylhexadeca-2,6,10,14-tetraenal (4) ($C_{20}H_{32}O_2$), (S,2Z,6E,10E)-12-hydroxy-3,7,11, 15-tetramethylhexadeca-2,6,10,14-tetraenal (5) ($C_{20}H_{32}O_2$), and 6,7,9,10,11,12,14,15-tetrahydrophytol (42) ($C_{20}H_{32}O$) by HRMS (Table S1), observing the molecular ions $[M]^+$ at m/z 334.2506, 304.2408, 304.2410, and 288.2450, respectively [46]. Furthermore, electron ionization mass spectrometry (EIMS) (70 eV) analysis was carried out to complement the identification, in which the molecular ions $[M]^+$ were confirmed. In addition, other characteristic product ions were also observed, for instance, in the MS spectrum of compound 3 the presence of the ions at m/z 316 $[M - H_2O]^+$, 265, 233, 215, 187,137, 123, 107, 93, 81, 69, 55 was verified [46].

Eleganolone (15) was identified by Gallé et al. [21] through high resolution electron ionization mass spectrometry (HREIMS) and ^{1}H (400 MHz, CDCl$_3$), ^{13}C (100 MHz, CDCl$_3$), and DEPT NMR, by comparison with the data described in literature [20,31]. NMR spectral data are described in Tables S2 and S3. The HREIMS of compound 15 present an ion peak for the sodium adduct ($[M + Na]^+$) at m/z 327.23193, indicating the molecular formula $C_{20}H_{32}O_2$ [21].

Smyrniotopoulos et al. identified a new linear diterpene, bifurcatriol (14), from an Irish sample of B. bifurcata, using the spectroscopic techniques mentioned above (IR, 1D and 2D NMR, HRMS) and also experimental and computational vibrational circular dichroism (VCD) spectroscopy, which was used to determine the structure and absolute configuration of the compound [50]. Taking into account its HRMS, the ion $[M + Na]^+$ was observed at m/z 347.2559, being assigned to the molecular formula $C_{20}H_{36}O_3$ [50].

Furthermore, chromatographic systems coupled to spectroscopic techniques, such as gas chromatography-mass spectrometry (GC-MS) have been also applied, with the advantage to simultaneously allowing identification and quantification [38]. Santos et al. identified and quantified the linear diterpenes present in a DCM extract from B. bifurcata, accounting 0.189% ± 0.013% of dw, which corresponded to about 57% of the total amount of lipophilic compounds detected [38]. The direct GC-MS analysis of the extract, using a DB-1 column (Agilent) and without any previous fractionation or derivatization, allowed them to identify six linear diterpenes. Hereof, this study stands out from the others here reviewed, which involved mostly NMR analysis, often accomplished by previous fractionation and/or purification steps. It must be highlighted the mass spectrum obtained for neophytadiene (46), in which the molecular ion $[M]^+$ at m/z 278, and also some major product ions at m/z 43 ($[C_3H_7]^+$), 57 ($[C_4H_9]^+$), 68, 82, 95 ($[C_7H_{11}]^+$), 109, and 123 ($[C_9H_{15}]^+$), were observed. In the same way, geranylgeraniol (39) mass spectrum presented the molecular ion $[M]^+$ at m/z 290, and characteristic products ions at m/z 69 ($[C_5H_9]^+$), 81 ($[C_6H_9]^+$), 121 ($[C_{11}H_{19}]^+$), 272 ($[M - H_2O]^+$)[38].

A more detailed discussion of the spectroscopic features of these compounds is beyond the scope of the present review, however its availability in a systematized way is undoubtedly important for the readers in the field. Therefore, an exhaustive compilation of NMR and MS data for linear diterpenes from B. bifurcata is systematized in supplementary Tables S1, S2, and S3.

4. Biological Activities of B. bifurcata Diterpenes-Enriched Extracts: In vitro and In Chemico Assays

The interest in B. bifurcata linear diterpenes-enriched extracts has increased in recent years due to the vast range of biological activities already associated with these compounds. Despite being very rare in nature, they are present in high amounts in B. bifurcata lipidic extracts, as shown above. An overview of the biological activities already reported for B. bifurcata linear diterpenes-enriched extracts or purified components is present in Table 2 (studies involving isolated diterpenes from B. bifurcata and those involving B. bifurcata extracts previously found to be rich in linear diterpenes were considered).

Most of the studies have evaluated the biological activities of B. bifurcata linear diterpenes and extracts through in vitro or *in chemico* assays. Therefore, the future development of in vivo assays to corroborate these results may be crucial to their exploitation for high-value applications.

4.1. Antimicrobial Activity

Biard et al. firstly reported that the Et$_2$O extract of *B. bifurcata* showed antimicrobial activity against *Mycobacterium smegmatis* [20] Subsequently, they proceeded to the isolation of the major compound, namely eleganolone (**15**), which also inhibited the bacteria growth at 75 µg mL^{-1} (expressed as minimal inhibitory concentration (MIC)), as well as that of *Bacillus subtilis* (MIC = 2.5 mg mL^{-1}), *Mycobacterium aquae* (MIC = 400 µg mL^{-1}), *Mycobacterium ranae* (MIC = 100 µg mL^{-1}), *Mycobacterium xenoqui* (MIC = 200 µg mL^{-1}), and *Mycobacterium avium* (MIC = 100 µg mL^{-1}) [20]. Hellio et al. also reported the antibacterial activity of eleganediol (**9**) and eleganolone (**15**) against a strain of *Bacillus sp.* (MIC = 8 µg mL^{-1}) [23].

Furthermore, Hellio et al. reported the antimicrobial activity of two eleganolone (**15**) derivatives, ((10E,14E)-16-hydroxy-2,10,14-trimethyl-6-methylenehexadeca-2,10,14-triene-4,7-dione (**22**) and (6E,14E)-16-hydroxy-2,6,14-trimethyl-10-methylenehexadeca-2,6,14-triene-4,11-dione (**25**), against a gram-positive bacteria, namely *Bacillus sp.* (MIC = 8 µg mL^{-1}), as well as against marine fungi, namely *Corollospora maritima, Lulworthia sp.*, and *Dendryphiella salina*, MIC = 8 µg mL^{-1} [23].

Santos et al. demonstrated that a DCM *B. bifurcata* extract rich in linear diterpenes (48.29 mg g^{-1} of extract) exhibited antibacterial activity against both gram-positive (namely, *Staphylococcus aureus* ATCC®6538 (MIC = 1024 µg mL^{-1}) and ATCC®43300 (MIC = 2048 µg mL^{-1})) and gram-negative (in particular, *Escherichia coli* ATCC®25922 (MIC = 2048 µg mL^{-1})) bacteria. In addition, this extract was shown to reinforce the antimicrobial activity of several antibiotics. The combination of the extract with gentamicin or tetracycline resulted in a severe decrease of the antibiotic MIC against the three strains. Rifampicin MIC also decreased about 87% and 50% in the presence of the extract toward *Staphylococcus aureus* ATCC®43300 and *Escherichia coli* ATCC®25922, respectively. Thus, this synergism of *B. bifurcata* extracts with antibiotics could be further exploited in a way to overcome the antibiotic-resistant bacteria strains, which is a serious public health problem [38].

Alves et al. studied the antibacterial activity (expressed in zone of inhibition (ZI)) of MeOH and DCM extracts of *B. bifurcata*. Both extracts were revealed to be active against *Escherichia coli* ATCC 10536 (ZI: 7.0 ± 0.0 mm and 8.3 ± 0.6 mm for MeOH and DCM extracts, respectively), while MeOH extract was also shown to inhibit *Staphylococcus aureus* ATCC 25923 (7.0 ± 0 mm ZI) [55]. The MeOH extract also presented antibacterial activity against *Bacillus subtilis* ATCC 6633 (6.7 ± 0.6 mm ZI) and *Escherichia coli* ATCC 25922 (6.7 ± 0.6 mm ZI) [55]. In fact, antimicrobial activity of both MeOH and DCM *B. bifurcata* extracts was also demonstrated against another gram-negative bacteria, *Pseudomonas aeruginosa* ATCC 27853 (11.3 ± 1.5 mm ZI and 8.3 ± 1.2 mm ZI, respectively), and toward *Saccharomyces cerevisiae* ATCC 9763, which was expressed in the inhibitory concentration of the extract required to decrease microbial concentration by 50% (IC$_{50}$), IC$_{50}$ = 26.68 µg mL^{-1} and IC$_{50}$ = 17.06 µg mL^{-1}, for MeOH and DCM extracts, respectively [55]. According to these results, a higher potential antibacterial activity against *Pseudomonas aeruginosa* ATCC 27853 in the MeOH extract was observed while the DCM extract showed a higher antifungal activity against *Saccharomyces cerevisiae* ATCC 9763 [55].

Antiprotozoal activity has been one of the most studied biological activities for linear diterpenes from *B. bifurcata*. Protozoal infections, in particular malaria, leishmaniosis, and sleeping sickness, among others, are fatal diseases [35]. Recently, Smyrniotopoulos et al. proved the antiprotozoal activity of bifurcatriol (**14**), obtained after several purification steps [50]. This linear diterpene also revealed antimalarial activity toward a resistant K1 strain of the malaria parasite, *Plasmodium falciparum* (IC$_{50}$ = 0.65 ± 0.05 µg mL^{-1}), with a good selectivity, and protozoal activity against *Trypanosoma brucei rhodesiense* (IC$_{50}$ = 11.8 ± 0.01 µg mL^{-1}), *Trypanosoma cruzi* (IC$_{50}$ = 47.8 ± 0.59 µg mL^{-1}), and *Leishmania donovani* (IC$_{50}$ = 18.8 ± 0.12 µg mL^{-1}) [50]. After the evaluation of the antiprotozoal activity of an EtOAc extract, through a bio-guided fractionation, Gallé et al. proved that eleganolone (**15**) was responsible for the antimalarial (or anti-plasmodial) activity of the extract toward *Plasmodium falciparum* (IC_{50} = 2.6 µg mL^{-1}), with a good selectivity index (SI = 21.6). However, this component presented lower trypanocidal activity against *Trypanosoma brucei rhodesiense* (IC_{50} = 13.7 µg mL^{-1}) and *Trypanosoma cruzi* (IC_{50} = 17.7 µg mL^{-1}) than the crude extract, which exhibited a promising trypanocidal activity with a mild selectivity index (IC_{50} = 0.53 µg mL^{-1}; selectivity index (SI) = 11.6) [21]. In fact, the enhanced activities of crude (thus more complex) extracts may be due to synergism effects, highlighting their potential without laborious and expensive fractionation/purification steps, often involving hazardous solvents. The exploitation of the trypanocidal activity of *B. bifurcata* extracts enriched in linear diterpenes may be important considering the gaps associated with sleeping sickness (trypanosomiasis) therapy, namely the fact that available drugs are outdated, causing severe adverse reactions [21].

Leishmaniosis, which is a common disease worldwide, affecting several mammal species, including humans [52], has been also the focus of different studies concerning the bioprospection of linear diterpenes from *B. bifurcata*. Antiprotozoal activity of EtOAc:MeOH soluble extract against *Leishmania donovani* (IC_{50} = 6.4 µg mL^{-1}) was also shown [61]. Although, the EtOAc (10% *w/v*) extract was shown to be the most active against amastigotes of this strain, presenting an IC_{50} of 3.8 µg mL^{-1} [35]. Vonthron-Sé et al. also tested this active extract against erythrocytes infected by a resistant K1 strain of *Plasmodium falciparum* (100% of growth inhibition (GI) at 9.7 µg mL^{-1}) and *Trypanosoma cruzi* trypamastigotes (78% of GI at 9.7 µg mL^{-1}). These activities seem to be induced by toxicity [35]. Antiprotozoal activity of a *B. bifurcata* extract against *Trypanosoma brucei rhodeisense* (IC_{50} = 1.9 µg mL^{-1}), *Trypanosoma cruzi* (IC_{50} = 34.7 µg mL^{-1}), and *Mycobacterium tuberculosis* (MIC = 64.0 µg mL^{-1}) (antitubercular activity) was also reported [61].

4.2. Antifouling Activity

Antifouling activity has been also proven in *B. bifurcata* extracts with high contents of linear diterpenes. The exploitation of this capacity of *B bifurcata* diterpenes could be an environmentally safe alternative for modern marine engineering and shipping operations, for offshore structures, and for aquaculture equipment [23,36]. In fact, the control of biofouling is an important problem of marine technology [23], with the use of heavy metal-based paints being already restricted due to the toxicity of organotin compounds to marine organisms [23,36]. Bacteria are commonly responsible for biofouling, forming a biofilm with other micro- and macrofoulers, such as algae or invertebrates, adhering to surfaces [14].

The antifouling activity of an Et$_2$O *B. bifurcata* extract, in which two linear diterpenes were identified, was also tested against *Balanus amphitrite* cyprid, and was shown to be highly active (efficient concentration of extract to decrease microbial concentration by 50%, EC_{50} = 0.43 (0.88 – 1.26, conf. lim. 95%) µg mL^{-1}), whereas eleganolone (15) (EC_{50} = 2.14 (0.88 – 3.9, conf. lim. 95%) µg mL^{-1}) and eleganediol (9) (EC_{50} = 40.37 (11.89 – 62.93, conf. lim. 95%) µg mL^{-1}) were shown to be moderate and low active, respectively. This study also proved that *B. bifurcata* extracts are toxic against *Balanus amphitrite* nauplius II after 24 h of treatment (lethal concentration (LC) = 0.64 (0.26 – 1.14, conf. lim. 95%) µg mL^{-1})). Compounds **9** (LC = 7.31 (3.84 – 8.78, conf. lim. 95%) µg mL^{-1}) and **15** (LC = 3.48 (2.53 – 4.52, conf. lim. 95%) µg mL^{-1}) showed lower toxicity [26]. The antiadhesion activity of compounds **9** and **15** were also studied against a strain of *Polibacter sp.* (EC_{50} = 63.5 ± 8.3 µg mL^{-1}; EC_{50} = 58.4 ± 1.7 µg mL^{-1}) and of *Paracoccus sp.* (EC_{50} = 103.9 ± 12.8 µg mL^{-1}; EC_{50} = 40.3 ± 13.5 µg mL^{-1}), with the component **15** being more active toward these two strains [25,44].

The antifouling activity of *B. bifurcata* linear diterpenes, considering the biofouling promoted by macroalgae and blue mussel, were also evaluated. The antifouling activity of eleganediol (9) was tested by Hellio et al., who proved that this linear diterpene is able to inhibit macroalgal spore and zygote development, particularly of *Enteromorpha intestinalis* (65.2% ± 1.2% GI) and *Sargassum muticum* (81.5% ± 3.4% GI), and to inhibit diatom growth (*Amphora coffeaformis* (37.3% ± 1.9% GI), *Phaeodartylum tricornutum* (42.8% ± 1.5% GI), and *Cylindrotheca closterium* (39.5% ± 1.6% GI)) [23]. Other linear diterpenes from *B. bifurcata*, such as 12-(S)-hydroxygeranylgeraniol (**1**) and geranylgeraniol (**39**) also showed antifouling activity toward macroalgal spores and zygotes. Compound **1** was shown to inhibit the development of *Sargassum muticum* (72.0% ± 2.2% GI) spore and zygote, whereas compound **39** was active against *Enteromorpha intestinalis* (67.3% ± 2.1% GI) and *Ulva lactuca* (83.1% ± 3.4% GI), as well as inhibiting the blue mussel *Mytilus edulis* adhesion (77.0% ± 2.8% inhibition of phenoloxidase activity (IPA)) [23].

Maréchal et al. studied the seasonal variation on the antifouling activity of crude *B. bifurcata* Et$_2$O extracts (from Brittany, France) against cyprids of *Balanus amphitrite* and the marine bacteria *Cobetia marina* (MIC: 12.2 ± 0.4 to 26.3 ± 1.3 µg mL^{-1}) and *Pseudoalteromonas haloplanktis* (MIC: 6.5 ± 0.6 to 15.5 ± 0.8 µg mL^{-1}) [36].

Furthermore, the antifouling activity of ether extracts of *B. bifurcata* from different sampling sites was also tested. An extract of *B. bifurcata* from Quiberon, France was found to be active against *Ulva lactuca* spore and zygote development (78.7% ± 2.8% GI), whereas the Port Sall (France) and Oualidia (Morocco) *B. bifurcata* extracts inhibit the growth of diatoms (*Amphora coffeaformis* (83.9% ± 4.2% GI), *Phaeodartylum tricornutum* (86.2% ± 3.4% GI), *Cylindrotheca closterium* (69.2% ± 2.4% GI)) and inhibit the adhesion of the blue mussel *Mytilus edulis* (80.6% ± 2.3% IPA), respectively [23].

4.3. Antiproliferative Activity

The cytotoxic activity of two bifurcadiol derivatives ((2E,10E,12R)-3,11,15-trimethyl-7-methylenehexadeca-2,10,14-triene-1,6,12-triol (**6**), and (2E,10E,12R)-3,7,11,15-tetramethylhexadeca-2,10,14-triene-1,7,12-triol (**7**) isolated from *B. bifurcata* were evaluated. These linear diterpenes were shown to be active against the NSCLC-N6 cell line (a human non–small-cell bronchopulmonary carcinoma line), presenting IC$_{50}$ values of 12.3 and 9.5 µg mL^{-1}, respectively) [44]. Eleganediol (**9**) and bifurcane (**10**), isolated from a *B. bifurcata* extract, showed anti-proliferative activity at 100 µg mL^{-1}, toward MDA-MB-231 tumor cells (mammary gland/breast adenocarcinoma), resulting in 1.8% and 2.9% of cell viability, respectively [48].

Some studies also evaluated the in vitro antiproliferative activity of *B. bifurcata* extracts. Zubia et al. tested the cytotoxic activity of DCM:MeOH extracts of this brown macroalga against three tumoral cell lines (Daudi, Jurkat and K562), which resulted in, approximately, 40% of cell viability reduction with Daudi and K562 and about 20% of cell viability reduction with Jurkat cell lines [8]. Two carcinoma models (Caco-2 and HepG-2) were used to evaluate the in vitro antitumor activity of *B. bifurcata* extracts. In this research, Alves et al. showed high cell proliferation inhibition of both DCM and MeOH extracts (at 1 mg mL^{-1}) against these tumoral cell lines. The IC$_{50}$ values obtained with MeOH extract was 437.1 (266.0 – 718.1) µg mL^{-1} for Caco-2 and 252.0 (162.0 – 392.2) µg mL^{-1} for HepG-2. Although, DCM extract exhibited promising cell proliferation inhibition and cytotoxicity, against Caco-2 (IC$_{50}$ = 82.31 (54.7 – 123.8) µg mL^{-1}; IC$_{50}$ = 90.09 (70.82 – 114.6) µg mL^{-1}) and HepG-2 (IC$_{50}$ = 95.63 (69.66 – 131.3) µg mL^{-1}; IC$_{50}$ = 123.9 (95.47 – 160.8) µg mL^{-1}), when compared with the results obtained for cisplatin and tamoxifen, which are two commercial drugs [55].

In addition, Moreau et al. showed irreversible arrest of well-differentiated pathologic cells (such as NSCLC-N6) proliferation induced by a *B. bifurcata* MeOH extract rich in diterpenes. This antiproliferative effect is a mechanism of action that overcomes the limited effectiveness of many cycle-dependent anticancer drugs on such slowly developing tumors. After 72 h of treatment with *B. bifurcata* extract (2.5 µg L hours^{-1}), the cell growth in the G1 phase of the cell cycle was inhibited, and kinetic assays in pretreated cells proved that this growth arrest was irreversible [37].

Besides these results regarding anti-proliferative activity of *B. bifurcata* linear diterpenes and extracts, bioaccessibility and bioavailability assays were not yet performed. In fact, most of the in vitro studies have not used gut cell lines, which allow consideration of the absorption and distribution stages. Thus, other in vitro assays are required in the future to complement these results.

4.4. Antioxidant Activity

The prospection of natural components from macroalgae with antioxidant activity has been object of several studies, since oxidative stress is known to be related with several diseases, such as cancer, chronic inflammation, atherosclerosis, and cardiovascular disorder, among others [8]. Furthermore, consumers have, currently, preference for products from natural sources and are conscious about the toxicity associated with synthetic antioxidants [8]. The industrial implementation of natural antioxidants, whether at the level of food industry or the cosmetic or therapeutic industry (i.e., nutraceuticals), appears as a promising alternative to synthetic antioxidants [54]. This may be one of the reasons why antioxidant activity has been one of the most studied biological activities in B. bifurcata extracts [8,38,54,55].

The antioxidant potential of B. bifurcata linear diterpenes and extracts has been evaluated by different assays, such as 2,2-diphenyl-1-picrylhydrazyl (DPPH), 2,2'-azino-bis(3-ethylbenzothiazoline-6-sulphonic acid (ABTS), and oxygen radical absorbent capacity (ORAC). The results of DPPH and ABTS assays are commonly expressed as IC_{50} values, defined as the inhibitory concentration of the extract required to decrease by 50% the initial radical concentration. Nonetheless, the comparison of the different IC_{50} values between published studies is not always possible, since the IC_{50} value depends on the methodology used by each author, as well as on the standards used. For example, Santos et al. used ascorbic acid and 3,5-di-tert-4-butylhydroxytoluene (BHT) as positive control whereas Pinteus et al. used only BHT [38,54]. Despite earlier studies, namely from Santos et al. and Alves et al., using the same standards as positive control, the DPPH assay conditions were different, which make the results incomparable [38,55].

Zubia et al. determined the antioxidant activity of B. bifurcata crude DCM:MeOH extract by three methods: DPPH (efficient concentration of extract to decrease reagent concentration by 50%, $EC_{50} = 0.56 \pm 0.00$ mg mL^{-1}), reducing activity (90.97% at 500 mg L^{-1}), and β-carotene-linoleic acid system (76.13% of inhibition at 500 mg L^{-1}) [8]. A DCM extract, obtained from a B. bifurcata sample of Ria de Aveiro, Portugal, was evaluated by DPPH and ABTS assays, exhibiting IC_{50} values of 365.57 ± 10.04 μg mL^{-1} and 116.25 ± 2.54 μg mL^{-1} for DPPH and ABTS, respectively [38]. Alves et al. also carried out DPPH assay in both MeOH (IC_{50} = 58.82 (50.65 – 68.31) μg mL^{-1}) and DCM (IC_{50} = 344.70 (246.10 – 482.80) μg mL^{-1}) extracts of a B. bifurcata from Peniche Coast, Portugal, however with MeOH extract showing a higher antioxidant activity than DCM extract [54,55]. Notwithstanding, the DCM extract showed an IC_{50} value close to that obtained in a similar study [38,54,55]. In addition to DPPH assay, the ORAC of MeOH (3151.35 ± 119.33 μmol trolox equivalents (TE) g^{-1} extract (ext)) and DCM (589.98 ± 7.33 μmol TE g^{-1} ext) extracts were determined [54,55].

4.5. Anti-Inflammatory Activity

The anti-inflammatory activity of a B. bifurcata extract enriched in linear diterpenes was described by Santos et al., who analyzed a DCM extract from a Portuguese sample [38]. The capacity of this extract to modulate nitric oxide (NO) was evaluated through an in vitro model of inflammation consisting of macrophages stimulated with lipopolysaccharides (LPS) and, simultaneously, the cell viability was analyzed by the resazurin-based assay, which allowed researchers to select concentrations with bioactivity and without cytotoxicity. The accumulation of nitrites in the culture medium, using the Griess assay, was measured to determine the extract effect on NO production. Thus, LPS-induced NO production was 6% inhibited in the presence of the extract at a concentration of about 50 μg mL^{-1} [38].

Table 2. *B. bifurcata* linear diterpenes and crude extracts' biological activities.

Compounds/Crude Extract (Yield)	Biological Activities	Ref.
12-(S)-hydroxygeranylgeraniol (1)	Antimitotic activity (assay of cytotoxicity activity—inhibition of development of fertilized eggs of the common sea urchin *Paracentrotus lividus*—EC_{50} = 18 µg mL^{-1}	[43]
	Antifouling activity toward macroalgae spore and zygote development (*Sargassum muticum* (72.0% ± 2.2% GI))	[23]
(S)-12-hydroxygeranylgeranic acid (2)	Antimitotic activity (assay of cytotoxicity activity—inhibition of development of fertilized eggs of the common sea urchin *Paracentrotus lividus*—EC_{50} = 60 µg mL^{-1}	[43]
(2E,10E,12R)-3,11,15-trimethyl-7-methylenehexadeca-2,10,14-triene-1,6,12-triol (6)	Cytotoxic activity: inhibit in vitro proliferation of pathogenic cells (NSCLC-N6—derived from a human non–small-cell bronchopulmonary carcinoma) by terminal differentiation. IC_{50} = 12.3 µg mL^{-1}	[44]
(2E,10E,12R)-3,7,11,15-tetramethylhexadeca-2,10,14-triene-1,7,12-triol (7)	Cytotoxic activity: inhibit in vitro proliferation of pathogenic cells (NSCLC-N6—derived from a human non–small-cell bronchopulmonary carcinoma) by terminal differentiation. IC_{50} = 9.5 µg mL^{-1}	[44]
Eleganediol (9)	Antibacterial activity (against *Bacillus* sp. (MIC = 8 µg mL^{-1})	
	Antifouling activity toward macroalgal spore and zygote development (*Enteromorpha intestinalis* (65.2 ± 1.2% GI), *Sargassum muticum* (81.5 ± 3.4% GI)), and against diatom growth (*Amphora coffeaformis* (37.3% ± 1.9% GI), *Phaeodartylum tricornutum* (42.8% ± 1.5% GI), *Cylindrotheca closterium* (39.5% ± 1.6% GI))	[23]
	Antimitotic activity (assay of cytotoxicity activity—inhibition of development of fertilized eggs of the common sea urchin *Paracentrotus lividus*—EC_{50} = 36 µg mL^{-1}	[43]
	Antiadhesion activity (against a strain of *Polibacter* sp. (EC_{50} = 63.5 ± 8.3 µg mL^{-1}) and of *Paracoccus* sp. (EC_{50} = 103.9 ± 12.8 µg mL^{-1})	[25]
	Antifouling activity (against *Balanus amphitrite* cyprid (EC_{50} = 40.37 (11.89 – 62.93, conf. lim. 95%) µg mL^{-1})	[26]
	Toxicity (against *Balanus amphitrite* nauplius (LC = 7.31 (3.84 – 8.78, conf. lim. 95%) µg mL^{-1}))	
Bifurcane (10)	Antiproliferative activity toward MDA-MB-231 tumor cells (1.8% cell viability at 100 µg mL^{-1})	[48]
	Antimitotic activity (assay of cytotoxicity activity - inhibition of development of fertilized eggs of the common sea urchin *Paracentrotus lividus* - EC_{50} = 12 µg mL^{-1}).	[29]
Bifurcatriol (14)	Antiproliferative activity toward MDA-MB-231 tumor cells (2.9% cell viability at 100 µg mL^{-1})	[48]
	Antimalarial activity (against resistant K1 strain of the malaria parasite, *Plasmodium falciparum* – IC_{50} = 0.65 ± 0.05 µg mL^{-1})	
	Antiprotozoal activity: *Trypanosoma brucei rhodesiense* (IC_{50} = 11.8 ± 0.01 µg mL^{-1}), *Trypanosoma cruzi* (IC_{50} = 47.8 ± 0.59 µg mL^{-1}), *Leishmania donovani* (IC_{50} = 18.8 ± 0.12 µg mL^{-1}) Cytotoxicity against the L6 rat myoblast cell line (IC_{50} = 56.6 ± 0.004 µg mL^{-1})	[50]

Table 2. Cont.

Compounds/Crude Extract (Yield)	Biological Activities	Ref.
Eleganolone (15)	Antimicrobial activity (against *Mycobacterium smegmatis* (75 μg mL^{-1}), *Bacillus subtilis* (2.5 mg mL^{-1}), *Mycobacterium aquae* (400 μg mL^{-1}), *Mycobacterium ranae* (100 μg mL^{-1}), *Mycobacterium xenopi* (200 μg mL^{-1}), *Mycobacterium avium* (100 μg mL^{-1}))	[20]
	Antiprotozoal activity (against *Trypanosoma brucei rhodesiense* (IC$_{50}$ = 13.7 μg mL^{-1}), *Trypanosoma cruzi* (IC$_{50}$ = 17.7 μg mL^{-1}), *Plasmodium falciparum*, IC$_{50}$ = 2.6 μg mL^{-1} (SI = 21.6))	[21]
	In vitro antiplasmodial activity (against *Plasmodium falciparum* 7G8 strain – antimalarial activity – In fraction: 47% of growth inhibition at 10 μg mL^{-1})	[22]
	Antibacterial activity (against *Bacillus* sp. (MIC = 8 μg mL^{-1})	[23]
	Anti-adhesion activity (against a strain of *Polibacter* sp. (EC$_{50}$ = 58.4 ± 1.7 μg mL^{-1}) and of *Paracoccus* sp. (EC$_{50}$ = 40.3 ± 13.5 μg mL^{-1})	[25]
	Antifouling activity (against *Balanus amphitrite* cyprid (EC$_{50}$ = 2.14 (0.88 – 3.9, conf. lim 95%) μg mL^{-1})	[26]
	Toxicity (against *Balanus amphitrite* nauplius (LC = 3.48 (2.53 – 4.52, conf. lim 95%) μg mL^{-1}))	
	Cytotoxicity (against mouse fibroblast cell line (L929), IC$_{50}$ = 22 μg mL^{-1})	[30]
	Antioxidant potential (ORAC—1663.83 ± 25.35 μmol TE g^{-1} of compound, FRAP—8341.18 ± 177.72 μM FeSO$_4$ g^{-1} compound)	[51]
(6E,10E,14E)-16-hydroxy-2,6,10,14-tetramethylhexadeca-2,6,10,14-tetraen-4-one (21)	Cytotoxicity (against mouse fibroblast cell line (L929), IC$_{50}$ = 18 μg mL^{-1})	[30]
(10E,14E)-16-hydroxy-2,10,14-trimethyl-6-methylenehexadeca-2,10,14-triene-4,7-dione (22)	Antimicrobial activity against gram-positive bacteria (*Bacillus*, MIC = 8 μg mL^{-1}) and marine fungi (MIC = 8 μg mL^{-1}) (such as *Corollospora maritima*, *Lulworthia* sp., and *Dendryphiella salina*)	[23]
Eleganolal (23)	Antioxidant potential (ORAC—667.48 ± 10.96 μmol TE g^{-1} of compound, FRAP—8635.37 ± 389.54 μM FeSO$_4$ g^{-1} compound)	[51]
(6E,14E)-16-hydroxy-2,6,14-trimethyl-10-methylenehexadeca-2,6,14-triene-4,11-dione (25)	Antimicrobial activity against gram-positive bacteria (*Bacillus*, MIC = 8 μg mL^{-1}) and marine fungi (MIC = 8 μg mL^{-1}) (such as *Corollospora maritima*, *Lulworthia* sp., and *Dendryphiella salina*)	[23]
Eleganolonebutenolide (32)	Cytotoxicity (against mouse fibroblast cell line (L929), IC$_{50}$ = 27 μg mL^{-1})	[30]
14,15-dihydro-eleganonic acid (33)	Cytotoxicity (against mouse fibroblast cell line (L929), IC$_{50}$ = 20 μg mL^{-1})	[30]
Geranylgeraniol (39)	Antifouling activity—macroalgal spore and zygote development (*Enteromorpha intestinalis* (67.3 ± 2.1% GI); *Ulva lactuca* (83.1% ± 3.4% GI)) and inhibition of adhesion of the blue mussel *Mytilus edulis* (77.0% ± 2.8% IPA)	[23]
Bifurcanol (41)	Antimitotic activity (assay of cytotoxicity activity—inhibition of development of fertilized eggs of the common sea urchin *Paracentrotus lividus*—EC$_{50}$ = 4 μg mL^{-1}).	[43]
	Cytotoxicity (against mouse fibroblast cell line (L929), IC$_{50}$ = 24 μg mL^{-1}).	[30]

Table 2. Cont.

Compounds/Crude Extract (Yield)	Biological Activities	Ref.
DCM extract (3.92 ± 0.09% (w/w))	Antioxidant activity (in vitro: DPPH assay: IC$_{50}$ = 365.57 ± 10.04 µg mL^{-1}, ABTS assay: IC$_{50}$ = 116.25 ± 2.54 µg mL^{-1}) Anti-inflammatory activity (NO production (% of LPS): 6% at 50 µg mL^{-1}) Antibacterial activity (against both gram-positive (*Staphylococcus aureus* ATCC®6538 (MIC = 1024 µg mL^{-1}), *Staphylococcus aureus* ATCC®43300 (MIC = 2048 µg mL^{-1}) and gram-negative (*Escherichia coli* ATCC®25922 (MIC = 2048 µg mL^{-1})) strains) Synergistic effects with antibiotic:Against *S. aureus* ATCC®6538 (Gent (MIC = 32 µg mL^{-1}); Gent + Ext (MIC = 16 µg mL^{-1}); Tetra (MIC = 16 µg mL^{-1}); Tetra + Ext (MIC = 8 µg mL^{-1}))Against *S. aureus* ATCC®43300 (Rif (MIC = 16 µg mL^{-1}); Rif + Ext (MIC < 2 µg mL^{-1}); Gent (MIC > 256 µg mL^{-1}); Gent+Ext (MIC = 16 µg mL^{-1}); Tetra (MIC > 256 µg mL^{-1}); Tetra + Ext (MIC < 2 µg mL^{-1}))Against *E. coli* ATCC®25922 (Rif (MIC = 32 µg mL^{-1}); Rif + Ext (MIC = 16 µg mL^{-1}); Gent (MIC > 256 µg mL^{-1}); Gent+Ext (MIC < 2 µg mL^{-1}); Tetra (MIC = 18 µg mL^{-1}); Tetra + Ext (MIC < 2 µg mL^{-1}))	[38]
EtOAc extract *	Antiprotozoal activity (against erythrocytes infected by a resistant K1 strain of *Plasmodium falciparum* (100% of GI at 9.7 µg mL^{-1}), *Trypanosoma cruzi* trypamastigotes (78% of GI at 9.7 µg mL^{-1}), and *Leishmania donovani* amastigotes (100% of GI at 9.7 µg mL^{-1}), IC$_{50}$ = 3.8 µg mL^{-1}) Cytotoxicity activity (against L6 cells, rat skeletal myoblasts, IC$_{50}$ = 6 µg mL^{-1})	[35]
EtOAc:MeOH (1:1) soluble extract*	Anti-tubercular activity (against *Mycobacterium tuberculosis*, MIC = 64.0 µg mL^{-1}) Antiprotozoal activity (against *Trypanosoma brucei rhodsiense* (IC$_{50}$ = 1.9 µg mL^{-1}), *Trypanosoma cruzi* (IC$_{50}$ = 34.7 µg mL^{-1}), and *Leishmania donovani* (IC$_{50}$ = 6.4 µg mL^{-1})) Cytotoxicity (IC$_{50}$ = 32.7 µg mL^{-1})	[61]
DCM-MeOH ASE extract*	Antioxidant activity (DPPH assay: EC$_{50}$ = 0.56 ± 0.00 mg mL^{-1}, reducing activity: 90.97% at 500 mg L^{-1}, β-carotene-linoleic acid system assay: 76.13% ± 0.55% of inhibition at 500 mg L^{-1}, TPC 0.96% dw) Antitumoral activity (tested with Daudi (Human Burkitt's lymphoma), K562 (Human chronic myelogenous leukemia) (~40% of viable cells), and Jurkat (Human leukemic T cell lymphoblast) (~20% of viable cells) cells)	[8]
MeOH clean and enrich extract *	Antioxidant activity (TPC: 129.17 ± 0.002 mg GAE g^{-1} ext, ORAC: 3151.35 ± 119.33 µmol TE g^{-1} ext, DPPH: IC$_{50}$ = 58.82 (50.65 – 68.31) µg mL^{-1}) Antimicrobial activity (against *Pseudomonas aeruginosa* ATCC 27853 (11.3 ± 1.5 mm ZI), *Escherichia coli* ATCC 105366 (7.0 ± 0.0 mm ZI), *Escherichia coli* ATCC 25922 (6.7 ± 0.6 mm ZI), *Staphylococcus aureus* ATCC 25923 (7.0 ± 0.0 mm ZI), and *Saccharomyces cerevisiae* ATCC 9763 (IC$_{50}$ = 26.68 µg mL^{-1})) Antitumor activity: cell proliferation inhibition (tested in 2 in vitro carcinoma models, a human colorectal adeno-carcinoma (Caco-2) (IC$_{50}$ = 437.1 (266.0 – 718.1) µg mL^{-1}), and a human hepatocellular liver cancer (HepG-2) (IC$_{50}$ = 252.0 (162.0 – 392.2) µg mL^{-1}))	[54,55]

Table 2. Cont.

Compounds/Crude Extract (Yield)	Biological Activities	Ref.
DCM extract *	Antioxidant activity (TPC: 43.21 ± 0.043 mg GAE g^{-1} ext, ORAC: 589.98 ± 7.33 μmol TE g^{-1} ext, DPPH: IC$_{50}$ = 344.70 (246.10 – 482.80) μg mL^{-1})	[54, 55]
	Antimicrobial activity (against gram-negative bacteria (*Pseudomonas aeruginosa* ATCC 27853 (8.3 ± 1.2 mm ZI), *Escherichia coli* ATCC 105366 (8.3 ± 0.6 mm ZI)), and *Saccharomyces cerevisiae* ATCC 9763 (IC$_{50}$ = 17.06 μg mL^{-1}))	
	Antitumor activity: cell proliferation inhibition and cytotoxicity (tested in 2 in vitro carcinoma models, a human colorectal adeno-carcinoma (Caco-2) (IC$_{50}$ = 82.31 (54.7 – 123.8) μg mL^{-1}) (IC$_{50}$ = 90.09 (70.82 – 114.6) μg mL^{-1}), and a human hepatocellular liver cancer (HepG-2) (IC$_{50}$ = 95.63 (69.66 – 131.3) μg mL^{-1}) (IC$_{50}$ = 123.9 (95.47 – 160.8) μg mL^{-1}))	
Et$_2$O extract(2.2%–2.9% of dw)	Antifouling activity (against 2 marine bacteria, *Cobetia marina* (MIC between 12.2 ± 0.4 to 26.3 ± 1.3 μg mL^{-1}) and *Pseudoalteromonas haloplanktis* (MIC between 6.5 ± 0.6 to 15.5 ± 0.8 μg mL^{-1}), and cypris larvae of the barnacle, *Balanus amphitrite* (EC$_{50}$ = 10 μg mL^{-1}))	[36]
MeOH clean and enriched extract(6.92% of dw)	Anti-proliferative effect (of well-differentiated pathologic cells, such as a human non-small-cell bronchopulmonary carcinoma line (NSCLC-N6) (IC$_{50}$ = 4 μg mL^{-1}), by terminal differentiation)	[37]
EtOAc extract(4.80% of dw)	Antiprotozoal activity (against *Trypanosoma brucei rhodesiense* trypomastigotes—crude extracts and the most active fraction)	[21]
Et$_2$O extract	Antifouling activity (against *Balanus amphitrite* cyprid (EC$_{50}$ = 0.43 (0.88 – 1.26, conf. lim. 95%) μg mL^{-1})	[26]
	Toxicity (against *Balanus amphitrite* nauplius (LC = 0.64 (0.26 – 1.14, conf. lim. 95%) μg mL^{-1}))	
Et$_2$O extract(3.15% of dw)	Antifouling activity toward macroalgal spore and zygote development (*Ulva lactuca* (78.7% ± 2.8% GI), against diatom growth (*Amphora coffaeformis* (83.9% ± 4.2% GI), *Phaeodactylum tricornutum* (86.2% ± 3.4% GI), *Cylindrotheca closterium* (69.2% ± 2.4% GI)), and inhibition of adhesion of the blue mussel *Mytilus edulis* (80.6% ± 2.3% IPA)	[23]
Fraction of DCM extract(0.95% of cw)	Neuroprotective effect (prevent changes in mitochondrial potential (218.10% ± 14.87% of control), reduction of H$_2$O$_2$ levels production (204.50% ± 15.12% of control), revert neurotoxic effect on cell viability to about 20%–25%).	[51]

ABTS - 2,2′-azino-bis(3-ethylbenzothiazoline-6-sulphonic acid; ASE—accelerated solvent extraction; DCM—dichloromethane; DPPH—2,2-diphenyl-1-picrylhydrazyl assay; EC$_{50}$—efficient concentration of extract to decrease microbial concentration by 50%; Ext—extract; FRAP—ferric reducing antioxidant power; Gent—gentamicin; GI—growth inhibition; IC$_{50}$—inhibitory concentration of the extract required to decrease microbial concentration by 50%; LC—lethal concentration; LPS—lipopolysaccharides; MIC—minimal inhibitory concentration; ORAC—oxygen radical absorbent capacity; Rif—rifampicin; SI—selectivity index; TE—trolox equivalents; Tetra—tetracycline; TPC—total phenolic content; ZI—zone of inhibition; *—linear diterpenes were not identified, however the authors justify theoretically that these components may be responsible for the determined biological activities.

4.6. Other Biological Activities

Two components widely reported in *B. bifurcata* samples, namely eleganediol (**9**) and eleganolone (**15**), were studied regarding antihypertensive and relaxing activities. These components were isolated from *Cystoseira balearica*. These pharmacological assays were performed on different guinea pig intestinal preparations, and allowed researchers to identify bioactive effects of compounds **9** and **15**, such as blocking the isoprenaline inotropic activity and inhibiting the contractile activities of acetylcholine (pIC_{50} = 4.71 ± 0.18 µg mL^{-1}; pIC_{50} = 4.60 ± 0.03 µg mL^{-1}, respectively) and histamine (pIC_{50} = 5.18 ± 0.01 µg mL^{-1}; pIC_{50} = 4.84 ± 0.20 µg mL^{-1}, respectively) on ileum musculature. In addition, compounds **9** and **15** relaxed, in a dose-dependent manner, the same preparations precontracted with 300 mM BaCl$_2$ (pIC_{50} = 4.34 ± 0.02 µg mL^{-1}; pIC_{50} = 4.34 ± 0.02 µg mL^{-1}, respectively) or with 600 mM KCl (pIC_{50} = 4.47 ± 0.06 µg mL^{-1}; pIC_{50} = 4.73 ± 0.18 µg mL^{-1}, respectively) [53,64].

Silva et al. proved that a *B. bifurcata* DCM extract also presents neuroprotective potential. Neuroprotective effects were highlighted in a neurotoxic model induced in a human neuroblastoma cell line (SH-SY5Y), whereas the neuroprotection mechanisms were evaluated by the determination of mitochondrial membrane potential, H_2O_2 production, among others. After fractionation, the cyclohexane-EtOAc (1:2) fraction was shown to have a promising neuroprotective performance, due to its ability to prevent changes in mitochondrial potential (218.10% ± 14.87% of control), and to induce the reduction of H_2O_2 levels of production (204.50% ± 15.12% of control), as well as to revert neurotoxic effect on cell viability (about 20%–25%). Considering these results, Silva et al. investigated the composition of this fraction, through purification steps, in order to isolate the potential bioactive molecules. Eleganolone (**15**) and eleganolal (**23**) were the two major compounds of this fraction. Then, their antioxidant activity was evaluated, demonstrating lower ability to reduce the DPPH radical, when compared to the fraction from which they were isolated. Although, taking into account the results of FRAP and ORAC assays, compounds **15** (8341.18 ± 177.72 µM FeSO$_4$ g^{-1} compound and 1663.83 ± 25.35 µmol TE g^{-1} compound, respectively) and **23** (8635.37 ± 389.54 µM FeSO$_4$ g^{-1} compound and 667.48 ± 10.96 µmol TE g^{-1} compound, respectively) expressed antioxidant capacity, since these linear diterpenes exhibited a high potential in reducing peroxyl radicals and have a strong iron reduction capacity, compared to the BHT. In this sense, these components might be promising candidates for further neuroprotection studies [51].

4.7. In Vitro Estimation of Toxicity

The evaluation of biological dose effects should be combined with the respective assessment of toxicity, since this is a crucial parameter to ensure that bioactive compounds and/or extracts are safe for humans.

The cytotoxicity of linear diterpenes obtained from a *B. bifurcata* sample, collected in Brittany, France, was evaluated using sea urchin eggs, which have been considered a model for studies on cell division and embryologic development and commonly used to obtain a general screening of cytotoxicity [14]. The ability of some linear diterpenes to inhibit the development of fertilized eggs of the common sea urchin *Paracentrotus lividus* was evaluated through a cytotoxicity activity test [29,43]. The test showed that 12-(S)-hydroxygeranylgeraniol (**1**), bifurcane (**10**), and bifurcanol (**41**) were active, with EC$_{50}$ values of 18 µg mL^{-1}, 12 µg mL^{-1}, and 4 µg mL^{-1}, respectively. Whereas, (S)-12-hydroxygeranylgeranic acid (**2**) and eleganediol (**9**) exhibited moderate antimitotic activity with EC$_{50}$ values of 60 µg mL^{-1} and 36 µg mL^{-1}, respectively [29,43].

The cytotoxicity of nine linear diterpenes isolated from *B. bifurcata* were tested by Göthel et al. [30]. Bifurcane (**10**), bifurcanone (**18**), eleganonic acid (**31**), and bibiolone (**34**) were shown to be inactive (when IC$_{50}$ > 40 µg mL^{-1}) against mouse fibroblast cell line (L929), whereas eleganolone (**15**) (IC$_{50}$ = 22 µg mL^{-1}), (6E,10E,14E)-16-hydroxy-2,6,10,14-tetramethylhexadeca-2,6,10,14-tetraen-4-one (**21**) (IC$_{50}$ = 18 µg mL^{-1}), eleganolonebutenolide (**32**) (IC$_{50}$ = 27 µg mL^{-1}), 14,15-dihydro-eleganonic acid (**33**) (IC$_{50}$ = 20 µg mL^{-1}), and bifurcanol (**41**) (IC$_{50}$ = 24 µg mL^{-1}) exhibited very low toxicity [30]. In the case of compound **15**, for example, the cytotoxicity IC$_{50}$ value was higher than the EC$_{50}$ found for antifouling activity (against *Trypanosoma brucei rhodesiense* (IC_{50} = 13.7 µg mL^{-1}), *Trypanosoma cruzi* (IC_{50} = 17.7 µg mL^{-1}), *Plasmodium falciparum* (IC_{50} = 2.6 µg mL^{-1}), and *Balanus amphitrite* cyprid (EC_{50} = 2.14 (0.88–3.9, conf. lim. 95%) µg mL^{-1}) [21,26].

For instance, Smyrniotopoulos et al. [50] analyzed the cytotoxicity of bifurcatriol (**14**), showing that this linear diterpene had cytotoxicity against the L6 rat myoblast cell line, IC_{50} = 56.6 ± 0.004 µg mL^{-1} [50]. Actually, this value is considerably higher that the IC_{50} values observed for antimalarial and antiprotozoal activities, compromising, therefore, the use of this compound for such purposes.

In fact, other studies have shown biological activities and cytotoxicity of *B. bifurcata* extracts, with both expressed at µg mL^{-1} [35,61]. Notwithstanding, these toxicities corresponded to EtOAc and EtOAc:MeOH extracts, with the toxicity of the most relevant and studied extracts, namely DCM and EtOH extracts, remaining unknown. In addition, considering bioactive extracts in which a high toxicity is present, the hypothesis that bioactive and toxic components are not the same must be carefully taken into account. Therefore, it is crucial to investigate the compounds responsible for the biological activities found, as well as evaluating their toxic nature. Thus, strategies to separate the bioactive compounds from those with high toxicity must be developed. In vitro cytotoxicity studies must be accomplished for interspecies correlations. Hence, to ponder a potential application of a bioactive compound and/or extract, it is essential to ensure that the magnitude order of bioactivity is significantly higher than those of toxicity.

In vitro toxicity assays involving marine bacteria should also be considered in the future, since equations for interspecies dose correlations have already been established, allowing researchers to correlate the bacteria data with rat or mouse toxicity, which avoids mammalian laboratory tests [65,66].

Finally, the safe use of these components must be verified by additional studies, in particular in vivo assays, considering the different range of possible applications, in order to confirm that they are safe to humans.

5. Potential Applications for *B. bifurcata* Extracts

Taking into account the diverse biological activities already attributed to *B. bifurcata* linear diterpenes, different studies have already exploited specific applications for these components or enriched extracts. Miranda et al. studied the effect of a preliminary dipping treatment containing a *B. bifurcata* extract in the fish quality during chilled storage. The choice of this brown macroalga was due to its content on antioxidant and antimicrobial compounds, i.e., diterpenes, among others [67]. Through microbial analysis, the inhibitory effects against Enterobacteriaceae, lipolytic, and psychotropic bacteria were proven. These results can be explained by two combined effects: the removal through the washing effect of blood, digestive juices, slime, and feces from the fish surface; and the presence of a high content of antimicrobial diterpenes from the algae extract. Chemical assays, in particular, trimethylamine and free fatty acids formation, allowed researchers to prove the enhancement of fish quality in the presence of algae extracts. Although, these effects were found in specimens submitted to the most concentrated algae extract, at advanced storage time (in most cases), which means that the combined treatment, including washing in an ethanolic-aqueous solution and the inclusion of a bioactive *B. bifurcata* extract, had beneficial effects on fish quality. In fact, the quality during chilled storage is a major concern of the food industry. Wild marine species are often exposed to several handling and technological processes, which determine the quality of the final product [67]. A water dipping step is often applied before storage to remove blood, slime, and other undesirable components and to partially prevent microbial contamination. This preliminary step is also carried out to avoid the development of different damage pathways, resulting from microbial activity, autolysis and lipid oxidation, among others [67]. Thus, the inclusion of a bioactive *B. bifurcata* extract may be a practical application for both on-board and in-land fish storage strategies [67].

The use of a *B. bifurcata* extract in the green synthesis of copper oxide nanoparticles (CONPs) was also reported. This strategy aimed to overcome some drawbacks of conventional processes (such as the use of toxic chemicals as reducing and capping agents of nanoparticles), which limit the use of nanoparticles in applications related to clinical fields. The synthesis of CONPs using this marine brown macroalga was focused on "green" chemistry and bioprocess approaches [68]. In addition to being an environmental friendly bioprocess (no chemical reagents or surfactant templates were applied), these CONPs showed good antibacterial activity against gram-negative (*Enterobacter aerogenes*) (ZI = 14 mm) and gram-positive (*Staphylococcus aureus*) (ZI = 16 mm) bacteria [68].

6. Conclusions and Future Perspectives

Macroalgae are one of the most promising sources of secondary metabolites, which have already been associated to several biological activities. For this reason, an increase in the investment and research on these marine resources has been observed. The focus of this review was the bioprospection of linear diterpenes from *B. bifurcata*, including the methodologies of extraction and structural elucidation and the biological activities already associated to these brown macroalga components. A detailed collection of NMR and MS data is provided, which will be of utmost importance in future studies of bioprospection of linear diterpenes from *B. bifurcata*.

B. bifurcata has earned special emphasis, due to their special ability to biosynthesize linear diterpenes, which are rarely found in brown macroalgae species outside the Sargassaceae family. In fact, some studies have proven that these secondary metabolites are responsible for several biological activities, such as antibacterial, antiprotozoal, antifouling, and antitumoral, among others. Linear diterpenes from *B. bifurcata*, particularly eleganolone (**15**) and eleganediol (**9**), showed significant antifouling, antibacterial, and antihypertensive activities in the range of $\mu g\ mL^{-1}$.

Notwithstanding, extraction methodologies have been identified as one of the major challenges to develop viable and safe high-value applications, namely in food, nutraceutical, or pharmaceutical fields. The conventional extraction methodologies normally used to extract these compounds involve the use of organic solvents, often toxic to humans and environmentally hazardous. Furthermore, these extraction methodologies also raise other concerns, namely, the long operation times, consumption of high volumes of expensive solvents, and high energetic demand. Thus, new and eco-friendly methodologies should be applied, taking into account their overall feasibility. In particular, emergent extraction methodologies able to use small amounts of organic solvents, or even offering the possibility for their replacement by water, should be considered.

The purification and/or fractionation steps have been already applied by some authors, frequently for identification purposes, for *B. bifurcata*, although there are also studies reporting biological activities of *B. bifurcata* extracts without isolating the bioactive compounds. The isolation, or at least the fractionation, should be considered in order to enhance the bioactivity and also eliminate some antagonistic effects, for instance, bio-guided fractionation or a faster strategy that has already been tested, known as "pharmacophoric deconvolution", should be further exploited. Another strategy could be the development and optimization of more selective extraction methodologies. Additionally, before any possible application, the cytotoxicity of the extracts, fractions, or isolated compounds should be evaluated.

In vivo assays for the determination of dose effect and the consumer security evaluation may be also considered to confirm the potential of *B. bifurcata* linear diterpenes in pharmaceutical, cosmetic, or nutraceutical applications. In addition, the incorporation of these extracts in biomaterials should be considered. Finally, for possible food industry applications, the legislation may be revised in order to evaluate *B. bifurcata* as an edible species.

Finally, and despite the use of metabolic engineering and synthetic biology in macroalgae's bioactive components, production is still in its infancy and largely unexploited in *B. bifurcata*, although the new advances in these fields should be undoubtably considered in future works. Actually, the increasing development of multi-omics techniques, including genomics, transcriptomics, proteomics, and metabolomics have enabled the creation of libraries and models that can predict the behavior of biological systems as well as allow the optimization of cellular processes in order to produce target compounds. This could be a valuable and key strategy in the exploitation of B. bifurcata as a source of linear diterpenes for high-value applications.

Supplementary Materials: The following are available online at http://www.mdpi.com/1660-3397/17/10/556/s1, Table S1: MS data of linear diterpenes identified in B. bifurcata; Table S2: 1H NMR spectral data for linear diterpenes identified in B. bifurcata; Table S3: 13C NMR spectral data of linear diterpenes identified in B. bifurcata.

Author Contributions: A.C.S.P., J.A.S., S.M.R., A.J.D.S., and S.A.O.S wrote and edited the manuscript.

Funding: This research was funded by the project AgroForWealth: Biorefining of agricultural and forest by-products and wastes: integrated strategic for valorization of resources towards society wealth and sustainability (CENTRO-01-0145-FEDER-000001), funded by Centro2020, through FEDER and PT2020, by FCT/MCTES which financed the project CICECO-Aveiro Institute of Materials, FCT Ref. UID/CTM/50011/2019 and QOPNA research Unit (FCT UID/QUI/00062/2019).

Conflicts of Interest: The authors declare no conflict of interest.

References

1. Balina, K.; Romagnoli, F.; Blumberga, D. Seaweed biorefinery concept for sustainable use of marine resources. *Energy Procedia* **2017**, *128*, 504–511. [CrossRef]
2. Fernand, F.; Israel, A.; Skjermo, J.; Wichard, T.; Timmermans, K.R.; Golberg, A. Offshore macroalgae biomass for bioenergy production: Environmental aspects, technological achievements and challenges. *Renew. Sustain. Energy Rev.* **2017**, *75*, 35–45. [CrossRef]
3. European Commission. COM(2012) 494—Communication from the Commission to the European Parliament, the Council, the European Economic and Social Committee and the Committee of the Regions: Blue Growth Opportunities for Marine and Maritime Sustainable Growth; Publications Office of the European Union: Luxemburg, 2012.
4. Stengel, D.B.; Connan, S. *Natural Products From Marine Algae*; Methods in Molecular Biology; Stengel, D.B., Connan, S., Eds.; Springer: New York, NY, USA, 2015; Volume 1308, ISBN 978-1-4939-2683-1.
5. Wijesinghe, W.A.J.P.; Jeon, Y.J. Biological activities and potential cosmeceutical applications of bioactive components from brown seaweeds: A review. *Phytochem. Rev.* **2011**, *10*, 431–443. [CrossRef]
6. Klnc, B.; Cirik, S.; Turan, G.; Tekogul, H.; Koru, E. Seaweeds for Food and Industrial Applications. In *Food Industry*; InTechOpen: London, UK, 2013.
7. Freitas, A.C.; Rodrigues, D.; Rocha-Santos, T.A.P.; Gomes, A.M.P.; Duarte, A.C. Marine biotechnology advances towards applications in new functional foods. *Biotechnol. Adv.* **2012**, *30*, 1506–1515. [CrossRef] [PubMed]
8. Zubia, M.; Fabre, M.S.; Kerjean, V.; Lann, K.L.; Stiger-Pouvreau, V.; Fauchon, M.; Deslandes, E. Antioxidant and antitumoural activities of some Phaeophyta from Brittany coasts. *Food Chem.* **2009**, *116*, 693–701. [CrossRef]
9. Holdt, S.L.; Kraan, S. Bioactive compounds in seaweed: Functional food applications and legislation. *J. Appl. Phycol.* **2011**, *23*, 543–597. [CrossRef]
10. Okuzumi, J.; Takahashi, T.; Yamane, T.; Kitao, Y.; Inagake, M.; Ohya, K.; Nishino, H.; Tanaka, Y. Inhibitory effects of fucoxanthin, a natural carotenoid, on N-ethyl-N'-nitro-N-nitrosoguanidine-induced mouse duodenal carcinogenesis. *Cancer Lett.* **1993**, *68*, 159–168. [CrossRef]
11. Koyanagi, S.; Tanigawa, N.; Nakagawa, H.; Soeda, S.; Shimeno, H. Reviewed the Structured and Bioactive Compound of Fucoidan. *Biochem. Pharmacol.* **2003**, *65*, 173–179. [CrossRef]
12. Wijesekara, I.; Yoon, N.Y.; Kim, S.K. Phlorotannins from *Ecklonia cava* (Phaeophyceae): Biological activities and potential health benefits. *BioFactors* **2010**, *36*, 408–414. [CrossRef] [PubMed]
13. Blunt, J.W.; Carroll, A.R.; Copp, B.R.; Davis, R.A.; Keyzers, R.A.; Prinsep, M.R. Marine natural products. *Nat. Prod. Rep.* **2018**, *35*, 8–53. [CrossRef]
14. Muñoz, J.; Culioli, G.; Köck, M. Linear diterpenes from the marine brown alga *Bifurcaria bifurcata*: A chemical perspective. *Phytochem. Rev.* **2013**, *12*, 407–424. [CrossRef]
15. Le Lann, K.; Jégou, C.; Stiger-Pouvreau, V. Effect of different conditioning treatments on total phenolic content and antioxidant activities in two Sargassacean species: Comparison of the frondose *Sargassum muticum* (Yendo) Fensholt and the cylindrical *Bifurcaria bifurcata* R. Ross. *Phycol. Res.* **2008**, *56*, 238–245. [CrossRef]
16. Guiry, M.D.; Guiry, G.M. *Bifurcaria bifurcata* R. Ross. Available online: https://www.algaebase.org/search/genus/detail/?genus_id=78&-session=abv4:AC1F25E1169cb0028AQS8B54C575 (accessed on 3 May 2019).

17. Le Lann, K.; Rumin, J.; Cérantola, S.; Culioli, G.; Stiger-Pouvreau, V. Spatiotemporal variations of diterpene production in the brown macroalga *Bifurcaria bifurcata* from the western coasts of Brittany (France). *J. Appl. Phycol.* **2014**, *26*, 1207–1214. [CrossRef]
18. Culioli, G.; Ortalo-Magné, A.; Richou, M.; Valls, R.; Piovetti, L. Seasonal variations in the chemical composition of *Bifurcaria bifurcata* (Cystoseiraceae). *Biochem. Syst. Ecol.* **2002**, *30*, 61–64. [CrossRef]
19. Biard, J.F.; Verbist, J.F.; Floch, R.; Letourneux, Y. Epoxyeleganolone et eleganediol, deux nouveaux diterpenes de *Bifurcaria bifurcata* ross (cystoseiracees). *Tetrahedron Lett.* **1980**, *21*, 1849–1852. [CrossRef]
20. Biard, J.F.; Verbist, J.F.; Letourneux, Y. Cétols Diterpeniques à Activite Antimicrobienne de *Bifurcaria bifurcata*. *J. Med. Plant Res.* **1980**, *40*, 288–294. [CrossRef] [PubMed]
21. Gallé, J.; Attitoua, B.; Kaiser, M.; Rusig, A.; Lobstein, A.; Vonthron-Sénécheau, C. Eleganolone, a Diterpene from the French Marine Alga *Bifurcaria bifurcata* Inhibits Growth of the Human Pathogens *Trypanosoma brucei* and *Plasmodium falciparum*. *Mar. Drugs* **2013**, *11*, 599–610. [CrossRef] [PubMed]
22. Nardella, F.; Margueritte, L.; Lamure, B.; Martine, J.; Viéville, P.; Bourjot, M. Targeted discovery of bioactive natural products using a pharmacophoric deconvolution strategy: Proof of principle with eleganolone from *Bifurcaria bifurcata* R. Ross. *Phytochem. Lett.* **2018**, *26*, 138–142. [CrossRef]
23. Hellio, C.; Thomas-Guyon, H.; Culioli, G.; Piovettt, L.; Bourgougnon, N.; le Gal, Y. Marine antifoulants from Bifurcaria bifurcata (Phaeophyceae, Cystoseiraceae) and other brown macroalgae. *Biofouling* **2001**, *17*, 189–201. [CrossRef]
24. Ortalo-Magné, A.; Culioli, G.; Valls, R.; Pucci, B.; Piovetti, L. Polar acyclic diterpenoids from *Bifurcaria bifurcata* (Fucales, Phaeophyta). *Phytochemistry* **2005**, *66*, 2316–2323. [CrossRef]
25. Camps, M.; Briand, J.F.; Guentas-Dombrowsky, L.; Culioli, G.; Bazire, A.; Blache, Y. Antifouling activity of commercial biocides vs. natural and natural-derived products assessed by marine bacteria adhesion bioassay. *Mar. Pollut. Bull.* **2011**, *62*, 1032–1040. [CrossRef] [PubMed]
26. Geraci, S.; Faimali, M.; Piovetti, L.; Cimino, G. Antifouling from Nature: Laboratory Test with Balanus amphitrite Darwin on Algae and Sponges. In *10th International Congress on Marine Corrosion and Fouling, University of Melbourne, February 1999*; Lewis, J.A., Ed.; DSTO Aeronautical and Maritime Research Laboratory: Melbourne, VIC, Australia, 2001; pp. 88–97.
27. Combaut, G.; Piovetti, L. A novel acyclic diterpene from the brown alga *Bifurcaria bifurcata*. *Phytochemistry* **1983**, *22*, 1787–1789. [CrossRef]
28. Hougaard, L.; Anthoni, U.; Christophersen, C.; Nielsen, P.H. Eleganolone derived diterpenes from *Bifurcaria bifurcata*. *Phytochemistry* **1991**, *30*, 3049–3051. [CrossRef]
29. Valls, R.; Piovetti, L.; Banaigs, B.; Archavlis, A.; Pellegrini, M. (S)-13-hydroxygeranylgeraniol-derived furanoditerpenes from *Bifurcaria bifurcata*. *Phytochemistry* **1995**, *39*, 145–149. [CrossRef]
30. Göthel, Q.; Lichte, E.; Köck, M. Further eleganolone-derived diterpenes from the brown alga *Bifurcaria bifurcata*. *Tetrahedron Lett.* **2012**, *53*, 1873–1877. [CrossRef]
31. Culioli, G.; Daoudi, M.; Mesguiche, V.; Valls, R.; Piovetti, L. Geranylgeraniol-derived diterpenoids from the brown alga *Bifurcaria bifurcata*. *Phytochemistry* **1999**, *52*, 1447–1454. [CrossRef]
32. Culioli, G.; Mesguiche, V.; Piovetti, L.; Valls, R. Geranylgeraniol and geranylgeraniol-derived diterpenes from the brown alga *Bifurcaria bifurcata* (Cystoseiraceae). *Biochem. Syst. Ecol.* **1999**, *27*, 665–668. [CrossRef]
33. Culioli, G.; Di Guardia, S.; Valls, R.; Piovetti, L. Geranylgeraniol-derived diterpenes from the brown alga *Bifurcaria Bifurcata*: Comparison with two other Cystoseiraceae species. *Biochem. Syst. Ecol.* **2000**, *28*, 185–187. [CrossRef]
34. Göthel, Q.; Muñoz, J.; Köck, M. Formyleleganolone and bibifuran, two metabolites from the brown alga *Bifurcaria bifurcata*. *Phytochem. Lett.* **2012**, *5*, 693–695. [CrossRef]
35. Vonthron-sé, C.; Kaiser, M.; Devambez, I.; Vastel, A.; Mussio, I.; Rusig, A. Antiprotozoal Activities of Organic Extracts from French Marine Seaweeds. *Mar. Drugs* **2011**, *9*, 922–933. [CrossRef] [PubMed]
36. Maréchal, J.P.; Culioli, G.; Hellio, C.; Thomas-Guyon, H.; Callow, M.E.; Clare, A.S.; Ortalo-Magné, A. Seasonal variation in antifouling activity of crude extracts of the brown alga *Bifurcaria bifurcata* (*Cystoseiraceae*) against cyprids of Balanus amphitrite and the marine bacteria Cobetia marina and Pseudoalteromonas haloplanktis. *J. Exp. Mar. Bio. Ecol.* **2004**, *313*, 47–62. [CrossRef]
37. Moreau, D.; Thomas-Guyon, H.; Jacquot, C.; Jugé, M.; Culioli, G.; Ortalo-Magné, A.; Piovetti, L.; Roussakis, C. An extract from the brown alga *Bifurcaria bifurcata* induces irreversible arrest of cell proliferation in a non-small-cell bronchopulmonary carcinoma line. *J. Appl. Phycol.* **2006**, *18*, 87–93. [CrossRef]

38. Santos, S.; Trindade, S.; Oliveira, C.; Parreira, P.; Rosa, D.; Duarte, M.; Ferreira, I.; Cruz, M.; Rego, A.; Abreu, M.; et al. Lipophilic fraction of cultivated *Bifurcaria bifurcata* R. Ross: Detailed composition and in vitro prospection of current challenging bioactive properties. *Mar. Drugs* **2017**, *15*, 340. [CrossRef] [PubMed]
39. Balboa, E.M.; Conde, E.; Moure, A.; Falqué, E.; Domínguez, H. In vitro antioxidant properties of crude extracts and compounds from brown algae. *Food Chem.* **2013**, *138*, 1764–1785. [CrossRef] [PubMed]
40. Hu, J.; Yang, B.; Lin, X.; Zhou, X.-F.; Yang, X.-W.; Liu, Y. *Handbook of Marine Macroalgae*; Kim, S.-K., Ed.; John Wiley & Sons, Ltd.: Chichester, UK, 2011; ISBN 9781119977087.
41. Gross, H.; König, G.M. Terpenoids from marine organisms: Unique structures and their pharmacological potential. *Phytochem. Rev.* **2006**, *5*, 115–141. [CrossRef]
42. Dhar, M.K.; Koul, A.; Kaul, S. Farnesyl pyrophosphate synthase: A key enzyme in isoprenoid biosynthetic pathway and potential molecular target for drug development. *N. Biotechnol.* **2013**, *30*, 114–123. [CrossRef] [PubMed]
43. Valls, R.; Banaigs, B.; Piovetti, L.; Archavlis, A.; Artaud, J. Linear diterpene with antimitotic activity from the brown alga *Bifurcaria bifurcata*. *Phytochemistry* **1993**, *34*, 1585–1588. [CrossRef]
44. Culioli, G.; Ortalo-Magné, A.; Daoudi, M.; Thomas-Guyon, H.; Valls, R.; Piovetti, L. Trihydroxylated linear diterpenes from the brown alga *Bifurcaria bifurcata*. *Phytochemistry* **2004**, *65*, 2063–2069. [CrossRef]
45. Valls, R.; Banaigs, B.; Francisco, C.; Codomier, L.; Cave, A. *An Acyclic Diterpene from the Brown Alga Bifurcaria bifurcata*; Pergamon: Oxford, UK, 1986; Volume 25.
46. Culioli, G.; Daoudi, M.; Ortalo-Magné, A.; Valls, R.; Piovetti, L. (S)-12-Hydroxygeranylgeraniol-derived diterpenes from the brown alga *Bifurcaria bifurcata*. *Phytochemistry* **2001**, *57*, 529–535. [CrossRef]
47. Semmak, L.; Zerzouf, A.; Valls, R.; Banaigs, B.; Jeanty, G.; Francisco, C. Acyclic diterpenes from *Bifurcaria bifurcata*. *Phytochemistry* **1988**, *27*, 2347–2349. [CrossRef]
48. Smyrniotopoulos, V.; Firsova, D.; Rae, M.; Heesch, S.; Fearnhead, H.; Tasdemir, D. Linear diterpenes with anticancer activity from the irish brown alga *Bifurcaria bifurcata*. *Planta Med.* **2014**, *80*. [CrossRef]
49. El Hattab, M.; Ben Mesaoud, M.; Daoudi, M.; Ortalo-Magné, A.; Culioli, G.; Valls, R.; Piovetti, L. Trihydroxylated linear diterpenes from the brown alga *Bifurcaria bifurcata*. *Biochem. Syst. Ecol.* **2008**, *36*, 484–489. [CrossRef]
50. Smyrniotopoulos, V.; Merten, C.; Kaiser, M.; Tasdemir, D. Bifurcatriol, a new antiprotozoal acyclic diterpene from the brown alga *Bifurcaria bifurcata*. *Mar. Drugs* **2017**, *15*, 245. [CrossRef]
51. Silva, J.; Alves, C.; Freitas, R.; Martins, A.; Pinteus, S.; Ribeiro, J.; Gaspar, H.; Alfonso, A.; Pedrosa, R. Antioxidant and Neuroprotective Potential of the Brown Seaweed Bifurcaria bifurcata in an in vitro Parkinson's Disease Model. *Mar. Drugs* **2019**, *17*, 85. [CrossRef] [PubMed]
52. Ainane, T.; Abourriche, A.; Bennamara, A.; Charrouf, M.; Lemrani, M. Antileishmanial activity of extracts from a brown seaweed *Bifurcaria bifurcata* the atlantic coast of Casablanca (Morocco). *BioTechnology* **2015**, *11*, 7–11.
53. Della Pieta, F.; Bilia, A.R.; Breschi, M.C.; Cinelli, F.; Morelli, I.; Scatizzi, R. Crude extracts and two linear diterpenes from Cystoseira balearica and their activity. *Planta Med.* **1993**, *59*, 135–138. [PubMed]
54. Pinteus, S.; Silva, J.; Alves, C.; Horta, A.; Fino, N.; Rodrigues, A.I.; Mendes, S.; Pedrosa, R. Cytoprotective effect of seaweeds with high antioxidant activity from the Peniche coast (Portugal). *Food Chem.* **2017**, *218*, 591–599. [CrossRef]
55. Alves, C.; Pinteus, S.; Simões, T.; Horta, A.; Silva, J.; Tecelão, C.; Pedrosa, R. *Bifurcaria bifurcata*: A key macro-alga as a source of bioactive compounds and functional ingredients. *Int. J. Food Sci. Technol.* **2016**, *51*, 1638–1646. [CrossRef]
56. Jun, X. High-Pressure processing as emergent technology for the extraction of bioactive ingredients from plant materials. *Crit. Rev. Food Sci. Nutr.* **2013**, *53*, 837–852. [CrossRef]
57. Alexandre, E.M.C.; Castro, L.M.G.; Moreira, S.A.; Pintado, M.; Saraiva, J.A. Comparison of emerging technologies to extract high-added value compounds from fruit residues: Pressure- and electro-based technologies. *Food Eng. Rev.* **2017**, 1–23. [CrossRef]
58. Ibtissam, C.; Hassane, R.; José, M.; Francisco, D.S.J.; Antonio, G.V.J.; Hassan, B.; Mohamed, K. Screening of antibacterial activity in marine green and brown macroalgae from the coast of Morocco. *African J. Biotechnol.* **2009**, *8*, 1258–1262.

59. Agregán, R.; Munekata, P.E.; Domínguez, R.; Carballo, J.; Franco, D.; Lorenzo, J.M. Proximate composition, phenolic content and in vitro antioxidant activity of aqueous extracts of the seaweeds *Ascophyllum nodosum*, *Bifurcaria bifurcata* and *Fucus vesiculosus*. Effect of addition of the extracts on the oxidative stabi. *Food Res. Int.* **2017**, *99*, 986–994. [CrossRef] [PubMed]
60. Azmir, J.; Zaidul, I.S.M.; Rahman, M.M.; Sharif, K.M.; Mohamed, A.; Sahena, F.; Jahurul, M.H.A.; Ghafoor, K.; Norulaini, N.A.N.; Omar, A.K.M. Techniques for extraction of bioactive compounds from plant materials: A review. *J. Food Eng.* **2013**, *117*, 426–436. [CrossRef]
61. Spavieri, J.; Allmendinger, A.; Kaiser, M.; Casey, R.; Hingley-wilson, S.; Lalvani, A.; Guiry, M.D.; Blunden, G.; Tasdemir, D. Antimycobacterial, Antiprotozoal and Cytotoxic Potential of Twenty-one Brown Algae (Phaeophyceae) from British and Irish Waters. *Phyther. Res.* **2010**, *24*, 1724–1729. [CrossRef] [PubMed]
62. Huang, H.W.; Hsu, C.P.; Yang, B.B.; Wang, C.Y. Advances in the extraction of natural ingredients by high pressure extraction technology. *Trends Food Sci. Technol.* **2013**, *33*, 54–62. [CrossRef]
63. Barba, F.J.; Zhu, Z.; Koubaa, M.; Sant'Ana, A.S.; Orlien, V. Green alternative methods for the extraction of antioxidant bioactive compounds from winery wastes and by-products: A review. *Trends Food Sci. Technol.* **2016**, *49*, 96–109. [CrossRef]
64. Della Pieta, F.; Breschi, M.C.; Scatizzi, R.; Cinelli, F. Relaxing activity of two linear diterpenes from Cystoseira brachycarpa var. balearica on the contractions of intestinal preparations. *Planta Med.* **1995**, *61*, 493–496. [CrossRef]
65. Salvador, Â.; Król, E.; Lemos, V.; Santos, S.; Bento, F.; Costa, C.; Almeida, A.; Szczepankiewicz, D.; Kulczyński, B.; Krejpcio, Z.; et al. Effect of Elderberry (*Sambucus nigra* L.) Extract Supplementation in STZ-Induced Diabetic Rats Fed with a High-Fat Diet. *Int. J. Mol. Sci.* **2017**, *18*, 13. [CrossRef]
66. Devillers, J.; Pandard, P.; Thybaud, E.; Merle, A. Interspecies correlations for predicting the acute toxicity of xenobiotics. In *Ecotoxicology Modeling*; Emerging Topics in Ecotoxicology; Devillers, J., Ed.; Springer US: Boston, MA, USA, 2009; Volume 2, pp. 85–115.
67. Miranda, J.M.; Trigo, M.; Barros-Velázquez, J.; Aubourg, S.P. Quality Enhancement of Chilled Lean Fish by Previous Active Dipping in *Bifurcaria bifurcata* Alga Extract. *Food Bioprocess Technol.* **2018**, *11*, 1662–1673. [CrossRef]
68. Abboud, Y.; Saffaj, T.; Chagraoui, A.; El Bouari, A.; Brouzi, K.; Tanane, O.; Ihssane, B. Biosynthesis, characterization and antimicrobial activity of copper oxide nanoparticles (CONPs) produced using brown alga extract (*Bifurcaria bifurcata*). *Appl. Nanosci.* **2014**, *4*, 571–576. [CrossRef]

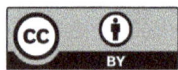

© 2019 by the authors. Licensee MDPI, Basel, Switzerland. This article is an open access article distributed under the terms and conditions of the Creative Commons Attribution (CC BY) license (http://creativecommons.org/licenses/by/4.0/).

MDPI
St. Alban-Anlage 66
4052 Basel
Switzerland
Tel. +41 61 683 77 34
Fax +41 61 302 89 18
www.mdpi.com

Marine Drugs Editorial Office
E-mail: marinedrugs@mdpi.com
www.mdpi.com/journal/marinedrugs

www.ingramcontent.com/pod-product-compliance
Lightning Source LLC
LaVergne TN
LVHW071937080526
838202LV00064B/6626